The Neurology of Consciousness: Cognitive Neuroscience and Neuropathology

The Neurology of Consciousness: Cognitive Neuroscience and Neuropathology

Edited by

Steven Laureys and Giulio Tononi

AMSTERDAM • BOSTON • HEIDELBERG • LONDON • NEW YORK • OXFORD
PARIS • SAN DIEGO • SAN FRANCISCO • SINGAPORE • SYDNEY • TOKYO
Academic Press is an imprint of Elsevier

Academic Press is an imprint of Elsevier
32 Jamestown Road, London NW1 7BY, UK
30 Corporate Drive, Suite 400, Burlington, MA 01803, USA
525 B Street, Suite 1900, San Diego, CA 92101-4495, USA

First edition 2009

British Library Cataloguing in Publication Data
A catalogue record for this book is available from the British Library

Library of Congress Cataloging-in-Publication Data
A catalog record for this book is available from the Library of Congress

ISBN: 978-0-12-374168-4

For information on all Academic Press publications
visit our website at www.books.elsevier.com

Typeset by Charon Tec Ltd (A Macmillan Company), Chennai, India
www.charontec.com.

Printed and bound in China

09 10   10 9 8 7 6 5 4 3 2 1

To our families and loved ones;
to our students, fellows and teachers.

Contents

Preface

Thinking must never submit itself, neither to a dogma, nor to a party, nor to a passion, nor to an interest, nor to a preconceived idea, nor to anything whatsoever, except to the facts themselves, because for it to submit to anything else would be the end of its existence.

Henri Poincaré (1854–1912;
French mathematician and theoretical physicists)

'Truth is sought for its own sake. And those who are engaged upon the quest for anything for its own sake are not interested in other things. Finding the truth is difficult, and the road to it is rough.' wrote Ibn al-Haytham (965–1039; Persian polymath), a pioneer of the scientific method. This book tackles one of the biggest challenges of science; understanding the biological basis of human consciousness. It does so through observation and experimentation in neurological patients, formulating hypotheses about the neural correlates of consciousness and employing an objective and reproducible methodology. This scientific method, as first proposed by Isaac Newton (1643–1727; English polymath), has proven utterly successful in replacing dark-age, 'magical thinking' with an intelligent, rational understanding of nature. Scientific methodology, however, also requires imagination and creativity. For example, methodologically well-described experiments permitted Louis Pasteur (1822–1895; French chemist and microbiologist) to reject the millennia-old Aristotelian (384–322 BC; Greek philosopher) view that living organisms could spontaneously arise from non-living matter. Pasteur's observations and genius gave rise to germ theory of medical disease which would lead to the use of antiseptics and antibiotics, saving innumerable lives.

The progress of science also largely depends upon the invention and improvement of technology and instruments. For example, the big breakthroughs of Galileo Galilei (1564–1642; Tuscan astronomer) were made possible thanks to eyeglass makers' improvements in lens-grinding techniques, which permitted the construction of his telescopes. Similarly, advances in engineering led to space observatories such as the Hubble Telescope to shed light on where we come from. Rigorous scientific measurements permitted to trace back the birth of the universe to nearly 14.000 million years; the age of the earth to more than 4.500 million years; the origin of life on earth to (very) approximately 3.500 million years and the apparition of the earth's first simple animals to about 600 million years. Natural evolution, as brilliantly revealed by Charles Darwin (1809–1882), over these many million years gave rise to nervous systems as complex as the human brain, arguably the most complex object in the universe. And somehow, through the interactions among its 100 billion neurons, connected by trillions of synapses, emerges our conscious experience of the world and of ourselves.

Neurology is the study of mankind itself, said Wilder Penfield (1891–1976; Canadian neurosurgeon). You are your brain. This book offers neurological facts on consciousness and impaired consciousness. While philosophers have pondered upon the mind–brain conundrum for millennia, without making much if any progress, scientists have only recently been able to explore the connection analytically through measurements and perturbations of the brain's activity. This ability again stems from recent advances in technology and especially from emerging functional neuroimaging modalities. As demonstrated in the chapters of this book, the mapping of conscious perception and cognition in health (e.g., conscious waking, sleep, dreaming, sleepwalking and anaesthesia) and in disease (e.g., coma, near-death, vegetative state, seizures, split-brains, neglect, amnesia, dementia, etc.) is providing exiting new insights into the functional neuroanatomy of human consciousness. Philosophers might argue that the subjective aspect of the mind will never be sufficiently accounted for by the objective methods of reductionistic science. We here prefer a more pragmatic approach and see no reason that scientific and technological advances will not ultimately lead to an understanding of the neural substrate of consciousness.

This book originated partly to satisfy our own curiosity about consciousness. We thank our funding agencies including the National Institutes of Health, the European Commission, the McDonnell Foundation, the Mind Science Foundation Texas, the Belgian National Funds for Scientific Research (FNRS), the French Speaking Community Concerted Research Action, the Queen Elisabeth Medical Foundation, the Liège Sart Tilman University Hospital, the University of Liège and the University of Wisconsin School of Medicine and Public Health. We learned a lot while working on *The Neurology of Consciousness* and hope you do too while reading it.

March 2008
Steven Laureys (Liège) and Giulio Tononi
(Madison)

Prologue

CONSCIOUSNESS AND THE BRAIN

Suddenly it is spring.

We have survived the long winter of behaviourism. We have tripped over the traces of reflexology. We are about to walk out of the long shadow of psychoanalysis. This, surely, is cause for celebration. Consciousness, like sleep, is of the Brain, by the Brain, and for the Brain. A new day is dawning.

The brain is not, after all, a black box. We can now look into it as its states produce a rainbow array of colours to admire and contemplate. We can distinguish waking, sleeping, and, yes, even dreaming. We can compare these normal states of consciousness with each other and with abnormal states of the brain and consciousness caused by disease and disorder. Of course we will still use behaviourism to help us understand our habits and in the design of cognitive science tools but we will look beyond all that, to the brain, and to consciousness itself.

The brain is still a collection of reflexes but neuronal clocks and oscillators alter reflex excitability as they undergo spontaneous changes in the temporal phase of their intrinsic cyclicity. The timing mechanisms of these clocks can be established using the tools of neuroscience that served reflexology so well. Single neurons and single molecules of their chemical conversation can be resolved, mapped, and compared with the coloured pictures of the brain in action.

The brain still keeps most of its activity out of consciousness but what it excludes and admits is governed more by rules of activation, input–output gating, and neuromodulation than by repression. The unconscious is now seen as a vast and useful look-up system for the conscious brain rather than a seething source of devils aiming at the disruption of consciousness. Consciousness itself is thus a tool for investigation of itself as well as for the study of that small part of the unconscious that is dynamically repressed.

This is all to the good. So why not simply dance with glee? We must be chagrined because we are now faced with recognition of the impoverishment of our psychology. It has not grown as fast as our neurobiology. Some say that we do not need psychology anyway. But these eliminative materialists will never satisfy the subjectivist in all of us. We refuse to believe that conscious choice is truly or completely illusory. We refuse to believe that consciousness is without function. Rather than refurbish psychoanalysis, which is now so scientifically discredited as to be an embarrassment, we need to construct a responsible introspectionism to take full advantage of the opportunities presented by the new dawn. In my opinion, we need to take ourselves far more seriously as expert self-observers. We need to take closer account of how consciousness works. We need to use the fruits of third person accounts to better inform and direst first person enquiries. Consciousness, we are relieved to admit, is finally a bona fide subject of enquiry. Let us take the next obvious step and teach it to study itself.

For starters, consider the mental status exam which has long been so useful a part of patient examination in neurology and psychiatry. It does inform most of the modules of modern cognitive science such as sensation, perception, attention, emotion, and so on but it does not go into adequate detail in characterizing each aspect of mentation. For example, dreaming is said to be bizarre but 5 years of scrupulous work were required to show that dream bizarreness reduced to plot discontinuity and incongruity. Hence dream bizarreness is microscopic disorientation. Since disorientation is a component of delirium, it was natural to ask the question: in what other ways is dreaming like delirium? The visuomotor hallucinations, the confabulation, and the memory loss all assume new meaning in the light of this formulation. Dreaming is delirium by definition.

Cognitive science does already use the quantifiability of behaviouristic paradigms to study the modules of consciousness experimentally. But sentient human subjects, including brain-damaged ones, are privy to detailed experiential data that we need to heed and harness. 'Did your dreaming change after your stroke' is a question only recently asked. It opens a whole new area for clinical neuropsychology. The creation of a responsible introspective approach to the subjective awareness of altered mental states is a task for which sophisticated hardware is no substitute. The fact that paper and pencils are cheap does not mean they should not be used to study consciousness.

In all the excitement, we may also be chastened by the relatively low spatial resolving power of current imaging techniques, which are still two orders of magnitude less sensitive than cellular and molecular neuroscience probes. An important antidote to this defect is brain imaging of those animal species that are such useful models of human consciousness. And while we are about it we might just take such animal models of consciousness a bit more seriously. We will always be limited in what experiments are possible in humans. What can and what can we not expect to learn from animals. Moreover, speaking of models, is it not time for an improvement on two dimensional diagrams showing brain regions and alterations of consciousness. Since it is spring, we should let a thousand flowers bloom. The visual and mathematical talents of brain scientists may now awaken and provide us with brain images of our own devising.

For the research scientists and clinicians who share a passion for understanding the brain basis of mind, this book provides a rich offering of observations that will be essential; building blocks of the new synthesis. Here, at last, is a survey of the way that damage to the brain alters consciousness. This volume is a well-equipped hardware shop with most of the pieces that are needed to build a state-of-the-art model of how the brain performs its most magical function, the creation of a self that sees, perceives, knows that it does so, and dares to ask how.

Allan Hobson
Harvard Medical School, Boston, Massachusetts

List of Contributors

Michael T. Alkire* Department of Anesthesiology and Center for Neurobiology of Learning and Memory, University of California, Irvine, Orange, CA, USA. Phone: +1 714 456 5501, Fax: +1 714 456 7702, E-mail: malkire@ucl.uci.edu

Claudio L. Bassetti* Department of Neurology, University Hospital Zurich, Zurich, Switzerland. Phone: +41 44 255 5503, Fax: +41 44 255 4649, E-mail: claudio.bassetti@nos.usz.ch

James L. Bernat* Neurology Section, Dartmouth-Hitchcock Medical Center, Lebanon, NH, USA. Phone: +1 603 650 8664, Fax: +1 603 650 6233, E-mail: bernat@dartmouth.edu

Olaf Blanke* Laboratory of Cognitive Neuroscience, Brain Mind Institute, Ecole Polytechnique Fédérale de Lausanne (EPFL), Swiss Federal Institute of Technology, Lausanne, Switzerland. Phone: +41 21 6939621, Fax: +41 21 6939625, E-mail: olaf.blanke@epfl.ch

Hal Blumenfeld* Department of Neurology, Neurobiology and Neurosurgery, Yale University School of Medicine, New Haven, CT, USA. Phone: +1 203 785 3928, Fax: +1 203 737 2538, E-mail: hal.blumenfeld@yale.edu

Melanie Boly Coma Science Group, Neurology Department and Cyclotron Research Center, University of Liège, Liège, Belgium

Marie-Aurélie Bruno Coma Science Group, Neurology Department and Cyclotron Research Center, University of Liège, Liège, Belgium

Chris Butler Department of Clinical Neurosciences, Western General Hospital, Edinburgh, UK. E-mail: chris.butler@ed.ac.uk

Antonio Damasio* University of Southern California, College of Letters, Arts and Sciences, Los Angeles, CA, USA. Phone: +1 213 740 3462, E-mail: damasio@usc.edu

Sebastian Dieguez Department of Neurology, University Hospital, Geneva, Switzerland

Joseph Fins* Division of Medical Ethics, Weill Medical College of Cornell University, New York, NY, USA. Phone: +1 212 746 4246, Fax: +1 212 746 8738, E-mail: jjfins@mail.med.cornell.edu

Michael S. Gazzaniga* Sage Center for the Study of the Mind, University of California, Santa Barbara, CA, USA. Phone: +1 805 893 5006, Fax: +1 805 893 4303, E-mail: gazzaniga@psych.ucsb.edu

Joseph T. Giacino* JFK Johnson Rehabilitation Institute, Edison and New Jersey Neuroscience Institute, Edison, NJ, USA. Phone: +1 732 205 1461, Fax: +1 732 632 1584, E-mail: jgiacomo@solarishs.org

Olivia Gosseries Coma Science Group, Neurology Department and Cyclotron Research Center, University of Liège, Liège, Belgium

Christof Koch* Koch Laboratory, Division of Biology and Division of Engineering and Applied Science, California Institute of Technology, Pasadena, CA, USA. Phone: +1 626 395 6054, Email: koch@klab.caltech.edu

Andrea Kübler* Institute of Medical Psychology and Behavioral Neurobiology, University of Tübingen, Tübingen, Germany. Phone: +49 7071 297 4221, E-mail: andrea.kuebler@uni-tuebingen.de

Ron Kupers PET Center, Rigshospitalet, Copenhagen, Denmark

Steven Laureys* Neurology Department, University Hospital CHU and Research Associate, Belgian National Funds for Scientific Research, Cyclotron Research Center, University of Liege, Liège, Belgium. Phone: +32 4 366 23 04, Fax: +32 4 366 29 46, E-mail: steven.laureys@ulg.ac.be

Kaspar Meyer Brain and Creativity Institute, University of Southern California, Los Angeles, CA, USA

Michael B. Miller University of California, Santa Barbara, CA, USA

Lionel Naccache* Fédération de Neurophysique Clinique, Hôpital de la Pitié-Salpêtrière, Paris, France. Phone: +31 1 40779799, E-mail: lionel.nagacche@wanadoo.fr

Paolo Nichelli Dip.di Patologia Neuropsicosensoriale Sezione di Neurologia, Università di Modena,

Modena, Italy. Phone: +39 059 3961659, E-mail: nichelli@unimo.it

Adrian M. Owen* MRC Cognition and Brain Sciences Unit and Wolfson Brain Imaging Centre, University of Cambridge, Cambridge, UK. Phone: +44 1223 355294, Fax: +44 1223 359062, E-mail: adrian.owen@mrc-cbu.cam.ac.uk

Pietro Pietrini* Laboratory of Clinical Biochemistry, University of Pisa, Pisa, Italy. Phone: +39 50 993410, Fax: +39 50 2218660, E-mail: pietro.pietrini@med.unipi.it

Bradley R. Postle* Department of Psychology and Psychiatry, University of Wisconsin-Madison, Madison, USA. Phone: +1 608 2624330, Fax: +1 608 262 4029, E-mail: postle@wisc.edu

Maurice Ptito Ecole d'optométrie, Université de Montréal, Montréal, Canada; Danish Research Center on Magnetic Resonance, Hvidovre Hospital, Copenhagen, Denmark

Marcus E. Raichle* Washington University School of Medicine, St Louis, MO, USA. Phone: +1 314 362 6907, Phone: +1 314 362 6907 (lab.), Fax: +1 314 362 6110, E-mail: marc@npg.wustl.edu

Geraint Rees* Institute of Cognitive Neuroscience and Wellcome Trust Centre for Neuroimaging, University College London, London, UK. Phone: +44 20 7679 5496, Fax: +44 20 7813 1420, E-mail: g.rees@fil.ion.ucl.ac.uk

Eric Salmon Cyclotron Research Centre and Department of Neurology, University of Liege, Liege, Belgium. Phone: +32 4 366 2316, E-mail: eric.salmon@ulg.ac.be

Nicholas D. Schiff Department of Neurology and Neuroscience, Weill Medical College of Cornell University, New York, NY, USA. Phone: +1 212 7468532, E-mail: nds2001@med.cornell.edu

Caroline Schnakers Coma Science Group, Neurology Department and Cyclotron Research Center, University of Liège, Liège, Belgium

Wolf Singer* Max Planck Institut für Hirnforschung, Frankfurt/Main, Germany. Phone: +49 69 96769218, Fax: +49 69 96769327, E-mail: singer@mpih-frankfurt.mpg.de

Abraham Z. Snyder Department of Radiology and Neurology, Washington University School of Medicine, St Louis, MO, USA. Phone: +1 314 362 6907, Fax: +1 314 362 6110, E-mail: avi@npg.wustl.edu

Giulio Tononi* Department of Psychiatry, University of Wisconsin, Madison, WI, USA. Phone: +1 608 2636063, Fax: +1 608 2639340, E-mail: gtononi@wisc.edu

Naotsugu Tsuchiya Division of the Humanities and Social Sciences, California Institute of Technology, Pasadena, CA, USA. E-mail: naotsugu@gmail.com

Audrey Vanhaudenhuyse Coma Science Group, Neurology Department and Cyclotron Research Center, University of Liège, Liège, Belgium

Patrik Vuilleumier* Laboratory for Behavioral Neurology and Imaging of Cognition, Clinic of Neurology and Department of Neurosciences, University Medical Center, Geneva, Switzerland. Phone: +41 22 3795 381, Fax: +41 22 379 5402, E-mail: patrik.vuilleumier@medicine.unige.ch

G. Bryan Young Department of Clinical Neurological Sciences, London Health Sciences Centre, London, Ontario, Canada. Phone: +1 519 6632911, Fax: +1 519 6633115, E-mail: bryan.young@lhsc.on.ca

Adam Zeman* Peninsula Medical School, Mardon Centre, Exeter, UK. Phone: +44 1392 208583 or Phone: +44 1392 208581 (secretary), E-mail: adam.zeman@pms.ac.uk

Note: *Senior author.

BASICS

Consciousness: An Overview of the Phenomenon and of Its Possible Neural Basis[1]

Antonio Damasio and Kaspar Meyer

OUTLINE

ABSTRACT

The first part of this chapter provides a phenomenological description of consciousness from a dual perspective. From the observer's perspective, a conscious subject (1) is awake; (2) displays background emotions; (3) exhibits attention; and (4) shows evidence of purposeful behaviour. From the subject's perspective, consciousness emerges when the brain generates (a) neural patterns about objects in sensorimotor terms; (b) neural patterns about the changes those objects cause in the internal state of the organism; and (c) a second-order account that interrelates (a) and (b). The second-order account describing the relationship between the organism and the object is the neural basis of subjectivity; it portrays the organism as the protagonist to which objects are referred and establishes 'core consciousness'. 'Extended consciousness' occurs when objects are related to the organism not only in the 'here and now' but in a broader context encompassing the organism's past and its anticipated future. In the second part of the chapter, we describe the neural structures required to generate consciousness according to the preceding hypothesis, drawing on (a) extant neuroanatomical and neurophysiological data and (b) a number of conditions in which wakefulness, core consciousness, and extended consciousness are selectively impaired, such as coma, vegetative state, and anaesthesia. We conclude that a number of cortical midline structures, especially in the medial parietal region (the so-called posteromedial cortices), are essential to the generation of both core and extended consciousness.

[1]This work was financially supported by the Mathers Foundation (A.D.) and by the Swiss National Science Foundation (K.M.).

The topic of consciousness remains controversial both within and outside neuroscience. In addition to the problems posed by explaining biologically any aspect of mental activity, the difficulties also stem from the range of concepts associated with the term consciousness and from the need to specify the particular meaning attached to each of them. In approaching consciousness and its possible neuroanatomical basis, we shall begin by outlining what we mean by consciousness and providing a working definition of the phenomenon. Following that, we present a neurobiological account of consciousness compatible with the definition, and describe the neuroanatomical structures required to realize consciousness in that perspective.

DEFINING CONSCIOUSNESS

It would be convenient if consciousness could be defined very simply as the mental property we acquire when we wake up from dreamless sleep, and lose when we return to it. This definition might help if we were explaining consciousness to a newly arrived extraterrestrial, or to a child, but it would fail to describe what consciousness is, mentally speaking.

The commonplace dictionary definitions of consciousness tend to fare better since they often state that consciousness is the ability to be aware of self and surroundings. These definitions are circular – given that awareness is often seen as a synonym of consciousness itself, or at least as a significant part of it – but in spite of the circularity, such definitions capture something essential: consciousness does allow us to know of our own existence and of the existence of objects and events, inside and outside our organism. However, although an improvement, these definitions do not go far enough. In particular, they do not recognize the need for a dual perspective in consciousness studies. One perspective is internal, first-person, subjective, and mental. Another perspective is external, third-person, objective, and behavioural. The latter, of course, is the observer's perspective, an observer who, incidentally, may be a clinician or a researcher.

What does a conscious person look like to an observer? What are the telltale behavioural signs of consciousness? The sign of consciousness we should consider first is wakefulness. If we disregard the somewhat paradoxical situation of dream sleep, one cannot be conscious and asleep. Wakefulness is easy to establish on the basis of a few objective signs: subjects should open their eyes upon request; the muscular tone should be compatible with movements against gravity; and there should be a characteristic awake electroencephalography (EEG) pattern. However, although normal consciousness requires wakefulness, the presence of wakefulness does not guarantee consciousness. Patients with impaired consciousness in conditions such as vegetative state, epileptic automatisms, and akinetic mutism, are technically awake but cannot be considered conscious (see below for a behavioural description of these disorders).

Second, conscious persons exhibit background emotions. The term emotion usually conjures up the primary emotions (e.g., fear, anger, sadness, happiness, disgust) or the social emotions (e.g., embarrassment, guilt, compassion), but the phenotypes of emotion also include background emotions, which occur in continual form when the organism is not engaged in either primary or social emotions. Background emotions are expressed in configurations of body movement and suggest to the observer states such as fatigue or energy; discouragement or enthusiasm; malaise or well-being; anxiety or relaxation. Telltale signals include the overall body posture and the range of motion of the limbs relative to the trunk; the spatial profile of limb movements; the speed of motion; the congruence of movements occurring in different body tiers; and, perhaps most importantly, the animation of the face. When we observe someone with intact consciousness, well before any words are spoken or major gestures produced, we find ourselves presuming the subject's state of mind. Correct or not, those presumptions are largely based on preverbal emotional signals available in the subject's behaviour. The absence of background emotions usually betrays impairments of consciousness.

Third, conscious subjects exhibit attention. They orient themselves towards objects and concentrate on them as needed. Eyes, head, neck, torso, and arms move about in a coordinated pattern which establishes an unequivocal relationship between subjects and certain stimuli in their surround. The mere presence of attention towards an external object usually signifies the presence of consciousness, but there are exceptions. Patients in states of akinetic mutism, whose consciousness is impaired, can pay *transient* attention to a *salient* object or event, for example, a phone ringing, a tray with food, an observer calling their name. Attention only denotes the presence of consciousness when it can be *sustained* over a substantial period of time and is focused on the objects or events that must be considered for behaviour to be appropriate in a given context. This period of time is measured in the order of minutes rather than seconds.

Another important qualification is needed. Lack of attention towards an external object may indicate that attention is being directed towards an internally represented mental object and does not necessarily denote impaired consciousness, as in absentmindedness. However, sustained failure of attention as happens in drowsiness, confusional states, or stupor, is associated with the dissolution of consciousness. Attention is disrupted in coma, VS, and general anaesthesia.

Neither attention nor consciousness are monoliths but rather occur in levels and grades, from simple (core consciousness) to complex (extended consciousness). Low-level attention is needed to engage core consciousness; in turn, the process of core consciousness permits higher-level attention.

Fourth, conscious persons exhibit purposeful behaviour. The presence of adequate and purposeful behaviour is easy to establish in patients who can converse with the observer. When there are impairments of communication, however, the observation requires more detail. Purposeful behaviour towards a stimulus suggests a recognizable plan that could only have been formulated by an organism cognizant of its immediate past, of its present, and of anticipated future conditions. The sustained purposefulness and adequateness of behaviour require consciousness even if consciousness does not guarantee purposeful and adequate behaviour. Sustained adequate behaviour is accompanied by a flow of emotional states as it unfolds background emotions that continuously underscore the subject's actions. Conscious human behaviour exhibits a continuity of emotions induced by a continuity of thoughts. (Of note, terms such as alertness and arousal are often incorrectly used as synonyms of wakefulness, attention, and even consciousness. The term 'alertness' should be used to signify that the subject is both awake and disposed to perceive and act, the proper meaning of 'alert' being somewhere between 'awake' and 'attentive'. The term 'arousal' denotes the presence of signs of autonomic nervous system activation such as changes in skin colour (rubor or pallor), behaviour of skin hair (piloerection), diameter of the pupils, sweating, sexual erection, all of which correspond to the lay term 'excitement'. Thus, subjects can be awake, fully conscious, and alert without being aroused; on the other hand, they can be aroused during sleep and even coma, when they are obviously not awake, attentive, or conscious.)

What does consciousness look like from the internal perspective?

The answer to this question is tied to what we regard as a central problem in the study of consciousness: subjectivity and the process that generates subjectivity. From the internal standpoint, consciousness consists of a multiplicity of mental images of objects and events, located and occurring inside or outside the organism, and formulated in the perspective of the organism. Those images are automatically related to mental images of the organism in which they occur, thus appearing to be 'owned by' the organism and 'perceived' in its perspective. (By 'object' we mean entities as diverse as a person, a place, a state of localized pain, or a state of feeling; by 'event' we mean the actions of objects and the relationships among objects. Note that both objects and events may be part of the current occurrences or, alternatively, may be recalled from memory. By 'image' we mean a mental pattern in any of the sensory modalities, for example sound images, tactile images, or images of pain or well-being conveyed by somatic sensation. We do not regard the issue of generating mental images as an insurmountable problem in consciousness research. We believe that mental images correspond to neural patterns and acknowledge that further understanding of the relationship between neural and mental descriptions is required. We also note that, in this review, we shall not address the qualia problem at all.)

From the internal perspective, the first step in the making of consciousness consists of generating neural patterns representing objects or events. The mental images which arise from these neural patterns, and whose ensemble constitutes a mental event, i.e. mind, are integrated across sensory modalities in space and time; for example, the visual and auditory images of a person who is speaking to us, along with images of facts related to that person, are synchronized and spatially coherent. However, consciousness requires something beyond the production of such multiple images. It requires the creation of a sense of self in the act of knowing, a second step that follows that of creating mental images for objects and events. This second step delivers information about our own mind and organism. It creates knowledge to the effect that we have a mind and that the contents of our mind are shaped in a particular perspective, namely that of our own organism. This second step in the generation of consciousness allows us to construct not just the mental images of objects and events, for example the temporally and spatially unified images of persons, places, and of their components and relationships, but also the mental images which automatically convey the sense of a self in the act of knowing. In other words, the second step consists of generating the appearance of an owner and observer of the mind, *within* that very same mind [1, 2].

How is this sense of self constructed by the brain? In answering this question, it is indispensable to note that consciousness is not only about the representation of objects and events, but also about the representation of the organism it belongs to, as the latter interacts with objects and events. The sense of our organism in the act of knowing endows us with the feeling of ownership of the objects to be known. We have suggested that this sense of self is newly created for each moment in time; conscious individuals continuously generate 'pulses of consciousness' which bring together organism and object, multiple and consecutive periods of mental knowledge along with the external behaviours that accompany this process. (For other views on the phenomena of consciousness from philosophical, cognitive and neurobiological angles see [3–12].)

Taking into account all of the above, our working definition describes consciousness as *a momentary creation of neural patterns which describe a relation between the organism, on the one hand, and an object or event, on the other.* This composite of neural patterns describes a state that, for lack of a better word, we call the *self.* That state is the key to subjectivity. The mental states which inhere in the processing of neural patterns related to all sorts of objects and events are now imbued with neural patterns and corresponding mental states which correspond to the relationship between the organism and objects/events. The definition also specifies that *the creation of self neural patterns is accompanied by characteristic observable behaviours.*

In conclusion, consciousness must be considered from two standpoints: the external (behavioural) and the internal (cognitive, mental). From the external standpoint, the human organism is said to be conscious when it exhibits signs of wakefulness, background emotions, sustained attention towards objects and events in its environment, and sustained, adequate, and purposeful behaviour relative to those objects and events. From the internal standpoint, a human organism is said to be conscious when its mental state represents objects and events in relation to itself, that is when the representation of objects and events is accompanied by the sense that the organism is the perceiving agent.

In the absence of the above collection of behavioural signs, it is not permissible to say that a person is conscious unless the person reports by gesture, words, or some other behavioural manifestation that in spite of the absence of such signs, there is in fact a conscious mind at work. This is precisely the situation of locked-in patients, who exhibit, via a minimal amount of movement, unequivocal evidence of conscious mental activity. In the absence of *any* conventional form of communication, the assumption that the individual is conscious is unlikely to be correct although, at the moment, it cannot be verified one way or another. Accordingly, we caution against interpreting signs of coherent brain activity in either resting or activation imaging scans as evidence for consciousness. Unless we are prepared to reject the current understanding of the phenomenon, consciousness is associated with behaviours that communicate the contents of a mind aware of self and surroundings. On the other hand,

we applaud the attempts to identify conditions of disturbed consciousness in which particular patterns of stimulation may temporarily restore some aspects of consciousness [13].

VARIETIES OF CONSCIOUSNESS

The evidence from neurological patients makes it clear that there are simple and complex kinds of consciousness. The simplest kind, which we call 'core consciousness', conforms to the concept of consciousness described just above, and provides the organism with a sense of self about one moment, now, and about one place, here. The complex kind of consciousness, which we call 'extended consciousness', provides the organism with an elaborate sense of self and places that self in individual historical time, in a perspective of both the lived past and the anticipated future. Core consciousness is a simple biological phenomenon, and its mental aspect is comparably simple; it operates in stable fashion across the lifetime of the organism; and it is not dependent on conventional memory, working memory, reasoning, or language. Extended consciousness is a complex biological phenomenon and is mentally layered across levels of information; it evolves during the lifetime of the organism; it depends on memory; and it is enhanced by language.

The sense of self which emerges in core consciousness is the 'core self', a transient form of knowledge, recreated for each and every object with which the organism interacts. The traditional notion of self, however, is associated with the idea of identity and personhood, and corresponds to a more complex variety of consciousness we call extended consciousness. The self that emerges in extended consciousness is a relatively stable collection of the unique facts that characterize a person, the 'autobiographical self'. The autobiographical self depends on memories of past situations. Those memories were acquired because core consciousness allowed the experience of the respective situations, in the first place.

Impairments of core consciousness compromise extended consciousness, indicating that extended consciousness depends on core consciousness. The disturbance of core consciousness compromises all aspects of mental activity, because core consciousness establishes a basic sense of self, thereby allowing the mind of the organism to take possession of the objects it interacts with, and to add them to the autobiographical self. Any object or event, current or recalled from memory, can only become conscious when the basic self is generated. Core consciousness is a central resource and serves the entire compass of neural patterns generated in the brain.

It is noteworthy that impairments of neural pattern processing (and thus mental image generation) within one sensory modality only compromise the conscious appreciation of one aspect of an object (e.g., visual or auditory) but do not compromise consciousness of the same object through a different sensory channel (e.g., olfactory or tactile). Image-making within a sensory modality may be lost entirely, as in cortical blindness, or just in part. For example, achromatopsia is a circumscribed defect of the ability to imbue images with colour. Patients so affected have a disturbance of object processing for certain attributes of an object, but they generate normal images for other visual aspects of that object (as, for example, its form), and also for all other modalities. From the fact that they are aware of their lack of ability, it can be derived that they even create a mental image for the fact that their object processing is abnormal. In brief, outside of the area of defective knowledge, those patients have normal core consciousness and normal extended consciousness. Their circumscribed defect underscores the fact that core consciousness and its resulting sense of self are a central resource.

Core consciousness is fundamentally different from, but not unrelated to, other cognitive processes. On the contrary, core consciousness is a prerequisite for the focusing and enhancement of attention and working memory; enables the establishment of explicit memories; is indispensable for language and normal communication; and renders possible the intelligent manipulations of images (e.g., planning, problem solving, and creativity). Furthermore, although core consciousness is not equivalent to wakefulness or low-level attention, it requires both to operate normally, as already mentioned.

Core consciousness is also not equivalent to working memory although it is related to it. As we have seen, core consciousness is newly and individually generated for each object or event. On the other hand, working memory is vital for the process of extended consciousness, because a percept has to be held active over a certain amount of time in order to be placed into the rich context extended consciousness endows it with.

Core consciousness does not depend on the processes of conventional learning and memory, either, that is, it does not depend on creating a stable memory for an image or recalling it. Also, core consciousness is not based on language, is not equivalent to manipulating images in planning, problem solving, and creativity. Patients with profound defects of reasoning and planning often exhibit normal core consciousness although the higher levels of extended consciousness may be impaired. In other words, wakefulness, image-making, attention, working memory, conventional memory, language, and intelligence can be separated by cognitive component analysis. Some of these functions (wakefulness, image-making, attention) operate in concert to permit core consciousness; others (working memory, conventional memory, language, and reasoning) assist extended consciousness.

Finally, yet another note is pertinent on the relation between emotion and consciousness. Patients whose core consciousness is impaired do not reveal emotion by facial expression, body expression, or vocalization. The entire range of emotion, from background emotions to secondary emotions, is usually missing in these patients. By contrast, patients with preserved core consciousness but impaired extended consciousness have normal background and primary emotions. In the very least, this association suggests that some of the neural devices on which both emotion and core consciousness depend are co-located.

THE NEURAL BASIS OF CONSCIOUSNESS

As outlined above, consciousness is not one single, uniform phenomenon. Core consciousness depends on wakefulness. Extended consciousness, in turn, depends on core consciousness. In other words, the phenomenon has levels of organizational complexity, neurally and mentally speaking, and those levels are nested. The search for their neural correlates yields different results in each case.

Establishing the neural grounds for consciousness can be approached from two directions. One is to draw on current knowledge from neurophysiology and neuroanatomy in order to identify a roster of structures suitable to carry out the operations we regard as necessary. The other is to consider structural and functional imaging as well as neuropathological studies of conditions in which the critical components we outlined – wakefulness, core consciousness, and extended consciousness – are selectively altered, either because of brain injury or by the action of pharmaceutical agents. We shall begin this section with the first approach.

Neuroanatomical and Neurophysiological Considerations

Wakefulness

Varied cell groups in the brainstem modulate wakefulness by ascending projections to the cerebral cortex. The nuclei of the reticular formation have been divided by Parvizi and Damasio [14] into four groups: the classical reticular nuclei; the monoaminergic nuclei (noradrenergic, serotoninergic, and dopaminergic); the cholinergic nuclei; and the autonomic nuclei. There is evidence that several of these cell groups can modulate cortical activity. For example, there are presumably glutaminergic projections from the classical reticular nuclei to the intralaminar nuclei of the thalamus, which in turn project to large areas of the cerebral cortex (e.g., [15, 16]; for an overview see [14]). Also, the projections from the cholinergic nuclei to the nucleus reticularis of the thalamus impede the generation of thalamic sleep spindles which hallmark deep sleep [17]. Recently, Vogt and Laureys [18] have suggested that cortical arousal may also be mediated by mesopontine cholinergic projections to the antero-ventral thalamic nucleus, which, in turn, has a prominent projection to the retrosplenial cortex and may be responsible for the high rate of glucose metabolism commonly observed in the latter region. In addition to these reticulothalamocortical projections, the nuclei of the reticular formation may exert their influence on the cerebral cortex also via direct cortical pathways or via the basal forebrain and the basal ganglia.

Core Consciousness

We have noted above that core consciousness requires two players, the organism and the object, and concerns their relationship: the fact that the organism is relating to an object, and that the object–organism relationship causes a change in the organism. Elucidating the neurobiology of core consciousness requires the discovery of a composite neural map which brings together in time the pattern for the object, the pattern for the organism, and establishes the relationship between the two [2].

We propose that consciousness begins to occur *when the brain generates a non-verbal account of how the organism's representation is affected by the organism's processing of an object, and when this process enhances the image of the causative object, thus placing it saliently in a spatial and temporal context* [2].

The neural pattern at the basis of the non-verbal account is generated by structures capable of receiving signals from maps which represent both the organism and the object. We call this a 'second-order map' to distinguish it from 'first-order maps' which describe the organism and the object, respectively. The non-verbal account describes the relationship between the reactive changes in the internal milieu, the viscera, the vestibular apparatus, and the musculoskeletal

frame, on the one hand, and the object that causes those changes, on the other hand. We propose that the mental image which inheres in the second-order neural pattern describing the object–organism relationship is tantamount to 'knowing about' the subject's involvement with the object, the central aspect of conscious experience. We also propose that the creation of this neural pattern causes a modulation of the neural patterns which describe the object, leading to the enhancement of its representation, at the same time that the representation of the organism may lose saliency, especially in the case of external objects and events. The mental state of 'perceiving an object', its experience, emerges from the contents of the non-verbal organism/object relationship account, and from the enhancement of the object.

Thus, the neural pattern which underlies core consciousness for an object is a large-scale, multiple-site neural pattern involving activity in three interrelated sets of structures: the set whose cross-regional activity generates an integrated view of the organism; the set whose cross-regional activity generates the representation of the object; and the set which is responsible for interrelating the two others. The object representation set is critical twice: it is both the initiator of the changes and the recipient of modulating influences.

It is well known that the organism is represented in the brain, although the idea that such a representation is relevant to consciousness and to the notion of self has not received much attention (for an exception see [1, 2, 19], and more recently [20]). The brain represents varied aspects of the structure and current state of the organism in a large number of neural maps from the level of the brainstem and hypothalamus to that of the primary and association somatosensory cortices (e.g., SI, S2, insular cortex, parietal cortex), and, for example, the cingulate cortex. The state of the internal milieu, the viscera, the vestibular apparatus, and the musculoskeletal system are thus continuously represented as a set of activities we call the 'proto-self' [2, 14].

On the other hand, extensive studies of perception, learning and memory, and language, have provided evidence for how the brain processes an object, in sensorimotor terms, and how knowledge about an object can be stored in memory, categorized in conceptual or linguistic terms, and retrieved. In the relationship process we have proposed above, the object – either coming from the environment or recalled from memory – is exhibited as neural patterns in the sensory association cortices appropriate for its nature. The association cortices, with respect to consciousness, are involved in various functions: first, they represent the object; second, they change the state of the body and, consequently, the neural maps representing it; third, they signal to second-order maps; and fourth, they receive modulatory signals from the second-order maps which will lead to the enhancement of the object's representation.

As will become evident from several lines of data described in following sections, the so-called posteromedial cortex (PMC), in particular, seems to play an important role in generating the second-order multiple-site neural map which represents the relationship between object and organism. The PMC is the conjunction of the posterior cingulate cortex, the retrosplenial cortex, and the precuneus (Brodmann areas 23a/b, 29, 30, 31, and 7m) and has been shown to possess connections to most all cortical regions (except for primary sensory and primary motor cortices) and to numerous thalamic nuclei [21]. Most of these connections are reciprocal. Damasio [2] hypothesized that this region played a critical role in the generation of the self process.

The generation of all the neural patterns described above is not achieved by the cerebral cortex alone. Rather, it is assisted by thalamocortical interactions [22–27].

Extended Consciousness

Extended consciousness requires working memory and explicit long-term memory (including both semantic and episodic memories). Working memory is a prerequisite to extended consciousness because it allows holding active, simultaneously and for a substantial amount of time, the images which define the object and the many images whose collection defines the autobiographical self. Long-term memory, on the other hand, is needed for the build-up of autobiographical memories in the first place. The recall of those memories replicates images, just like those of any external object, which prompt their own pulse of core consciousness. Thus, it becomes apparent that extended consciousness depends on core consciousness in two ways: first, core consciousness is needed for the creation of the autobiographical self, and second, the contents of the autobiographical self can be experienced generating their own pulse of core consciousness. It is apparent that the structures necessary for extended consciousness encompass an extremely wide array of brain regions. Extended consciousness cannot operate, for example, when the higher-order association cortices are compromised because the availability of past records and the reenactment of their categorization and spatial–temporal structuring is precluded.

Other Relevant Evidence

An intriguing series of functional neuroimaging studies has recently demonstrated that, at rest, the brain is not really at rest (e.g., [28–30]). A network of brain regions, comprising among others the posteromedial, the medial prefrontal, and the lateral parietal cortices, displays three interesting properties: first, it shows a considerable amount of activity when subjects are at rest, not performing any task in particular; second, when subjects engage in a wide variety of goal-directed tasks, the level of activity decreases; and third, this decrease may fail to appear when the ongoing process concerns the self and the states of others, including, for example, certain emotions ([31]; unpublished observations). The overlap of large sections of this network with the areas displaying functional impairment during various states of altered consciousness (see below) is striking, especially with regard to the PMC.

What are the functional implications of this somewhat enigmatic intrinsic brain activity? Several authors have pointed to a variety of self-related functions (e.g., [32–34]; for a review see [35]). In particular, differential activation in the precuneus could be observed in various paradigms involving reflection on the subjects' own personality traits or retrieval of autobiographic events (e.g., [36–39]), thus during task strongly engaging the autobiographical self.

Deriving Neuroanatomy from Clinical Neurological Evidence

The distinction among wakefulness, core consciousness, and extended consciousness requires that we address varied situations in which these operations are selectively impaired. For each situation, we will provide a short behavioural description, followed by an overview of pertinent neuropathological and functional imaging findings.

Impaired Wakefulness, Impaired Core Consciousness

States in which both wakefulness and awareness are impaired include general anaesthesia, coma, and slow-wave sleep. These conditions permit limited external analysis because nearly all behavioural manifestations of consciousness are abolished. The notion that consciousness is also suspended from the internal viewpoint is based on the commonplace experience of ourselves when we sleep and when we undergo general anaesthesia. It is also based on reports from patients who returned to consciousness after being in coma. Whereas these patients can usually recall both the loss of consciousness and the return to knowingness, little if anything is recalled of the intervening period, which can span weeks or months. In all likelihood, this is so because a compromise of consciousness entails a disturbance of learning and memory such that mental contents are either not recorded properly or are recorded but not accessible.

As a common feature in all three conditions at issue, there is, in many cases, structural damage to, or altered metabolism of, brainstem structures. The cases of coma caused by structural lesions reveal that the primary site of dysfunction is in structures of the upper brainstem, hypothalamus, and thalamus [40], although diffuse bihemispheric cortical or white-matter damage may also be the cause (e.g., [41]). Parvizi and Damasio [42] showed that in coma caused by brainstem stroke, the lesions most often affected the tegmentum bilaterally and were located in upper pons and midbrain or upper pons alone. Functional imaging shows metabolic impairment in the brainstem and the thalamus during coma resulting from brain trauma [41].

In general anaesthesia, there was considerable overlap of the metabolic suppression effect of several anesthetic agents (such as propofol, various inhalative agents, benzodiazepines, and centrally acting α-2-receptor agonists) in the thalamus [43]. Since a large part of the positron emission tomography (PET) signal originates from synaptic activity, this effect may in fact represent a site of action different from the thalamus, alternatively in brainstem arousal centres or in the cerebral cortex [43]. For example, the effect of propofol was in part attributed to the 'reticulothalamic system' based on a strong covariation between thalamic and midbrain blood flow [44, 45].

Similarly, during slow-wave sleep, the tegmental sector of the pons and the mesencephalon as well as the thalamus showed marked deactivations [46].

Persistent Wakefulness, Impaired Core Consciousness

Conditions in which wakefulness persists, but core consciousness is absent, include vegetative state (VS), akinetic mutism, and certain types of epileptic seizures. Of note, in these conditions, as opposed to those discussed in the preceding section, findings from neuropathology and functional imaging suggest a relative sparing of the brainstem ([2], Chapter 8; [41]), a possible exception being complex-partial seizures in which an increase of brainstem and thalamic metabolism could be identified during or after the seizure [47, 48].

From a behavioural point of view, the VS is distinguished from coma in that patients exhibit cycles of sleep and wakefulness, as evidenced by the opening and closing of the eyes and, on occasion, by their EEG.

Another state of preserved wakefulness but minimal attention and behaviour is akinetic mutism, a term suggestive of what goes on externally, but which fails to suggest the fact that consciousness is severely diminished or suspended. Patients remain mostly motionless and speechless for long periods which may last weeks or months. They lie in bed with eyes open but with a blank facial expression, never expressing any emotion. They may track an object in motion for a few instants but non-focused staring is rapidly resumed. Occasionally, they make purposeful movements with arm and hand, but in general, their limbs are in repose. When asked about their situation, the patients are invariably silent, although, after much insistence, they may offer their name. They generally do not react to the presence of relatives or friends. As the patients emerge from this state and gradually begin to answer some questions, they have no recall of any particular experience during their long period of silence; they do not report having fear or anxiety or wishing to communicate.

Epileptic automatisms most often occur as part of, or immediately after, absence seizures or complex-partial seizures [49, 50]. In absence seizures, consciousness is momentarily suspended along with emotion, attention, and purposeful behaviour. The disturbance is accompanied by a characteristic EEG pattern. The typical absence seizure is among the most pure examples of loss of consciousness, the term absence being shorthand for 'absence of consciousness'.

All of the conditions discussed so far, including the ones in the preceding section (coma, general anaesthesia, slow-wave sleep, VS, akinetic mutism, and epileptic seizures), that is all states in which core consciousness is compromised, share an important characteristic: they typically have damage and/or altered metabolism in a number of midline structures such as the PMC, the medial prefrontal cortex, the anterior cingulate cortex, and the thalamus.

The VS can evolve from coma, and so, not surprisingly, it may also be associated with diffuse cortical or white-matter damage, or with focal, bilateral damage to the thalamus (e.g., [40, 51]). Functional neuroimaging studies reveal similar cortical correlates in coma and VS, specifically, decreased activity in medial and lateral prefrontal, temporo-parietal, and posteromedial cortices (e.g., [52]). A special role of the PMC is suggested by the fact that this region displays the most marked increase of activity when patients recover from the VS [53]. Also, the activity in this region differentiates between the VS and the so-called minimally conscious state [41, 52].

At the level of the cerebral cortex, general anaesthesia induced by a variety of anesthetic agents is also associated with decreases of activity in the PMC and, to lesser extent, in the medial prefrontal cortex [43]. The same two regions (among others) also display metabolic decreases during slow-wave sleep [46, 54].

Akinetic mutism is most often produced by bilateral cerebrovascular lesions in the mesial frontal regions. The anterior cingulate cortex, along with nearby regions such as the basal forebrain, is almost invariably damaged, but the condition may also result from dysfunction in the PMC ([2], Chapter 8).

Imaging results from epileptic seizures are controversial, but there is evidence for metabolic abnormalities in some of the midline structures mentioned above [48, 55–58].

Persistent Wakefulness, Persistent Core Consciousness, Impaired Extended Consciousness

Although extended consciousness is impaired in many disorders, there does not seem to be any condition in which core consciousness persists while extended consciousness is completely abolished. Patients suffering from transient global amnesia have significantly reduced extended consciousness; however, their verbal reports and behaviour clearly indicate that their mental state is not limited to core consciousness. In advanced Alzheimer's disease, extended consciousness is nearly abolished but eventually, in late stages of the condition, so is core consciousness. Thus, distinctive neuropathological correlates are unavailable.

Concluding Remarks

Based on the foregoing, the following conclusions appear reasonable. Bilateral lesions of the brainstem tegmentum compromise wakefulness as well as core and extended consciousness. This is due, in part, to disruption of the activating influence of several brainstem nuclei on the thalamus and on the cerebral cortex. However, because lesions of the tegmentum also disrupt afferent relays of the somatosensory system and deprive the brain of information about the current state of the organism, we suggest that by so doing they compromise the proto-self. We thus attribute a dual function to the normal brainstem tegmentum,

concerning both wakefulness and core consciousness. (Extensive damage to the hypothalamus probably contributes to impairments of core consciousness via the role of hypothalamic nuclei in the proto-self process.)

Damage to the thalamus has varied effects on wakefulness, core consciousness, and extended consciousness, depending on the exact location of the lesion. Damage to the intralaminar thalamic system causes lethargy or coma whereas lesions of specific nuclei as, for example, the lateral geniculate body, only affect the corresponding sensory modality (e.g., [25]; and see [59, 60]). From a theoretical point of view, the major impact of damage to the intralaminar thalamic nuclei has two explanations. First, as noted, the intralaminar nuclei play an important role in relaying the modulating influences of the reticular formation to the cerebral cortex. Second, according to Llinás [22–26], the intralaminar nuclei play an important role in the temporal conjunction of neural patterns. In terms of our proposal, we assume that the neural patterns representing the object and the organism, the second-order map interrelating them, and all the neural patterns representing the contents of extended consciousness require thalamocortical interactions.

Damage to, or impaired function in, cortical midline structures such as the superior and medial prefrontal cortices, the anterior cingulate cortices, and, especially, the PMC, disrupt consciousness to varying degrees but do not affect wakefulness. We attribute the critical involvement of the PMC and other midline structures in the maintenance of consciousness to their role in establishing the wide-ranging second-order map which interrelates the first-order maps representing the object and the organism, respectively.

Structural damage or malfunction in a wide variety of cortical areas can compromise different aspects of extended consciousness while leaving core consciousness unaffected. This effect can be attributed to the dependence of extended consciousness on both working memory and conventional memory which, in turn, depend on the proper functioning of association cortices in all sectors of the telencephalon and on the hippocampal system. On the other hand, a complete disruption of extended consciousness only seems to occur when the brain structures implementing core consciousness are damaged or display decreased activity.

Given the above, we suggest that extended consciousness fundamentally relies on the same midline structures as core consciousness. Midline cortices, and the PMC in particular, would not only relate the representation of the object to the representation of the physical organism but also to various aspects of the autobiographical self of the same organism.

AN EVOLUTIONARY PERSPECTIVE

In brief, we propose that, in evolution, core consciousness came to exist when second-order maps first brought together the representation of the organism modified by perceptual engagement, with the representation of the object that caused the modifications. We attribute a key role in generating these second-order maps to the PMC and we note, again, that myriad brain regions are required to represent organism and object. It seems conceivable that extended consciousness eventually emerged as a growing number of brain areas became interlinked to the PMC, gradually endowing the core-conscious organism with a broader scope of nearly simultaneous associations. A neural architecture with convergence/divergence properties would be suitable to carry out this task, and the massive afferent and efferent connectivities we have gleaned in the monkey identify the PMC as a suitable executor (see [21]). If core consciousness establishes the relationship between an object and the organism, extended consciousness enriches the relationship by creating additional links between the object and the organism, not just with respect to the presence of the latter in the here and now, but also to its past and anticipated future.

What is the evolutionary advantage of consciousness? In prior work we have addressed this question by describing consciousness as a sophisticated means of upholding the integrity of the organism by contributing importantly to homeostasis [2]. All organisms possess efficient automatic regulatory mechanisms, internal as well as behavioural, which keep various biological parameters within the narrow range compatible with the continuity of life. Consciousness permits an extension of these automatic homeostatic mechanisms by allowing for flexibility and planning, important functions in complex and unpredictable environments. Conscious organisms know about their past and can make guesses about their future. They can implement this knowledge and manipulate it through planning, in an endeavour to approach that which is beneficial and avoid the harmful.

There is a remarkable overlap of biological functions within the structures which support the integrated maps of the organism state (the proto-self) and the second-order maps interrelating the organism and the object. For example, they are implicated in (a) regulating homeostasis and signalling body structure and state, including the processing of signals related to pain, pleasure, and drives; (b) participating in the processes of emotion and feeling; (c) participating in processes of attention; (d) participating in the processes of wakefulness and sleep; and (e) participating in the learning process.

The meaning of these functional overlaps may be gleaned by focusing on the brainstem, where distinct 'families' of nuclei are closely contiguous and highly interconnected. It makes good evolutionary and functional sense that structures governing attention and emotion should be in the vicinity of those which signal and regulate body states since the causes and consequences of emotion and attention are related to the fundamental process of managing life, and it is not possible to manage life and maintain homeostatic balance without data on the current state of the organism's body proper. When we regard consciousness as another contributor to the regulation of homeostasis, it also appears functionally expedient to place its critical neural machinery within, and in the vicinity of, the neural machinery involved in basic homeostasis, that is, the machinery of emotion, attention, and regulation of body state.

The role that has been traditionally assigned to the brainstem's 'ascending reticular activating system' and to its extension in the thalamus, namely wakefulness, as described in the classical work of Moruzzi and Magoun [61], Penfield and Jasper [49], and in recent work by Llinás (e.g., [22, 23]), Hobson [62], Steriade [17, 63–65], Munk et al. [66], and Singer [67] is compatible with this interpretation. The 'ascending reticular activating system' allows cortical circuits to operate at the level of wakefulness necessary for consciousness to occur, and may perhaps contribute to the organization of activities that correspond to the actual contents of consciousness. However, the activating system's contribution is not sufficient to explain consciousness comprehensively.

References

1. Damasio, A.R. (1998) Investigating the biology of consciousness. *Phil Trans R Soc Lond B* 353:1879–1882.
2. Damasio, A.R. (1999/2000) *The Feeling of What Happens: Body and Emotion in the Making of Consciousness*, New York: Harcourt Brace.
3. Baars, B.J. (1988) *A Cognitive Theory of Consciousness*, Cambridge: Cambridge University Press.
4. Chalmers, D.J. (1995) Facing up to the problem of consciousness. *J Conscious Stud* 2:200–219.
5. Crick, F. (1994) *The Astonishing Hypothesis: The Scientific Search for the Soul*, New York: Charles Scribner's Sons.
6. Crick, F. and Koch, C. (2003) A framework for consciousness. *Nat Neurosci* 6:119–126.
7. Dennett, D. (1991) *Consciousness Explained*, Boston, MA: Little Brown.
8. Edelman, G.M. (1989) *The Remembered Present*, New York: Basic Books.
9. Edelman, G.M. and Tononi, G. (2000) *A Universe of Consciousness: How Matter Becomes Imagination*, New York: Basic Books.

10. Koch, C. (2004) *The Quest for Consciousness – A Neurobiological Approach*, Greenwood Village: Roberts and Company Publishers.

11. Metzinger, T. (2003) *Being No One. The Self Model Theory of Subjectivity*, Cambridge, MA: MIT Press.

12. Searle, J. (1992) *The Rediscovery of the Mind*, Cambridge, MA: MIT Press.

13. Schiff, N.D., Giacino, J.T., Kalmar, K., Victor, J.D., Baker, K., Gerber, M., Fritz, B., Eisenberg, B., O'Connor, J., Kobylarz, E.J., Farris, S., Machado, A., McCagg, C., Plum, F., Fins, J.J. and Rezai, A.R. (2007) Behavioral improvements with thalamic stimulation after severe traumatic brain injury. *Nature* 448:600–603.

14. Parvizi, J. and Damasio, A.R. (2001) Consciousness and the brainstem. *Cognition* 49:135–160.

15. Kinomura, S., Larsson, J., Gulyas, B. and Roland, P.E. (1996) Activation by attention of the human reticular formation and thalamic intralaminar nuclei. *Science* 271:512–515.

16. Steriade, M. (1996) Arousal: Revisiting the reticular activating system. *Science* 272:225–226.

17. Steriade, M. (1993) Central core modulation of spontaneous oscillations and sensory transmission in thalamocortical systems. *Curr Opin Neurobiol* 3:619–625.

18. Vogt, B.A. and Laureys, S. (2005) Posterior cingulate, precuneal and retrosplenial cortices: Cytology and components of the neural network correlates of consciousness. *Prog Brain Res* 150:205–217.

19. Damasio, A.R. (1994) *Descartes' Error: Emotion, Reason, and the Human Brain*, New York: Grosset/Putnam.

20. Damasio, A.R. and Damasio, H. (2006) Minding the Body. *Daedalus (J Am Acad Arts Sci)* 135 (3):15–22.

21. Parvizi, J., Van Hoesen, G.W., Buckwalter, J. and Damasio, A. (2006) Neural connections of the posteromedial cortex in the macaque. *Proc Natl Acad Sci USA* 103:1563–1568.

22. Llinás, R.R. and Paré, D. (1991) Of dreaming and wakefulness. *Neuroscience* 44:521–535.

23. Llinás, R.R. and Ribary, U. (1993) Coherent 40-Hz oscillation characterizes dream state in humans. *Proc Natl Acad Sci USA* 90:2078–2081.

24. Llinás, R.R., Ribary, U., Contreras, D. and Pedroarena, C. (1998) The neuronal basis for consciousness. *Phil Trans R Soc Lond B* 353:1841–1849.

25. Llinás, R.R., Leznik, E. and Urbano, F.J. (2002) Temporal binding via cortical coincidence detection of specific and nonspecific thalamocortical inputs: A voltage-dependent dye-imaging study in mouse brain slices. *Proc Natl Acad Sci USA* 99:449–454.

26. Llinás, R.R. and Steriade, M. (2006) Bursting of thalamic neurons and states of vigilance. *J Neurophysiol* 95:3297–3308.

27. Ribary, U. (2005) Dynamics of thalamo-cortical network oscillations and human perception. *Prog Brain Res* 150:127–142.

28. Gusnard, D.A. and Raichle, M.E. (2001) Searching for a baseline: Functional imaging and the resting human brain. *Nat Rev Neurosci* 2:685–694.

29. Raichle, M.E., MacLeod, A.M., Snyder, A.Z., Powers, W.J., Gusnard, D.A. and Shulman, G.L. (2001) A default mode of brain function. *Proc Natl Acad Sci USA* 98:676–682.

30. Raichle, M.E. and Mintun, M.A. (2006) Brain work and brain imaging. *Annu Rev Neurosci* 29:449–476.

31. Damasio, A.R., Grabowski, T.J., Bechara, A., Damasio, H., Ponto, L.L.B., Parvizi, J. and Hichwa, R.D. (2000) Subcortical and cortical brain activity during the feeling of self-generated emotions. *Nat Neurosci* 3:1049–1056.

32. Gusnard, D.A., Akbudak, E., Shulman, G.L. and Raichle, M.E. (2001) Medial prefrontal cortex and self-referential mental activity: Relation to a default mode of brain function. *Proc Natl Acad Sci USA* 98:4259–4264.

33. Lou, H.C., Luber, B., Crupain, M., Keenan, J.P., Nowak, M., Kjaer, T.W., Sackeim, H.A. and Lisanby, S.H. (2004) Parietal cortex and representation of the mental self. *Proc Natl Acad Sci USA* 101:6827–6832.

34. Vogeley, K. and Fink, G.R. (2003) Neural correlates of the first-person perspective. *Trends Cogn Sci* 7:38–42.

35. Cavanna, A.E. and Trimble, M.R. (2006) The precuneus: A review of its functional anatomy and behavioural correlates. *Brain* 129:564–583.

36. Addis, D.R., McIntosh, A.R., Moscovitch, M., Crawley, A.P. and McAndrews, M.P. (2004) Characterizing spatial and temporal features of autobiographical memory retrieval networks: A partial least squares approach. *Neuroimage* 23:1460–1471.

37. Gilboa, A., Winocur, G., Grady, C.L., Hevenor, S.J. and Moscovitch, M. (2004) Remembering our past: Functional neuroanatomy of recollection of recent and very remote personal events. *Cereb Cortex* 14:1214–1225.

38. Kircher, T.T.J., Brammer, M., Bullmore, E., Simmons, A., Bartels, M. and David, A.S. (2002) The neural correlates of intentional and incidental self-processing. *Neuropsychologia* 40:683–692.

39. Kjaer, T.W., Nowak, M. and Lou, H.C. (2002) Reflective self-awareness and conscious states: PET evidence for a common midline parietofrontal core. *Neuroimage* 17:1080–1086.

40. Plum, F. and Posner, J.B. (1980) *The Diagnosis of Stupor and Coma*, Philadelphia, PA: F. A. Davis Company.

41. Laureys, S., Owen, A.M. and Schiff, N.D. (2004) Brain function in coma, vegetative state, and related disorders. *Lancet Neurol* 3:537–546.

42. Parvizi, J. and Damasio, A.R. (2003) Neuroanatomical correlates of brainstem coma. *Brain* 126:1524–1536.

43. Alkire, M.T. and Miller, J. (2005) General anesthesia and the neural correlates of consciousness. *Prog Brain Res* 150:229–244.

44. Fiset, P., Paus, T., Daloze, T., Plourde, G., Meuret, P., Bonhomme, V., Hajj-Ali, N., Backman, S.B. and Evans, A.C. (1999) Brain mechanisms of propofol-induced loss of consciousness in humans: A positron emission tomographic study. *J Neurosci* 19:5506–5513.

45. Fiset, P., Plourde, G. and Backman, S.B. (2005) Brain imaging in research on anesthetic mechanisms: Studies with propofol. *Prog Brain Res* 150:245–250.

46. Maquet, P., Degueldre, C., Delfiore, G., Aerts, J., Peters, J.-M., Luxen, A. and Franck, G. (1997) Functional neuroanatomy of human slow wave sleep. *J Neurosci* 17:2807–2812.

47. Lee, K.H., Meador, K.J., Park, Y.D., King, D.W., Murro, A.M., Pillai, J.J. and Kaminski, R.J. (2002) Pathophysiology of altered consciousness during seizures: Subtraction SPECT study. *Neurology* 59:841–846.

48. Blumenfeld, H., McNally, K.A., Vanderhill, S.D., LeBron Paige, A., Chung, R., Davis, K., Norden, A.D., Stokking, R., Studhome, C., Novotny, E.J.Jr., Zubal, I.G. and Spencer, S.S. (2004) Positive and negative network correlations in temporal lobe epilepsy. *Cereb Cortex* 14:892–902.

49. Penfield, W. and Jasper, H. (1954) *Epilepsy and the Functional Anatomy of the Human Brain*, Boston, MA: Little, Brown.

50. Penry, J.K., Porter, R. and Dreifuss, F. (1975) Simultaneous recording of absence seizures with video tape and electro-encephalography, a study of 374 seizures in 48 patients. *Brain* 98:427–440.

51. Graham, D.I., Maxwell, W.L., Hume, A.J. and Jennett, B. (2005) Novel aspects of the neuropathology of the vegetative state after blunt head injury. *Prog Brain Res* 150:445–453.

52. Laureys, S., Faymonville, M.-E., Ferring, M., Schnakers, C., Elincx, S., Ligot, N., Majerus, S., Antoine, S., Mavroudakis, N., Berre, J., Luxen, A., Vincent, J.-L., Moonen, G., Lamy, M.,

Goldman, S. and Maquet, P. (2003) Differences in brain metabolism between patients in coma, vegetative state, minimally conscious state and locked-in syndrome. *Eur J Neurol* 10 (Suppl 1):224–225.

53. Laureys, S., Boly, M. and Maquet, P. (2006) Tracking the recovery of consciousness from coma. *J Clin Invest* 116:1823–1825.

54. Maquet, P. (2000) Functional neuroimaging of normal human sleep by positron emission tomography. *J Sleep Res* 9:207–231.

55. Archer, J.S., Abbott, D.F., Wates, A.B. and Jackson, G.D. (2003) fMRI "deactivation" of the posterior cingulate during generalized spike and wave. *Neuroimage* 20:1915–1922.

56. Blumenfeld, H. (2005) Consciousness and epilepsy: Why are patients with absence seizures absent? *Prog Brain Res* 150:271–286.

57. Salek-Haddadi, A., Lemieux, L., Merschhemke, M., Friston, K.J., Duncan, I.S. and Dish, D.R. (2003) Functional magnetic resonance imaging of human absence seizures. *Ann Neurol* 53:663–667.

58. Aghakhani, Y., Bagshaw, A.P., Benar, C.G., Hawco, C., Andermann, F., Dubeau, F. and Gotman, J. (2003) fMRI activation during spike- and wave-discharges in idiopathic generalized epilepsy. *Brain* 127:1127–1144.

59. Façon, E., Steriade, M. and Wertheim, N. (1958) Prolonged hypersomnia caused by bilateral lesions of the medial activator system; thrombotic syndrome of the bifurcation of the basilar trunk. *Rev Neurol (Paris)* 98:117–133.

60. Castaigne, P., Buge, A., Escourolle, R. and Masson, M. (1962) Ramollissement pédonculaire médian, tegmento-thalamique avec ophthalmoplégie et hypersomnie. *Rev Neurol (Paris)* 106:357–367.

61. Moruzzi, G. and Magoun, H.W. (1949) Brain stem reticular formation and activation of the EEG. *Electroencephalogr Clin Neurophysiol* 1:455–473.

62. Hobson, A. (1994) *The Chemistry of Conscious States*, New York: Basic Books.

63. Steriade, M. (1988) New vistas on the morphology, chemical transmitters and physiological actions of the ascending brainstem reticular system. *Archives Italiennes de Biologie* 126:225–238.

64. Steriade, M. (1993) Basic mechanisms of sleep generation. *Neurology* 42:9–17.

65. Steriade, M. (1995) Brain activation, then (1949) and now: Coherent fast rhythms in corticothalamic networks. *Archives Italiennes de Biologie* 134:5–20.

66. Munk, M.H.J., Roelfsema, P.R., Konig, P., Engel, A.K. and Singer, W. (1996) Role of reticular activation in the modulation of intracortical synchronization. *Science* 272:271–274.

67. Singer, W. (1998) Consciousness and the structure of neuronal representations. *Phil Trans R Soc Lond B* 353:1829–1840.

The Neurological Examination of Consciousness

Hal Blumenfeld

ABSTRACT

Disorders of consciousness present a diagnostic challenge to the clinician, with crucial implications for treatment and prognosis. Despite spectacular advances in neuroimaging and other cutting-edge technologies, a carefully performed general and neurological examination remains critical in the evaluation of these patients. In this chapter, we will review the neurological examination findings in the major states of impaired consciousness ranging from brain death, coma, vegetative state, and minimally conscious state to other disorders of consciousness, and conditions which can mimic impaired consciousness including psychological disorders and the locked-in syndrome. When possible, specific positive and negative examination findings defining each condition will be discussed based on recent multi-disciplinary reviews and consensus statements. Continued study of the neurological examination in states of impaired consciousness will provide improved font-line tools for patient diagnosis and management. In addition, the anatomical basis for examination findings in states of impaired consciousness sheds important light on the fundamental mechanisms of normal and abnormal consciousness.

INTRODUCTION

In the era of advanced life support, and continually improving intensive and long-term care, the number of surviving patients with impaired consciousness is increasing. Evaluation of patients with impaired consciousness requires a comprehensive multidisciplinary approach including patient history, examination, and various diagnostic tests. However, the lynch pin of this assessment is the neurological examination. The neurological examination provides the most direct and interactive assessment of the patient's level of functioning. Put simply, the neurological examination is critical since it reveals what the patient can or cannot do.

The findings on neurological examination are most useful in determining the diagnosis, and in tracking the course of recovery in patients with disorders of consciousness. For example, the neurological examination is the main tool used to determine if a patient is brain dead, comatose, or in a different state of impaired consciousness, and can help formulate initial hypotheses about localizing lesions and diagnosing the underlying cause of the patient's condition. Interpretation of the neurological examination has been greatly aided in recent years by advances in neuroimaging. Computerized tomography (CT), magnetic resonance imaging (MRI), and functional neuroimaging (PET, fMRI) now allow unprecedented clinical–anatomical correlations to be made *in vivo*. In addition, the significance of these clinical–anatomical relationships in patients with impaired consciousness has been greatly enhanced by recent large multi-center studies of patient outcome and prognosis.

In this chapter, we will first introduce the neurological examination, and discuss special considerations required for patients with disorders of consciousness. We will next provide an anatomical model for normal consciousness, and review the neuroanatomical basis of the major states of impaired consciousness. The majority of this chapter will then be dedicated to a discussion of the neurological examination findings that define each of the main states of impaired consciousness, including brain death, coma, vegetative state, minimally conscious state, other states of impaired consciousness, and disorders that resemble impaired consciousness. When possible, we will discuss specific positive and negative findings that define each of these states, and relate these findings to anatomical localization based on clinical series, pathology, neuroimaging, and recent consensus statements.

THE NEUROLOGICAL EXAMINATION

The neurological examination as a diagnostic tool gained mythical proportions in the pre-CT/MRI era when great clinicians could pinpoint a lesion in the nervous system with often astounding accuracy. Decisions for surgery and other interventions were frequently made based entirely on the neurological history and physical findings. Today, with the availability of modern imaging techniques the neurological examination takes on a new and equally important role in diagnosis and management. Rather than serving as an end in and of itself, the neurological examination today is a critical way station in the clinical decision making process.

Although many individual variations exist based on clinical style and the patient setting, the neurological examination is generally described using the following six subdivisions: (1) mental status; (2) cranial nerves; (3) motor examination; (4) reflexes; (5) coordination and gait; and (6) sensory examination. There are many excellent resources for review of the neurological examination including several textbooks, and interactive websites (see for example http://neuroexam.com and http://medlib.med.utah.edu/neurologicexam/index.html).

In patients with impaired consciousness, there are a number of special considerations when performing the neurological examination. Prior to neurological examination, as in all patients, a detailed general physical examination is imperative, and may reveal evidence of head trauma, meningeal irritation, elevated intracranial pressure, or other findings related to the cause of altered consciousness. On neurological examination, many of the tests used in awake patients are limited or impossible due to reduced cooperation (Table 2.1). For example, the mental status examination is often limited to assessing level of consciousness through simple questions/commands or observing the response to different stimuli. Other parts of the examination are also often limited to passive testing. For example, on cranial nerve examination, visual fields can be tested by blink to threat, pupils by light response, eye movements by tracking and vestibular stimulation, facial sensation and movements by corneal reflex, nasal tickle, and grimace response. Hearing evaluation may require speaking directly into the patient's ear (checking first for obstruction, and for history of hearing loss), using the patient's first name when appropriate as a potent stimulus. Gag reflex can be tested by moving the endotracheal tube, and cough reflex by tracheal suctioning. Sensory and

I.   Mental status
     Document level of consciousness with a *specific statement* of what the patient did in response to particular stimuli.

II. Cranial nerves
     1. Ophthalmoscopic examamination (CN II)
     2. Pupillary responses (CN II, III)
     3. Vision (CN II)
         Blink to threat, visual tracking, optokinetic nystagmus
     4. Extraocular movements and vestibulo-ocular reflex (CN III, IV, VI, VIII)
         Spontaneous extraocular movements, nystagmus, dysconjugate gaze, or deviation of both eyes to one side, oculocephalic maneuver (doll's eyes test), caloric testing
     5. Corneal blink reflex, facial asymmetry, grimace response (CN V, VII)
     6. Pharyngeal (gag) and tracheal (cough) reflexes (CN IX, X)

III. Sensory/motor examination
     1. Spontaneous movements
     2. Withdrawal or posturing reflexes with painful stimulus

IV. Reflexes
     1. Deep tendon reflexes
     2. Plantar responses
     3. Special reflexes in cases of suspected spinal cord lesions

V.   Coordination/gait
     Usually not testable

Source: Modified with permission from [1].

motor examinations are often combined using vigorous sensory stimulation to elicit motor responses. Spinal reflexes are tested in the same manner as in the awake patient, but coordination and gait often cannot be tested at all (Table 2.1).

Because the neurological examination evaluates function, it is crucial to tailor the examination to the individual patient's strengths and limitations. If all tests are too difficult (e.g., asking a minimally conscious patient to indicate on their left hand the number of fingers corresponding the first letter of the city they are in) then residual function and improvements will be missed. Conversely, if all tests are too easy (e.g., asking a mildly aphasic patient to close and open their eyes on command) then subtle deficits will be missed. Therefore, to accurately titrate the patient's level of function, each part of the examination should be performed using several tests with varying levels of difficulty, beginning with easy and moving to more difficult. In equivocal cases, it is also helpful to use several different tests of the same function to confirm results, and to return and retest the patient at different times.

Sensitivity to patients and families should remain paramount in examining patients with impaired consciousness. Although noxious stimuli can be useful in localization and prognosis, the use of noxious stimuli should be minimized whenever possible, to avoid unnecessary suffering. Family members should be informed through ongoing discussions of the patient's condition, and may not want to be present for some parts of the examination. It should also be kept in mind that some patients are more aware than is obvious, and the content and tone of discussions taking place in the presence of the patient should be carried out with consideration of their potential emotional responses.

Examination of patients with impaired consciousness can also be very challenging to avoid misdiagnosis. It has been reported, for example, that patients in chronic care are often misdiagnosed as being vegetative when in fact some degree of consciousness or awareness can be demonstrated on more careful examination [2, 3]. Practical suggestions for the evaluation of patients with impaired consciousness have been proposed by several authors [2, 4]. Patients should ideally be examined in the seated position, since upright posture can enhance arousal [2]. Each test should be performed repeatedly to distinguish coincidental from voluntary responses, and the entire examination should be repeated at several different times of the day. Sedating medications should be avoided if possible. Special care should be taken in patients with impaired sensory or motor function due to neurological or orthopaedic disorders, impaired hearing, or impaired vision since these deficits can mask an underlying preserved awareness. Similarly, in infancy and early childhood cognitive and sensory–motor systems are not fully developed, so criteria for evaluating impaired consciousness are different from in adults. Input from family members or other staff members can be helpful in observing inconsistent or low-frequency behaviours, and in designing tests that are within the capabilities of the patient.

Despite these precautions, diagnosing consciousness or awareness based on the presence of 'meaningful responses' or 'purposeful responses' can be subjective. A number of standardized tests have, therefore, been developed for evaluating consciousness in brain damaged patients. These standardized tests are the subject of several recent excellent reviews [2, 5], and will not be discussed further here. However, we will emphasize the use of objective criteria, derived from consensus reviews whenever possible, in an effort to accurately diagnose the different states of impaired consciousness.

CONSCIOUSNESS

Consciousness includes several distinct functions which are implemented in specific neuroanatomical networks in the brain (see also the preceding chapter in this volume). Classically, consciousness can be separated into systems necessary for controlling the *level* of consciousness, and systems involved in generating the *content* of consciousness ([6], p. 11). We recently summarized the interactions of these systems ([7, 8]; Chapter 19 in this volume), and briefly review an anatomical model of consciousness again here. The *content*

of consciousness may be considered the substrate upon which level-of-consciousness systems act. Therefore, the anatomical structures important for the content of consciousness include: (i) multileveled cortical and subcortical hierarchies involved in sensory–motor functions, (ii) medial temporal and medial diencephalic structures interacting with cortex for generation of memory, and (iii) limbic system structures involved in emotions and drives. The *level of consciousness* in turn, also depends on multiple systems acting together. These include systems necessary for maintaining: (i) the alert, awake state, (ii) attention, and (iii) awareness of self and the environment. Anatomical

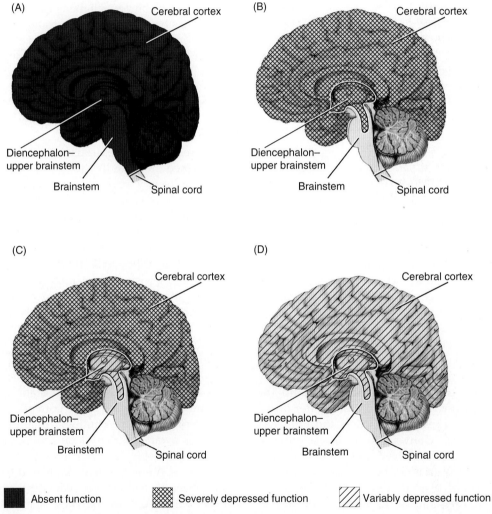

FIGURE 2.1   Schematic representation of brain impairment in major states of impaired consciousness. (A) Brain death. All cortical, subcortical, and brainstem function is irreversibly lost. Spinal cord function may be preserved. No responses can be elicited except for spinal cord reflexes. (B) Coma. There is severe impairment of cortical function and of the diencephalic/upper brainstem activating systems. Patients are unarousable with eyes closed, and have no purposeful responses, but brainstem reflex activity is present. (C) Vegetative state. Cortical function is severely impaired, but there is some preserved diencephalic/upper brainstem activating function. Like in coma, patients are unconscious at all times, with no purposeful responses, but they can open their eyes spontaneously or with stimulation, exhibit primitive orienting responses, and sleep–wake cycles. (D) Minimally conscious state or better. Impaired function of the cerebral cortex and diencephalic/upper brainstem activating systems is variable. Patients exhibit some purposeful responses, along with deficits, depending on the severity of brain dysfunction.

structures which control the level of consciousness constitute what could, in analogy to sensory, motor and other systems, be called the 'consciousness system' (see also Chapter 19 this volume). The consciousness system at minimum includes regions of the frontal and parietal association cortex, cingulate cortex, precuneus, thalamus, and multiple activating systems located in the basal forebrain, hypothalamus, midbrain, and upper pons. Some would also include the basal ganglia and cerebellum due to their possible roles in controlling attention.

Lesions in certain regions of the consciousness system can cause coma. This is particularly true for bilateral lesions of the association cortex, medial thalamus (including the intralaminar regions), or upper brainstem tegmentum. Lesions in other areas controlling the level of consciousness, or unilateral lesions, may cause more subtle impairments in arousal, attention, or awareness of self and the environment. Finally, lesions in systems generating the content of consciousness can cause selective deficits in perception, known as agnosias, deficits in motor planning known as apraxias, language disorders, memory deficits, and emotional or motivational disorders.

In this chapter we will discuss the neurological examination in states of impaired consciousness, including those which affect the level or the content of consciousness. We will first provide a brief overview of the major states of impaired consciousness, before discussing the neurological examination of each state in more detail.

STATES OF IMPAIRED CONSCIOUSNESS

The major states of impaired consciousness are summarized in Figure 2.1 and Table 2.2. These disorders can be classified based on the severity and extent of brain structures affected. For example, brain death occurs when the entire forebrain, midbrain, and hindbrain irreversibly cease to function. The spinal cord and peripheral nerves may be spared in brain death. In coma, the forebrain and diencephalic/upper brainstem activating systems have severely depressed function, leading to loss of consciousness, but the brainstem and spinal cord can carry out various reflex responses. The vegetative state is distinguished from coma by the recovery of sufficient diencephalic/upper brainstem function to allow sleep–wake cycles, and simple orienting responses to occur to external stimuli, however consciousness is still absent. In addition to these three classic states of impaired consciousness, there are numerous other states in which consciousness is only partially or variably affected (Figure 2.1D; Table 2.2).

TABLE 2.2   States of Impaired Consciousness

	Cortex: Purposeful responses to stimuli	Diencephalon/upper brainstem: Behavioural arousal, sleep–wake cycles	Brainstem[a]: Brainstem reflexes	Spinal cord: Spinal reflexes
Classic states of impaired consciousness				
Brain death	No	No	No	Yes
Coma	No	No	Yes	Yes
Vegetative state	No	Yes	Yes	Yes
Other states of impaired consciousness				
Minimally conscious state	Yes, at times	Yes	Yes	Yes
Stupor, obtundation, lethargy, delirium	Yes, at times	Variable	Yes	Yes
Status epilepticus	Variable	Variable	Yes	Yes
Akinetic mutism, abulia, catatonia	Yes, at times	Yes	Yes	Yes
Neglect and other disorders of attention	Yes, at times	Yes	Yes	Yes
Sleep, normal and abnormal	Yes, at times	Yes	Yes	Yes
States resembling impaired consciousness				
Locked-in syndrome	No[b]	Yes	Yes	Yes
Dissociative disorders, somatoform disorders	Yes, at times	Yes	Yes	Yes

[a] Refers to other brainstem systems and pathways aside from those participating directly in behavioural arousal.
[b] Some patients may have preserved vertical eye movements, eye blinking, or other slight movements under volitional control.

Finally, in some conditions such as the locked-in syndrome, or psychogenic pseudocoma, patients may be fully conscious, yet appear to be in a coma. Careful neurological examination is a crucial step in evaluating patients with impaired consciousness, and together with other diagnostic tests, can provide essential information about the localization, diagnosis, and prognosis for patients with these disorders. We will now discuss the neurological examination findings in each of these states of impaired consciousness in greater detail.

NEUROLOGICAL EXAMINATION IN CLASSIC STATES OF IMPAIRED CONSCIOUSNESS

Brain Death

In brain death there is irreversible cessation of all functions of the brain including the brainstem (Figure 2.1A). Consciousness is, therefore, permanently lost in brain death. Neurological examination of the patient with brain death demonstrates no response to any stimulation, aside from reflexes mediated by the spinal cord. Because brain death is the legal equivalent of death in many societies, detailed criteria have been established for the determination of brain death [9–13]. These criteria include the requirement that (i) CNS depressants and neuromuscular blockade are absent, (ii) blood testing is done to detect reversible causes such as toxic or metabolic abnormalities, (iii) hypothermia or hypotension are absent, and (iv) the evaluation is repeated at least twice, separated by an appropriate time interval [9–13]. Brain death is a clinical diagnosis, and the neurological examination is the most important test used to establish brain death. In cases where the diagnosis remains uncertain, additional confirmatory tests (e.g., cerebral angiography, electroencephalography (EEG), transcranial Doppler, or nuclear medicine scan) can be done [10, 12]. However, because confirmatory tests may produce similar results in patients with severe brain injury who do not yet meet clinical criteria for brain death [10], the clinical examination remains the central part of the evaluation of brain death.

The neurological examination in brain death (Table 2.3) reveals no responses to any stimuli aside from

TABLE 2.3   Neurological Examination in States of Impaired Consciousness

Test[a]	Brain death	Coma	Vegetative state	Minimally conscious or better
Mental status				
Sleep–wake cycles	No	No	Yes	Yes
Responds appropriately to questions/commands	No	No	No	Yes, variable
Says single words (may be inappropriate)	No	No	No	Yes
Orienting movements (eyes, head, body) towards visual, tactile, or auditory stimuli	No	No	Yes	Yes
Noxious stimuli (loud voice, nasal tickle, endotracheal suctioning, pressure to orbital ridge, mandible, sternum, or nail bed)				
Speaks, purposeful movements	No	No	No	Yes, at times
Opens eyes, basic orienting movements	No	No	Yes	Yes
Grunts, moans	No	Yes	Yes	Yes
Grimaces	No	Yes	Yes	Yes
Noxious stimuli → limb movements (see sensory/motor examination below)				
Cranial nerves				
Pupil light reflex	No	Yes	Yes	Yes
Eye closure to bright light	No	No	Caution advised[b]	Yes
Blink to threat	No	No	Caution advised[b]	Yes
Optokinetic nystagmus	No	No	No[c]	Yes
Visual tracking	No	No	No	Yes
Orienting movement of eyes and head towards visual, auditory, or tactile[d] stimuli	No	No	Yes	Yes
Spontaneous roving or other eye movements	No	Yes	Yes	Yes
Eyes move in response to oculocephalic maneuver or cold water calorics	No	Yes	Yes	Yes (but may be masked by voluntary eye movements)
Corneal reflex	No	Yes	Yes	Yes

Table 2.3 (*Continued*)

Test[a]	Brain death	Coma	Vegetative state	Minimally conscious or better
Jaw jerk reflex	No	Can occur	Can occur	Can occur
Grimace to painful stimulus	No	Yes	Yes	Yes
Gag reflex	No	Yes	Yes	Yes
Sneeze, cough, hiccough, yawn	No	Yes	Yes	Yes
Spontaneous chewing movements	No	Yes	Yes	Yes
Swallowing reflex	No	Yes	Yes	Yes
Coordinated chewing and swallowing	No	No	No	Yes
Moans or makes other non-word sounds	No	Yes	Yes	Yes
Sensory and motor examinations				
Spontaneous purposeful limb movement	No	No	No	Yes
Spontaneous non-purposeful limb movement	No	Yes	Yes	Yes
Non-directed scratching, rubbing movements	No	Yes[e]	Yes[e]	Yes
Shivering	No	Yes	Yes	Yes
Grasp reflex	No	Yes	Yes	Yes
Limb movements to noxious stimuli				
Localizes (moves another limb to point of stimulation)	No	No	No[d]	Yes
Purposeful, non-stereotyped withdrawal (moves in different directions away from stimuli on different sides of same limb)	No	No	No[c]	Yes
Upper extremity flexor or extensor posturing, lower extremity extensor posturing	No[f]	Yes	Yes	Can occur, but usually see more purposeful response
Spinal reflexes and movements				
Deep tendon reflexes in extremities	Yes	Yes	Yes	Yes
Abdominal cutaneous reflexes	Yes	Yes	Yes	Yes
Plantar response (flexor or extensor)	Yes	Yes	Yes	Yes
Lower extremity triple flexion	Yes	Yes	Yes	Can occur, but usually see more purposeful response
Spontaneous finger jerks or toe undulation	Yes	Yes	Yes	Yes
Lazarus sign[g]	Yes	Not seen	Not seen	Not seen

[a] Some tests appear more than once, for example grimace response under Mental Status and under Cranial nerves.

[b] Caution has been advised in making the diagnosis of vegetative state if blink to threat is present [14, 15], however others consider blink to threat compatible with the vegetative state [2, 16, 17]. Similar considerations likely apply to eye closure in response to bright light.

[c] No formal studies have been done and exceptions may exist.

[d] Orienting towards (but not actually reaching and touching) painful or other tactile stimuli have been described in vegetative state, but unlike visual and auditory stimuli, were not listed in the Multi-Society Task Force consensus statement [14].

[e] Automatic scratching or similar movements have been described in coma [18] and the vegetative state [16] however, this may be controversial since recent criteria include these movements in the minimally conscious state [4].

[f] Extensor posturing-like movements of the upper extremity have been reported in some cases of brain death [19, 20]; see text for discussion.

[g] Lazarus sign is a particular sequence of spinal cord-mediated limb movements seen in brain death upon disconnection of the ventilator, or flexion of the neck (see text for details).

reflexes mediated by the spinal cord. Brainstem function must be absent, and patients are apneic. Special tests are often performed on the neurological examination when assessing for brain death to ensure that no brainstem function remains. These include response to noxious stimuli (see Table 2.3), ice water calorics (a test for preserved pontine function), and the apnea test (a test for preserved medullary function), all described in detail elsewhere [9–13].

Some spontaneous or reflex movements can occur in brain death due to preserved function of the spinal cord [19, 21]. For example, deep tendon reflexes in the upper and lower extremities, plantar cutaneous flexor or extensor responses (Babinski sign), abdominal cutaneous reflexes, triple flexion of the lower extremities, and autonomic changes such as sweating, blushing, and tachycardia upon stimulation are not incompatible with brain death since they are mediated by the spinal cord [10, 20, 22, 23]. Shoulder and intercostal movements resembling respiratory movements (but without significant tidal volumes) can occur in brain death, and are presumably also mediated by the spinal cord [10]. Undulating toe flexion, and finger jerks (myoclonus-like) have also been reported in brain death [20, 22, 24, 25].

In occasional patients with brain death, a complex and sometimes startling set of spinal cord reflexes may be seen, referred to as the Lazarus sign [26–28]. The

Lazarus sign is usually elicited when the respirator is disconnected or by passive neck flexion, and consists of arm flexion at the elbows, shoulder adduction, arm elevation, hand crossing and dystonia (as if reaching for the endotracheal tube, or praying), followed by movement of the hands downward to rest alongside the torso [20, 22, 25]. Leg movements and trunk flexion have also been reported. These reflexes are thought to be mediated by stimulation of the cervical spinal cord, either by movement or hypoxia upon disconnection of the ventilator. In typical cases, the Lazarus sign does not contradict the diagnosis of brain death; however, caution is advised if unusual features are present.

It should be emphasized that the presence of any brainstem or cranial nerve function is not compatible with the diagnosis of brain death. For example, the presence of flexor or extensor posturing, a cough reflex, respiratory movements with significant tidal volumes, or any cranial nerve functions imply that some brainstem function remains, and therefore, are not compatible with brain death. Facial myokymia, presumably mediated peripherally, can be seen in some patients; however, caution is advised since any brainstem function would preclude brain death, and confirmatory testing may be appropriate in these cases [20]. Other examples where caution is appropriate are thoracic contraction reflexes in response to endotracheal suction (resembling cough or respiratory movements), upper limb extension–pronation reflex (resembling brainstem-mediated extensor posturing), and other unusual reflexes or spontaneous movements [19, 25, 29, 30]. Although there are well documented cases where such movements can be mediated by the spinal cord, confirmatory testing may be appropriate when the diagnosis of brain death is uncertain.

In summary, all brain function irreversibly stops in brain death, so consciousness is lost permanently. Residual movements can be seen, mediated by the spinal cord.

Coma

The most commonly accepted definition of coma, as proposed by Plum and Posner is unarousable unresponsiveness in which the patient lies with the eyes closed ([6], p. 5). Duration is at least 1 hour to distinguish coma from transient loss of consciousness such as concussion or syncope [14]. Coma rarely lasts longer than 2–4 weeks, since nearly all patients either deteriorate or emerge into vegetative state or better within this time [6]. In coma, the functions of the cerebral cortex, diencephalon, and upper brainstem activating systems are markedly depressed (Figure 2.1B). However, function is preserved in other brainstem areas capable of mediating various reflex responses (Table 2.2). Cerebral metabolism in coma is usually globally decreased by ~50%, although it can be increased in occasional cases of axonal shear injury (reviewed in [17]). Patients in coma are fully unconscious. However, in contrast to brain death, during coma many simple or even complex reflex activities may occur via the brainstem. In addition, unlike in brain death, coma can be reversible.

On examination, patients in coma do not open their eyes or arouse even with vigorous noxious stimulation (Table 2.3) [6]. Some patients may grimace or make unintelligible sounds in coma [6, 18], but they do not orient towards stimuli, or exhibit any psychologically meaningful or purposeful responses, since these behaviours are mediated by the cortex. Brainstem responses, on the other hand, can occur. Since coma is often associated with brainstem lesions, the brainstem responses which occur are frequently abnormal. For example, patients in coma may show pupillary light responses, but the pupils may be abnormal in size and/or shape, with large or irregular pupils seen in midbrain compression (e.g., tentorial herniation with compression of oculomotor parasympathetic fibers), and small pupils seen in pontine lesions (damage to descending sympathetic fibers in lateral tegmentum). A variety of abnormal spontaneous eye movements occur, including ocular bobbing (associated with pontine lesions), and slow roving eye movements [18, 31–33]. Vestibulo-ocular reflex eye movements can be induced either by oculocephalic or caloric stimulation, although the rapid phases are usually suppressed in coma. Pontine and medullary circuits may enable corneal, jaw jerk, gag, cough, and swallowing reflexes to occur in some patients. Brainstem control of circulatory and respiratory function can be preserved, but may also be abnormal, especially if the lower brainstem is involved. A variety of abnormal breathing patterns can be observed in coma, including Cheynes-Stokes respiration, central hyperventilation, apneustic, and ataxic breathing [6, 18]. Patients in coma often require intubation both for ventilatory support and for airway protection. Cranial nerve responses that are thought to depend on cortical function, such as blink to visual threat, eye closure to bright light, and optokinetic nystagmus, are absent in coma.

Patients in coma may have characteristic flexor or extensor posturing reflexes of the upper and lower extremities (Table 2.3), mediated by descending brainstem pathways. Flexor or extensor posturing can be stimulus induced or spontaneous, and is sometimes mistaken for seizures. Other spontaneous purposeless movements of the limbs and myoclonus are not uncommon in coma. Patients may have purposeless, coordinated automatisms including repetitive scratching, rubbing, squeezing, or patting movements [18], although this may be controversial since recent criteria include such movements in the minimally conscious state [4]. Shivering movements can certainly be seen in coma [18], and may arise from the brainstem reticulospinal tract [34]. However, purposeful (as opposed to reflex) withdrawal from noxious stimuli, or other responses demonstrating volition, do not occur in coma. Distinguishing purposeful withdrawal from reflex responses requires some skill, and repeated careful observations, although as already discussed, repeated noxious stimuli should be avoided when possible, and performed with sensitivity to the patient and family. Purposeful responses can be distinguished from reflex if the direction of movement is different for pinch to the flexor and extensor (or medial and lateral) surfaces of a limb, and if the movement changes to avoid the stimulus. In addition, abduction of the arm at the shoulder or of the leg at the hip joint is not usually seen during reflex responses [18]. In contrast, reflex responses tend to be stereotyped, and to have the same pattern regardless of how elicited. The same stereotyped posturing reflexes can often be elicited even by stimuli in a different part of the body. In addition to brainstem reflexes, spinal cord reflexes (e.g., tendon reflexes, lower extremity triple flexion) can also be seen in coma and need to be distinguished from purposeful responses.

A major feature of coma which distinguishes it from vegetative state is the lack of sleep–wake cycles. Also, unlike the vegetative state, patients in coma do not open their eyes or arouse even with vigorous noxious stimulation (Table 2.3) [6]. As has already been discussed, coma usually does not last longer than 2–4 weeks since within this time most patients either deteriorate, or emerge into vegetative state or better stages of recovery.

In summary, patients in coma are deeply unconscious, and have no signs of arousal even with vigorous stimulation. Some responses can be seen, mediated by brainstem and spinal cord reflexes.

Vegetative State[1]

Like coma, patients in a vegetative state do not have meaningful responses to any external stimuli, but can exhibit brainstem and spinal reflexes [16]. The major distinction from coma is the presence of rudimentary arousal/orienting responses and sleep–wake

cycles in the vegetative state. Cortical function is markedly depressed in vegetative patients, like in coma, as evidenced by ~50% reduction in cerebral metabolism [35]. However, in the vegetative state, metabolic function of the brainstem, hypothalamus, and basal forebrain are reported to be relatively spared [17]. Unlike coma, sufficient diencephalic and upper brainstem activating function is present in the vegetative state to generate periods of eye opening, as well as primitive orienting reflexes (Figure 2.1C; Table 2.2). Vegetative state can occur after patients emerge from an acute catastrophic brain insult causing coma, or can also be seen in degenerative or congenital nervous system disorders, or after an acute insult without a preceding interval of coma. Vegetative state lasting more than 1 month is called a persistent vegetative state [14]. Prognosis is discussed in a later chapter of this volume. The two most common findings on pathology in vegetative state are necrosis of the cerebral cortex, thalamus and brainstem (usually seen after anoxic injury) and diffuse axonal shear injury (usually seen after trauma), although other pathological findings can be seen in degenerative, developmental, and other disorders [5, 14, 36]. Less commonly, vegetative state can occur with involvement mainly of the thalamus, as in the highly publicized case of Karen Ann Quinlan [37]. Patients in the vegetative state, like in coma, are completely unconscious of themselves and their surroundings.

The diagnosis of the vegetative state requires special attention, since both false positive and false negative diagnoses can occur relatively easily [2, 3, 38]. Repeat examination is often necessary at different times of the day, and input from family members can be helpful [2].

Examination of patients in the vegetative state reveals no purposeful responses to verbal, visual, auditory, tactile, or noxious stimulation (Table 2.3). In addition, patients in the vegetative state have bowel and bladder incontinence [15, 14]. Unlike coma, patients in the vegetative state may open their eyes in response to stimulation, and exhibit spontaneous sleep–wake cycles. They also have spontaneous opening of the eyes, purposeless eye movements, blinking, and trunk or limb movements during the awake portion of sleep–wake cycles [15, 14]. Patients may grunt, moan, or make other unintelligible sounds, but produce no meaningful language. They can smile, shed tears, cry, and some patients in the vegetative state will grimace in response to a painful stimulus, or exhibit startle myoclonus [15, 14]. These responses all occur in a stereotyped but not in a contextually appropriate manner [17]. Rarely, well documented cases have been observed of patients with isolated preserved

---

[1]Terms such as coma vigil, neocortical death, or apallic syndrome were used in the past for vegetative and similar states, but are imprecise, and are no longer used today.

functions (e.g., saying a single word unrelated to external stimuli) in patients who otherwise fit all criteria for vegetative state, and showed no evidence of long-term recovery [17]. These cases are exceptional, however, and any intelligible speech is usually considered incompatible with the vegetative state.

Like in coma, brainstem and cranial nerve reflex responses can occur in the vegetative state (Table 2.3). An important feature of vegetative state is the absence of sustained tracking eye movements (visual pursuit). The return of tracking eye movements is one of the earliest signs of recovery from the vegetative state [14]. Care must be taken, since ability to track may depend on the inherent interest or other features of the stimulus used [39]. Some patients in the vegetative state can have primitive orienting reflexes, consisting of eyes and head turning towards a visual or auditory stimulus, presumably mediated by brainstem circuits; however, sustained or consistent visual pursuit or fixation is usually considered incompatible with the vegetative state [14]. Optokinetic nystagmus is also thought to depend on the cortex and is often absent; however, no formal studies have been done in the vegetative state, and anecdotal observations suggest it may occur in some cases. Care is necessary in the examination, since roving eye movements in the vegetative state can sometimes be mistaken for visual tracking. In addition, although vegetative patients may occasionally have basic orienting movements towards a stimulus, they do not localize a noxious stimulus by moving another limb to remove it (i.e., they may move grossly towards a stimulus, but do not actually reach the target by touching the stimulated point).

Blink to visual threat suggests neocortical function, and caution has been advised in diagnosing vegetative state in the presence of this response [14]. However, some consider response to visual threat to be compatible with the diagnosis of vegetative state [2, 16, 17]. Conversely, absence of blink to threat does not prove lack of awareness, since patients with brain injury often have severe visual impairment [3]. Similar considerations to blink to visual threat likely also apply to testing eye closure in response to bright light.

Patients in the vegetative state do not have coordinated chewing and swallowing, however, they may have preserved gag, cough, suck, and swallow reflexes, and may exhibit some spontaneous chewing movements [15, 5, 14]. Some studies report that a significant number of vegetative patients are capable of receiving nutrition by the oral route following a careful swallowing evaluation [40, 41]. However, because aspiration risk is high [42, 43], the majority of vegetative patients are fed by enteral tube feeds [44].

Brainstem and hypothalamic autonomic functions are preserved in the vegetative state. This often allows sufficient digestive, cardiac, respiratory, thermoregulatory, and salt and water homeostasis for patients to survive for long periods of time if nutrition and nursing care are provided.

On sensory–motor examination of the limbs (Table 2.3), patients in the vegetative state can show reflex responses or posturing mediated by the brainstem and spinal cord, but do not exhibit purposeful limb withdrawal, or localization of stimuli using another limb. Like in coma, limb abduction or non-stereotyped withdrawal in response to stimuli on different sides of the same limb is thought to not occur in vegetative state; however, this has not been formally studied and exceptions may exist. A variety of spontaneous purposeless trunk or limb movements can be seen during the awake portion of sleep–wake cycles in the vegetative state [14, 15]. Fragments of undirected coordinated movements such as scratching were described in early studies of vegetative state [16] and coma [18], however, in more recent work such movements are considered evidence for the minimally conscious state [4]. Although a primitive grasp reflex may be seen in the vegetative state [16], reaching for objects or holding them in a manner to accommodate their size and shape is considered evidence for consciousness [4], and is not part of the vegetative state.

In summary, patients in the vegetative state can open their eyes and exhibit basic orienting responses, but show no conscious, purposeful activity. Reflexes and other movements are seen, mediated by the brainstem, spinal cord, and brainstem–diencephalic arousal systems.

NEUROLOGICAL EXAMINATION IN OTHER STATES OF IMPAIRED CONSCIOUSNESS

Minimally Conscious State

The minimally conscious state was defined relatively recently in an effort to promote research and understanding of patients with severely impaired consciousness, but who do not meet diagnostic criteria for coma or vegetative state because they demonstrate some inconsistent but clear evidence of consciousness [4, 5, 17]. Prognosis, diagnosis, and treatment of the minimally conscious state are still under investigation in this relatively newly defined category of impaired consciousness, but recommended criteria for diagnosis were established by the multi-disciplinary Aspen Workgroup [4]. In the minimally conscious state, there is variable impaired function of the cerebral cortex, diencephalon, and upper brainstem (Figure 2.1D). This allows occasional conscious behaviours to occur, unlike in vegetative state or coma. Patients may enter the minimally conscious state as they emerge from coma or vegetative state, or they can become minimally conscious as a result of acute injury, or chronic degenerative or congenital conditions.

Examination of patients in the minimally conscious state (Table 2.3) reveals severely impaired consciousness, along with some inconsistent or variable evidence of preserved consciousness. This may include one or more of the following: following of simple commands, vocalization or gestures that depend on linguistic content of questions (e.g., indicate yes/no by either gestures or verbal response to questions, regardless of accuracy), smiling or crying in appropriate response to emotional but not to neutral stimuli, intelligible verbalization or gestures, sustained visual fixation or pursuit, localization of noxious or non-noxious stimuli, purposeful reaching for objects, and holding or touching objects in a manner that accommodates size and shape [4]. Note that all of these responses are absent in coma or vegetative state (Table 2.3), but can be seen in the minimally conscious state. These responses in minimally conscious state are inconsistent, but are reproducible enough to distinguish them from reflex or coincidental spontaneous movements. Prolonged and repeated evaluation is often necessary to make this distinction, and to determine with confidence whether some preserved consciousness is present [2, 4, 5]. As in the vegetative state (but unlike in coma), patients in the minimally conscious state do have sleep–wake cycles [4].

Patients are considered to no longer be in the minimally conscious state if they display functional interactive communication, or functional use of two different objects [4]. Functional interactive communication was defined by the Aspen Workgroup as 'accurate yes/no responses to six of six basic situational orientation questions on two consecutive evaluations' (e.g., 'Are you sitting down?' or 'Am I pointing to the ceiling?'). Functional object use was defined as 'generally appropriate use of at least two different objects on two consecutive evaluations' (e.g., bringing a comb to the head, or a pencil to a sheet of paper) [4]. Functional interactive communication need not occur verbally for these criteria, but could also take place through writing, yes/no signals, or other forms of communication [4].

As in other states of impaired consciousness, repeated testing is often necessary to confirm the diagnosis of minimally conscious state [2, 5, 17]. It is also important to exclude impaired responses due to factors other than diminished level of consciousness, such as sensory or motor impairment, aphasia, agnosia, apraxia, or impaired motor initiation as in akinetic mutism [4].

Stupor, Obtundation, Lethargy, Delirium, Dementia

There is a wide continuum of levels of consciousness between coma and the fully awake state. Aside from the vegetative state, and minimally conscious states, a variety of more poorly defined terms are sometimes used to describe different states along this continuum, including lethargy, hypersomnia, obtundation, stupor, semi-coma, etc. Although these terms can sometimes be useful shorthand for patients with partially impaired consciousness, they are imprecise, and further details are needed to more fully describe the patient's level of consciousness [18]. Generally, it is best in these cases to document the patient's level of alertness with a specific statement of what the patient did in response to particular stimuli, instead of relying on jargon. For example, the term stupor has been applied to patients who arouse briefly with vigorous stimulation [6]. However, it is much more informative to other clinicians if instead of using this term, a description is provided, for example 'nail bed pressure, or pressure to the supraorbital ridge caused the patient to briefly open their eyes, moan, and push away the examiner with one hand before lapsing back into unresponsiveness'. Similarly, patients who are obtunded, lethargic, or hypersomnolent are all awake at times but have diminished responses, and are much better described by using specific examples, than by these labels.

Much has been written about delirium, confusional state, encephalopathy, and organic brain syndrome, which are all terms for an acute or subacute disorder of attention and self-monitoring, in which there is usually a waxing and waning level of consciousness. Classically, this is caused by toxic or metabolic disturbances, but can also be seen in febrile illnesses, head trauma, or following seizures. Examination of these patients requires care to distinguish a general deficit in arousal and attention, from focal neurobehavioural deficits.

In dementia, which includes Alzheimer's and other disorders in which there is a decline in cognitive ability, the level of consciousness is not typically affected until the end stages, although the content of consciousness clearly is.

Transient States of Impaired Consciousness

Several disorders can cause relatively brief episodes of impaired consciousness. These include syncope, seizures, transient ischemic attack, narcolepsy, migraine, hypoglycemia, and psychiatric disorders. The neurological examination of patients during and after transient episodes of impaired consciousness can provide crucial information about the localization and differential diagnosis. We will discuss these transient disorders of impaired consciousness only briefly here, as they are covered extensively in standard neurology texts. In vasovagal syncope, patients may report a darkening of vision ("blacking out") and then typically become limp and unresponsive, with skin often pale, cool, and sweaty to the touch. Patients are usually flaccid, although in some cases jerking movements (convulsive syncope) can occur. Duration is brief (less than 1–2 minutes). Afterwards, patients classically have an immediate return of normal mental status with no deficits, although some mild lethargy is fairly common following syncope. Other cardiac disorders, hypotension, and arrhythmias can also cause transient impaired consciousness with similar features, but may have longer duration and if sustained can lead to anoxic brain injury. Seizures have variable effects on consciousness depending on the seizure type (see Chapter 19). Unlike syncope, seizures or transient ischemic attacks often produce mental status changes or other neurological deficits which persist for a period of time after the episode has ended. Vertebrobasilar transient ischemic attack, or migraine involving the vertebrobasilar system can cause transient impairment of consciousness, often with associated brainstem abnormalities on neurological examination. Intermittent obstruction of cerebrospinal fluid flow, as in colloid cyst of the third ventricle, can sometimes cause transient impairment of consciousness, as can hypoglycemia, narcolepsy, and psychiatric disorders (e.g. dissociative episodes, conversion disorder), each with their own distinctive features on neurological examination.

Status Epilepticus

An important consideration in the differential diagnosis of non-transient disorders of consciousness is status epilepticus, meaning continuous seizure activity. Although seizures are often easy to recognize, in some cases of non-convulsive status epilepticus only subtle twitching or no motor activity at all may be present. Case series of electroencephalograms (EEG)

performed in patients with disorders of consciousness have found a high incidence of non-convulsive status epilepticus [45, 46], and persistent non-convulsive status epilepticus is also fairly common after treatment of overt status epilepticus [47, 48]. EEG is therefore advisable in all patients for which a clear cause of impaired consciousness is not known. It is important also to note that some cases of status epilepticus may cause only subtle alterations of consciousness, particularly with prolonged spike-wave discharges [49, 50]. Additional discussion of impaired consciousness in epileptic seizures can be found in Chapter 19 of this volume.

Sleep and Narcolepsy

Consciousness is altered during sleep, whether occurring normally, or as part of a sleep disorder such as narcolepsy. Although both coma and sleep involve lying with eyes closed and unresponsiveness to the environment, they can usually be distinguished relatively easily since comatose patients are unarousable regardless of the stimulus, and patients in coma do not undergo cyclical variations of state as seen during sleep. Fisher has described similarities between sleep and coma in some detail, and noted that in some stages of sleep patients may be nearly unarousable, have roving eye movements, small pupils despite the darkness, flaccid immobile limbs, decreased or absent tendon reflexes, and unilateral or bilateral Babinski signs [18]. In lighter stages of sleep (stages I and II), there may be occasional spontaneous limb movements and slow roving eye movements. Most awareness of the surrounding environment is lost in stages I and II of sleep. During slow-wave sleep (stages III and IV), muscle tone is diminished, breathing is slow and deep, individuals are unaware of external events, and may be difficult to arouse. After slow-wave sleep, muscle tone decreases further, but the eyes exhibit fast movements, and dreaming commonly occurs in so-called rapid eye movement (REM) sleep. Individuals can be aroused from REM sleep relatively easily. In narcolepsy, fragments of REM sleep intrude during waking, which can cause sudden onset of REM sleep, and loss of awareness of the surroundings, resembling other transient states of impaired consciousness.

Akinetic Mutism, Abulia, Catatonia

There are several states of profound apathy that, in the extreme, can resemble vegetative or minimally conscious states. These include akinetic mutism, abulia, and catatonia. These disorders have in common dysfunction of circuits involving the frontal lobes, diencephalon, and ascending dopaminergic projections, important to initiation of motor and cognitive activity. In akinetic mutism [6, 51, 52] the patient appears fully awake, and unlike the vegetative state, they will visually track the examiner. However, they usually do not respond to any commands. Akinetic mutism can be viewed as an extreme form of abulia, often resulting from frontal lesions, in which patients usually sit passively, but may occasionally respond to questions or commands after a long delay. In some patients, abulia or akinetic mutism can be reversed with dopaminergic agonists. Some consider akinetic mutism to be a subcategory of the minimally conscious state [53], however, the Aspen Workgroup considered akinetic mutism to be primarily a defect in motor initiation rather than in consciousness [4]. Catatonia is a similar akinetic state that can occasionally be seen in advanced cases of schizophrenia. Again, frontal and dopaminergic dysfunction have been implicated. Other, related akinetic–apathetic states include advanced parkinsonism, severe depression, and the neuroleptic malignant syndrome.

Neglect, Agnosia and Other Neurobehavioural Deficits

Although not usually considered among the disorders of consciousness, a variety of focal brain lesions can cause neurobehavioural deficits which impair the content, if not the level of consciousness. For example, in agnosias perception occurs but is stripped of its usual meaning, leading to loss of awareness in a specific realm. Thus, patients with prosopagnosia are unconscious of the connection between a particular face and that person's identity, and patients with anosognosia are unaware of their own illness. Aphasia can cause lack of awareness of language meaning and formulation, and disruption of the 'inner voice' forming the usual narrative of our conscious experience. Patients with neglect, typically caused by large non-dominant hemisphere lesions, are more obviously unaware of the contralateral environment and even of their own bodies. Large non-dominant hemisphere lesions often cause deficits in arousal, in addition to hemispatial neglect and inattention [54]. Other disorders of attention, similarly, lead to impaired awareness of certain stimuli, and in that sense could be considered a disorder of consciousness.

STATES RESEMBLING IMPAIRED CONSCIOUSNESS

Locked-in Syndrome

Patients who have absent motor function, but maintain intact sensation and cognition are said to be 'locked-in'. The locked-in syndrome can sometimes be mistaken for coma [53, 55]. Unlike coma, however, these patients are conscious, and may be able to communicate through vertical eye movements or eye blinks. The usual cause of locked-in syndrome is an infarct in the ventral pons (basilar artery territory) affecting the bilateral corticospinal and corticobulbar tracts. Less common causes include other lesions of the pons (haemorrhage, tumour, encephalitis, multiple sclerosis, central pontine myelinolysis), lesions in the bilateral cerebral peduncles or internal capsules, or severe disorders of peripheral nerve (most commonly acute inflammatory demyelinating polyneuropathy), muscle, or the neuromuscular junction.

In the locked-in syndrome, the spinal cord and cranial nerves do not receive signals from the cortex, and the patient is unable to move. Sensory pathways and the diencephalic/upper brainstem activating systems are spared. The patient is therefore, fully aware, and able to feel, hear, and understand everything in their environment. Brain metabolism is relatively normal in the locked-in syndrome [17, 35].

Examination of patients with the locked-in syndrome requires special attention to detect residual subtle movements they may use to signal conscious awareness through responses to questions or commands. Horizontal eye movements depend on pontine circuits, and are usually absent in the locked-in syndrome. However, vertical eye movements and eyelid elevation are controlled by a region in the tegmentum of the rostral midbrain, which is often spared in the locked-in syndrome. Patients with locked-in syndrome, therefore, often have sparing of vertical eye movements and eye opening, and can communicate using these eye movements. Responses to yes–no questions or communication using a letter board are laborious but possible under these circumstances. Special computer interfaces based on eye movements have been developed for patients with locked-in syndrome. One French journalist even wrote an entire book after becoming locked-in (The Diving Bell and the Butterfly). Consideration and sensitivity are appropriate in these profoundly disabled individuals who may retain full awareness of their surroundings, along with very active emotional and intellectual responses.

Establishment of the ability to communicate is the most critical part of the neurological examination in the locked-in syndrome. Other portions of the examination may reveal, as in coma, brainstem and spinal cord reflexes that occur without volitional control, and abnormal reflexes can be present depending on the specific lesion location.

Dissociative Disorders, Somatoform Disorders

Several psychological disorders can cause patients to appear as if in a coma. In addition to catatonia and severe depression mentioned above, patients may be unresponsive when in a dissociative state, often resulting from severe emotional trauma. Somatoform disorders such as conversion disorder, somatization disorder, or factitious disorder can also sometimes produce states resembling coma, sometimes called 'pseudocoma' [56, 57]. Often these can be distinguished from coma by a carefully performed neurological examination, which usually reveals responses that are not consistent with coma, decreased consciousness, or the locked-in syndrome. Well-known examples include the hand drop test (patients in pseudocoma will avoid striking their own face when their hand is released over their face) and optokinetic nystagmus (absent in coma; however, the response may also be suppressed in patients who do not focus on the visual stimulus). However, in some cases of possible psychiatric disorders resembling impaired consciousness vs. organic disorders causing some degree of lethargy, the diagnosis may not be obvious.

SUMMARY AND CONCLUSIONS

The neurological examination is crucial in the evaluation of patients with disorders of consciousness. We have discussed special considerations in performing the neurological examination in this population, including strategies for improving diagnostic yield, and the importance of sensitivity to patients and families facing these challenging disorders. We have reviewed the neuroanatomical basis of the major disorders of consciousness, including brain death, coma, vegetative state, minimally conscious state, and other conditions (Figure 2.1). Findings on neurological examination were discussed for each of these conditions (Tables 2.1–2.3), making it clear that apparently small details can make a big difference in patient diagnosis, treatment, and outcome. For example, subtle eye movements or other minimal movements may be the only indication that an apparently comatose

patient is in fact fully conscious, but 'locked-in'. Limb movements occur in all disorders of consciousness, but depending on the details, these movements could indicate that the patient is either responding purposefully, or exhibiting brainstem reflexes, or is capable of only spinal reflexes consistent with brain death. Patients in the minimally conscious state or with akinetic mutism may appear on casual observation to have no purposeful responses, but on more careful and protracted examination reveal evidence of consciousness. These examples, and many others, demonstrate that crucial distinctions can made upon careful neurological examination of patients with disorders of consciousness.

Much additional work is needed to better define the examination findings in disorders of consciousness, and to relate specific deficits and preserved functions to long-term outcome based on large studies, ideally performed in a prospective manner. In addition, the anatomical basis of specific deficits and preserved functions in disorders of consciousness require further study. Improvements in structural neuroimaging have greatly facilitated the ability to correlate impaired function with specific anatomical brain regions in a manner that was only possible previously with postmortem studies. Furthermore, functional neuroimaging has the potential to revolutionize how patients with disorders of consciousness are evaluated, since these methods could ultimately reveal internal conscious mental activity not apparent based on external behaviour [58–60]. Additional investigations will likely lead to a very different future understanding of neurological examination findings in patients with disorders of consciousness.

ACKNOWLEDGEMENTS

I am very grateful to Steven Laureys, Joseph Giacino, Shirley H. Wray, Grant T. Liu, and Howard Pomeranz for helpful discussions, and to Michael J. Purcaro for the illustrations. This work was supported by NIH R01 NS055829, R01 NS049307, the Donaghue Foundation, and the Betsy and Jonathan Blattmachr family.

References

1. Blumenfeld, H. (2002a) *Neuroanatomy Through Clinical Cases*, Sunderland, MA: Sinauer Assoc. Publ., Inc.
2. Majerus, S., Gill-Thwaites, H., Andrews, K. and Laureys, S. (2005) Behavioral evaluation of consciousness in severe brain damage. *Prog Brain Res* 150:397–413.

3. Andrews, K., Murphy, L., Munday, R. and Littlewood, C. (1996) Misdiagnosis of the vegetative state: Retrospective study in a rehabilitation unit [see comment]. *BMJ* 313:13–16.

4. Giacino, J.T., Ashwal, S., Childs, N., Cranford, R., Jennett, B., Katz, D.I., Kelly, J.P., Rosenberg, J.H., Whyte, J., Zafonte, R. D. and Zasler, N.D. (2002) The minimally conscious state: Definition and diagnostic criteria [see comment]. *Neurology* 58:349–353.

5. Giacino, J. and Whyte, J. (2005) The vegetative and minimally conscious states: Current knowledge and remaining questions. *J Head Trauma Rehabil* 20:30–50.

6. Plum, F. and Posner, J.B. (1982) *The Diagnosis of Stupor and Coma*, 3rd Edition Philadelphia, PA: Davis.

7. Blumenfeld, H. (2002b) *Neuroanatomy through Clinical Cases, Chapter 20, Epilogue: A Simple Working Model of the Mind*, Sunderland, MA: Sinauer Assoc. Publ., Inc.

8. Blumenfeld, H. and Taylor, J. (2003) Why do seizures cause loss of consciousness? *The Neuroscientist* 9:301–310.

9. Task Force for the determination of brain death in children (1987) Guidelines for the determination of brain death in children. Task Force for the determination of brain death in children. *Neurology* 37:1077–1078.

10. American Academy of Neurology (1995) Practice parameters for determining brain death in adults (summary statement). The Quality Standards Subcommittee of the American Academy of Neurology [see comment]. *Neurology* 45:1012–1014.

11. Wijdicks, E.F. (1995) Determining brain death in adults [see comment]. *Neurology* 45:1003–1011.

12. Wijdicks, E.F. (2001) The diagnosis of brain death [see comment]. *New Engl J Med* 344:1215–1221.

13. Wijdicks, E.F. (2006) The clinical criteria of brain death throughout the world: Why has it come to this? [see comment]. *Can J Anaesth* 53:540–543.

14. The Multi-Society Task Force on PVS (1994) Medical aspects of the persistent vegetative state (1). The Multi-Society Task Force on PVS [see comment]. *New Engl J Med* 330:1499–1508.

15. Working Group of the Royal College of Physicians (1996) The permanent vegetative state. Review by a working group convened by the Royal College of Physicians and endorsed by the Conference of Medical Royal Colleges and their faculties of the United Kingdom. *J Roy Coll Phys Lond* 30:119–121.

16. Jennett, B. and Plum, F. (1972) Persistent vegetative state after brain damage. A syndrome in search of a name. *Lancet* 1:734–737.

17. Laureys, S., Owen, A.M. and Schiff, N.D. (2004) Brain function in coma, vegetative state, and related disorders. *Lancet Neurol* 3:537–546.

18. Fisher, C.M. (1969) The neurological examination of the comatose patient. *Acta Neurol Scand* 45 (Suppl 36):31–56.

19. Jorgensen, E.O. (1973) Spinal man after brain death. The unilateral extension–pronation reflex of the upper limb as an indication of brain death. *Acta Neurochir* 28:259–273.

20. Saposnik, G., Bueri, J.A., Maurino, J., Saizar, R. and Garretto, N.S. (2000) Spontaneous and reflex movements in brain death. *Neurology* 54:221–223.

21. Ivan, L.P. (1973) Spinal reflexes in cerebral death. *Neurology* 23:650–652.

22. Bueri, J.A., Saposnik, G., Maurino, J., Saizar, R. and Garretto, N.S. (2000) Lazarus' sign in brain death. *Mov Disord* 15:583–586.

23. Saposnik, G., Maurino, J. and Bueri, J. (2001) Movements in brain death [see comment]. *Eur J Neurol* 8:209–213.

24. Saposnik, G., Maurino, J., Saizar, R. and Bueri, J.A. (2004) Undulating toe movements in brain death. *Eur J Neurol* 11:723–727.

25. Jain, S. and DeGeorgia, M. (2005) Brain death-associated reflexes and automatisms. *Neurocrit Care* 3:122–126.

26. Mandel, S., Arenas, A. and Scasta, D. (1982) Spinal automatism in cerebral death. *New Engl J Med* 307:501.

27. Ropper, A.H. (1984) Unusual spontaneous movements in brain-dead patients. *Neurology* 34:1089–1092.

28. Heytens, L., Verlooy, J., Gheuens, J. and Bossaert, L. (1989) Lazarus sign and extensor posturing in a brain-dead patient. Case report. *J Neurosurg* 71:449–451.

29. Marti-Fabregas, J., Lopez-Navidad, A., Caballero, F. and Otermin, P. (2000) Decerebrate-like posturing with mechanical ventilation in brain death. *Neurology* 54:224–227.

30. Spittler, J.F., Wortmann, D., vonDuring, M. and Gehlen, W. (2000) Phenomenological diversity of spinal reflexes in brain death. *Eur J Neurol* 7:315–321.

31. Fisher, C.M. (1967) Some neuro-ophthalmological observations. *J Neurol Neurosurg Psychiatr* 30:383–392.

32. Liu, G.T. (1999) Coma. *Neurosurg Clin N Am* 10:579–586.

33. Liu, G.T. and Galetta, S.L. (2001) The neuro-ophthalmologic examination (including coma). *Ophthalmol Clin N Am* 14:23–39.

34. Gilbert, G.J. (2007) Unilateral shivering: A result of lateral medullary infarction. *South Med J* 100:540–541.

35. Levy, D.E., Sidtis, J.J., Rottenberg, D.A., Jarden, J.O., Strother, S.C., Dhawan, V., Ginos, J.Z., Tramo, M.J., Evans, A.C. and Plum, F. (1987) Differences in cerebral blood flow and glucose utilization in vegetative versus locked-in patients. *Ann Neurol* 22:673–682.

36. Adams, J.H., Graham, D.I. and Jennett, B. (2000) The neuropathology of the vegetative state after an acute brain insult. *Brain* 123:1327–1338.

37. Kinney, H.C., Korein, J., Panigrahy, A., Dikkes, P. and Goode, R. (1994) Neuropathological findings in the brain of Karen Ann Quinlan. The role of the thalamus in the persistent vegetative state [see comment]. *New Engl J Med* 330:1469–1475.

38. Childs, N.L., Mercer, W.N. and Childs, H.W. (1993) Accuracy of diagnosis of persistent vegetative state [see comment]. *Neurology* 43:1465–1467.

39. Vanhaudenhuyse, A., Schnakers, C., Bredart, S. and Laureys, S. (2008) Assessment of visual pursuit in post-comatose states: Use a mirror. *J Neurol Neurosurg Psychiatr* 79:223.

40. O'Neil-Pirozzi, T.M., Momose, K.J., Mello, J., Lepak, P., McCabe, M., Connors, J.J. and Lisiecki, D.J. (2003) Feasibility of swallowing interventions for tracheostomized individuals with severely disordered consciousness following traumatic brain injury. *Brain Injury* 17:389–399.

41. Lin, L.-C., Hsieh, P.-C., Wu, S.-C. (2008) Prevalence and associated factors of pneumonia in patients with vegetative state in Taiwan. *J Clin Nurs* 17(7): 861–868.

42. Mackay, L.E., Morgan, A.S. and Bernstein, B.A. (1999) Swallowing disorders in severe brain injury: Risk factors affecting return to oral intake. *Arch Phys Med Rehabil* 80:365–371.

43. Morgan, A.S. and Mackay, L.E. (1999) Causes and complications associated with swallowing disorders in traumatic brain injury. *J Head Trauma Rehabil* 14:454–461.

44. Whyte, J., Laborde, A. and Dipasquale, M.C. (1999) Assessment and treatment of the vegetative and minimally conscious patient. In Rosenthal, M., Kreutzer, J.S., Griffith, E.R. and Pentland, B., (eds.) *Rehabilitation of the Adult and Child with Traumatic Brain Injury*, pp. 435–452. philadelphia, PA, FA Davis.

45. Privitera, M., Hoffman, M., Moore, J.L. and Jester, D. (1994) EEG detection of nontonic-clonic status epilepticus in patients with altered consciousness. *Epilepsy Res* 18:155–166.

46. Claassen, J., Mayer, S.A., Kowalski, R.G., Emerson, R.G. and Hirsch, L.J. (2004) Detection of electrographic seizures with continuous EEG monitoring in critically ill patients. *Neurology* 62:1743–1748.

47. DeLorenzo, R.J., Waterhouse, E.J., Towne, A.R., Boggs, J.G., Ko, D., DeLorenzo, G.A., Brown, A. and Garnett, L. (1998) Persistent nonconvulsive status epilepticus after the control of convulsive status epilepticus. *Epilepsia* 39:833–840.

48. Treiman, D.M., Meyers, P.D., Walton, N.Y., Collins, J.F., Colling, C., Rowan, A.J., Handforth, A., Faught, E., Calabrese, V.P., Uthman, B.M., Ramsay, R.E. and Mamdani, M.B. (1998) A comparison of four treatments for generalized convulsive status epilepticus. Veterans Affairs Status Epilepticus Cooperative Study Group [comment]. *New Engl J Med* 339:792–798.

49. Gokygit, A. and Caliskan, A. (1995) Diffuse spike-wave status of 9-year duration without behavioral change or intellectual decline. *Epilepsia* 36:210–213.

50. Vuilleumier, P., Despland, P.A. and Regli, F. (1996) Failure to recall (but not to remember): Pure transient amnesia during nonconvulsive status epilepticus. *Neurology* 46:1036–1039.

51. Fisher, C.M. (1983) Honored guest presentation: Abulia minor vs. agitated behavior. *Clin Neurosurg* 31:9–31.

52. Wijdicks, E.F. and Cranford, R.E. (2005). Clinical diagnosis of prolonged states of impaired consciousness in adults [see comment]. *Mayo Clin Proc* 80:1037–1046.

53. American Congress of Rehabilitation Medicine (1995) Recommendations for use of uniform nomenclature pertinent to patients with severe alterations in consciousness. American Congress of Rehabilitation Medicine [see comment] [erratum appears in *Arch Phys Med Rehabil* 1995 Apr, 76(4):397]. *Arch Phys Med Rehabil* 76:205–209.

54. Heilman, K.M., Valenstein, E. and Watson, R.T. (2000) Neglect and related disorders. *Semin Neurol* 20:463–470.

55. Laureys, S., Pellas, F., VanEeckhout, P., Ghorbel, S., Schnakers, C., Perrin, F., Berre, J., Faymonville, M.E., Pantke, K.H., Damas, F., Lamy, M., Moonen, G. and Goldman, S. (2005) The locked-in syndrome: What is it like to be conscious but paralyzed and voiceless? *Prog Brain Res* 150:495–511.

56. Henry, J.A. and Woodruff, G.H. (1978) A diagnostic sign in states of apparent unconsciousness. *Lancet* 2:920–921.

57. Shaibani, A. and Sabbagh, M.N. (1998) Pseudoneurologic syndromes: Recognition and diagnosis [see comment]. *Am Family Physician* 57:2485–2494.

58. Laureys, S., Giacino, J.T., Schiff, N.D., Schabus, M. and Owen, A.M. (2006) How should functional imaging of patients with disorders of consciousness contribute to their clinical rehabilitation needs? *Curr Opin Neurol* 19:520–527.

59. Owen, A.M., Coleman, M.R., Boly, M., Davis, M.H., Laureys, S. and Pickard, J.D. (2006) Detecting awareness in the vegetative state [see comment]. *Science* 313:1402.

60. Di, H.B., Yu, S.M., Weng, X.C., Laureys, S., Yu, D., Li, J.Q., Qin, P.M., Zhu, Y.H., Zhang, S.Z. and Chen, Y.Z. (2007) Cerebral response to patient's own name in the vegetative and minimally conscious states [see comment]. *Neurology* 68:895–899.

Functional Neuroimaging

Steven Laureys, Melanie Boly and Giulio Tononi

ABSTRACT

While philosophers have for centuries pondered upon the relation between mind and brain, neuroscientists have only recently been able to explore the connection analytically – to peer inside the black box. This ability stems from recent advances in technology and emerging neuroimaging modalities. It is now possible to produce not only remarkably detailed images of the brain's structure (i.e., anatomical imaging) but also to capture images of the physiology associated with mental processes (i.e., functional imaging). We are able to 'see' how specific regions of the brain 'light up' when activities such as reading this book are performed and how our neurons and their elaborate cast of supporting cells organize and coordinate their tasks. As demonstrated in the other chapters of this book, the mapping of cognitive processes (mostly by measuring regional changes in blood flow, initially by positron emission tomography or PET and currently by functional magnetic resonance imaging or fMRI) is providing insight into the functional neuroanatomy of consciousness.

The idea that regional cerebral blood flow (rCBF) is intimately related to brain function goes back more than a century ago. As often the case in science, this idea was initially the result of unexpected observations

(see Box 3.1). In what follows we will introduce the area of functional brain imaging (i.e., positron emission tomography or PET, single photon emission tomography or SPECT, functional magnetic resonance

MEASURING BLOOD FLOW AS AN INDEX OF NEURAL ACTIVITY

The Italian physiologist Angelo Mosso studied pulsations of the living human brain that keep pace with the heartbeat [1]. These pulsations can be observed on the surface of the fontanelles in newborn children. Mosso believed that they reflected blood flow to the brain. He observed similar pulsations in an adult with a post-traumatic skull defect over the frontal lobes. While studying this subject, a peasant named Bertino, Mosso observed a sudden increase in the magnitude of the 'brain's heartbeats' when the ringing church bells signalled the time for a required prayer (indicated by arrow in Figure 3.1). The changes in brain pulsations occurred independently of any change in pulsations in the forearm. Mosso understood that the bells had reminded Bertino of his obligation to say a silent Ave Maria. Intrigued by this observation, Mosso then asked

Bertino to perform a mental calculation and again he observed an increase in pulsations and, presumably, in blood flow as the subject began the calculation and a second rise just as he answered. This was the first study ever to suggest that measurement of cerebral blood flow might be a way of assessing human cognition.

Charles Roy and Charles Sherrington further characterized this relationship. They suggested that 'the brain possesses an intrinsic mechanism by which its vascular supply can be varied locally in correspondence with local variations of functional activity'. One of the most extraordinary examples of this relationship was observed in Walter K., a German American sailor who consulted Dr John Fulton for a humming noise in his head. Fulton, when listening with a stethoscope at the back of his patient's head, confirmed this bruit and organized an exploratory intervention. During neurosurgery, a large arteriovenous malformation overlying the visual cortex was observed. An attempt to remove the malformation failed and left Walter with a bony defect. His physicians could now hear the bruit even more clearly. The patient mentioned that the noise in his head became louder when he was using his eyes. As Dr Fulton later published in *Brain*, 'It was not difficult to convince ourselves that when the patient suddenly began to use his eyes after a prolonged period of rest in a dark room, there was a prompt and noticeable increase in the intensity of his bruit' [3]. Fulton's studies made him postulate that it was the effort of trying to discern objects that were just at the limit of his patient's acuity which brought on the increases of the bruit. Merely shining light into his eyes when he was making no mental effort had no effect. This was a remarkable observation, the significance of which would not be appreciated for many years. It was probably the first ever recorded result of top-down influences on sensory processing [2].

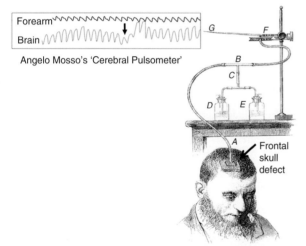

FIGURE 3.1 The 'brain's heartbeats' recorded during inner speech (saying a silent Ave Maria indicated by the arrow) (1881). *Source*: Adapted from Posner and Raichle [2].

imaging or fMRI, electroencephalography or EEG, event-related potentials or ERPs, magnetoencephalography or MEG, magnetic resonance spectroscopy or MRS and transcranial magnetic stimulation or TMS). Each technique provides different information and has its own advantages and disadvantages in terms of cost, safety and temporal and spatial resolution (Figure 3.2). After briefly discussing the functional neuroimaging techniques, we will present a short overview of study design and methods to process and analyse the

data. We will here not discuss structural neuroimaging (i.e., x-ray computed tomography or CT and magnetic resonance imaging or MRI – see Box 3.2).

POSITRON EMISSION TOMOGRAPHY

PET has its roots in tissue autoradiography, a method used for many years in animal studies to investigate organ metabolism and blood flow. Researchers in the field of tissue autoradiography became fascinated when CT was introduced in the 1970s. They realized that if the anatomy of an organ could be reconstructed by passing an x-ray beam

through it, the distribution of a previously administered radioisotope could also be reconstructed *in vivo*. They simply had to measure the emission of radioactivity from the body section. With this insight was born the idea of autoradiography of living human subjects. A crucial element was the choice of the radioisotope. A class of radioisotopes was selected that emitted positrons (i.e., particles identical to electrons except that they carry a positive charge). A positron will immediately combine with a nearby electron. They will annihilate each other, emitting two gamma rays in the process. Because each gamma ray travels in opposite directions, detectors around the sample can detect the gamma rays and locate their origin. The crucial role of positrons in human autoradiography gave rise to the name positron emission tomography or PET [5].

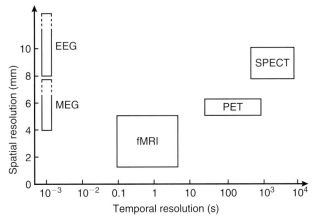

FIGURE 3.2   Approximation of the resolution in time and space of the most commonly employed functional neuroimaging techniques based on measurements of haemodynamic (fMRI, PET and SPECT) and electrical (EEG and MEG) activity of the brain. *Source*: Adapted from [4].

Throughout the late 1970s and early 1980s, PET was rapidly developed to measure various activities in the brain, such as glucose metabolism, blood flow, oxygen consumption and uptake of drugs. Although PET is primarily a research tool for brain imaging, its increasing availability in medical centres for oncology makes likely more widespread application to neurological diseases. The most frequently performed PET studies measure resting regional cerebral metabolic rates

---

BOX 3.2

STRUCTURAL NEUROIMAGING

The modern era of medical imaging began in the early 1970s with the introduction of a remarkable technique called x-ray computed axial tomography, now known as CAT, x-ray CT or just CT. It changed forever the practice of neurology because, for the first time, clinicians could non-invasively view the living brain (standard x-rays only reveal bone and some surrounding tissues). Second, it stimulated engineers and scientists to consider alternative ways of creating images of the body's interior using similar mathematical and computerized strategies for image reconstruction (e.g., SPECT and PET) [2]. Despite its wide availability, CT has been replaced by the more sensitive MRI as the procedure of choice for cerebral imaging. MRI stands for a vast and varied array of techniques that use no ionizing radiation and provides an enormous range of information. From an established ability to provide high-quality structural information, MR techniques are rapidly advancing and provide other clinically relevant physiological information as spectroscopic studies illuminating

the details of biochemical status (MR spectroscopy or MRS), blood oxygenation level allowing functional activation studies (functional MRI or fMRI), cerebral blood compartment (MR angiography or MRA), perfusion (perfusion-weighted MRI or PWI), water molecular diffusion (diffusion-weighted imaging or DWI), cerebral microstructure and fiber tracking (using diffusion anisotropy effects measured by diffusion tensor imaging or DTI), magnetization transfer (MT) imaging, etc.

At present, MRI is the procedure of choice for the structural imaging of the brain. However, it is susceptible to movement artifacts and patients who are on life support systems, have gunshot wounds or who have implanted MRI incompatible material (pacemakers, prostheses…), still represent problems. The main limit on the wealth of diagnostic information that can be obtained for each patient is in the duration of the procedure. Ongoing refinements of fMRI, MRA, MRS, PWI, DWI, DTI and other MR techniques are allowing them to fit into routine clinical practice.

for glucose (rCMRGlu) or changes in rCBF as indirect index of neural synaptic activity [6]. Recent developments are PET/CT combined imaging (offering improved attenuation correction and co-registration or fusion of the functional PET image with a high anatomical resolution CT image).

PET scanning involves the administration of positron-emitting radionuclides with short half-lives in which particle disintegration is captured by multiple sensors positioned around the head. The radiotracer is administered into a vein in the arm and is taken up by the brain through the bloodstream. After a course of a few millimetres the positron will interact with an electron in the brain tissue and produce two high-energy photons, at approximately 180 degrees apart from each other. In the PET scanner, a ring of detectors around the patient's head can detect these coincident photons. As the radioactive compound accumulates in different regions of the brain and positron annihilations occur, the scanner detects the coincident rays produced at all positions outside the head and reconstructs an image that depicts the location and concentration of the radioisotope within a plane of the brain. This emission scan is then corrected by comparison with the attenuation image made from a transmission scan of the subject's head. PET studies involve the use of a cyclotron to produce the radioactive tracers. The type of information of the PET image is determined by the administered radiolabeled compound. Oxygen-15, fluorine-18, carbon-11 and nitrogen-13 are common radioisotopes, which can combine with other elements to create organic molecules that can substitute for natural substances, such as water, glucose, the L-DOPA, benzodiazepine receptor ligands, etc. Using different compounds, PET can assess regional blood flow, oxygen and glucose metabolism, neurotransmitter and drug uptake in the tissues of the working brain. PET can sample all parts of the brain with equal resolution and sensitivity. Typically, it can locate changes in activity with an accuracy of about 6 mm.

In the past decade, PET was the most widely used technique to assess the neural substrates of cognitive processes at the macroscopic level, but it is now superseded by fMRI. PET remains a powerful tool in receptor imaging (e.g., assessment of neurotransmitter or drug uptake) and molecular imaging (e.g., assessment of gene expression or protein synthesis) in both normal and pathological states [7].

Cerebral Metabolic Rate for Glucose

To study regional cerebral glucose utilization, a positron-labelled deoxyglucose tracer is used (i.e.,

[^{18}F]fluorodeoxyglucose-FDG) [8]. This tracer is taken up by active brain regions as if it was glucose. However, once inside the cell, FDG is phosphorylated by hexokinase to FDG-6-phosphate which is not a substrate for glucose transport and cannot be metabolized by phosphohexoseisomerase, the next enzyme in the glucose metabolic pathway. Thus, labelled FDG-6-phosphate becomes metabolically trapped within the intracellular compartment. The amount of radioactive label that eventually remains in each discrete region of the brain is related to the glucose uptake and metabolism of that particular region. An FDG-PET scan summates approximately 30 minutes of cerebral glucose metabolism and allows assessment of regional variations. However, given the half-life of ^{18}F (2 hours), it is less suited for brain activation studies.

Cerebral Blood Flow

Most PET activation studies rely on the administration of radioactively labelled water – specifically, hydrogen combined with oxygen 15, a radioactive isotope of oxygen (H$_2$^{15}O). The labelled water emits copious numbers of positrons as it decays (hydrogen isotopes cannot be used, because they do not emit positrons). In just over a minute after intravenous injection, the radioactive water accumulates in the brain, forming an image of blood flow. The radioactivity of the water produces no deleterious effects. Oxygen 15 has a half-life of only 2 minutes; an entire sample decays almost completely in about 10 minutes (five half-lives) into a non-radioactive form. The rapid decay substantially reduces the exposure of subjects to the potentially harmful effects of radiation. Moreover, only low doses of the radioactive label are necessary. The fast decay and small amounts permit many measures of blood flow to be made in a single experiment. In this way, H$_2$^{15}O-PET can take multiple pictures of the brain at work in different experimental conditions. Each picture represents the average neural activity of about 45 seconds. The total number of scans that can be made per subject (typically about 12 images) is limited by the exposure to radiation.

SINGLE PHOTON EMISSION COMPUTED TOMOGRAPHY

In general, SPECT tracers are more limited than PET tracers in the kinds of brain activity they can monitor, but they are longer lasting. Thus, SPECT does not require an onsite cyclotron. However, most

SPECT technology is relatively non-quantitative, does not permit measured attenuation correction and has a spatial resolution inferior to that of PET. On the other hand, SPECT is less expensive and more widely available.

Similar to PET, SPECT uses also radioactive tracers, but it involves the detection of individual photons (low-energy gamma rays) rather than positrons emitted at random from the radionuclide to be imaged. Typical radionuclides include technetium-99m (^{99m}Tc) and iodine-123 (^{123}I) with half-lives of respectively 6 and 13 hours. On average, SPECT acquisition times are 20–30 minutes.

Frequently used radiolabeled agents for brain perfusion SPECT are Tc-99m-hexamethyl propylamine oxime (Tc-99m-HMPAO; a lipid soluble macrocyclic amine) and Tc-99m-bicisate ethyl cysteinate dimer (Tc-99m-ECD). Long half-life, rapid brain uptake and slow clearance of most radiolabeled agents for brain perfusion SPECT offer the opportunity to inject the tracer at a time when scanning is impossible (e.g., during an epileptic crisis) and to scan (post-event) the associated distribution of activated brain regions. In addition to their use in determining perfusion, radiotracers can also be used to determine biochemical interactions such as receptor binding. For example, iodine-123 labelled ligands such as IBZM, iodo-hydroxy-methoxy-N-[(ethyl-pyrrolidinyl) methyl]-benzamide, have been developed for imaging the dopamine receptor system (IBZM is a D2 receptor agonist that shows high uptake in the striatum).

FUNCTIONAL MAGNETIC RESONANCE IMAGING

fMRI can detect an increase in blood oxygen concentration that occurs in an area of heightened neuronal activity. The basis for this capacity comes from the way neurons make use of oxygen. Functionally induced increases in blood flow are accompanied by alterations in the amount of glucose the brain consumes but not in the amount of oxygen it uses. Indeed, despite the presence of abundant oxygen, the normal brain resorts to anaerobic metabolism during spurts of neuronal activity. Apparently, this physiological behaviour relies on tactics similar to that present in sprinter's muscles. It is not yet fully understood why the brain acts this way. Additional blood to the brain without a concomitant increase in oxygen consumption leads to a heightened concentration of oxygen in the small veins draining the active neural centres. The reason is that supply has increased, but the demand

has not. Therefore, the extra oxygen delivered to the active part of brain simply returns to the general circulation by way of the draining veins.

The commonest form of functional MRI is blood oxygenation level dependent (BOLD) imaging [9]. The BOLD signal depends on the ratio of oxygenated to deoxygenated haemoglobin. In regions of neuronal activity this ratio changes as increased flow of oxygenated blood temporarily surpasses consumption, decreasing the level of paramagnetic deoxyhaemoglobin. These localized changes cause increases in magnetic resonance signal, which are used as markers of functional activation. Ultrafast scanning can measure these changes in signal, which are mapped directly onto a high-resolution scan of the subject's anatomy. fMRI studies require magnets with field strengths superior to one tesla (recent fMRI magnets are 7 T). Some concerns have been raised about the intensity of the magnetic field to which the tissues are exposed in MRI, but so far there are no known harmful biological effects. The largest limiting factor is the claustrophobia some subjects may suffer as in most instrument designs the entire body must be inserted into a relatively narrow tunnel. Other limiting drawbacks are its susceptibility to subjects' movement artifacts and artifacts related to the use of metal-containing devices in the magnet (i.e., EEG wires…).

ELECTROENCEPHALOGRAPHY

EEG detects spontaneous brain electrical activity from the scalp. It provides temporal resolution in the millisecond range. However, traditional EEG technology and practice provide insufficient spatial detail to identify relationships between brain electrical events and structures and functions visualized by fMRI. Recent advances help to overcome this problem by recording EEGs from more electrodes (experimental laboratories may use 256 electrodes), by registering EEG data with anatomical images, and by correcting the distortion caused by volume conduction of EEG signals through the skull and scalp. In addition, statistical measurements of sub-second interdependences between EEG time series recorded from different locations can help to generate hypotheses about the instantaneous functional networks that form between different cortical regions during mental processing. Physiological and instrumental artifacts (e.g., subject's eye or head movements, heartbeats or poor electrode contacts) can contaminate the EEG (and MEG). Care must be taken to correct or eliminate such artifacts before further analyses are performed.

Scalp-recorded EEGs in the waking state in healthy adults normally range from several to about 75 μV. The EEG signal is largely attributable to graded post-synaptic potentials of the cell body and large dendrites of vertically oriented pyramidal cells in cortical layers 3–5. These are synchronized by rhythmic discharges from thalamic nuclei, with the degree of synchronization of the underlying cortical activity reflected in the amplitude of the EEG. Most of the EEG signal originates in cortical regions near the recording electrode. The columnar structure of the cerebral cortex facilitates a large degree of their electrical summation rather than mutual cancellation. Thus, the EEG recorded at the scalp represents the passive conduction of currents produced by summating activity over large neuronal aggregates. Regional desynchronization of the EEG reflects increased mutual interaction of a subset of the population engaging in 'cooperative activity' and is associated with decreases in amplitude.

To measure the EEG, electrodes are attached to the scalp with a conducting paste. Each electrode is connected with an electrically 'neutral' lead attached to the ear, nose, chin or chest (i.e., reference montage) or with an 'active' lead located over a different scalp area (i.e., bipolar montage). Differential amplifiers are used to record voltage changes over time at each electrode. These signals are then digitized with 12 or more bits of precision and are sampled at a rate high enough to prevent aliasing of the signals of interest. EEGs are conventionally described as patterns of activity in five frequency ranges: delta (less than 4 Hz), theta (4–7 Hz), alpha (8–12 Hz), beta (13–35 Hz; sometimes subdivided in beta1 at 13–20 Hz and beta2 at 21–35 Hz) and gamma activity (above about 35 Hz).

EVOKED POTENTIALS

An evoked potential (EP) or ERP is the time-locked average of the EEG in response to a specific sensory, motor or cognitive event. Because of their low amplitude, especially in relation to the background EEG activity, a number of stimuli have to be recorded and averaged with a computer in order to permit their recognition and definition. The background EEG activity, which has no fixed temporal relationship to the stimulus, will be averaged out by this procedure.

Sensory evoked or 'exogenous' potentials are recordings of cerebral or spinal potentials elicited by stimulation of specific sensory pathways (e.g., visual evoked potentials elicited by monocular stimulation with a reversing checkerboard pattern; brainstem auditory evoked potentials elicited by monaural stimulation with repetitive clicks; and somatosensory evoked potentials elicited by electrical stimulation of a peripheral nerve). They are a routinely used means of monitoring the functional integrity of these pathways in neurology.

Certain EP components depend upon the mental attention of the subject and the setting in which the stimulus occurs, rather than simply on the physical characteristics of the stimulus. Such 'event-related' or 'endogenous' potentials (ERPs) are related in some manner to the cognitive aspects of distinguishing an occurring target stimulus [10]. For clinical purposes, attention has been directed particularly at the so-called P300 or P3 component of the ERP (named after its positive polarity and latency of approximately 300–400 ms after onset of an auditory target stimulus – e.g., an infrequent tone or the subject's own name [11]).

As a research tool, ERPs can provide valuable information about the timing and cortical distribution of the neuroelectrical activity generated during mental activity. An averaged EP waveform consists of a series of positive and negative waves; a significant difference in latency, amplitude, duration or topography of one or more of these waves between experimental conditions which differ in one specific cognitive factor is assumed to reflect the mass neural activity associated with that cognitive factor [10]. Measurements of changes in the amplitude and timings of peaks in the series of EP waves allow inferences to be made about the sequence and timing of task-associated processes, such as pre-stimulus preparation, encoding of stimulus features, conscious perception, operations such as matching or comparison of stimulus codes and memory codes, evaluation of the meaning of the stimulus, response selection and execution. Classical averaged EP method assumes that the component subprocesses comprising a cognitive behaviour do not vary in time from trial to trial [12].

MAGNETOENCEPHALOGRAPHY

MEG measures the magnetic fields generated by electrical activity within the brain. Magnetic field tomography (MFT; a technique based on distributed source analysis of MEG data) makes possible the three-dimensional reconstruction of dynamic brain activity in humans with a temporal resolution better than 1 ms and a spatial accuracy of 2–5 mm at the cortical level (which deteriorates to 1–3 cm at depths of 6 cm or more). Electrical currents generate magnetic fields. Biomagnetic fields directly reflect electrophysiological events of the brain and pass through the skull

BOX 3.3

THE INVERSE PROBLEM

Like for EEG, MEG data have to be subjected to an inverse problem algorithm to obtain an estimate for the distribution of the activity in the brain [13]. Similar to PET, fMRI and EEG these can then be displayed on cross-sectional anatomical images (obtained by MRI) of the same subject. The inverse problem relates to the difficulty to determine internal sources on the basis of measurements performed outside the head. The most common way to tackle this problem is to determine the single source current element (dipole) that most completely explains the EEG or MEG pattern. This can be done with a computer algorithm that starts from a random dipole position and orientation and keeps changing these parameters as long as the field pattern computed from the dipole keeps approaching the observed EEG or MEG pattern. When no further improvement is obtained, a minimum in the cost function has been reached; a source corresponding to this solution is called the equivalent current dipole (ECD). In most cases, however, the EEG or MEG data pattern cannot be accurately explained by a single source. In these cases, two or more dipoles could be used to explain the data, but this easily leads to computational difficulties in trying to determine the best multi-source solution. Alternatively, continuous solutions such as the minimum norm estimate might also be constructed [14]. When interpreting EEG or MEG results it should be born in mind that the inverse problem is fundamentally non-unique. This means that even if the complete electric and magnetic field around the head could be measured precisely, an infinite number of current distributions in the brain could still be constructed that would explain the measured fields. It is always possible that some sources are missed, whatever the measurement setup. For example, MEG alone is insensitive to radially oriented sources, but even when combined with EEG, silent sources are possible. Full use of available techniques requires the use of estimation theory to derive optimal solutions based on all available information, including MRI, PET and fMRI.

without distortion. Hence, currents initiated at the synapses, and guided post-synaptically by cell structure produce the magnetic field detectable outside the head. MEG is most sensitive to activity in the fissural cortex, where the current is oriented parallel to the skull, whereas it does not detect sources that are oriented exactly radially to the skull.

The average electromagnetoencephalogram is about ten picotesla (10^{-12} T) in amplitude, this is nine orders of magnitude smaller than the earth's steady magnetic field. The magnetic field produced by a single post-synaptic potential is too weak to be detected outside the head. Instead, what is detected is the macroscopic coherent activity of thousands of neurons. Measurements are performed inside magnetically shielded rooms. Sensitivity to such weak signals requires the use of cryogenic technologies. MEG instruments consist of superconducting quantum interference devices (SQUIDs), operating at liquid helium temperatures of $-269°C$ [15]. Recording neuromagnetic signals has been compared to listening for the footsteps of an ant in the middle of a rock concert.

The major advantage of techniques based on the measurements of cerebral electrical activity (i.e., EEG and MEG) is their uncompromised time resolution. Their major drawback, however, is their limited spatial resolution. Indeed, accurate localization of the source of brain activity remains difficult (see Box 3.3). Furthermore, the resolution becomes poorer the deeper into the brain we attempt to image. The main advantages of MEG compared with EEG are its superior spatial accuracy and ease of use, particularly when a large number of channels are involved (currently over 300). On the other hand, EEG complements MEG in detecting source components not detected by MEG (i.e., radially oriented sources) [16]. For the time being, MEG and MFT remain experimental research tools, unavailable to most clinical settings.

TRANSCRANIAL MAGNETIC STIMULATION

TMS is a tool for the non-invasive stimulation of the superficial cortex. TMS is now commonly used in clinical neurology to study central motor conduction time. Depending on stimulation parameters, TMS can excite or inhibit the arbitrary sites of the superficial cortex, allowing functional mapping and creation of transient functional lesions [17].

For TMS, a brief, high-current pulse is produced in a coil of wire, which is placed above the scalp. A magnetic field is produced with lines of flux passing perpendicularly to the plane of the coil. An electric field is induced perpendicularly to the magnetic field. The extent of neuronal activation varies with the intensity of stimulation. TMS ordinarily does not activate corticospinal neurons directly; rather it activates them indirectly through synaptic inputs. Intracortical inhibition and facilitation are obtained using paired-pulse studies and reflect the activity of interneurons in the cortex. Safety guidelines have been published in order to prevent induction of seizures [18]. Repetitive TMS can produce effects that last after the stimulation period.

In neuropsychology, the classical paradigm is that of studying the effects of brain lesions on behaviour. With TMS, this paradigm can be applied in spatially and temporally restricted fashion to healthy volunteers. It is now widely used as a research tool to study aspects of human brain physiology including motor function, vision, language and the pathophysiology of brain disorders. Combined with other brain-imaging techniques such as PET, EEG and fMRI, it can be used to evaluate cortical excitability and connectivity [19, 20]. TMS allows investigating the relationship between focal cortical activity and behaviour, to trace the timing at which activity in a particular cortical region contributes to a given task, and to map the functional connectivity between brain regions [21].

MAGNETIC RESONANCE SPECTROSCOPY

MRI is generally associated with the signals from hydrogen nuclei (i.e., protons) because of the large amounts of hydrogen atoms in human tissue and brain and the strong signals they provide. MRS also makes measurements of protons, but also of nuclei such as phosphorus (31P), carbon (13C) and fluorine (19F) [22]. It offers the potential of assessing brain function at metabolic and molecular levels. The technique uses natural emissions from atomic nuclei activated by magnetic fields to measure concentration of endogenous molecules. Potential nuclei include 31P, 13C, 23Na, 7Li, in addition to 1H. The 31P MR spectrum can detect tissue concentrations of the phosphomonoesters phosphocholine and inorganic orthophosphate, the phosphodiesters glycerol-3-phosphoethanolamine and glycerol-3-phosphocholine, the triphosphate ATP and other phosphorus-containing molecules including phosphocreatinine. 1H spectroscopy offers the ability to measure lactate concentrations and neuronal markers such as N-acetyl aspartate. MRS permits quantitative analysis of these compounds *in vivo* with the potential of three-dimensional resolution within the brain.

FUNCTIONAL NEUROIMAGING STUDY DESIGN

Mapping the human brain is distinct from the assumptions held by phrenologists of the 19th century. According to the German physician Franz Josef Gall, thought processes are localized in single brain areas identified by bumps on the skull. Gall posited that complex behavioural traits (e.g., ideality, cautiousness, imitation, self-esteem, calculation…) could be related to the size of these bumps. Although the 'bumps theory' was fanciful, the idea of a functional segregation of the brain was not. In 1861, by carefully studying the brain of a man who had lost the faculty of speech after a left inferior frontal lesion, Paul Broca became convinced that different functions could be localized in different parts of the cerebrum. At present, more than a century of neuropsychological investigations in brain damaged patients has confirmed that a cortical area can be specialized for some aspects of perceptual or sensorimotor processing and that this specialization is anatomically segregated in the cortex. In our current vision on brain function however, functional segregation holds for simple processes rather than for complex behaviours or traits such as those described by phrenologists. By now, the view is that the cortical infrastructure supporting a single function (and a fortiori a complex behaviour) may involve many specialized areas that combine resources by functional integration between them. Hence, functional integration is mediated by the interactions between functionally segregated areas, and functional segregation is meaningful only in the context of functional integration and vice versa.

In this framework, the foundation for most of functional neuroimaging studies is that complex behaviours can be broken down into a set of constituent mental operations. In order to read this text, for example, you must recognize that a string of letters is a word; then recognize the meaning of words, phrases and sentences; and finally create mental images. The methodological challenge is first to separate each of these tasks from a cognitive perspective and second to determine those parts of the brain that are active and those that are dormant during their performance. In the past, cognitive neuroscientists have relied on studies of laboratory animals and patients with localized brain lesions to gain insight into the brain's functions. Imaging techniques, however, permit us to visualize safely the anatomy and the function of the human brain, both in normal and in pathological conditions.

It is amazing that the most widely used strategy for functional neuroimaging of the past 15 years is based on an idea first introduced to psychology in 1868. Indeed, Franciscus C. Donders, a Dutch ophthalmologist and physiologist, then proposed a general method to estimate cognitive processes based on a simple logic. He subtracted the time needed to respond to a light (with, say, a press of a key) from the time needed to respond to a particular colour of light. He found that discriminating colour required about 50 ms more than simply responding to the light. In this way, Donders was the first to isolate a basic mental process and to obtain a measure of the time needed by the brain to perform this specific process [23].

The classical strategy in functional neuroimaging is designed to accomplish a similar subtraction but in terms of the brain areas implementing the mental process. In particular, images of neural activity (being it blood flow measured by fMRI or electrical activity measured by EEG or MEG) taken before a task is begun can be compared with those obtained when the brain is engaged in that task – but also see Chapter 7, on 'resting state' studies. The two periods are referred to as control state and task state. It is important to carefully choose each state so as to isolate as best as possible a limited number of operations. Subtracting neural activity measurements made in the control state from each task indicates those parts of the brain active during a particular task. To achieve reliable data, averages are made of many experimental trials in the same person or of responses across many individual subjects. Averaging enables the detection of changes in neural activity associated with mental activity that would otherwise be easily confused with spurious shifts resulting from noise.

It is important to stress that this methodological approach, known as the cognitive subtraction paradigm, has an important drawback. Indeed, in order to isolate the neural substrate of a given cognitive component of interest, it must be assumed that the only difference between the control state and task state is the component of interest to the exception of any other stimulus- or task-related processes. Unfortunately, this cannot always be easily and fully guaranteed. Analytic strategies, however, have been devised to circumvent this problem (see below), and cognitive subtraction designs remain the foundation of a large amount of functional neuroimaging experiments.

ANALYSING BRAIN IMAGING DATA

Regional differences among brain scans have long been characterized thanks to hand-drawn regions of interest (ROIs). This approach reduced the information from hundreds of thousands of voxels (volume elements that in three dimensions correspond to a pixel with a given slice thickness) to a handful of ROI measurements, with a somewhat imprecise anatomical validity. The development of more powerful voxel-based statistical methods has made these ROI analyses become obsolete. Although several solutions are in use in neuroscience laboratories, one of the most popular methods for the analysis of neuroimaging data is statistical parametric mapping (SPM). SPM is a standardized method that refers to the construction and assessment of spatially extended statistical processes used to test hypotheses about neuroimaging data (mainly PET, SPECT and fMRI). Statistical parametric maps can be thought of as 'x-rays' of the significance of an effect, which can be projected on a three-dimensional representation of the brain. These ideas have been instantiated in a software (last version called SPM5) by Karl Friston and coworkers at the Welcome Department of Cognitive Neurology in London (http//www.fil.ion.ucl.ac.uk/spm). SPM has become the most widely used and validated method to analyse functional neuroimaging data. There are two basic approaches when analysing and interpreting functional neuroimaging data. They are based upon the distinction between functional segregation and integration.

Functional Segregation

Using a functional specialization concept of the brain, the following sets of approaches are based on detecting focal differences. They generally fall into one of three broad categories: (1) the subtractive or categorical designs are predicated on the assumption that the difference between two tasks can be formulated as a separable cognitive or sensorimotor component and that the regionally specific differences in brain activity identify the corresponding functional area (i.e., the cognitive subtraction paradigm). Its utilization ranges from the functional anatomy of word processing to the functional specialization in visual cortex, an application that has been validated by electrophysiological studies in monkeys [24]. (2) The parametric or dimensional design assumes that regional physiology will vary systematically with the degree of cognitive or sensorimotor processing. Parametric designs may avoid many of the shortcomings of 'cognitive subtraction'. A fundamental difference between subtractive and parametric designs lies in treating a cognitive process not as a categorical invariant but as a dimension that can be expressed to a greater or lesser extent in relation to the brain's regional activity. (3) Factorial or interaction designs are also well suited to avoid the drawbacks of simple subtraction paradigms. Two or more factors can be combined in the same experiment, and the interaction term will assess the effect of one factor while excluding the effect of the other.

Functional Integration

The functional role played by any component (e.g., a neuron or a specific brain area) of a connected system (e.g., the brain) is largely defined by its connections. Connectionist approaches to understanding the integration of brain functions are well established [25]. The nature and organizational principles of intra-cortical [26] and subcortical [27] connections have provided a basis for mechanistic descriptions of brain function, referring to parallel, massively distributed and interconnected (sub)cortical areas. Anatomical connectivity, mainly determined by neuroanatomical tracer experiments in animals, is a necessary underpinning for these models. The concepts of functional and effective connectivity were developed in the analysis of separable spike trains obtained from multi-unit electrode recordings. However, the neurophysiological measurements obtained from functional neuroimaging have a very different timescale (seconds vs. milliseconds) and nature (metabolic or haemodynamic vs. spike trains) than those obtained from electrophysiological studies.

At present, analytical tools are available to assess the functional or effective connectivity between distant cerebral areas [28]. *Functional connectivity* is defined as the temporal correlation of a neurophysiological index (i.e., blood flow) measured in different remote brain areas, whereas *effective connectivity* is defined as the influence one neural system exerts over another [29]. In this context, a *psychophysiological interaction* can be assessed in the framework of the general linear model as employed by SPM [28] to explain the activity in one cortical area in terms of an interaction between the influences of another area in a given experimental context. Put simply, the statistical analysis will identify brain regions that show condition dependent differences in the way their activity relates to the activity in another (chosen) area. Alternatively, exploratory data driven approaches based on independent component analysis can be employed [30].

Preprocessing of the Data

Voxel-based analyses require the data to be in the same anatomical space. This is obtained by realigning the data. Indeed, in functional neuroimaging experiments movement-related variance components represent one of the most serious confounds. Therefore, scans from each subject are realigned using an optimization procedure minimizing the residual sum of squares [31]. In a second step, the realigned images are normalized. They are subject to non-linear warping so that they match a template that already conforms to a standard anatomical space [32]. Indeed, pooling neuroimaging data from grossly different individual brains requires a procedure to spatially normalize the individual brains to an idealized or standard brain for the purpose of achieving overlap between corresponding anatomical and functional areas in different subjects. The Talairach and Tournoux atlas was initially developed – and has proven very useful – for anatomical normalization required for neurosurgical procedures, particularly those at brain sites close to the origin of the reference system (i.e., the anterior and posterior commissures). Each point within Talairach space into which brains are transformed is defined using three coordinates (expressed in mm). The first coordinate defines the position in x, that is, from left (negative) to right (positive) with 0 mm corresponding to the interhemispheric line. The second defines the position in y, that is, from posterior (negative) to anterior (positive) with 0 mm corresponding to the anterior commissure. The third defines the position in z, that is, from bottom (negative) to top (positive) with 0 mm corresponding to the plane through anterior and posterior commissures. This standard coordinate system facilitates the reporting of results in a conventional way and facilitates comparisons between peak voxels obtained in experiments from different laboratories.

After spatial normalization, images need to be smoothed (i.e., convolved with an isotropic Gaussian kernel). Smoothing individual images prior to a statistical analysis offers: (1) an improved signal to noise ratio, (2) a conditioning of the data so that they conform more closely to the Gaussian field model which lies at the basis of the correction procedure for multiple statistical comparisons, (3) a better overlap between the localization of anatomical and functional brain areas from different subjects which permits intersubject averaging.

Statistical Analysis

The data obtained after preprocessing consist of a matrix of many hundredth thousandths of voxels for each subject and for each condition. Each of these voxels is characterized by the x, y and z spatial coordinates in the standard space and a value representing the functional activity in that voxel (i.e., BOLD signal, blood flow, glucose metabolism,...). The statistical analysis corresponds to modelling the data in order to partition observed neurophysiological states or responses into components of interest, confounds of no interest and an error term. This partitioning is effected using the framework of the general linear model to estimate the components in terms of parameters associated with the design matrix. The *analysis* of regionally specific effects uses the general linear model to assess differences among parameter estimates (specified by a contrast) in a univariate sense, by referring to the error variance. The significance of each contrast is assessed with a statistic with a student's t distribution under the null hypothesis for each and every voxel (i.e., SPM{t}). The SPM {t} is transformed to the unit normal distribution to give a Gaussian field or SPM{Z}.

Statistical Inference

The final stage is to make statistical inferences on the basis of the SPM and characterize the responses observed using the fitted responses or parameter estimates. On one hand, with an *a priori* anatomically constrained hypothesis about effects in a particular brain location, the Z value in that region in the SPM{Z} can be used to test the hypothesis (i.e., uncorrected P value; or (better) a small volume corrected P value calculated). On the other hand, if an anatomical site cannot be predicted *a priori*, a correction for multiple non-independent comparisons is required. Therefore, the theory of Gaussian fields [33] provides a way for correcting the P value for the multiple non-independent comparisons implicit in the analysis. This correction depends on the search volume, the residual degrees of freedom due to error and the final image smoothness estimate. The obtained corrected and uncorrected P values pertain to different levels of inference in terms of (1) the significance of the effect in a particular voxel, (2) the significance of the coactivation of a cluster of voxels in a specific region and (3) the significance of the coactivation of several clusters in the whole brain. Only in cases of well-documented prior neuroanatomical knowledge about the expected result, small volume corrected or uncorrected P values can be accepted. By specifying different contrasts, one can test for the variety of effects described above, and the significance values above a chosen threshold are comprehensively represented in an SPM map where each voxel is represented at its proper location on the brain template and where the T value in this voxel for a given contrast is represented by use of a colour intensity code.

MULTI-MODALITY AND REAL-TIME INTEGRATION

fMRI (and previously $H_2^{15}O$-PET) measures local changes in brain haemodynamics induced by cognitive or perceptual tasks. These measures have a uniformly high spatial resolution of millimetres or less, but poor temporal resolution (about 1s at best). Conversely, EEG and MEG measure instantaneously the current flows induced by synaptic activity, but the accurate localization of these current flows remains an unsolved problem. Techniques have been developed that, in the context of brain anatomy visualized with structural MRI, use both haemodynamic and electromagnetic measures to get estimates of brain activation with higher spatial and temporal resolution. These methods range from simple juxtaposition to simultaneous integrated techniques. Multi-modality integration requires an improved understanding of the coupling between the physiological phenomena underlying the different signal modalities [34]. Acquisition of simultaneous EEG during fMRI provides an additional monitoring tool for the analysis of brain state fluctuations. The exploration of brain responses following inputs or in the context of state changes is crucial for a better understanding of the basic principles governing large-scale neuronal dynamics [35].

The combination of TMS with EEG or PET permits the assessment of connectivity and excitability of the human cerebral cortex. PET and fMRI, working in a combination yet to be determined, can define the anatomy of the circuits underlying a behaviour of interest; electrical recording techniques can reveal the course of temporal events in these spatially defined circuits. Parallel information from different imaging modalities is beginning to be used to constrain the EEG or MEG inverse solutions (see Box 3.3) to limited regions of the cerebrum. This approach provides optimal combined spatial and temporal resolution by exploiting the best aspects of each technology. Combining various techniques offers a more complete characterization of the different aspects of brain activity during cognitive processing. This is even more so regarding our understanding of transitory phenomena (e.g., single hallucinations).

Finally, advances in acquisition techniques, computational power and algorithms increased the speed of fMRI significantly, making real-time fMRI feasible. Real-time fMRI allows for brain–computer interfaces (see Chapter 17) with a high spatial and temporal resolution. Recent studies have shown that such approaches can be used to provide online feedback of the BOLD signal and to learn the self-regulation of local brain activity [36]. This local self-regulation is being used as a new paradigm in cognitive neuroscience to study brain plasticity and the functional relevance of brain areas.

Functional neuroimaging experiments provide a vast amount of information. Recent efforts to create neuroscience databases could organize and quickly disseminate such a repository of data. As demonstrated in many chapters of this book, wise use of these powerful tools and the information they produce can aid our understanding and management of disorders of consciousness. Clearly, neuroimaging is heading us towards a much richer grasp of the relation between the human mind and the brain.

ACKNOWLEDGEMENTS

Steven Laureys and Melanie Boly are respectively Senior Research Associate and Research Fellow at the Belgian Fonds National de la Recherche Scientifique (FNRS) and are supported by the European Commission, the Centre Hospitalier Universitaire Sart Tilman, Liège, the University of Liège, the Concerted Research Action of the French Speaking Community of Belgium, and the Mind Science Foundation, San Antonio, Texas.

References

1. Mosso, A. (1881) *Ueber den Kreislauf des Blutes in Men*schlichen Gehirn, Leipzig: Verlag von Viet and Company, pp. 60–67.
2. Posner, M.I., and Raichle, M.E. (1994). Images of the Brain. In Images of Mind, pp. 53–81. New York, Scientific American Library.
3. Fulton, J.F. (1928) Observations upon the vascularity of the human occipital lobe during visual activity. Brain 51:310–320.
4. Laureys, S., Peigneux, P. and Goldman, S. (2002) Brain imaging. In D'haenen, H., den Boer, J.A. and Willner, P. (eds.), Biological Psychiatry, New York: pp. 155–166. John Wiley & Sons Ltd.
5. Ter-Pogossian, M.M., Raichle, M.E. and Sobel, B.E. (1980) Positron-emission tomography. Sci Am 243 (4):170–181.
6. Magistretti, P.J. and Pellerin, L. (1999) Cellular mechanisms of brain energy metabolism and their relevance to functional brain imaging. Philos Trans R Soc Lond B Biol Sci 354 (1387):1155–1163.
7. Phelps, M.E. (2000) Inaugural article: Positron emission tomography provides molecular imaging of biological processes. Proc Natl Acad Sci USA 97 (16):9226–9233.
8. Huang, S.C., et al. (1980) Noninvasive determination of local cerebral metabolic rate of glucose in man. Am J Physiol 238:69–82.
9. Ogawa, S., et al. (1990) Brain magnetic resonance imaging with contrast dependent on blood oxygenation. *Proc Natl Acad Sci USA* 87 (24):9868–9872.
10. Kotchoubey, B. (2005) Event-related potential measures of consciousness: Two equations with three unknowns. *Prog Brain Res* 150:427–444.
11. Perrin, F., et al. (2006) Brain response to one's own name in vegetative state, minimally conscious state, and locked-in syndrome. *Arch Neurol* 63 (4):562–569.
12. Gevins, A. (1998) The future of electroencephalography in assessing neurocognitive functioning. *Electroencephalogr Clin Neurophysiol* 106 (2):165–172.

13. Darvas, F., et al. (2004) Mapping human brain function with MEG and EEG: Methods and validation. *Neuroimage* 23 (Suppl 1):S289–S299.
14. Nenonen, J.T., Hamalainen, M.S. and Ilmoniemi, R.J. (1994) Minimum-norm estimation in a boundary-element torso model. *Med Biol Eng Comput* 32 (1):43–48.
15. Brenner, D., Williamson, S.J. and Kaufman, L. (1975) Visually evoked magnetic fields of the human brain. *Science* 190 (4213):480–482.
16. Naatanen, R., Ilmoniemi, R.J. and Alho, K. (1994) Magnetoencephalography in studies of human cognitive brain function. *Trends Neurosci* 17 (9):389–395.
17. Hallett, M. (2000) Transcranial magnetic stimulation and the human brain. *Nature* 406 (6792):147–150.
18. Wassermann, E.M. (1998) Risk and safety of repetitive transcranial magnetic stimulation: Report and suggested guidelines from the International Workshop on the Safety of Repetitive Transcranial Magnetic Stimulation, June 5–7, 1996. *Electroencephalogr Clin Neurophysiol* 108 (1):1–16.
19. Paus, T. (1999) Imaging the brain before, during, and after transcranial magnetic stimulation. *Neuropsychologia* 37 (2):219–224.
20. Massimini, M., et al. (2005) Breakdown of cortical effective connectivity during sleep. *Science* 309 (5744):2228–2232.
21. Pascual-Leone, A., Walsh, V. and Rothwell, J. (2000) Transcranial magnetic stimulation in cognitive neuroscience – virtual lesion, chronometry, and functional connectivity. *Curr Opin Neurobiol* 10 (2):232–237.
22. Dacey, R., et al. (1991) Relative effects of brain and non-brain injuries on neuropsychological and psychosocial outcome. *J Trauma* 31 (2):217–222.
23. Donders, F.C. (1969) On the speed of mental processes (translation). *Acta Psychol* 30:412–431.
24. Zeki, S. (1993) *A Vision of the Brain*, Oxford, Boston: Blackwell Scientific Publications, pp. xi, 366.
25. Hebb, D.O. (1964) *Organisation of Behavior*, New York: John Wiley & Sons Inc.
26. Goldman-Rakic, P.S. (1988) Topography of cognition: Parallel distributed networks in primate association cortex. *Annu Rev Neurosci* 11:137–156.
27. Mesulam, M.M. (1990) Large-scale neurocognitive networks and distributed processing for attention, language, and memory. *Ann Neurol* 28 (5):597–613.
28. Friston, K.J., et al. (1997) Psychophysiological and modulatory interactions in neuroimaging. *Neuroimage* 6:218–229.
29. Buchel, C. and Friston, K.J. (1997) Modulation of connectivity in visual pathways by attention: Cortical interactions evaluated with structural equation modelling and fMRI. *Cereb Cortex* 7 (8):768–778.
30. McKeown, M.J., et al. (1998) Analysis of fMRI data by blind separation into independent spatial components. *Hum Brain Mapp* 6 (3):160–188.
31. Friston, K., et al. (1995) Spatial realignment and normalization of images. *Hum Brain Mapp* 2:165–189.
32. Talairach, J. and Tournoux, P. (1998) *Co-planar Stereotaxis Atlas of the Human Brain*, Stuttgart: Georges Thieme Verlag.
33. Friston, K.J. (1997) Analysing brain images: Principles and overview. In Frackowiak, R.S.J. et al. (eds.), *Human Brain Function*, San Diego, CA: pp. 25–41. Academic Press.
34. Dale, A.M. and Halgren, E. (2001) Spatiotemporal mapping of brain activity by integration of multiple imaging modalities. *Curr Opin Neurobiol* 11 (2):202–208.
35. Ritter, P. and Villringer, A. (2006) Simultaneous EEG-fMRI. *Neurosci Biobehav Rev* 30 (6):823–838.
36. Weiskopf, N., et al. (2007) Real-time functional magnetic resonance imaging: Methods and applications. *Magn Reson Imaging* 25 (6):989–1003.

Consciousness and Neuronal Synchronization

Wolf Singer

ABSTRACT

A promising approach for the investigation of neuronal correlates of consciousness consists of comparing brain states associated with conscious and non-conscious processing of the same stimulus material, respectively. Because of the distributed organization of the primate brain and because of the inability to identify singular cortical or subcortical structures responsible for conscious experience, it is likely that the neuronal substrate that supports the functional states required for the constitution of conscious experience is distributed in nature. Based on the evidence that precise synchronization of oscillatory neuronal responses is likely to serve the binding of distributed computational results into coherent representations, we hypothesized that brain states compatible with conscious processing should be characterized by a high degree of synchrony, that is temporal coherence of activity. To this end we investigated the electrophysiological correlates of binocular rivalry in animals and of subliminal and conscious perception in human subjects. Both approaches suggest the conclusion that precise synchronization of oscillatory neuronal responses in the high frequency range (beta, gamma) plays an important role in gating the access of sensory signals to the workspace of consciousness. Thus, the data support Sherrington's conjecture: 'Pure conjunction in time without necessarily cerebral conjunction in space lies at the root of the solution of the problem of the unity of mind'.

Consciousness is commonly equated with the ability to be aware of one's perceptions, feelings and intentions. In human subjects, characteristic features of the contents of consciousness are their unity and reportability. Search for the neuronal substrate of awareness therefore requires identification of the neuronal mechanisms through which brains generate unified representations of cognitive contents. Because brains can perform complete cognitive and executive functions without being aware of them, it is further necessary to explore the neuronal signatures that distinguish non-conscious from conscious processes. Here, data are reviewed that address both questions. It is proposed that contents that can in principle access consciousness are represented as dynamical spatio-temporal activity patterns evolving in extended assemblies of interacting cortical neurons. In order to actually enable access to consciousness, the assemblies encoding the respective contents need in addition engage in precisely synchronized oscillatory activity.

The term 'consciousness' has a number of different connotations ranging from awareness of one's perceptions and sensations to self-awareness, the perception of oneself as a responsible agent that is endowed with intentionality and free will. Reductionistic explanations of the various aspects of self-consciousness will probably not be possible without including the phenomena that result from interpersonal discourse and emerge only from social interactions, while phenomenal awareness, the ability to be aware of one's perceptions and intentions may be explainable without having to invoke social realities. One necessary prerequisite for the analysis of the neuronal correlates of consciousness (NCC) is to understand how brains perceive and represent the contents of cognition because one is always conscious of something. The respective contents of consciousness can be derived from extero- or enteroceptive sensory input or from information stored in memories. Thus, being conscious of something appears to involve a cognitive process that monitors neuronal activation patterns irrespective of whether these result from sensory input or are internally generated. Because sensory signals can be readily processed and influence motor responses without being consciously perceived, the cognitive operations leading to conscious experience are likely to differ from straightforward sensory-motor processing. Likewise, motor acts can be initiated in the absence of external stimuli and without conscious intention, suggesting different mechanisms for the initiation of consciously intended or unconsciously executed self-paced movements. A promising strategy for the analysis of the NCC could thus be the identification of the differences between neuronal processes associated with these respective conditions. Conscious processing could involve additional structures, for example particular cortical areas, or it could be associated with specific dynamical states of the involved networks. In any case, one expects a final common path for the access to consciousness because the contents of

conscious experience can be derived from many different external and internal sources and then be combined into a unitary experience. In other words, the neuronal activation patterns representing the contents of conscious experience should have certain signatures in common, irrespective of whether they are due to sensory input or self-generated activity.

Two non-exclusive possibilities may be considered. Conscious and non-conscious processes could involve the same anatomical substrate but differ with respect to certain state variables such as temporal coherence or synchrony or they could require recruitment of additional structures, conscious processing necessitating the engagement of particular cortical areas or a minimum number of cooperating cortical areas. Evidence from comparative behavioural studies suggests that the ability for conscious processing increases with the graded expansion of the cerebral cortex during evolution and with the graded maturation of cortical areas during ontogeny. The evolutionary changes of the mammalian brain consist essentially of an apposition of new cortical areas. These phylogenetically more recent areas are remote from primary sensory input and communicate mainly with one another and areas of lower order [1]. During ontogenetic development the increasing differentiation of conscious processing from rudimentary awareness of sensations to the fully expressed self-consciousness of the adult goes in parallel with the gradual maturation of the phylogenetically more recent cortical areas. Taken together, this evidence suggests that the cognitive functions supporting conscious processing involve higher order cortical areas that have been added in the course of evolution. Because phylogenetically ancient and recent areas have a very similar internal organization, it is likely that they perform similar computations. Because the more recent areas receive their input no longer from the sense organs but mainly from the older, lower order cortical areas, it can be assumed that they treat the results of lower order processes in the same way as these treat input from the sensory periphery. Part of the inner eye function of consciousness could thus rely on an iteration of self-similar cortical processes.

The ability of brains to become aware of their own operations and states could, thus, be due to an iteration of the same cognitive operations that support primary sensory processing. If so, the explanatory gap in the study of NCC would be reducible to the question of how the cerebral cortex processes signals and generates representations. If this question is resolved for primary sensory functions, the discovered strategies should be generalizeable to the formation of the coherent and unified meta-representations that are believed to be the basis of conscious experience.

TWO REPRESENTATIONAL STRATEGIES

If the argument is valid that the internal monitoring functions that lead to consciousness rely on similar cognitive operations as those applied to signals conveyed by the sense organs, the search for the neuronal substrate of phenomenal awareness converges with the search for the nature of the neuronal codes used by the cerebral cortex to extract, represent and store information about perceptual objects.

Evidence from single-unit analysis, non-invasive imaging studies and clinical observations suggests that evolved brains use two complementary strategies in order to represent contents (see also [2, 3]). The first strategy is thought to rely on individual neurons that are tuned to particular constellations of input activity. Through their selective responses, these neurons establish explicit representations of particular constellations of features. It is commonly held that the specificity of these neurons is brought about by selective convergence of input connections in hierarchically structured feed-forward architectures. This representational strategy allows for rapid processing and is ideally suited for the representation of frequently occurring stereotyped combinations of features; but this strategy is expensive in terms of the number of required neurons and not suited to cope with the virtually infinite diversity of possible feature constellations encountered in real world objects. The second strategy appears to consist of the temporary association of large numbers of widely distributed neurons into functionally coherent assemblies which as a whole represent a particular content whereby each of the participating neurons represents only some aspects of composite perceptual objects. This representational strategy is more economical with respect to neuron numbers because, as already proposed by Hebb [4], a particular neuron can, at different times, participate in different assemblies just as particular features can be part of many different perceptual objects. Moreover, this representational strategy is more flexible. It allows for the rapid *de novo* representation of constellations that have never been experienced before because there are virtually no limits to the dynamic association of neurons in ever changing constellations. In addition, assembly coding allows for the representation of nested relations between multiple objects, a function that is difficult to realize, if objects are represented by individual, semantically unrelated neurons. Thus, for the representation of contents consisting of multiple, interrelated components whose nature and constellation are permanently changing, the second strategy

of distributed coding appears to be better suited than the first.

The meta-representations postulated as substrate for conscious experience have to accommodate contents that are particularly unpredictable and rich in combinatorial complexity. In order to support the unity of consciousness, the computational results of a large number of subsystems have to be bound together in ever changing constellations and at the same rapid pace as the contents of awareness change. It appears then as if the second representational strategy that is based on the formation of dynamic assemblies would be more suitable for the implementation of the meta-representations that support consciousness than the explicit strategy. Further support for this view comes from considerations on the state dependency and the non-locality, that is the distributed nature of mechanisms supporting conscious experience. If conscious experience depends on the ability to dynamically bind the results of subsystem computations into a unified meta-representation, conditions required for the dynamic configuration of assemblies ought to be the same as those required for awareness to occur. Neuronal codes that are readily observable in deep anaesthesia, or during slow wave sleep, or in the absence of attention should not be accepted as sufficient correlates of awareness or consciousness although they are likely to be necessary components of the more global states required for the manifestation of consciousness. In this sense the local codes, many of which can be deciphered even in light anaesthesia, would be a subset but not the full set of correlates of consciousness. At low processing levels, the response properties of individual neurons tend to differ only little in awake and anaesthetized brains. Therefore, it is unlikely that the explicit representations encoded by these neurons are the substrate of the meta-representations that support consciousness. However, the activation patterns of neurons in higher cortical areas undergo substantial changes when the brain shifts between states that are compatible or incompatible with conscious processing. This suggests that the activity of these neurons depends on cooperative interactions that only come into play when the brain is awake and attentive. As discussed later, such cooperativity could be the result of the coordinating mechanisms that are required for the dynamic binding of distributed neuronal responses into coherent representations.

One candidate mechanism for dynamic binding is the precise synchronization of neuronal responses that occurs when neuronal populations engage in well synchronized oscillatory activity in the beta- and gamma-frequency range (for review see [3, 5]).

These synchronized oscillations are strongly reduced or missing when the brain is in states that are incompatible with conscious processing, suggesting that the mechanisms involved in the organization of distributed representations play a role in conscious processing.

If the meta-representations postulated as substrate of conscious experience were indeed based on widely distributed assemblies rather than on responses of local groups of neurons then consciousness should be rather resistant to local lesions. While lesions in subsystems are expected to prevent conscious experience of the contents provided by the respective subsystem, consciousness *per se* should not be jeopardized. It should break down only if lesions interfere with the coordinating mechanisms that permit establishment of globally coherent cell assemblies. This prediction is by and large in agreement with the known consequences of circumscribed cortical lesions. They eliminate from conscious experience the specific contents processed by the lesioned areas but there is no distinct site of the neocortex whose destruction would lead to a loss of consciousness. It is only after lesions affecting the global coordination of cortical functions that consciousness is abolished.

These considerations suggest that the contents of conscious experience are represented by distributed codes. The following sections will, therefore, focus on the evidence for such coding strategies.

THE SIGNATURE OF DISTRIBUTED CODES

In distributed coding an important constraint needs to be met. A mechanism is required that permits dynamic association of selected neurons into distinct, functionally coherent assemblies and that labels grouped responses in a way that assures their joint processing. To achieve this goal neurons have to convey two messages in parallel. First, they have to signal whether the feature or the constellation of features which they encode is present, and it is commonly held that they do so by increasing their discharge rate. Second, they have to indicate with which other neurons they actually cooperate at any particular moment in time to form an assembly. Numerous theoretical studies have addressed the question how assemblies can self-organize through cooperative interactions among distributed but interconnected neurons [6–9]. Here, the focus will be on the question how responses of cells that have been grouped into an assembly can be tagged as related. Such tagging is equivalent with assuring that responses are processed together. One way to achieve

this is to jointly raise their saliency. In principle there are at least three non-exclusive options. First, non-grouped responses can be inhibited; second, the amplitude of the selected responses can be enhanced; and third, the selected cells can be made to discharge in precise temporal synchrony. All three mechanisms enhance the relative impact of the grouped responses. The first two strategies, which rely on the modulation of discharge rates, have been thoroughly investigated and appear to be common at all levels of processing. Evidence indicates that attentional mechanisms that select responses and bind them together for further joint processing act through such modulation of discharge rates [10, 11]. However, these selection mechanisms have certain disadvantages when used for the labelling of assemblies because they may introduce ambiguities [12] and reduce processing speed [13]. Ambiguities could arise because discharge rates of cells vary over a wide range as a function of stimulus energy and of the match between stimulus and receptive field properties. How these modulations can be distinguished from those signalling the relatedness of responses is unclear. Processing speed would be reduced because rate coded assemblies can only be identified after a sufficient number of spikes have been integrated to distinguish high from low rates. Therefore, rate coded assemblies need to be maintained for some time in order to be distinguishable, which reduces substantially the rate with which different assemblies can follow one another. Finally, conditions may arise where several different assemblies have to coexist during the interval of subjective presence. In this case, neurons belonging to different assemblies would exhibit equally enhanced discharge rates and it is hard to see how the necessary segregation could be achieved.

Both restrictions, the ambiguity and the slow processing speed, can be overcome if the selection and labelling of responses is achieved through synchronization of individual discharges and hence through a temporal rather than a rate code [12, 14, 15]. Expressing the relatedness of responses by rendering discharges coincident with a precision in the range of milliseconds resolves the ambiguities resulting from stimulus-dependent rate fluctuations because synchronization can be adjusted independently of rates. Synchronization also accelerates the rate at which different assemblies can follow one another because the selected event is the individual spike or a brief burst of spikes and saliency is enhanced only for those discharges that are precisely synchronized. The rate at which different assemblies can follow one another without getting confounded is then limited only by the duration of the interval over which cells act as coincidence detectors, that is the interval over which synchronized synaptic potentials summate substantially more effectively than temporally dispersed inputs (for a detailed discussion see [16, 17]).

EXPERIMENTAL EVIDENCE FOR GROUPING BY SYNCHRONY

Following the discovery of stimulus related response synchronization among neurons in the cat visual cortex [18, 19], numerous experiments have been performed in the search for a correlation between the occurrence of response synchronization and cognitive processes. One of the predictions to be tested was that synchronization probability should reflect some of the Gestalt criteria according to which the visual system groups related features during scene segmentation. Among the grouping criteria examined so far are continuity, vicinity, similarity and colinearity in the orientation domain, and common fate in the motion domain [14, 20–27]. So far, the results of these investigations are compatible with the hypothesis that the probability of response synchronization reflects the Gestalt criteria applied for perceptual grouping (see also [28]). Stimulus-specific response synchronization has been found within and across different areas, and even between hemispheres (for review see [3]). Most importantly, none of these synchronization phenomena were detectable by correlating successively recorded responses to the same stimuli. This indicates that synchronization was not due to stimulus locking of responses but to internal dynamic coordination of spike timing. The observed coincidences of discharges were much more frequent than expected from mere covariation of event related rate changes.

Studies involving lesions [29, 30] and developmental manipulations [31, 32] indicate that the interactions responsible for these dynamic synchronization phenomena are mediated to a substantial extent by cortico-cortical connections. The criteria for perceptual grouping should then be reflected in the architecture of these connections and this postulate agrees with the evidence that cortico-cortical connections preferentially link neurons with related feature preferences (for review see [33]).

RESPONSE SYNCHRONIZATION AND BEHAVIOURAL STATES

Evidence indicates that highly precise, internally generated synchrony is considerably more pronounced in the awake than in the anaesthetized brain (for review see [3]). Of particular interest in this context is the finding that response synchronization is especially pronounced when the global electroencephalography (EEG) desynchronizes and when subjects are attentive. Stimulating the mesencephalic reticular formation in anaesthetized animals leads to a transient desynchronization of the EEG, resembling the transition from slow wave sleep to rapid eye movement sleep. Munk et al. [34] and Herculano-Houzel et al. [35] have shown that stimulus-specific synchronization of neuronal responses is drastically facilitated when the EEG is in a desynchronized rather than in a synchronized state.

Direct evidence for an attention related facilitation of synchronization has been obtained from cats that had been trained to perform a visually triggered motor response [36]. Simultaneous recordings from visual, association, somatosensory and motor areas revealed that the cortical areas involved in the execution of the task synchronized their activity, predominantly with zero phase-lag, as soon as the animals prepared themselves for the task and focused their attention on the relevant stimulus. Immediately after the appearance of the visual stimulus, synchronization increased further over the recorded areas, and these coordinated activation patterns were maintained until the task was completed. However, once the reward was available and the animals engaged in consummatory behaviour, these coherent patterns collapsed and gave way to low frequency oscillatory activity that did not exhibit any consistent phase relations. This close correspondence between the execution of an attention demanding visuo-motor performance and the occurrence of zero phase-lag synchrony suggests a functional role of the temporal patterning in the large scale coordination of cortical activity. It appears as if attentional mechanisms imposed a coherent subthreshold modulation on neurons in cortical areas that need to participate in the execution of the anticipated task and thereby permit rapid synchronization of selected responses. According to this scenario, the attentional mechanisms would induce what one might call a state of expectancy in the respective cortical areas by imposing on them a specific, task related dynamic activation pattern. Once stimulus-driven input becomes available, this patterned activity would act like a dynamic filter that permits rapid synchronization of selected responses, thereby accomplishing the required grouping and binding of responses, facilitating rapid transmission of the synchronized activity and assuring selective routing of responses to the processing structures that need to be engaged to accomplish the task. For a more detailed discussion of the role of synchronized oscillatory activity for the attention-dependent selection of neuronal responses and the selective routing of activity across processing stages, the reader is referred to [17, 37–43].

PERCEPTION AND RESPONSE SYNCHRONIZATION

A close correlation between response synchronization and conscious perception has been found in experiments on binocular rivalry. When the two eyes are presented with patterns that cannot be fused into a single coherent percept, the two patterns are perceived in alternation rather than as a superposition of their components. This implies that there is a gating mechanism which selects in alternation the signals arriving from the two eyes for access to conscious processing. Interocular rivalry is thus a suitable paradigm for investigating the neuronal correlates of conscious perception.

Multiunit and field potential responses were recorded with chronically implanted electrodes from up to 30 sites in cat primary visual cortex while the animals were exposed to rivalrous stimulation conditions [39, 44]. In order to assure that the animals exhibited interocular rather than just figural rivalry they had been made strabismic shortly after birth as this is a condition that favours alternating use of the two eyes. Because the animal performs tracking eye movements only for the pattern that is actually perceived, patterns moving in opposite directions were presented dichoptically in order to determine from the tracking movements which signals were actually perceived by the animal. The outcome of these experiments was surprising as it turned out that the discharge rate of neurons in primary visual cortex failed to reflect the suppression of the non-selected signals. A close and highly significant correlation existed, however, between changes in the strength of response synchronization and the outcome of rivalry. Cells mediating responses of the eye that won in interocular competition and were perceived consciously increased the synchronicity of their responses upon introduction of the rivalrous stimulus while the reverse was true for cells driven by the eye that became suppressed. Thus, in this particular case of competition, selection of responses for further processing appears to be achieved by raising the saliency of responses through synchronization rather than enhancing discharge frequency. Likewise, suppression is not achieved by inhibiting responses but by desynchronization.

Thus, at least in primary visual areas, there is a remarkable dissociation between perception and the discharge rate of individual neurons. Cells whose responses are not perceived and are excluded from controlling behaviour respond as vigorously as cells whose responses are perceived and support behaviour. Another puzzling result of the rivalry study is that responses that win the competition increase their synchronicity upon presentation of the rivalrous stimulus. This suggests the action of a mechanism that enhances the saliency of the selected responses by improving their synchronicity in order to protect them against the interference caused by the rivalrous stimulus.

Further evidence that synchronization is used as a strategy complementary to rate increases in order to enhance the saliency of cortical responses has been obtained in a recent study on apparent brightness [45]. The apparent brightness (contrast) of a circular target grating is enhanced when it is embedded in a surrounding grating that differs either in orientation or in phase from the target grating. The greater the offset in orientation or in phase between the two gratings, the stronger the enhancement of perceived brightness of the target grating. Multisite recordings have revealed that the saliency of the responses to the target grating is enhanced by increased discharge rate in case of orientation offset and by increased synchrony in case of phase offset. Both changes correspond exactly with the psychophysical functions of perceived brightness and the resulting perceptual effects are indistinguishable.

In conclusion, there are numerous conditions in which evaluation of internally generated correlation patterns permits the extraction of information about stimulus configurations, global brain states, attention and neuronal correlates of perception that cannot be obtained by solely analysing the responses of individual neurons sequentially. The relevant variable containing this additional information is often the precise synchronization of a fraction of the discharges constituting the respective responses. The data indicate further that responses containing synchronized epochs are more salient, have a higher probability of being processed further and, eventually, of being perceived consciously.

THE GENERALITY OF SYNCHRONICITY

Studies in non-visual sensory modalities and in the motor system indicate that synchrony and oscillatory activity are ubiquitous phenomena in the nervous system. Synchronization occurs in a variety of distinct frequency bands and has been found in all sensory modalities. Synchronization in the high frequency range (beta- and gamma-oscillations) has been observed in the olfactory system, in virtually all of the cortical areas investigated so far, the hippocampus and the basal ganglia (for review see [46, 47]).

Synchronization also plays a role in the linkage between cortical assemblies and subcortical target structures such as the superior colliculus and the pool of motor neurons in the spinal cord. This is suggested by the existence of precise temporal relationships between the discharges of neurons in areas of the visual cortex and the superior colliculus [48]. In these experiments, it could be shown that corticotectal interactions are strongly dependent on the temporal coherence of cortical activity. If cortical neurons engage in synchronous oscillatory activity either with partners within the same cortical area or with cells in other cortical areas, their impact on tectal cells is enhanced, indicating that tectal cells are driven more effectively by synchronous than by asynchronous cortical activity. In magnetoencephalography (MEG) studies in human subjects engaged in a visuo-motor task [41] it was found that propagation of task relevant signals was greatly enhanced, as revealed by shortened reaction times, when sending and receiving structures got entrained through attentional mechanisms in synchronous oscillatory activity in the gamma-frequency range. These findings are consistent with the idea that the temporal organization of activity patterns plays an important role not only in the coordination of distributed cortical processes but also in the gating of cortical output activity (see also [43]).

SYNCHRONIZED GAMMA OSCILLATIONS AND CONSCIOUS PERCEPTION

In order to directly examine the relation between neuronal synchrony and conscious processing, we designed a paradigm that allowed us to identify the neuronal signatures that distinguish between conscious and unconscious processing of visual stimuli [49]. Subjects had to detect and identify words presented between masking stimuli and decide in a forced choice paradigm whether the sample words matched a later presented word or object. In half of the trials the masks were adjusted so that the subjects had no conscious recollection of having seen the sample word. Reaction time measurements revealed that

the 'invisible' words had been processed and semantically decoded. Analysis of simultaneously recorded EEG activity revealed a number of events associated only with conscious processing. Time–frequency plots of the power of oscillations across a wide frequency range revealed that consciously perceived stimuli induced theta oscillations in multiple cortical regions that were maintained until the test stimulus was presented and a decision reached. Moreover, there was an increase of the late component of the P300 evoked potential which has been interpreted as a correlate of the transfer of information into working memory. And finally, a burst of gamma activity occurred over central and frontal leads just prior and during the presentation of the test stimulus, whose time of appearance could be anticipated because the interval between sample and test stimuli was fixed. In agreement with other evidence [50–53] we interpreted this anticipatory gamma activity as correlate of a reactivation of contents stored in working memory. Of particular interest in the present context is the finding that the earliest event distinguishing conscious and unconscious processing was not visible in the *power* changes of oscillations but in their *phase locking*. About 180 ms after presentation of stimuli that were consciously perceived, there was an epoch, lasting around 100 ms, during which induced gamma oscillations recorded from a large number of regions exhibited precise *phase locking* both within and across hemispheres. Thus, not the power of the local stimulus induced gamma oscillations but their precise phase locking across a widely distributed cortical network was the earliest signature of conscious processing. Numerous studies revealed that encoding and processing of stimuli is associated with an increase of the power of both evoked (stimulus locked) and induced (not stimulus locked) gamma oscillations. In the present experiments stimuli had been processed also in the condition where they were not consciously perceived. Therefore, it is not too unexpected, that local gamma oscillations had the same power in the conscious and unconscious condition. What distinguished these two conditions was the global synchronization of local gamma oscillations. This suggests that conscious processing requires a particular dynamical state of cortical networks that is characterized by a brief episode of very precise phase locking of high frequency oscillatory activity. We propose that this particular state, because of its short latency and because of its global coherence, serves as trigger event for the access to conscious processing. This view is compatible with the hypothesis, that the global workspace for conscious processing is accessible only for activity patterns that fulfil certain threshold criteria [54–57]. Precise temporal coherence could be such a criterion (see also [58–61]). One attractive possibility is that this transient event of perfect synchrony resets the multiple parallel processes to a common time frame, allowing for a global integration and representation of information provided by sensory input and internal stores. The global theta rhythm that follows after this trigger event could provide the time frame for such integration. In the hippocampus [62], and more recently also in the neocortex, slow oscillations in the theta range have been found to be coupled to the coexisting beta- and gamma-oscillations. This suggests the hypothesis, that local coordination of computations within specific cortical areas is achieved by fast ticking clocks, such as beta- and gamma-oscillations while global and sustained integration of local results is achieved at a slower pace by low frequency oscillations. This would allow the brain to represent the results of the numerous parallel computations at different temporal and spatial scales, whereby the two dimensions would be intimately related. The more global the representation, the longer the time scale for the integration of distributed information. It is perhaps more than a mere coincidence that the duration of subjective presence corresponds approximately to the cycle time of theta rhythms.

AN ATTEMPT OF SYNTHESIS

It appears from the graded emergence both during evaluation and ontogeny of the different levels of consciousness, access consciousness, phenomenal awareness and self-consciousness, that consciousness depends on the availability of processing levels capable of creating meta-representations, that is on the iteration of the cognitive processes that have evolved to establish representations of sensory information. The required neuronal substrate for this iteration could be the higher order cortical areas that have been added in the course of evolution and that process the output of lower order areas in the same way as these process their respective sensory input. By necessity, the higher order areas need to integrate computational results of very different origin and in ever changing constellations. This requires a lingua franca for the communication between cortical areas and a high degree of flexibility for the recombination of computational results obtained in the various cortical subsystems. The first prerequisite appears to be fulfilled by the homogeneity of cortical processing modules. Phylogenetically old and new areas have very similar functional architectures, suggesting that they operate

according to similar principles and process and encode information in similar ways. The second prerequisite, the combinatorial flexibility of the meta-representations would be fulfilled if these consisted of the coordinated responses of neuronal assemblies rather than of the responses of individual specialized cells. As suggested by numerous studies based on invasive and non-invasive measurements of neuronal responses both in animals and human subjects, this coordination of assemblies appears to be accomplished by the transient synchronization of discharges with a precision in the millisecond range which is in turn supported by the synchronization of oscillations in the high frequency range. It follows from these premises that the formation of meta-representations encoding the coherent contents of conscious experience should be associated with the precise synchronization of oscillatory responses in widely distributed cortical networks – and this is what recent experiments appear to confirm.

For a content to be included in the meta-representations underlying conscious experience neurons coding for this content need of course be active. However, as the reviewed data suggest, these responses are only a necessary but not a sufficient condition for conscious experience. Hence, correlations between perceptual awareness and cellular responses can indicate at best that the discharges of cells at a particular processing stage are necessary for a particular content to reach the level of awareness. Consciousness, rather than being associated with the activation of a particular group of neurons in a particular region of the brain, appears to be an emergent property of a specific dynamical state of the cortical network – a state that is characterized by a critical level of precise temporal coherence among responses of a sufficiently large population of distributed neurons.

References

1. Krubitzer, L. (1998) Constructing the neocortex: Influence on the pattern of organization in mammals. In Gazzaniga, M.S. and Altman, J.S. (eds.), *Brain and Mind: Evolutionary Perspectives*, pp. 19–34. Strasbourg: HFSP.
2. Singer, W. (1995) Development and plasticity of cortical processing architectures. *Science* 270:758–764.
3. Singer, W. (1999) Neuronal synchrony: A versatile code for the definition of relations? *Neuron* 24:49–65, 111–125.
4. Hebb, D.O. (1949) *The Organization of Behavior*, New York: John Wiley & Sons.
5. Engel, A.K. and Singer, W. (2001) Temporal binding and the neural correlates of sensory awareness. *Trends Cogn Sci* 5 (1):16–25.
6. Braitenberg, V. (1978) Cell assemblies in the cerebral cortex. In Heim, R. and Palm, G. (eds.) *Architectonics of the Cerebral Cortex. Lecture Notes in Biomathematics 21, Theoretical Approaches in Complex Systems*, pp. 171–188. Springer-Verlag.

7. Edelman, G.M. (1987) *Neural Darwinism: The Theory of Neuronal Group Selection*, New York: Basic Books.

8. Palm, G. (1990) Cell assemblies as a guideline for brain research. *Concepts Neurosci* 1:133–147.

9. Gerstein, G.L. and Gochin, P.M. (1992) Neuronal population coding and the elephant. In Aersten, A. and Braitenberg, V. (eds.) *Information Processing in the Cortex, Experiments and Theory*, pp. 139–173. Springer-Verlag.

10. Cook, E.P. and Maunsell, J.H.R. (2004) Attentional modulation of motion integration of individual neurons in the middle temporal visual area. *J Neurosci* 24 (36):7964–7977.

11. Reynolds, J.H. and Desimone, R. (1999) The role of neural mechanisms of attention in solving the binding problem. *Neuron* 24:19–29.

12. Von der Malsburg, C. (1985) Nervous structures with dynamical links. *Ber Bunsenges Phys Chem* 89:703–710.

13. Singer, W., Engel, A.K., Kreiter, A.K., Munk, M.H.J., Neuenschwander, S. and Roelfsema, P.R. (1997) Neuronal assemblies: Necessity, signature and detectability. *Trends Cog Sci* 1 (7):252–261.

14. Gray, C.M., König, P., Engel, A.K. and Singer, W. (1989) Oscillatory responses in cat visual cortex exhibit inter-columnar synchronization which reflects global stimulus properties. *Nature* 338:334–337.

15. Singer, W. and Gray, C.M. (1995) Visual feature integration and the temporal correlation hypothesis. *Annu Rev Neurosci* 18:555–586.

16. Singer, W. (2000) Response synchronization: A universal coding strategy for the definition of relations. In Gazzaniga, M.S. (ed.) *The New Cognitive Neurosciences*, 2nd Edition Cambridge, MA: pp. 325–338. MIT Press.

17. Fries, P., Nikolic, D. and Singer, W. (2007) The gamma cycle. *Trends Neurosci* 30 (7):309–316.

18. Gray, C.M. and Singer, W. (1987) Stimulus-specific neuronal oscillations in the cat visual cortex: A cortical functional unit. *Soc Neurosci Abstr* 13:1449.

19. Gray, C.M. and Singer, W. (1989) Stimulus-specific neuronal oscillations in orientation columns of cat visual cortex. *Proc Natl Acad Sci USA* 86:1698–1702.

20. Engel, A.K., König, P. and Singer, W. (1991a) Direct physiological evidence for scene segmentation by temporal coding. *Proc Natl Acad Sci USA* 88:9136–9140.

21. Engel, A.K., Kreiter, A.K., König, P. and Singer, W. (1991c) Synchronization of oscillatory neuronal responses between striate and extrastriate visual cortical areas of the cat. *Proc Natl Acad Sci USA* 88:6048–6052.

22. Freiwald, W.A., Kreiter, A.K. and Singer, W. (1995) Stimulus dependent intercolumnar synchronization of single unit responses in cat area 17. *Neuroreport* 6:2348–2352.

23. Castelo-Branco, M., Goebel, R., Neuenschwander, S. and Singer, W. (2000) Neural synchrony correlates with surface segregation rules. *Nature* 405:685–689.

24. Kreiter, A.K. and Singer, W. (1996) Stimulus-dependent synchronization of neuronal responses in the visual cortex of awake macaque monkey. *J Neurosci* 16:2381–2396.

25. Samonds, J.M., Allison, J.D., Brown, H.A. and Bonds, A.B. (2003) Cooperation between area 17 neuron pairs enhances fine discrimination of orientation. *J Neurosci* 23 (6):2416–2425.

26. Samonds, J.M., Allison, J.D., Brown, H.A. and Bonds, A.B. (2004) Cooperative synchronized assemblies enhance orientation discrimination. *Proc Natl Acad Sci USA* 101 (17):6722–6727.

27. Samonds, J.M., Zhou, Z., Bernard, M.R. and Bonds, A.B. (2006) Synchronous activity in cat visual cortex encodes collinear and cocircular contours. *J Neurophysiol* 95:2602–2616.

28. Tallon-Baudry, C. and Bertrand, O. (1999) Oscillatory gamma activity in humans and its role in object representation. *Trends Cogn Sci* 3 (4):151–162.

29. Engel, A.K., König, P., Kreiter, A.K. and Singer, W. (1991b) Interhemispheric synchronization of oscillatory neuronal responses in cat visual cortex. *Science* 252:1177–1179.

30. Nowak, L.G., Munk, M.H.J., Nelson, J.I. and Bullier, J.A.C. (1995) Structural basis of cortical synchronization. I. Three types of interhemispheric coupling. *J Neurophysiol* 74:2379–2400.

31. Löwel, S. and Singer, W. (1992) Selection of intrinsic horizontal connections in the visual cortex by correlated neuronal activity. *Science* 255:209–212.

32. König, P., Engel, A.K., Löwel, S. and Singer, W. (1993) Squint affects synchronization of oscillatory responses in cat visual cortex. *Eur J Neurosci* 5:501–508.

33. Schmidt, K.E., Goebel, R., Löwel, S. and Singer, W. (1997) The perceptual grouping criterion of colinearity is reflected by anisotropies of connections in the primary visual cortex. *Eur J Neurosci* 9:1083–1089.

34. Munk, M.H.J., Roelfsema, P.R., König, P., Engel, A.K. and Singer, W. (1996) Role of reticular activation in the modulation of intracortical synchronization. *Science* 272:271–274.

35. Herculano-Houzel, S., Munk, M.H.J., Neuenschwander, S. and Singer, W. (1999) Precisely synchronized oscillatory firing patterns require electroencephalographic activation. *J Neurosci* 19 (10):3992–4010.

36. Roelfsema, P.R., Engel, A.K., König, P. and Singer, W. (1997) Visuomotor integration is associated with zero time-lag synchronization among cortical areas. *Nature* 385:157–161.

37. Bauer, M., Oostenveld, R., Peeters, M. and Fries, P. (2006) Tactile spatial attention enhances gamma-band activity in somatosensory cortex and reduces low-frequency activity in parieto-occipital areas. *J Neurosci* 26 (2):490–501.

38. Engel, A.K., Fries, P. and Singer, W. (2001) Dynamic predictions: Oscillations and synchrony in top-down processing. *Nat Rev Neurosci* 2:704–716.

39. Fries, P., Neuenschwander, S., Engel, A.K., Goebel, R. and Singer, W. (2001a) Rapid feature selective neuronal synchronization through correlated latency shifting. *Nat Neurosci* 4 (2):194–200.

40. Fries, P., Reynolds, J.H., Rorie, A.E. and Desimone, R. (2001b) Modulation of oscillatory neuronal synchronization by selective visual attention. *Science* 291:1560–1563.

41. Schoffelen, J.-M., Oostenveld, R. and Fries, P. (2005) Neuronal coherence as a mechanism of effective corticospinal interaction. *Science* 308:111–113.

42. Womelsdorf, T., Fries, P., Mitra, P.P. and Desimone, R. (2006) Gamma-band synchronization in visual cortex predicts speed of change detection. *Nature* 439:733–736.

43. Womelsdorf, T., Schoffelen, J.-M., Oostenveld, R., Singer, W., Desimone, R., Engel, A.K. and Fries, P. (2007) Modulation of neuronal interactions through neuronal synchronization. *Science* 316:1609–1612.

44. Fries, P., Roelfsema, P.R., Engel, A.K., König, P. and Singer, W. (1997) Synchronization of oscillatory responses in visual cortex correlates with perception in interocular rivalry. *Proc Natl Acad Sci USA* 94:12699–12704.

45. Biederlack, J., Castelo-Branco, M., Neuenschwander, S., Wheeler, D.W., Singer, W. and Nikolic, D. (2006) Brightness induction: Rate enhancement and neuronal synchronization as complementary codes. *Neuron* 52:1073–1083.

46. Singer, W. (2004) Synchrony, oscillations, and relational codes. In Chalupa, L.M. and Werner, J.S. (eds.) *The Visual Neurosciences*, Cambridge, MA: pp. 1665–1681. The MIT Press, A Bradford Book.

47. Jermakowicz, W.J. and Casagrande, V.A. (2007). Neural networks a century after Cajal. *Brain Res Rev* (Special Issue) Golgi & Cajal (in press).

48. Brecht, M., Singer, W. and Engel, A.K. (1998) Correlation analysis of corticotectal interactions in the cat visual system. *J Neurophysiol* 79:2394–2407.

49. Melloni, L., Molina, C., Pena, M., Torres, D., Singer, W. and Rodriguez, E. (2007) Synchronization of neural activity across cortical areas correlates with conscious perception. *J Neurosci* 27 (11):2858–2865.

50. Tallon-Baudry, C., Bertrand, O., Peronnet, F. and Pernier, J. (1998) Induced g-band activity during the delay of a visual short-term memory task in humans. *J Neurosci* 18 (11):4244–4254.

51. Tallon-Baudry, C., Kreiter, A.K. and Bertrand, O. (1999) Sustained and transient oscillatory responses in the gamma and beta bands in a visual short-term memory task in humans. *Vis Neurosci* 16:449–459.

52. Tallon-Baudry, C., Bertrand, O. and Fischer, C. (2001) Oscillatory synchrony between human extrastriate areas during visual short-term memory maintenance. *J Neurosci* 21:RC177. 1–5

53. Tallon-Baudry, C., Mandon, S., Freiwald, W.A. and Kreiter, A.K. (2004) Oscillatory synchrony in the monkey temporal lobe correlates with performance in a visual short-term memory task. *Cerebr Cortex* 14 (7):713–720.

54. Baars, B.J. (1997) In the theatre of consciousness. Global workspace theory, a rigorous scientific theory of consciousness. *J Conscious Stud* 4 (4):292–309.

55. Dehaene, S., Kerszberg, M. and Changeux, J.P. (1998) A neuronal model of a global workspace in effortful cognitive tasks. *Proc Natl Acad Sci USA* 95:14529–14534.

56. Sergent, C., Baillet, S. and Dehaene, S. (2005) Timing of the brain events underlying access to consciousness during the attentional blink. *Nat Neurosci* 8 (10):1391–1400.

57. Dehaene, S., Changeux, J.-P., Naccache, L., Sackur, J. and Sergent, C. (2006) Conscious, preconscious, and subliminal processing: A testable taxonomy. *Trends Cogn Sci* 10 (5):204–211.

58. Engel, A.K., Fries, P., König, P., Brecht, M. and Singer, W. (1999a) Temporal binding, binocular rivalry, and consciousness. *Conscious Cognit* 8:128–151.

59. Engel, A.K., Fries, P., König, P., Brecht, M. and Singer, W. (1999b) Does time help to understand consciousness? *Conscious Cognit* 8:260–268.

60. Tononi, G., Srinivasan, R., Russell, D.P. and Edelman, G.M. (1998) Investigating neural correlates of conscious perception by frequency-tagged neuromagnetic responses. *Proc Natl Acad Sci USA* 95:3198–3203.

61. Varela, F., Lachaux, J.-P., Rodriguez, E. and Martinerie, J. (2001) The brainweb: Phase synchronization and large-scale integration. *Nat Rev Neurosci* 2:229–239.

62. Csicsvari, J., Jamieson, B., Wise, K.D. and Buzsáki, G. (2003) Mechanisms of gamma oscillations in the hippocampus of the behaving rat. *Neuron* 37:311–322.

Neural Correlates of Visual Consciousness

Geraint Rees

ABSTRACT

Vision is our primary sense, and seeing is accompanied by visual awareness or subjective experience of the visual world around us. Changes in the visual world often lead to changes in the content of visual awareness, and this is accompanied by changes in neural activity. However, not all neural activity associated with vision is correlated with changes in the contents of visual awareness. Indeed, much of the neural activity underpinning our ability to see remains unconscious and inaccessible to introspection. For example, the detailed computations underlying our ability to see three-dimensional depth are not apparent in awareness; just the end result of those computations. Thus, determining the neural correlates of the contents of visual awareness requires an empirical distinction to be made between neural activity that is correlated with the contents of visual awareness and that correlated only with unconscious processes. This chapter focuses on how recent studies of the visual system in humans have contributed to our emerging knowledge and understanding of the neural correlates of the contents of visual awareness.

BRAIN ACTIVITY ASSOCIATED WITH VISUAL STIMULI THAT DO NOT REACH AWARENESS

Visual stimuli that remain invisible to the observer can nevertheless influence both behaviour and brain activity (though see [1] for a sceptical critique). For example, words presented briefly and immediately preceding a mask cannot be seen but nevertheless subsequent responses of the observer can be primed by these masked and invisible words in a fashion related to their meaning [2]. This shows that the words have been processed unconsciously to the point of semantic identification. Evidence for substantial processing of visual stimuli that do not enter awareness is not restricted to words. For example, orientation-selective aftereffects can result from exposure to grating stimuli that are too fine to be consciously perceived [3], suggesting orientation selective but unconscious activation of visual cortex. During binocular rivalry incompatible monocular images compete for perceptual dominance. Despite complete perceptual dominance of one monocular image, sensitivity to input from the suppressed eye is only moderately (but not fully) reduced [4, 5]. Indeed, selective adaptation by suppressed images can be of equal magnitude as for dominant images [6], suggesting that information about visual stimulation may reach at least early visual areas largely unattenuated.

Such behavioural findings are consistent with measurements of brain activity associated with the presentation of visual stimuli that do not reach awareness (Figure 5.1). Activation related to features of masked and invisible stimuli (including words) can be identified in early retinotopic visual cortex [7, 8], motion-selective areas [9], word-selective areas [10] and object-selective areas of both ventral [11] and dorsal [12] visual pathways. Such observations of brain activity associated with invisible stimuli are not restricted to masking paradigms, as unconscious activation of the ventral visual pathway during the attentional blink can reflect both object identity [13] and semantic processing of visual stimuli [14, 15]. Changes in an object that are not perceived due to introduction of visual flicker between changes nevertheless lead to category-specific activity in the ventral visual pathway [16] and this activity can precede conscious change detection [17]. Moreover, brain

activation associated with unconscious perception is not confined to the cortex. Subcortical structures associated with emotional processing such as the amygdala can be activated by fearful face stimuli that are rendered invisible through masking [18], in response to the emotional content of invisible words [19] or during suppression in binocular rivalry [20].

Visual cortex can also be activated by stimuli that do not reach awareness in patients with damage to parietal cortex causing visual extinction. Patients with visual extinction show deficient awareness for contralesional visual stimuli, particularly when a competing stimulus is also present ipsilesionally. When visual stimuli are presented to patients with visual extinction, areas of both primary and extrastriate visual cortex that are activated by a seen left visual field stimulus are also activated by an unseen and extinguished left visual field stimulus [21–23]. The unconscious processing of an extinguished face stimulus extends to face-selective cortex in the fusiform gyrus [23]; and the amygdala and orbitofrontal cortex can also be activated by unseen emotional stimuli [24].

Taken together, behavioural and brain imaging techniques therefore show that visual stimuli presented outside awareness can still be subject to considerable processing in many (if not all) areas of visual cortex plus associated subcortical structures. This renders a simple division of different areas of visual cortex into those supporting conscious or unconscious processing impossible. The empirical challenge is therefore to specify what aspects of processing are special about stimuli that enter visual awareness compared to those that remain invisible. This requires the

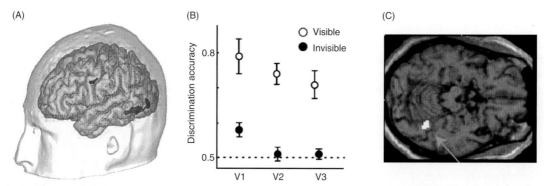

FIGURE 5.1   Activation of sensory cortices by stimuli that remain unconscious. (A) Masked and invisible words nevertheless evoke activation (shown in orange, superimposed on an anatomical image of the brain) of the fusiform gyrus. See Dehaene et al. [10] for further details. (B) Activity measured using BOLD contrast functional MRI in human V1–V3 can be used to discriminate the orientation (right or left-tilted) of a grating stimulus. Open symbols representing mean decoding accuracy for a group of subjects (error bars one SE) for visible stimuli; closed symbols for similarly oriented stimuli rendered invisible by masking. Note that the orientation of invisible stimuli can still be discriminated at a rate significantly better than chance in human V1. See Haynes and Rees (2005a) for further details. (C) Activity in the fusiform face area evoked by a face (vs. a house) stimulus presented in the neglected left hemifield of a patient with parietal neglect and left visual extinction. See Rees et al. [23] for further details.

5.1a Reprinted by permission from Macmillan Publishers Ltd, Nature Neuroscience, Dehaene, S., Nacache, L., Cohen, L., Bihan, D.L., Mangin, J.F., Poline, J.B. and Riviere, D. 'Cerebral mechanisms of word masking and unconscious repetition priming', 4:752–758, © 2001.

use of experimental paradigms where changes in the contents of visual awareness occur without corresponding changes in visual stimulation or behaviour [25]. Any consequent changes in brain activity are thus correlated directly with changes in the contents of visual awareness and not confounded by changes in unconscious processing associated with visual stimulation or behaviour. Such paradigms can be classified according to the nature of the changes in awareness that result [25].

UNPROMPTED (INVOLUNTARY) CHANGES IN THE CONTENTS OF VISUAL AWARENESS

Paradigms used to study the neural correlates of changes in the contents of visual awareness can be broadly divided into those that make use of situations where the contents of visual awareness change spontaneously in the absence of any changes in the sensory input; and deliberate changes in the contents of consciousness, associated with either a change in the context in which a stimulus is presented or associated with a deliberate act of will on the part of the observer. Examples of spontaneous changes in the contents of visual awareness include hallucinations, differences in visual perception when stimuli are presented near sensory thresholds or ambiguous figures where the same visual input can be interpreted in several different ways.

Near-Threshold Visual Stimulation

Varying the elementary features of a visual stimulus such as its contrast, luminance or duration of presentation can be used to define a perceptual threshold at which the stimulus becomes impossible to detect or discriminate. Presenting stimuli to observers just above such a threshold can be used to compare brain responses to physically identical stimuli that either enter awareness or remain unconscious. In primary visual cortex, when a simple low contrast grating is detected then the grating evokes significantly more activity than when it does not reach consciousness [26]. For more complex visual stimuli, activity in the ventral visual pathway evoked by objects correlates strongly with recognition performance, and successful detection of a face stimulus presented during the attentional blink evokes activity in the 'fusiform face area' (FFA), plus prefrontal cortex [27].

Conscious recognition of visually presented words is associated with both enhancement of activity in ventral visual cortex [10] and parietal cortical activation [28]. Successful identification evokes an event-related negativity [29, 30] and is associated with occipital magnetoencephalography (MEG) responses [31], spontaneous electrical oscillations at a frequency near 40 Hz [32] and modulation of the parieto-occipital alpha rhythm [33]. This electrophysiological evidence is consistent with interactions between visual and parietal cortex mediating successful identification. However brain activity associated with successful detection occurs very soon after the stimulus is presented, prior to the emergence of differences in activity over areas of parietal and prefrontal cortex.

The ability of observers to detect changes in a picture can also be rendered particularly difficult to detect by introducing a flicker between changes. Such physical changes to a picture that do not result in changes in visual awareness nevertheless evoke some activity in the ventral visual pathway [16, 34], and that activity can precede conscious change detection [17]. When the change is consciously perceived, there is further enhancement of activity in ventral visual cortical areas that represent the type of change, plus activation of parietal and prefrontal cortices [16, 35] and may reflect the deployment of attention [36].

Ambiguous Visual Stimuli

Binocular rivalry is a popular and enduring paradigm to study the neural correlates of consciousness [37]. When dissimilar images are presented to the two eyes, they compete for perceptual dominance so that each image is visible in turn for a few seconds while the other is suppressed. Such binocular rivalry is associated with suppression of monocular representations that can also be modulated by high-level influences such as perceptual grouping. Because perceptual transitions between each monocular view occur spontaneously without any change in the physical stimulus, neural correlates of the contents of awareness for each monocular percept may be distinguished from neural correlates attributable to stimulus characteristics (Figure 5.2).

Signals recorded using functional magnetic resonance imaging (fMRI) from the human lateral geniculate nucleus (LGN) exhibit such fluctuations during rivalry [38, 39]. Regions of the LGN that show strong eye preference also demonstrate strongly reduced activity during binocular rivalry when the stimulus presented in their preferred eye is perceptually suppressed. Primary visual cortex shows a similar pattern of changes in activity correlated with changes in the contents of consciousness [40–43]. In general (though

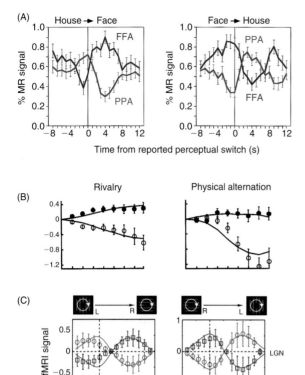

FIGURE 5.2   Fluctuations in activity in visual pathways associated with conscious perception during binocular rivalry. (A) Fusiform face area. Activity measured using functional magnetic resonance imaging (fMRI) from human FFA and parahippocampal place area (PPA) is plotted as a function of time relative to a perceptual switch from house to face (left panel) or face to house (right panel). It is apparent that activity in the FFA is higher when a face is perceived during binocular rivalry than when it is suppressed; and activity in the PPA is similarly higher when a house is perceived than when it is suppressed. For further details see Tong *et al.* [44]. (B) Binocular rivalry in primary visual cortex (V1). Activity measured using fMRI from human primary visual cortex is plotted as a function of time after a perceptual switch where the subsequent perception is of a high contrast stimulus (solid symbols) or low contrast stimulus (open symbols). The left hand panel plots activity following a perceptual switch due to binocular rivalry, while the right hand panel plots activity following a deliberate physical switch of monocular (non-rivalrous) stimuli. V1 activity therefore corresponds to perception during binocular rivalry and the amplitude changes are similar to those seen during physical alternation of corresponding monocular stimuli. For further details see Polonsky *et al.* [40]. (C) Rivalry in the lateral geniculate nucleus (LGN). Activity measured using fMRI is plotted as a function of time for voxels in the LGN selective for left eye stimuli (red symbols) or right eye stimuli (blue symbols) around the time (vertical dotted line) of a perceptual switch between left and right eye views (left panel) or right and left eye views (right panel). Reciprocal changes in signal in the different eye-selective voxels as a function of perceptual state can be readily seen. For further details see Haynes *et al.* [38].

5.2a Reprinted from *Neuron*, 21, Tong, F.., Nakayama, K., Vaughan, J.T. and Kanwisher, N., 'Binocular rivarly and visual awareness in human extrastriate cortex', pp 753–759, © 1998, with permission from Elsevier.
5.2b Reprinted by permission from Macmillan Publishers Ltd, *Nature Neuroscience*, Polonsky, A., Blake, R., Braun, J. and Heeger, D.J. 'Neuronal activity in human primary visual cortex correlates with perception during binocular rivalry', pp. 1153–1159, © 2000.

see [41]) such fluctuations in activity are about half as large as those evoked by non-rivalrous stimulus alternation. This indicates that the suppressed image during rivalry undergoes a considerable degree of unconscious processing. Further along the ventral stream, responses in the FFA during rivalry are equal in magnitude to responses evoked by non-rivalrous stimuli [44]. This suggests that neural competition during rivalry may have been resolved by these later stages of visual processing.

Other forms of bistable perception do not necessarily involve binocular competition. Nevertheless, a consistent finding is that these paradigms also result in activation of visual cortical structures that correspond to the attributes of whichever competing visual percept the observer currently reports [45–47].

In addition to showing that activity in ventral visual cortex is correlated with the contents of consciousness, studies of ambiguous figures have also provided evidence to suggest the involvement of areas of frontal and parietal cortex in visual awareness. These studies focused on activity that was time locked to the transitions between different perceptual states. Cortical regions whose activity reflects perceptual transitions include ventral extrastriate cortex, and also parietal and frontal regions previously implicated in the control of attention [48]. However, whereas extrastriate areas are also engaged by non-rivalrous perceptual changes, activity in frontal and parietal cortex is specifically associated with the perceptual alternations during rivalry. Similar parietal and frontal regions are active during perceptual transitions occurring while viewing a range of bistable figures (such as the Necker cube and Rubins face/vase) [45] and during stereo pop-out, as compared to those regions active during stable viewing [49]. Although frontal and parietal areas play a prominent role in the organization of behaviour, their involvement in rivalry is independent of motor report [50]. Activity is coordinated between ventral visual areas, parietal areas and prefrontal areas in a way that is not linked to external motor or sensory events but instead varies in strength with the frequency of perceptual events. This suggests that functional interactions between visual and frontoparietal cortex may make an important contribution to visual awareness.

The information encoded in early visual cortex during binocular rivalry is sufficient to reconstruct the dynamic stream of consciousness. Information that is contained in the multivariate pattern of responses to stimulus features in V1–V3 and recorded using fMRI can be used to accurately predict, and therefore track, changes in conscious contents during rivalry [51]. Accurate decoding is possible for extended periods of time during rivalry while awareness undergoes many spontaneous changes. Furthermore, accurate prediction during binocular rivalry can be established using signals recorded during stable monocular viewing, showing that prediction generalizes across different viewing conditions and does not require or rely on motor responses. It is therefore possible to predict the dynamically changing time course of subjective experience using brain activity alone. This raises the possibility that more complex dynamic changes in consciousness could be decoded from brain activity (see also Chapter 17 on brain–computer interfaces), though this in turn raises important questions about whether such an approach will be able to generalize to novel mental states [52].

Hallucinations

A hallucination is a sensory perception experienced in the absence of an external stimulus (as distinct from an illusion, which is a misperception of an external stimulus induced by context; see below). Hallucinations therefore dissociate neural processing associated with visual awareness from sensory stimulation, and are typically (though not exclusively) associated with damage to the visual system or psychiatric disorders. Patients with damage to the early visual system who experience hallucinations of colour, faces, textures and objects exhibit activity in functionally specialized areas of visual cortex corresponding to the contents of their hallucinations [53]. Similarly, patients with schizophrenia who experience visual and auditory hallucinations show activity in modality-specific cortex during hallucinatory episodes [54, 55]. Thus, changes in the content of visual awareness are correlated with content-specific modulation of visual cortex activity.

Summary

Common to these experimental paradigms are spontaneous changes in visual experience that are not accompanied by corresponding changes in visual input. Accordingly, neural activity correlated with the contents of consciousness can be dissociated from that associated with unconscious sensory processing. Both primary visual cortex and higher areas of the visual system show changes in activity strongly correlated with changes in the contents of visual awareness. In addition, changes in the contents of visual awareness associated with bistable perception are associated with time-locked activation of dorsolateral prefrontal and parietal cortex, implicating a network of cortical structures in visual awareness.

DELIBERATE CHANGES TO THE CONTENTS OF VISUAL AWARENESS

The second major group of experimental paradigms used to investigate visual awareness employ situations where deliberate changes are made either to the type of visual stimulation (e.g., the temporal or spatial context in which a stimulus is presented, giving rise to visual illusions) or where visual stimulation is constant but top-down signals associated with attention or imagery are varied.

Illusions

In contrast to hallucinations, illusions are misperceptions of external stimuli that are represented in awareness in an incorrect fashion. The content of the illusory perception typically depends on the context in which it occurs. For example, when a moving grating is divided by a large gap, observers report seeing a moving 'phantom' in the gap and there is enhanced activity in the locations in early retinotopic visual cortex that correspond to the visual field location where the illusion is perceived [56]. Moreover, when phantom-inducing gratings are paired with competing stimuli that induce binocular rivalry, spontaneous fluctuations in conscious perception of the phantom occur together with changes in early visual activity. Similarly, V1 activation can be found on the path of apparent motion [57] and is associated with strengthened feedback connections to that retinotopic location from cortical area V5/MT [58].

When a featureless achromatic target is placed on a textured pattern and steadily viewed in peripheral vision, after a few seconds it seems to fill-in with the surrounding texture, similar to the perceptual experience of patients with scotomas from damage to the visual pathways. Signals associated with such a target are reduced (but not entirely abolished) in contralateral visual cortex when it becomes invisible [59, 60], consistent with involvement of primary visual cortex in generating such an 'artificial scotoma' and with earlier findings that long-range colour filling-in is also associated with activity in primary visual cortex [61].

Primary visual cortex is also implicated in a number of other illusions (Figure 5.3). For example, when two objects subtending identical angles in the visual field are made to appear of different sizes by changing the particular three-dimensional context, the spatial extent of activation in V1 reflects the perceived rather than actual angular size of the objects [62]. These data thus show a rather close correspondence between either the level and spatial extent of V1 activation and the

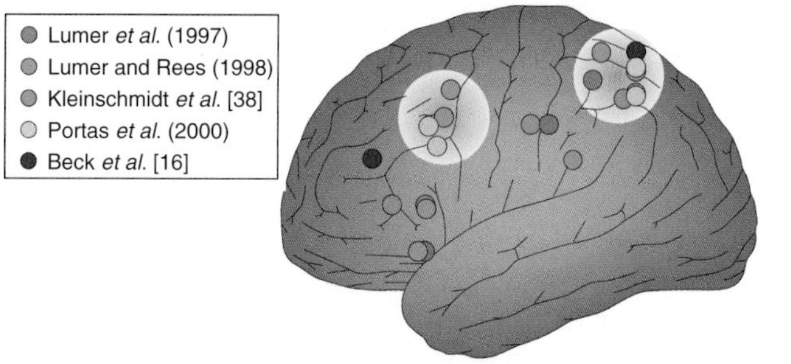

FIGURE 5.3 Parietal and prefrontal correlates of perceptual awareness. Foci of parietal and prefrontal activity measured using fMRI and associated with switches in the contents of consciousness independent of changes in physical stimulation are plotted on an anatomical brain image in a standard stereotactic space. Studies shown identify the neural correlates of perceptual switches during rivalry (Lumer et al., 1998; Lumer and Rees, 1999), during bistable perception generally [45], associated with stereo pop-out (Portas et al. 2000a) or change detection [16]. Clustering of activated foci (white circles) is apparent in superior parietal and dorsolateral prefrontal cortex.

perceived phenomenal properties of the visual world. Such a correspondence between V1 activity and the contents of visual awareness extends to cross-modal influences on visual perception. Irrelevant auditory stimulation can lead to illusory perception of a single flash as two flashes. In such circumstances, primary visual cortex shows enhanced activity compared to physically identical stimulation that is perceived correctly [63]. Moreover, this illusion is associated with very early modulation of MEG responses over posterior occipital sensors [64]. Responses in human V1 can therefore be altered by sound, and can reflect subjective perception rather than the physically present visual stimulus.

Illusions can also affect activity in higher visual areas. Perception of illusory or implied motion in a static visual stimulus results in activation of V5/MT [65, 66], while perception of illusory contours activates areas of early retinotopic extrastriate cortex [67–69]. Finally, sensory aftereffects are illusory sensory perceptions in the absence of sensory stimulation that typically occur following an extended period of adaptation to a sensory stimulus. Aftereffects that are contingent on prior adaptation to colour or motion activate either V4 [70–72] or V5/MT [73–75] respectively, and the time course of such activation reflects phenomenal experience [73, 74].

Attention

When subjects are engaged in a demanding task, irrelevant but highly salient stimuli outside the immediate focus of attention can go entirely unnoticed. This phenomenon is known as inattentional blindness, and suggests that visual awareness may depend on attention. Brain activity evoked by irrelevant sensory stimulation in ventral occipital and temporal cortex is reduced when attention is withdrawn [76–79]. Moreover, when inattentional blindness results for unattended words, then brain activity no longer differentiates between such meaningful words and random letters [80]. This suggests that attention is necessary both for brain activity associated with the higher processing of sensory stimuli, and for their subsequent representation in the contents of visual awareness. However, the availability of attention can strongly influence the processing of stimuli in early visual cortex that are rendered entirely invisible by binocular suppression [81]. Thus although attention might be necessary, it cannot be a sufficient condition for awareness (see Chapter 6 for further discussion of the relationship between attention and awareness).

Imagination

A conscious percept can be created by the act of imagination. In these circumstances there is a striking correspondence between the pattern of activation of visual cortices in response to sensory stimulation and to imagery resulting from top-down signals alone. In retinotopic visual cortex, patterns of activation evoked by visual imagery of flickering checkerboard correspond topographically to the patterns evoked by presentation of similar visual stimuli [82]. In extrastriate cortex, colour imagery activates colour-selective area V4 [83]. Neuronal populations further along the ventral visual pathway with stimulus specificity for faces or places are activated during imagery of these categories of object [84]. Finally, in patients with implanted electrodes for pre-surgical epilepsy mapping, single neurons in the human medial temporal lobe that fire selectively when particular visual stimuli are presented [85] are also activated when the individual imagines the same stimuli [86].

Sleep and Anaesthesia

Global alterations in the level of consciousness obviously lead to corresponding modifications in the ability to be aware of the environment. In contrast to the large number of studies in awake observers, there have been relatively few enquiries that address how activity in visual cortex is modified by global changes in level of consciousness (though see Chapter 10 for a more general discussion of anaesthesia plus Chapter 8 for a discussion of sleep). There is a dose dependent reduction in activation of V1 with thiopental [87], but that study did not measure depth of anaesthesia so could not correlate such findings with level of consciousness. Subanaesthetic isoflurane affects task-induced activation in frontal and parietal, but not visual cortices during performance of a visual search task [88]. Visual evoked potentials can still be obtained during anaesthesia, although somewhat unreliably in the operative environment [89], indicating some preservation of cortical processing.

Considering sensory processing more generally, primary auditory cortex activity can still be elicited when auditory stimuli are presented to subjects rendered unconscious through sleep [90] or coma [91], but activation of higher order multimodal association cortex in coma appears to be absent and any thalamo-cortical coupling is decreased relative to the conscious state [92]. Thus, it seems that primary auditory cortex continues to process stimuli when conscious state is perturbed, but activity in secondary sensory and higher cortical areas is strikingly reduced (see also Chapter 13 on brain activity in the vegetative state), consistent with a role for these areas in representing the contents of consciousness. However, whether such a generalization holds true for the visual modality remains to be established.

Summary

Common to these experimental paradigms are changes in visual experience induced by the presence (vs. absence) of a particular spatial and temporal context, or by the presence (vs. absence) of top-down signals, without corresponding physical stimulus changes. Activity in functionally specialized areas of the visual system changes in correspondence with the changes in visual awareness; and as for spontaneous changes in the contents of visual awareness, areas of dorsolateral prefrontal and parietal cortex are also activated.

NECESSARY AND SUFFICIENT CORRELATES OF CONSCIOUSNESS

fMRI and EEG/MEG studies in normal subjects, such as those discussed above, reveal the correlation between particular contents of consciousness and specific types of neural activity. However, they can neither ascertain whether this neural activity plays a causal role in determining the contents of consciousness, nor determine with certainty the necessary and sufficient correlates of consciousness. In order to do this, neural activity must be manipulated either experimentally (e.g., using transcranial magnetic stimulation (TMS)) or as a consequence of neurological disease causing brain damage (see also Chapters 11–27 for further discussion of pathological conditions and consciousness).

In individuals who are blind following retinal damage, phosphenes can be elicited by TMS of visual cortex. However, such stimulation does not elicit phosphenes when blindness results from damage to primary visual cortex [93]. This suggests that while retinal stimulation is not necessary for conscious visual experience of phosphenes, activity in primary visual cortex may be required. Indeed, visual experiences of varying complexity can be elicited by direct stimulation of the ventral visual pathway, confirming that retinal and subcortical processing may not be necessary for conscious visual experience, although it is not possible to entirely rule out their involvement through feedback loops [94]. This suggests that visual input from the retina and subcortical structures is not necessary for conscious visual experience. Whether V1 activity is necessary is more controversial. Activation of extrastriate cortex in the absence of awareness occurs when the blind visual field is stimulated in patients with damage to V1 [95, 96]. However, in at least some patients with V1 damage, residual conscious vision may return in the absence of functional ipsilesional V1 [97]. Reconciling these two observations is only possible if some specific functional aspect of V1 activity, such as its overall level or precise timing, plays a role in determining the contents of consciousness. Consistent with this, awareness of motion is impaired if feedback signals from V5/MT to V1 are disrupted by TMS [98, 99]. Similarly, using TMS to disrupt processing of a mask presented following a target can lead to unmasking and corresponding visibility of the original target [100]. These data suggest that signals in V1 representing feedback from other ventral visual (or higher cortical) areas may be required for awareness. Indeed, coupling is disrupted between the V1 representation of a visual stimulus and higher visual areas when that stimulus is rendered invisible by masking [7].

As previously discussed, damage to frontal and parietal cortex can lead to visual extinction and visual neglect in which awareness is lost for objects presented in one-half of the visual field, even though processing of visual stimuli in visual cortex may continue. This implies that signals in parietal and (possibly) frontal cortex are necessary for normal visual awareness. Consistent with such a notion, disruption of right parietal cortex using TMS leads to a greater rate of change blindness [101]. Parietal damage can also affect the rate of perceptual alternations in binocular rivalry [102], supporting a causal role for these structures in bistable perception. Moreover, when patients with parietal damage become aware of previously extinguished stimuli, such awareness is associated with enhanced covariation of activity in undamaged parietal, prefrontal and visual areas [22]. This suggests that interaction between frontal, parietal and stimulus-specific representations in visual cortices may be required for visual awareness.

OVERALL SUMMARY AND FUTURE DIRECTIONS

In the last decade, substantial progress has been made in establishing the patterns of brain activity in visual cortices associated with purely unconscious processing, and the changes in such activity that are correlated with different contents of visual awareness. Perhaps the most consistent finding is that activity in specific functionally specialized regions of visual cortex is necessary in order to experience particular contents of consciousness. For example, if the visual motion area V5/MT is damaged, or its activity disrupted, then motion will not be perceived. Thus, activity in functionally specialized areas of the visual system is necessary for awareness of the attribute that is represented in the neuronal specificities within that area. However, activity is also consistently observed in such areas in the absence of any awareness of the specific attribute represented. Thus activity in functionally specialized regions of visual cortex is necessary but not sufficient for awareness. Activity associated with unconscious processing is typically either weaker or has a different character (e.g., no 40 Hz oscillations; see Chapter 4 for further details) to that associated with conscious processing. But associations of parietal and frontal activity with awareness, plus long-range coupling of these structures with appropriate sensory representations during awareness, suggest that activated sensory representations may have to interact with higher areas to be represented in the contents of visual awareness. The challenge for the next decade is thus to more precisely delineate whether differences in the level or character of neuronal activity in functionally specialized areas are sufficient for awareness, or whether interactions with additional areas are also required.

ACKNOWLEDGEMENT

This work was supported by the Wellcome Trust.

References

1. Holender, D. and Duscherer, K. (2004) Unconscious perception: The need for a paradigm shift. *Percept Psychophys* 66:872–881. discussion 888–895.
2. Marcel, A.J. (1983) Conscious and unconscious perception: Experiments on visual masking and word recognition. *Cogn Psychol* 15:197–237.
3. He, S. and MacLeod, D.I. (2001) Orientation-selective adaptation and tilt after-effect from invisible patterns. *Nature* 411:473–476.
4. Wales, R. and Fox, R. (1970) Increment detection thresholds during binocular rivalry suppression. *Percept Psychophys* 8:827–835.
5. Watanabe, K., Paik, Y. and Blake, R. (2004) Preserved gain control for luminance contrast during binocular rivalry suppression. *Vision Res* 44:3065–3071.
6. Blake, R. and Fox, R. (1974) Adaptation to invisible gratings and the site of binocular rivalry suppression. *Nature* 249:488–490.
7. Haynes, J.D., Driver, J. and Rees, G. (2005b) Visibility reflects dynamic changes of effective connectivity between V1 and fusiform cortex. *Neuron* 46:811–821.
8. Haynes, J.D. and Rees, G. (2005a) Predicting the orientation of invisible stimuli from activity in human primary visual cortex. *Nat Neurosci* 8:686–691.
9. Moutoussis, K. and Zeki, S. (2006) Seeing invisible motion: A human fMRI study. *Curr Biol* 16:574–579.
10. Dehaene, S., Naccache, L., Cohen, L., Bihan, D.L., Mangin, J.F., Poline, J.B. and Riviere, D. (2001) Cerebral mechanisms of word masking and unconscious repetition priming. *Nat Neurosci* 4:752–758.
11. Moutoussis, K. and Zeki, S. (2002) The relationship between cortical activation and perception investigated with invisible stimuli. *Proc Natl Acad Sci USA* 99:9527–9532.
12. Fang, F. and He, S. (2005) Cortical responses to invisible objects in the human dorsal and ventral pathways. *Nat Neurosci* 8:1380–1385.
13. Marois, R., Chun, M.M. and Gore, J.C. (2000) Neural correlates of the attentional blink. *Neuron* 28:299–308.
14. Luck, S.J., Vogel, E.K. and Shapiro, K.L. (1996) Word meanings can be accessed but not reported during the attentional blink. *Nature* 383:616–618.
15. Vogel, E.K., Luck, S.J. and Shapiro, K.L. (1998) Electrophysiological evidence for a postperceptual locus of suppression during the attentional blink. *J Exp Psychol Hum Percept Perform* 24:1656–1674.
16. Beck, D.M., Rees, G., Frith, C.D. and Lavie, N. (2001) Neural correlates of change detection and change blindness. *Nat Neurosci* 4:645–650.
17. Niedeggen, M., Wichmann, P. and Stoerig, P. (2001) Change blindness and time to consciousness. *Eur J Neurosci* 14:1719–1726.
18. Morris, J.S., Ohman, A. and Dolan, R.J. (1999) A subcortical pathway to the right amygdala mediating 'unseen' fear. *Proc Natl Acad Sci USA* 96:1680–1685.
19. Naccache, L., Gaillard, R., Adam, C., Hasboun, D., Clemenceau, S., Baulac, M., Dehaene, S. and Cohen, L. (2005) A direct intracranial record of emotions evoked by subliminal words. *Proc Natl Acad Sci USA* 102:7713–7717.
20. Pasley, B.N., Mayes, L.C. and Schultz, R.T. (2004) Subcortical discrimination of unperceived objects during binocular rivalry. *Neuron* 42:163–172.
21. Rees, G., Wojciulik, E., Clarke, K., Husain, M., Frith, C. and Driver, J. (2000) Unconscious activation of visual cortex in the damaged right hemisphere of a parietal patient with extinction. *Brain* 123 (Pt 8):1624–1633.

22. Vuilleumier, P., Sagiv, N., Hazeltine, E., Poldrack, R.A., Swick, D., Rafal, R.D. and Gabrieli, J.D. (2001) Neural fate of seen and unseen faces in visuospatial neglect: A combined event-related functional MRI and event-related potential study. *Proc Natl Acad Sci USA* 98:3495–3500.

23. Rees, G., Wojciulik, E., Clarke, K., Husain, M., Frith, C. and Driver, J. (2002) Neural correlates of conscious and unconscious vision in parietal extinction. *Neurocase* 8:387–393.

24. Vuilleumier, P., Armony, J.L., Clarke, K., Husain, M., Driver, J. and Dolan, R.J. (2002) Neural response to emotional faces with and without awareness: Event-related fMRI in a parietal patient with visual extinction and spatial neglect. *Neuropsychologia* 40:2156–2166.

25. Frith, C., Perry, R. and Lumer, E. (1999) The neural correlates of conscious experience: An experimental framework. *Trends Cogn Sci* 3:105–114.

26. Ress, D. and Heeger, D.J. (2003) Neuronal correlates of perception in early visual cortex. *Nat Neurosci* 6:414–420.

27. Marois, R., Yi, D.J. and Chun, M.M. (2004) The neural fate of consciously perceived and missed events in the attentional blink. *Neuron* 41:465–472.

28. Kjaer, T.W., Nowak, M., Kjaer, K.W., Lou, A.R. and Lou, H.C. (2001) Precuneus-prefrontal activity during awareness of visual verbal stimuli. *Conscious Cogn* 10:356–365.

29. Ojanen, V., Revonsuo, A. and Sams, M. (2003) Visual awareness of low-contrast stimuli is reflected in event-related brain potentials. *Psychophysiology* 40:192–197.

30. Wilenius-Emet, M., Revonsuo, A. and Ojanen, V. (2004) An electrophysiological correlate of human visual awareness. *Neurosci Lett* 354:38–41.

31. Vanni, S., Revonsuo, A., Saarinen, J. and Hari, R. (1996) Visual awareness of objects correlates with activity of right occipital cortex. *Neuroreport* 8:183–186.

32. Summerfield, C., Jack, A.I. and Burgess, A.P. (2002) Induced gamma activity is associated with conscious awareness of pattern masked nouns. *Int J Psychophysiol* 44:93–100.

33. Vanni, S., Revonsuo, A. and Hari, R. (1997) Modulation of the parieto-occipital alpha rhythm during object detection. *J Neurosci* 17:7141–7147.

34. Huettel, S.A., Guzeldere, G. and McCarthy, G. (2001) Dissociating the neural mechanisms of visual attention in change detection using functional MRI. *J Cogn Neurosci* 13:1006–1018.

35. Koivisto, M. and Revonsuo, A. (2003) An ERP study of change detection, change blindness, and visual awareness. *Psychophysiology* 40:423–429.

36. Pessoa, L. and Ungerleider, L.G. (2004) Neural correlates of change detection and change blindness in a working memory task. *Cereb Cortex* 14:511–520.

37. Tong, F., Meng, M. and Blake, R. (2006). Neural bases of binocular rivalry. *Trends Cogn Sci* 10(11):502–511.

38. Haynes, J.D., Deichmann, R. and Rees, G. (2005a) Eye-specific effects of binocular rivalry in the human lateral geniculate nucleus. *Nature* 438:496–499.

39. Wunderlich, K., Schneider, K.A. and Kastner, S. (2005) Neural correlates of binocular rivalry in the human lateral geniculate nucleus. *Nat Neurosci* 8:1595–1602.

40. Polonsky, A., Blake, R., Braun, J. and Heeger, D.J. (2000) Neuronal activity in human primary visual cortex correlates with perception during binocular rivalry. *Nat Neurosci* 3:1153–1159.

41. Tong, F. and Engel, S.A. (2001) Interocular rivalry revealed in the human cortical blind-spot representation. *Nature* 411:195–199.

42. Lee, S.H. and Blake, R. (2002) V1 activity is reduced during binocular rivalry. *J Vis* 2:618–626.

43. Lee, S.H., Blake, R. and Heeger, D.J. (2005) Traveling waves of activity in primary visual cortex during binocular rivalry. *Nat Neurosci* 8:22–23.

44. Tong, F., Nakayama, K., Vaughan, J.T. and Kanwisher, N. (1998) Binocular rivalry and visual awareness in human extrastriate cortex. *Neuron* 21:753–759.

45. Kleinschmidt, A., Buchel, C., Zeki, S. and Frackowiak, R.S. (1998) Human brain activity during spontaneously reversing perception of ambiguous figures. *Proc Biol Sci* 265:2427–2433.

46. Sterzer, P., Russ, M.O., Preibisch, C. and Kleinschmidt, A. (2002) Neural correlates of spontaneous direction reversals in ambiguous apparent visual motion. *Neuroimage* 15:908–916.

47. Sterzer, P., Eger, E. and Kleinschmidt, A. (2003) Responses of extrastriate cortex to switching perception of ambiguous visual motion stimuli. *Neuroreport* 14:2337–2341.

48. Lumer, E.D., Friston, K.J. and Rees, G. (1998) Neural correlates of perceptual rivalry in the human brain. *Science* 280:1930–1934.

49. Portas, C.M., Strange, B.A., Friston, K.J., Dolan, R.J. and Frith, C.D. (2000a) How does the brain sustain a visual percept? *Proc Biol Sci* 267:845–850.

50. Lumer, E.D. and Rees, G. (1999) Covariation of activity in visual and prefrontal cortex associated with subjective visual perception. *Proc Natl Acad Sci USA* 96:1669–1673.

51. Haynes, J.D. and Rees, G. (2005b) Predicting the stream of consciousness from activity in human visual cortex. *Curr Biol* 15:1301–1307.

52. Haynes, J.D. and Rees, G. (2006) Decoding mental states from brain activity in humans. *Nat Rev Neurosci* 7:523–534.

53. Ffytche, D.H., Howard, R.J., Brammer, M.J., David, A., Woodruff, P. and Williams, S. (1998) The anatomy of conscious vision: An fMRI study of visual hallucinations. *Nat Neurosci* 1:738–742.

54. Silbersweig, D.A., Stern, E., Frith, C., Cahill, C., Holmes, A., Grootoonk, S., Seaward, J., McKenna, P., Chua, S.E., Schnorr, L., *et al.* (1995) A functional neuroanatomy of hallucinations in schizophrenia. *Nature* 378:176–179.

55. Oertel, V., Rotarska-Jagiela, A., van de Ven, V.G., Haenschel, C., Maurer, K. and Linden, D.E. (2007) Visual hallucinations in schizophrenia investigated with functional magnetic resonance imaging. *Psychiatr Res* 156:269–273.

56. Meng, M., Remus, D.A. and Tong, F. (2005) Filling-in of visual phantoms in the human brain. *Nat Neurosci* 8:1248–1254.

57. Muckli, L., Kohler, A., Kriegeskorte, N. and Singer, W. (2005) Primary visual cortex activity along the apparent-motion trace reflects illusory perception. *PLoS Biol* 3:e265, .

58. Sterzer, P., Haynes, J.D. and Rees, G. (2006) Primary visual cortex activation on the path of apparent motion is mediated by feedback from hMT + /V5. *Neuroimage* 32:1308–1316.

59. Mendola, J.D., Conner, I.P., Sharma, S., Bahekar, A. and Lemieux, S. (2006) fMRI measures of perceptual filling-in in the human visual cortex. *J Cogn Neurosci* 18:363–375.

60. Weil, R.S., Kilner, J.M., Haynes, J.D. and Rees, G. (2007) Neural correlates of perceptual filling-in of an artificial scotoma in humans. *Proc Natl Acad Sci USA* 104:5211–5216.

61. Sasaki, Y. and Watanabe, T. (2004) The primary visual cortex fills in color. *Proc Natl Acad Sci USA* 101:18251–18256.

62. Murray, S.O., Boyaci, H. and Kersten, D. (2006) The representation of perceived angular size in human primary visual cortex. *Nat Neurosci* 9:429–434.

63. Watkins, S., Shams, L., Tanaka, S., Haynes, J.D. and Rees, G. (2006) Sound alters activity in human V1 in association with illusory visual perception. *Neuroimage* 31:1247–1256.

64. Shams, L., Iwaki, S., Chawla, A. and Bhattacharya, J. (2005) Early modulation of visual cortex by sound: An MEG study. *Neurosci Lett* 378:76–81.

65. Zeki, S., Watson, J.D. and Frackowiak, R.S. (1993) Going beyond the information given: The relation of illusory visual motion to brain activity. *Proc Biol Sci* 252:215–222.

66. Kourtzi, Z. and Kanwisher, N. (2000) Activation in human MT/MST by static images with implied motion. *J Cogn Neurosci* 12:48–55.

67. Hirsch, J., DeLaPaz, R.L., Relkin, N.R., Victor, J., Kim, K., Li, T., Borden, P., Rubin, N. and Shapley, R. (1995) Illusory contours activate specific regions in human visual cortex: Evidence from functional magnetic resonance imaging. *Proc Natl Acad Sci USA* 92:6469–6473.

68. Mendola, J.D., Dale, A.M., Fischl, B., Liu, A.K. and Tootell, R.B. (1999) The representation of illusory and real contours in human cortical visual areas revealed by functional magnetic resonance imaging. *J Neurosci* 19:8560–8572.

69. Ritzl, A., Marshall, J.C., Weiss, P.H., Zafiris, O., Shah, N.J., Zilles, K. and Fink, G.R. (2003) Functional anatomy and differential time courses of neural processing for explicit, inferred, and illusory contours. An event-related fMRI study. *Neuroimage* 19:1567–1577.

70. Sakai, K., Watanabe, E., Onodera, Y., Uchida, I., Kato, H., Yamamoto, E., Koizumi, H. and Miyashita, Y. (1995) Functional mapping of the human colour centre with echo-planar magnetic resonance imaging. *Proc Biol Sci* 261:89–98.

71. Hadjikhani, N., Liu, A.K., Dale, A.M., Cavanagh, P. and Tootell, R.B. (1998) Retinotopy and color sensitivity in human visual cortical area V8. *Nat Neurosci* 1:235–241.

72. Barnes, J., Howard, R.J., Senior, C., Brammer, M., Bullmore, E.T., Simmons, A. and David, A.S. (1999) The functional anatomy of the McCollough contingent colour after-effect. *Neuroreport* 10:195–199.

73. Tootell, R.B., Reppas, J.B., Dale, A.M., Look, R.B., Sereno, M.I., Malach, R., Brady, T.J. and Rosen, B.R. (1995) Visual motion aftereffect in human cortical area MT revealed by functional magnetic resonance imaging. *Nature* 375:139–141.

74. He, S., Cohen, E.R. and Hu, X. (1998) Close correlation between activity in brain area MT/V5 and the perception of a visual motion aftereffect. *Curr Biol* 8:1215–1218.

75. Culham, J.C., Dukelow, S.P., Vilis, T., Hassard, F.A., Gati, J.S., Menon, R.S. and Goodale, M.A. (1999) Recovery of fMRI activation in motion area MT following storage of the motion aftereffect. *J Neurophysiol* 81:388–393.

76. Frith, C.D. and Allen, H.A. (1983) The skin conductance orienting response as an index of attention. *Biol Psychol* 17:27–39.

77. Rees, G., Frith, C.D. and Lavie, N. (1997) Modulating irrelevant motion perception by varying attentional load in an unrelated task. *Science* 278:1616–1619.

78. Rees, G., Frith, C. and Lavie, N. (2001) Processing of irrelevant visual motion during performance of an auditory attention task. *Neuropsychologia* 39:937–949.

79. Yi, D.J., Woodman, G.F., Widders, D., Marois, R. and Chun, M.M. (2004) Neural fate of ignored stimuli: Dissociable effects of perceptual and working memory load. *Nat Neurosci* 7:992–996.

80. Rees, G., Russell, C., Frith, C.D. and Driver, J. (1999) Inattentional blindness versus inattentional amnesia for fixated but ignored words. *Science* 286:2504–2507.

81. Bahrami, B., Lavie, N. and Rees, G. (2007) Attentional load modulates responses of human primary visual cortex to invisible stimuli. *Curr Biol* 17:509–513.

82. Slotnick, S.D., Thompson, W.L. and Kosslyn, S.M. (2005) Visual mental imagery induces retinotopically organized activation of early visual areas. *Cereb Cortex* 15:1570–1583.

83. Rich, A.N., Williams, M.A., Puce, A., Syngeniotis, A., Howard, M.A., McGlone, F. and Mattingley, J.B. (2006) Neural correlates of imagined and synaesthetic colours. *Neuropsychologia* 44:2918–2925.

84. O'Craven, K.M. and Kanwisher, N. (2000) Mental imagery of faces and places activates corresponding stimulus-specific brain regions. *J Cogn Neurosci* 12:1013–1023.

85. Kreiman, G., Koch, C. and Fried, I. (2000b) Category-specific visual responses of single neurons in the human medial temporal lobe. *Nat Neurosci* 3:946–953.

86. Kreiman, G., Koch, C. and Fried, I. (2000a) Imagery neurons in the human brain. *Nature* 408:357–361.

87. Martin, E., Thiel, T., Joeri, P., Loenneker, T., Ekatodramis, D., Huisman, T., Hennig, J. and Marcar, V.L. (2000) Effect of pentobarbital on visual processing in man. *Hum Brain Mapp* 10:132–139.

88. Heinke, W. and Schwarzbauer, C. (2001) Subanesthetic isoflurane affects task-induced brain activation in a highly specific manner: A functional magnetic resonance imaging study. *Anesthesiology* 94:973–981.

89. Wiedemayer, H., Fauser, B., Armbruster, W., Gasser, T. and Stolke, D. (2003) Visual evoked potentials for intraoperative neurophysiologic monitoring using total intravenous anesthesia. *J Neurosurg Anesthesiol* 15:19–24.

90. Portas, C.M., Krakow, K., Allen, P., Josephs, O., Armony, J.L. and Frith, C.D. (2000b) Auditory processing across the sleep-wake cycle: Simultaneous EEG and fMRI monitoring in humans. *Neuron* 28:991–999.

91. Laureys, S., Faymonville, M.E., Peigneux, P., Damas, P., Lambermont, B., Del Fiore, G., Degueldre, C., Aerts, J., Luxen, A., Franck, G., Lamy, M., Moonen, G. and Maquet, P. (2002) Cortical processing of noxious somatosensory stimuli in the persistent vegetative state. *Neuroimage* 17:732–741.

92. Laureys, S., Faymonville, M.E., Luxen, A., Lamy, M., Franck, G. and Maquet, P. (2000) Restoration of thalamocortical connectivity after recovery from persistent vegetative state. *Lancet* 355:1790–1791.

93. Cowey, A. and Walsh, V. (2000) Magnetically induced phosphenes in sighted, blind and blindsighted observers. *Neuroreport* 11:3269–3273.

94. Lee, H.W., Hong, S.B., Seo, D.W., Tae, W.S. and Hong, S.C. (2000) Mapping of functional organization in human visual cortex: Electrical cortical stimulation. *Neurology* 54:849–854.

95. Ptito, M., Johannsen, P., Faubert, J. and Gjedde, A. (1999) Activation of human extrageniculostriate pathways after damage to area V1. *Neuroimage* 9:97–107.

96. Goebel, R., Muckli, L., Zanella, F.E., Singer, W. and Stoerig, P. (2001) Sustained extrastriate cortical activation without visual awareness revealed by fMRI studies of hemianopic patients. *Vision Res* 41:1459–1474.

97. Kleiser, R., Wittsack, J., Niedeggen, M., Goebel, R. and Stoerig, P. (2001) Is V1 necessary for conscious vision in areas of relative cortical blindness? *Neuroimage* 13:654–661.

98. Pascual-Leone, A. and Walsh, V. (2001) Fast backprojections from the motion to the primary visual area necessary for visual awareness. *Science* 292:510–512.

99. Silvanto, J., Cowey, A., Lavie, N. and Walsh, V. (2005) Striate cortex (V1) activity gates awareness of motion. *Nat Neurosci* 8:143–144.

100. Ro, T., Breitmeyer, B., Burton, P., Singhal, N.S. and Lane, D. (2003) Feedback contributions to visual awareness in human occipital cortex. *Curr Biol* 13:1038–1041.

101. Beck, D.M., Muggleton, N., Walsh, V. and Lavie, N. (2006) Right parietal cortex plays a critical role in change blindness. *Cereb Cortex* 16:712–717.

102. Bonneh, Y.S., Pavlovskaya, M., Ring, H. and Soroker, N. (2004) Abnormal binocular rivalry in unilateral neglect: Evidence for a non-spatial mechanism of extinction. *Neuroreport* 15:473–477.

CHAPTER

6

The Relationship Between Consciousness and Attention

Naotsugu Tsuchiya and Christof Koch

OUTLINE

ABSTRACT

The relationship between selective attention and consciousness is a close one, leading many scholars to conflate the two. This chapter summarizes psychophysical and neurophysiological evidence arguing that top-down attention and consciousness are distinct phenomena that need not occur together and that can be independently manipulated. Subjects can become conscious of an isolated object, or the gist of the scene in the near-absence of top-down attention. Conversely, subjects can attend to perceptually invisible objects. Most remarkable, top-down attention and consciousness can have opposing effects. Neuroimaging studies are uncovering the distinct hemodynamic signatures of selective attention and consciousness. Untangling their tight relationship is a necessary step in the elucidation of consciousness and its material substrate.

INTRODUCTION

Commonly used in both everyday speech and in the scholarly literature, the terms 'attention' and 'consciousness' have resisted clear and compelling definitions. As argued elsewhere [1, 2] this unfortunate state of affairs will remain until the mechanistic basis of these phenomena has been thoroughly enunciated at the neuronal and molecular levels.

Few would dispute that the relationship between selective attention and perceptual consciousness is an intimate one. When we pay attention to an object, we become conscious of its various attributes; when we shift attention away, the object fades from consciousness. This has prompted many to posit that these two processes are inextricably interwoven, if not identical [3–9]. Others, going back to the 19th century [10], however, have argued that attention and consciousness are distinct phenomena, with distinct functions and neuronal mechanisms [2, 11–21].

Even if the latter proposition is true, what is the nature of their causal interaction? Is paying attention necessary and sufficient for consciousness? Or can conscious perception occur outside the spotlight of attention? Of course, this presupposes that consciousness is a unitary concept, which is not the case. Indeed, consciousness has been dissected on conceptual (access vs. phenomenal consciousness [18, 22]), ontological (hard vs. easy problem [23]), and psychological (explicit vs. implicit processes [24]) grounds. And attention has similarly been dissected into orienting, filtering, and searching functions, anterior and posterior brain circuits, exogenous (bottom-up) and endogenous (top-down) trigger mechanisms, and so forth [25].

We here summarize recent psychophysical and neurophysiological evidence in favour of a dissociation between selective attention and consciousness, and provide functional justifications for this reasoning. We argue that events or objects can be attended to without being consciously perceived. Furthermore, an event or object can be consciously perceived in the near-absence of top-down attentional processing. We review some remarkable evidence that top-down attention and consciousness can have opposing effects. We also refer to ongoing neuroimaging studies that are measuring attentional modulation of fMRI responses to invisible stimuli [26, 27]. We discuss empirical methods to manipulate the visibility of stimuli independently of top-down attention and refer to the post-decision wagering technique to measure consciousness [28, 29]. Finally, we speculate about the neuronal substrate of consciousness without attention.

Note that our usage of 'attention' always implies selective attention, rather than the processes that control the overall level of arousal and alertness. Furthermore, we restrict this review to visual attention and visual consciousness, as visual perception and the neurophysiology of vision is much better understood than other modalities.

FUNCTIONAL CONSIDERATIONS

Let us start by considering the functional roles of attention. Complex organisms, such as brains, suffer from informational overload. In primates, about one million fibers leave each eye and carry on the order of one megabyte per second of raw information. One way to deal with this deluge of data is to select a small fraction and process this reduced input in real time, while the non-attended portion of the input is processed at a reduced bandwidth. In this view, attention selects information of current relevance to the organism while the non-attended data suffer from benign neglect.

Since the time of Williams James, selection is known to be based on either bottom-up, exogenous or top-down, endogenous factors [30–32]. Exogenous cues are image-immanent features that transiently attract attention or eye gaze, independent of any particular task. Thus, if an object attribute (e.g., flicker, motion, colour, orientation, depth, or texture) differs significantly from its value in some neighbourhood, the object will be salient. This definition of bottom-up saliency has been implemented into a popular suite of neuromorphic vision algorithms that have at their core a topographic saliency map that encodes the saliency or conspicuity of locations in the visual field independent of the task [33] (see http://ilab.usc.edu for a C++ implementation and http://www.saliencytoolbox.net/ for a Matlab toolbox). Such algorithms account for a significant fraction of fixational eye movements [34, 35]. Candidates for such a map in the primate brain include the initial responses of neurons in the frontal eye field (FEF) and the lateral intraparietal sulcus (LIP) [36, 37] (see Box 6.1).

However, under many conditions, subjects can disregard salient, bottom-up cues when searching for particular objects in a scene by dint of top-down, task-dependent control of attention [38]. Bringing top-down, sustained attention to bear on an object or event in a scene takes time. Top-down attention selects input defined by a circumscribed region in space (*focal attention*), by a particular feature (*feature-based attention*), or by an object (*object-based attention*). It is the relationship between these volitionally controlled forms of selective, endogenous attention and consciousness that is the topic of this chapter.

Consciousness, on the other hand, is surmised to have quite different functions. These range from summarizing all relevant information pertaining to the current state of the organism and its environment and making this compact summary accessible to the planning stages of the brain, to detecting anomalies and errors, decision-making, language, inferring the internal state of other animals, setting long-term goals, making recursive models, and rational thought.

To the extent that one accepts that attention and consciousness have different functions, one has to accept that they cannot be the same process.

BOX 6.1

PSYCHOPHYSICAL TOOLS TO MANIPULATE TOP-DOWN ATTENTION

Top-down attention and consciousness are usually tightly coupled. To dissociate these two, experimental tools that manipulate either one independently in a specific manner with few side effects are called for.

There exist at least two forms of selective attention: stimulus-driven, bottom-up, saliency-mediated attention as well as task- and goal-dependent top-down attention, with some intermediate forms. Previously neutral stimuli (such as text or images of guns) can be associated with reward or punishment to acquire additional saliency. Biologically relevant stimuli may be preferred or disliked based on individual difference (e.g., snakes, spiders, and nude pictures).

A variety of techniques to manipulate these components of attention have been invented. It is not always easy to compare them, as each method interferes with attention at a different level of processing [39, 40].

In *Posner's cueing paradigm*, popular to study orienting [41], a target is preceded by an informative or a non-informative cue that appears at the target location or at fixation. Attentional effects are inferred in terms of reaction time and/or accuracy of target detection. Variants of this method demonstrated that an invisible cue can direct attention to the cued location [16, 42–47], clear support for attention without consciousness.

In *visual search*, subjects need to find a target among distractors; reaction time is related to the number of distractors. When the search slope is steep, the search process is said to be *serial*, and when flat, *parallel*. The former is usually taken as the evidence of processing by top-down attention. However, steep search may arise due to completely bottom-up factors [40]. This exemplifies a case where dual-tasks and visual search methods may yield inconsistent results.

The *dual-tasks paradigm* [31, 39, 46] manipulates top-down, focal attention without affecting bottom-up saliency: a central, attentional-demanding discrimination task is present at the centre of gaze, while a secondary stimulus is projected somewhere into the periphery (Figure 6.1A). Subjects either carry out the central, the

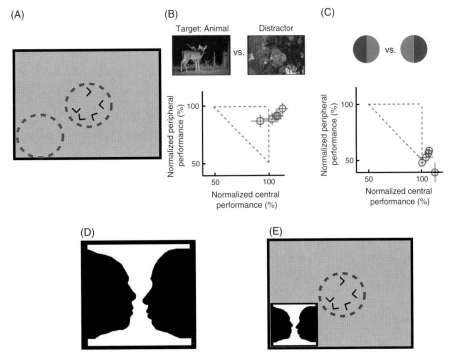

FIGURE 6.1 Manipulating top-down attention. (A) How performance of a secondary task in the periphery (empty red circle) is affected when a centrally presented attention-demanding task is performed simultaneously is studied with the aid of the dual-tasks paradigm. Deciding whether or not a natural scene includes an animal can be done at the same time as the central task – here a demanding letter discrimination – (panel B), while discriminating a red-green disk from a green-red one cannot be done when attention is engaged at the centre (panel C). (D) An example of a bistable conscious percept (Rubin vase: two silhouettes vs. a vase). (E) It would be interesting to characterize the effect of withdrawing top-down attention from Rubin's vase illusion by imbedding this bistable percept into a dual-tasks experiment [59, 60] (see Box 6.2). B and C modified from [48] and from [61] with permission.

peripheral, or both tasks simultaneously while the scene and its layout remain the same. Surprisingly, seemingly complex peripheral tasks can be done equally well under either single- or dual-tasks condition [48–50], while other, computationally simpler tasks deteriorate when performed simultaneously with the central task (Figure 6.1B and C). The dual-tasks paradigm quantifies what type of stimulus attributes can be signalled and consciously perceived in the near-absence of spatial attention [40].

Most importantly, the dual-tasks paradigm can be combined with a multitude of visual illusions that render stimuli invisible, allowing the independent manipulation of top-down attention and consciousness (Figure 6.1D and E), although a full factorial analysis for many popular experiments awaits the future (see Box 6.2).

The inference of attentional requirements from dual-tasks performance demands caution. High proficiency in such tasks is only achieved after extensive training of many hours. Such an extended training phase renders the task quite different from what naïve subjects experience [51, 52].

Finally, there are a class of neurological conditions as well as visual illusions in normal subjects where stimuli become invisible because of impairments in the mechanisms of top-down or bottom-up attention. Neglect and extinction [53], attentional blink [54, 55], inattentional blindness [56], and change blindness [57] are sometimes used as positive evidence for 'without attention, no consciousness' [3]. Although some attributes of the visual input need attentional amplification to rise to the level of consciousness, other aspects, such as the gist of the scene and its emotional content, are quite resistant to such attentional manipulations [56, 58].

Consider the four different ways in which a particular percept or behaviour can be classified depending on whether or not it requires top-down attention and whether it necessarily gives rise to consciousness (Table 6.1).

THE FOUR-FOLD WAY OF PROCESSING VISUAL EVENTS AND BEHAVIOURS

While many scholars agree that attention and consciousness are distinct, they insist that the former is necessary for the latter, and that non-attended events remain *sub rosa* from the point of view of consciousness. For example, Dehaene and colleagues [19] argue that without top-down attention, an event cannot be consciously perceived (preconscious). The evidence reviewed below argues otherwise.

More than a century of research efforts have quantified the ample benefits accrued to attended and consciously perceived events. For example, Mack and Rock [56] compellingly demonstrate that subjects must attend to become conscious of novel or unexpected stimuli. These occupy the lower right quadrant of our attention × consciousness design matrix (Table 6.1).

On the other end of the spectrum are objects or events that are not sufficiently salient to either attract bottom-up attention or a top-down attentional bias. Under these conditions, the net-wave of spiking activity moving from the retina into primary visual cortex and beyond will not trigger a conscious percept (but

TABLE 6.1   A Four-Fold Classification of Percepts and Behaviours

	May not give rise to consciousness	Gives rise to consciousness
Top-down attention is not required	Formation of afterimages Rapid vision (<120 ms) Zombie behaviours Accommodation reflex Pupillary reflex	Pop-out Iconic memory Gist Animal and gender detection in dual-tasks Partial reportability
Top-down attention is required	Priming Adaptation Processing of objects Visual search Thoughts	Working memory Detection and discrimination of unexpected and unfamiliar stimuli Full reportability

Note: This classification of percepts and behaviours depends on whether or not top-down attention is necessary and whether or not these percepts and behaviours necessarily give rise to phenomenal consciousness. Different percepts and behaviors are grouped together according to these two, psychophysically defined, criteria.

see further below). However, such non-attended or only minimally attended and non-conscious activity can still be causally effective and leave traces that can be picked up with sensitive behavioural techniques. For instance, such non-salient stimuli can cause negative afterimages [62–64]. These occupy the upper left quadrant of Table 6.1. Other likely examples include

BOX 6.2

HOW TO MEASURE VISUAL CONSCIOUSNESS

Visual consciousness can be manipulated using a multitude of illusions, such as backward masking, the standing wave of invisibility [65], crowding, bistable figures, binocular rivalry, flash suppression, continuous flash suppression [63, 66], motion-induced blindness and attentional blink (for a review see [67]). These techniques control the visibility of an object or part of thereof in both space and time. Yet how is visibility assayed? More generally, how can the degree of consciousness be probed?

The most lenient criterion is to accept what subjects subsequently report verbally; for example, 'I never saw the face'. Though widely used (such as when obtaining reports right after a fMRI session), this method is unsatisfactory because unattended items or task-irrelevant (implicit) features of stimuli may be inaccessible in subsequent recognition or recall tasks [68, 69, 70]. A more stringent criterion for non-conscious processing is to ask subjects about their experience directly at the time the stimulus is processed. When subjects deny seeing stimuli, the stimulus is processed at a *subjectively non-conscious* level. Although many studies involving non-conscious states adopt this convention, the definition suffers from the possibility of criterion shifts: for the same subjective experience of visibility, some subjects may deny seeing a stimulus while others may report seeing it, because their criterion of what to count as 'seen' differs [28].

The strictest procedure is to demonstrate null sensitivity using an appropriate overt behavioural measures, that is, $d' = 0$. For example, subjects can be given two alternative temporal intervals (or locations), each of which contains the stimulus equally often. If they are at chance in detecting/discriminating one from the other, they are (objectively) unaware of the stimulus (our use of 'subjective' and 'objective' here refers to the method used, not to the nature of the conscious experience, which is of course always subjective in terms of its phenomenology). Note that above-chance behavioural discrimination performance does not necessarily demonstrate conscious awareness, since patients with blindsight exhibit precisely such performance.

However, such an objective definition does not directly reflect phenomenal experience, which is the central issue. By applying the objective measure of signal discriminability to one's own judgement of whether the stimulus is seen or not, one can *objectively* measure *subjectivity*. That is, one can consider the discriminability (d') of one's own experience. For this method, subjects first make a detection/discrimination judgement, then rate the confidence in their decision. Defining 'hit' as proportion of high confident ratings given the decision was correct – p(high confidence | correct) – and 'false alarm' as the proportion of high confident ratings given the decision was incorrect – p(high confidence | incorrect) – one can calculate the signal discriminability (d' or area under the curve). In signal detection theory, this is called Type 2 analysis [71]. It has been applied to evaluation of above-chance behaviour in non-conscious perception [28, 72]. We believe that it is more fruitful to measure both objective and subjective thresholds simultaneously using confidence rating [73, 74] rather than debating which one is superior.

However, reflecting upon one's own judgement may require a substantial internal focus. Such an act itself can modify conscious experience significantly [75]. With a recently proposed method, *post-decision wagering*, this contamination due to introspection can be minimized [28, 29]. Following each response, subjects wager on their performance, betting either high or low. If the subject is confident that she saw the stimulus, reward maximization would presume that she would wager a higher amount than when she was unaware of the stimulus and was guessing (also see [76, 77]).

Here, subjects' awareness is gauged by their discriminability of their own judgement. This method proves to be easy and intuitive for subjects to use and very effective in reflecting one's subjective aspects of consciousness while minimizing interference to the quality of the experience. Persaud and colleagues [29] observed non-conscious, above-chance behaviours in blindsight patients, implicit learning, and the Iowa gambling task, while demonstrating non-conscious access to the information by post-decision wagering.

---

visuo-motor reflexes such as the accommodation and the pupillary reflexes.

What about the two remaining quadrants, covering events that require top-down attention but that do not give rise to conscious perception and events

that give rise to consciousness yet without top-down attention? These can be studied with techniques that independently manipulate top-down attention and visibility (Boxes 6.1 and 6.2).

ATTENTION WITHOUT CONSCIOUSNESS

Consider that subjects can attend to a location for many seconds and yet fail to see one or more attributes of an object at that location (lower left quadrant in Table 6.1). In lateral masking (*visual crowding*), the orientation of a peripherally presented grating is hidden from conscious sight but remains sufficiently potent to induce an orientation-dependent aftereffect [78]. Montaser-Kouhsari and Rajimehr [79] showed that an aftereffect induced by an invisible illusory contour required focal attention, even though the object at the centre of attention was invisible (see also [80, 81]). Naccache and colleagues [13] elicited priming for invisible words (suppressed by a combination of forward and backward masking) but only if the subject was attending to the invisible prime-target pair; without attention, the same word failed to elicit priming. Male/female nudes attracted attention when they were rendered completely invisible by continuous flash suppression [42]. Interestingly, in heterosexuals, these effects were only apparent for nudes of the opposite sex ([see also [43–45, 47]). Note that by themselves (i.e. without the mask), these stimuli are clearly visible.

Likewise, the blindsight patient GY has the usual reaction-time advantages for the detection of targets in his blind visual field when attentionally cued, even when the cues are located in his blind field and are therefore invisible to him [16, 82, 83].

Finally, feature-based attention can spread to invisible stimuli [84, 85]. Indeed, when searching for an object in a cluttered scene (e.g., keys in a messy room), attention is paid to an invisible object and its associated features.

In conclusion, attentional selection does not necessarily engender phenomenal sensations, although it may often do so.

CONSCIOUSNESS IN THE ABSENCE OF ATTENTION

Yet the converse can also occur and may be quite common (upper right quadrant in Table 6.1). When focusing intensely on one event, the world is not reduced to a tunnel, with everything outside the focus of attention gone. We are always aware of some aspects of the world surrounding us, such as its gist. Indeed, gist is immune from inattentional blindness [56]: when a photograph covering the entire background was briefly flashed, completely unexpectedly, onto a screen, subjects could accurately report a summary of what it contained. In the 30 ms necessary to apprehend the gist of a scene [86, 87], top-down attention cannot play much of a role (because gist is a property associated with the entire image, any process that locally enhances features is going to be only of limited use).

Take perception of a single object (say a bar) in an otherwise empty display, a non-ecological but common arrangement in many experiments. Here, what function would top-down, selective attention need to perform without any competing item in or around fixation? Indeed, the most popular neuronal model of attention, *biased competition* [88], predicts that in the absence of competition, no or little attentional enhancement occurs.

In a dual-tasks paradigm, the subject's attention is drawn to a demanding central task, while at the same time a secondary stimulus is flashed somewhere in the periphery (see Box 6.1). Using the identical retinal layout, the subject either performs the central task, or the peripheral task, or both simultaneously [31, 39, 46]. With focal attention busy at the centre, the subject can still distinguish a natural scene containing an animal (or a vehicle) from one that does not include an animal (or a vehicle) while being unable to distinguish a red-green bisected disk from a green-red one [48]. Likewise, subjects can tell male from female faces or even distinguish a famous from a non-famous face [49, 50], but are frustrated by tasks that are computationally much simpler (e.g., discriminating a rotated letter 'L' from a rotated 'T'). This is quite remarkable. Thus, while we cannot be sure that observers do not deploy some limited amount of top-down attention in these dual-tasks experiments that require training and concentration (i.e., high arousal), it remains true that subjects can perform certain discriminations but not others in the near-absence of top-down attention. And they are not guessing. They can be quite confident of their choices and 'see', albeit often indistinctly, what they can discriminate.

Can perception be studied in the complete absence of attention? This seems possible if, in the above-mentioned dual-task paradigm, subjects must perform a very demanding central task without needing to monitor the periphery. Such an experiment has been conducted to investigate the effects of attention on bistable perception [59]. A fundamental question in the perception of ambiguous figures is why they switch spontaneously despite constant retinal input. One influential theory posits that top-down attention triggers perceptual transitions [30]. To test this, Pastukhov and Braun [59] examined whether unattended and unreported bistable motion stimuli continued to switch. Consistent with other studies [60], they found that drawing attention away from the peripheral ambiguous percept slowed down the dominance periods but their statistical variability remained; even a complete withdrawal of attention failed to abolish transitions. In other words, top-down attention is not necessary for switches in the content of visual consciousness. Similar dual-tasks experiments can likewise be applied as a strict test for the necessity of top-down attention in learning, memory, adaptation, and other cognitive functions (see Box 6.1).

PROCESSING WITHOUT TOP-DOWN ATTENTION AND CONSCIOUSNESS

Visual input can be classified very rapidly. As famously demonstrated by Thorpe and colleagues [89, 90], around 120 ms following image onset, some brain processes begin to respond differentially to images containing one or more animals from pictures than contain none. At this speed, it is no surprise that subjects often respond without having consciously seen the image [91, 92]; consciousness for the image may come later or not at all. Dual-tasks and dual-presentation paradigms support the idea that such discriminations can occur in the near-absence of focal, spatial attention [48, 93] (but see [94]) implying that purely feed-forward networks can support complex visual decision-making in the absence of both attention and consciousness [91, 92]. Indeed, this has now been formally shown in the context of a purely feed-forward computational model of the primate's ventral visual system [95].

Animal experiments could prove this assertion. Imagine that all the cortico-cortical pathways from prefrontal cortex back to higher level visual cortex and from there on even further back to primary and secondary visual cortices would be transiently knocked out using a molecular silencing tool (without compromising feed-forward processing). That is, for a couple of hours, the brain of the monkey would only support feed-forward pathways. It is quite likely that such an animal could still carry out a previously learnt simple discrimination task with essentially the same level of performance as prior to the intervention (upper left quadrant in Table 6.1), without any top-down attention (since prefrontal cortex would have no means to modulate the processes in the visual brain), and without conscious perception.

ATTENTION AND CONSCIOUSNESS CAN OPPOSE EACH OTHER

Most remarkably, withdrawing top-down attention from a stimulus and cloaking it from consciousness can have opposing effects. When observers try to find two embedded targets within a rapidly flashed stream of stimuli, they often fail to see the second target, a phenomenon known as the *attentional blink* [54, 55]. Counter-intuitively, Olivers and Nieuwenhuis [96] found that observers can see both the first and the second targets better when they are distracted by a simultaneous auditory dual task or encouraged to think about task-irrelevant events.[1]

In most conditions, paying attention improves processing of stimulus. However, under certain conditions, low spatial frequency stimuli can be better discriminated without than with spatial attention [97–99]. During implicit learning, attentively trying to discover the underlying complex rule delays learning and impairs subsequent recognition [100]. Recent work on afterimages, stabilization of bistable figures, and complex decision-making hint at striking dissociations between top-down attention and consciousness (for more details, see Box 6.3). Such findings are nearly impossible to understand within a framework that aligns top-down attention closely with consciousness.

PHYSIOLOGICAL TECHNIQUES THAT DEMONSTRATE DISSOCIATIONS BETWEEN ATTENTION AND CONSCIOUSNESS

The neuronal footprints of non-conscious processing of visual information have been tracked using both event-related potentials (ERP), magnetoencephalography (MEG) and functional magnetic resonance imaging (fMRI) ([101–106]). Only recently have such tools been applied to separate the neuronal mechanisms of top-down attention from conscious and non-conscious processing [15, 26, 27, 107–109].

For example, in [15] a lateralized negativity that appears around 200 ms following image onset and that is linked to the action of attention, is still detected for

---

[1]Another example of attention hindering execution of a task is the tip-of-the-tongue phenomenon (H. Berlin, personal communication). Intense concentration on the missing name or word will often fail to recover it; instead it may suddenly 'pop into mind' when attention is focused on another task.

BOX 6.3

CAN TOP-DOWN ATTENTION BE OPPOSED TO CONSCIOUSNESS?

Attention and its neuronal correlate can be understood in the context of selection and biased competition [78]: attention acts as a winner-take-all, enhancing one coalition of neurons (representing the attended object) at the expenses of other coalitions (non-attended stimuli) [111]. Paradoxically though, reducing attention can enhance awareness [96] and certain behaviours [98–100, 112].

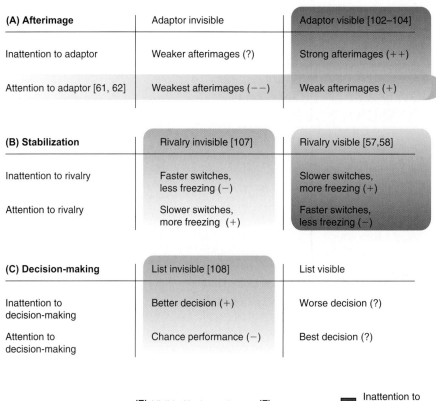

(A) Afterimage	Adaptor invisible	Adaptor visible [102–104]
Inattention to adaptor	Weaker afterimages (?)	Strong afterimages (++)
Attention to adaptor [61, 62]	Weakest afterimages (−−)	Weak afterimages (+)

(B) Stabilization	Rivalry invisible [107]	Rivalry visible [57,58]
Inattention to rivalry	Faster switches, less freezing (−)	Slower switches, more freezing (+)
Attention to rivalry	Slower switches, more freezing (+)	Faster switches, less freezing (−)

(C) Decision-making	List invisible [108]	List visible
Inattention to decision-making	Better decision (+)	Worse decision (?)
Attention to decision-making	Chance performance (−)	Best decision (?)

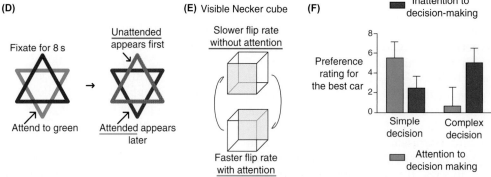

(D) Fixate for 8 s — Attend to green → Unattended appears first — Attended appears later

(E) Visible Necker cube — Slower flip rate without attention — Faster flip rate with attention

(F) Inattention to decision-making — Preference rating for the best car — Simple decision — Complex decision — Attention to decision making

FIGURE 6.2   Dissociation of the effects of attention and awareness. (A) and (D) When the adaptor is *invisible*, its afterimage is substantially *weakened* (pink gradation [63, 64]). Paradoxically, when the adaptor is *visible* and *attended*, the associated afterimage becomes weaker and appears *later* (blue gradation [113–115]). (B) and (E) When attention is *withdrawn* from a visible bistable/rivalry target (here, a Necker cube), the rate of perceptual flips *slows down* (blue gradation [59, 60]). When the target stimulus is intermittently presented (*stabilization*), the opposite may occur; *withdrawing* attention from the target reduces stabilization, that is, perceptual flips *speed up* (pink gradation [118]). (C) and (F) When confronted with a complex decision where many items must be remembered (*i.e.*, the list is *invisible*), distracting subjects from the decision-making process *improves* performance (pink gradation [119]). The last figure is modified from [119] and [61] with permission.

In the Rubin's ambiguous figure (see Figure 6.1D), the percept switches between two faces seen in profile and a vase. Discrimination of high-frequency stimuli, such as a line, presented on the face area when it is perceived as the figure is better than when it is perceived as the ground. If a blurred, low spatial frequency stimulus is presented in this region, it is better discriminated when the face is perceived as the ground. Something similar occurs when the target stimulus is presented on the vase area. In other words, a low spatial frequency stimulus is better detected on the unattended ground [97, 98]. Likewise, Yeshurun and Carrasco [99] showed that attention impairs the performance of texture segregation when the subject is required to process low spatial frequency information.

Consider the formation of afterimages (Figure 6.2A). If an item is attended during adaptation, the intensity of the subsequent afterimage becomes weaker and its duration shorter compared to an unattended item [113–115] (Figure 6.2D). If, however, the image is suppressed during adaptation, the afterimage is substantially weakened [63, 64]. Thus, focal attention and consciousness have opposing effects.

Next, consider *freezing* in bistable perception (Figure 6.2B) [116, 117]. During continuous viewing of an ambiguous stimulus, the percept flips stochastically. Yet if the bistable figure is briefly removed (leaving the display empty), the dominant percept at the start of the new display is the same as the one when the percept disappeared. This freezing is disrupted if spatial attention is distracted from the empty display [118], most likely by disrupting memory buildup. This can be thought of as

speeding up perceptual switching. Yet distracting focal attention during bistable perception slows down the switching rate [59, 60] (Figure 6.2E). In other words, withdrawing focal attention when the stimulus is invisible, not consciously seen, disrupts perceptual freezing, while withdrawing attention when the stimulus is visible slows down switching.

Finally, consider complex decision-making (Figure 6.2C). The Dijksterhuis' [119] study consisted of three phases: examination of items, deliberation, and decision. One of either 4 or 12 properties for each of 4 cars was shown one at a time during the examination phase. Subjects then deliberated for several minutes without the attributes being visible (i.e., subjects had to remember them; this can be thought of as an 'invisible' condition) before making a purchasing decision. Dijksterhuis and colleagues manipulated whether or not subjects were cognitively engaged during the deliberation period. They concluded that when faced with working memory overload, an explicit strategy based on deliberate and rational thought leads to poor decision-making for a complex decision, while distracting subjects when they decide which car to buy greatly increased the probability of a correct choice (Figure 6.2F). We surmise that if the list of items would have been present throughout the decision-making period – thereby reducing working memory load – an attentional distracting task would degrade purchasing performance. For a related finding in implicit learning, see [100].

Note that a complete orthogonal manipulation of attention and consciousness has not been performed in any of these examples.

a target that is rendered invisible via *object substitution masking* [110]. The authors conclude that this ERP component is the neuronal correlate of top-down attention even though the target is not consciously perceived.

More direct evidence comes from a recent fMRI study by Bahrami and colleagues [26], demonstrating that the processing of objects hidden from sight (with d′ = 0) via *continuous flash suppression* [63] depends on the availability of spatial attention (Figure 6.3). They varied the load of the central task in a dual-task design (Box 6.1). The hemodynamic blood-oxygen-level-dependent contrast (BOLD) response to the invisible objects in primary visual cortex, V1, was stronger when the central task was easy, that is, when spatial attention was available for processing the invisible, peripheral stimulus than when the central task was hard and more attentional resources were drawn to it. In other words, attention modulates the fMRI response of an invisible stimulus.

Taken together with related psychophysical findings [13, 79], these physiological experiments highlight the role of top-down attention in neuronal processing of invisible stimuli (see the bottom left in Table 6.1).

An even more paradoxical effect – that invisible stimuli can be more distracting than visible ones – was discovered by Tsushima and colleagues [27] (Figure 6.4). In this study, subjects had to detect foveally placed targets in a stream of characters – a *rapid serial visual presentation* (RSVP) task – surrounded by an annulus of moving dots. The fraction of dots moving coherently in one direction – the *motion coherence* – was varied from 0% (truly random dot motion) to 50% (half of the dots move in the same direction). When the central task was combined with the task-irrelevant surround motion, the central performance *dropped* when the coherent motion was perceptually below threshold (say at 5%, where the cloud of dots was not perceived

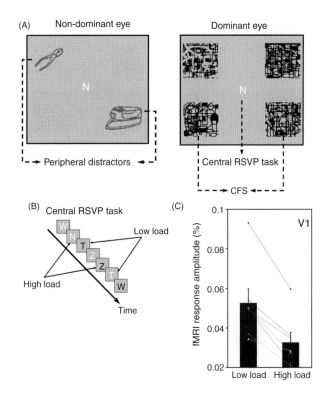

FIGURE 6.3 Neuronal activation by invisible stimuli is modulated by top-down attention. (A) Pictures of tools in the periphery of the non-dominant eye are rendered invisible by continuous flash suppression (CFS) at the corresponding and two other locations in the dominant eye. (B) At the centre of the display, subjects performed a rapid serial visual presentation (RSVP) task. In the low load condition, a target letter 'T' of white or black colour must be detected. In the high load condition, either a 'white N' or a 'black Z' must be detected, embedded within a stream of letters. (C) fMRI response amplitude in primary visual cortex to invisible objects is modulated by the attention load on the central task. *Source*: Modified from [26] with permission.

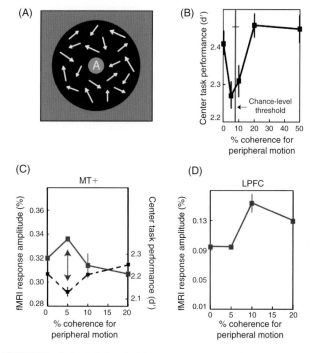

FIGURE 6.4 Subthreshold motion is more distracting than suprathreshold motion. (A) Subjects had to detect two target digits embedded in a rapid stream of letters (RSVP). Surrounding the letter stream, moving random dots of variable coherence were presented. (B) The central RSVP task performance (on the y-axis) dropped when the peripheral motion was below the threshold for detecting coherent motion. Note that stronger motion (i.e., higher coherency) did not interfere with the central task. (C) Activation of the cortical region MT+ was highest when peripheral motion was below threshold. (D) Activation of lateral prefrontal cortex (LPFC), which inhibits activity in MT+, was higher when motion coherence was above the threshold. Subthreshold motion does not activate LPFC. *Source*: Modified from [27] with permission.

to move coherently) compared to when the motion coherence was 0% or above threshold (e.g., 20%). This counterintuitive finding was explained by the parallel fMRI study in which the authors looked at BOLD activity in area MT+, which reflects the degree of distraction by the motion, and in the lateral prefrontal cortex (LPFC), which provides an attentional suppression signal to MT+ (Figure 6.4). Compatible with the behavioural findings, subthreshold motion did not elicit activity in the LPFC, resulting in higher distractor-related activity in MT+. On the other hand, suprathreshold motion evoked a stronger LPFC signal but a weaker MT+ one. The authors hypothesize that invisible motion activates MT+, impairing performance, but not the LPFC, which fails to inhibit MT+; thereby stimuli that are not consciously perceived can escape inhibitory control, a phenomenon more familiar from psychoanalysis than from sensory psychology [120].

RELATIONSHIP TO OTHER CONCEPTUAL DISTINCTIONS

The philosopher Block has argued for the existence of two different types of consciousness, phenomenal (*P*) and access (*A*) consciousness [18, 22]. *P* is the ephemeral feeling of seeing yellow, different from the feeling of seeing green. *A*, on the other hand, are the processes that access this information and do something with it, such as verbal or motor report or working memory.

Block [121] has argued that phenomenally conscious states may sometimes not be cognitively accessible, in the sense that they are consciously experienced but that subjects may only have limited access to their attributes as assayed by recall or alternative-forced choice judgements. We find this hypothesis plausible, a revision of our earlier position [2, 122]. In particular, within the framework espoused here, *P*-consciousness is close to what we have been calling consciousness without top-down attention, while *A*-consciousness is close to consciousness with attention (plus working memory and, in humans, verbal report) [123].

Consider Sperling's iconic memory experiment [68] or Landman's and colleagues [69] variant. Subjects report that they vividly and consciously see a field of letters or bars arranged on a circle. However, subjects only have very limited access to the detailed properties of the individual elements, unless top-down attention is directed to a subset of stimuli using appropriately timed cues. Our conjecture is that phenomenology without conscious access (*P* without *A*) is an example of consciousness without top-down attention processing. Note that the converse is not true; not every example of conscious perception in the (near-)absence of top-down attention is cognitive non-accessible, as is the case for face recognition in a dual-task paradigm [49, 50].

Dehaene and colleagues [19] propose a tripartite ontology, based on Baars' (for an updated view, see [17]) and Dehaene and colleagues' [124] global workspace hypothesis, whereby any physical stimulus triggers either *subliminal, preconscious,* or *conscious processing*. What decides the fate of any stimulus is its strength and whether or not top-down attention is deployed. Their distinction maps onto ours if subliminal processing is equated with the upper and lower left quadrants and preconscious with the upper right quadrant. One important difference is our assumption that consciousness can occur without top-down attention (upper right quadrant in Table 6.1). *A priori*, there is no fundamental reason why global workspace theory requires actively paying attention to a stimulus in order to be conscious of it. There might be many different routes by which the global workspace could be accessed, not only by virtue of top-down attention.

NEURONAL SUBSTRATE TO CONSCIOUSNESS WITHOUT ATTENTION

When we attend to a face or to an object within a cluttered scene, we usually become conscious of its attributes, with all of the attendant privileges of consciousness (e.g., access to working memory and, in people, verbal reportability). While the minimal neuronal mechanisms jointly sufficient for any one conscious visual percept remain elusive, a number of models posit that they must involve neuronal populations in extra-striate visual cortices having a reciprocal relationship – mediated by long-range cortico-cortical feedforward and feedback projections – with neurons

in parietal, premotor, and prefrontal cortices [1, 17, 124–126]. Furthermore, a number of elegant fMRI experiments [109, 127] are consistent with the hypothesis that primary visual cortex (V1) is necessary, but not sufficient for visual consciousness [128].

Decades of electrophysiological recordings in the monkey have proven that the spiking responses of neurons in the ventral visual stream (e.g., in areas V4 and IT) representing attended stimuli are boosted at the expense of the response to non-attended items [88, 129]. According to Crick and Koch [128], this enables these neurons to establish a reciprocal relationship with neurons in the dorsolateral prefrontal cortex and related regions that are involved in working memory and planning (and language in humans), leading to reverberatory neuronal activity that outlasts the initial stimulus duration. Critical to the formation of such a single and integrated coalition of neurons are the long-range axons of pyramidal neurons that project from the back to the front of cortex and their targets in the front that project back to the upper stages of the ventral pathway (possibly involving stages of the thalamus, such as the pulvinar [130], as well as the claustrum [131]. When such a wide-ranging coalition has established itself, the subject becomes conscious of its representational contents and gains access to short-term memory, planning, and language.

But what happens to those stimuli that do not benefit from attentional boosting? Depending on the exact circumstances (visual clutter in the scene, contrast, stimulus duration) these stimuli may likewise establish coalitions of neurons, aided by local (i.e. within the cortical area) and semi-local feedback (i.e. feedback projections that remain consigned to visual cortex) loops. However, as these coalitions of neurons lack coordinated support from feedback from prefrontal cortex, thalamus, and claustrum, their firing activity is less vigorous and may decay much more quickly. Yet aided by the neuronal representation of the entire scene, these weaker and more local coalitions may still be sufficient for some phenomenal percepts [132], even though the associated coalition does not reach into the front of the brain. In other words, for visual *P*-consciousness, coalitions in the back of cortex might be sufficient, while *A*-consciousness might require the associated coalition to reach into the frontal lobe.

DO THESE CONCLUSIONS HOLD FOR REAL LIFE?

It could be contested that top-down attention without consciousness and consciousness with little or no top-down attention are arcane laboratory curiosities, with little relevance to the real world. We believe otherwise.

A lasting insight into human behaviour – eloquently articulated by Friedrich Nietzsche and, later on, by Sigmund Freud – is that much action bypasses conscious perception and introspection. In particular, Goodale and Milner [133] isolated highly trained, automatic, stereotyped, and fluid visuo-motor behaviours that function in the absence of phenomenal experience. As anybody who runs mountain trails, climbs, plays soccer, or drives home on automatic pilot knows, such sensory–motor skills – dubbed *zombie behaviours* [134] – require rapid and sophisticated sensory processing. Confirming a long held belief among trainers, athletes performing their high-performance skills can do better under skill-irrelevant dual-tasks conditions (i.e., paying attention to tones) than when paying attention to their exhaustively trained behaviours [112].

The history of any scientific concept (e.g., energy, atom, gene) is one of increasing differentiation and sophistication until its essence can be explained in a quantitative and mechanistic manner in terms of elements operating at a lower, more elemental level. We are very far from this ideal in the inchoate science of consciousness. Yet functional considerations and the empirical and conceptual work of many scholars over the last decade make it clear that these psychological defined processes, top-down attention and consciousness, so often conflated, are not the same. One consequence of this distinction is that many of the neuronal correlates of consciousness (NCC) that have been reported are probably confounded by the neuronal correlates of attention [135, 136]. These empirical and functional considerations clear the deck for a neurobiological concerted attack on the core problem – that of identifying the necessary and sufficient neural causes of any one conscious percept.

QUESTIONS FOR FURTHER RESEARCH

1. When studying the NCC, great care must be taken to untangle the effects of top-down attention from those of consciousness [109, 137, 138]. Have the suggested NCC been confounded by attentional effects [131, 135, 136]?

2. Does perception of *gist*, a high-level semantic description of a scene (e.g., two people drinking, a man walking a dog), depend on focal, top-down attention? How good are people at describing the gist of novel, natural scenes under dual-tasks conditions?

3. What are the neuronal mechanisms that lead to improved zombie behaviours in the near-absence of top-down attention [112]? Do those aspects of reasoning, language processing and thinking that proceed in the absence of consciousness [7] function better without top-down attention?

4. Our arguments also apply for other modalities (e.g., hearing) although it might be more difficult to render tones perceptually silent. Are there robust techniques to manipulate consciousness in other modalities?

5. This review focuses on the selective filtering aspect of top-down attention and its relationship to consciousness. Another potential role for top-down attention is to bind features [139]. Some neurological evidence exists that binding can occur non-consciously [140]. It remains to be seen if normal subjects can bind features that are not consciously perceived.

6. Withdrawing attention reduces the rate of switching for ambiguous figures [59, 60]. What about the opposite direction of this causal relationship? Do subjects need to consciously perceive a bistable figure in order for it to switch back and forth?

ACKNOWLEDGEMENTS

We thank H. Berlin, R. Blake, N. Block, A. Cleeremans, S. He, Y. Jiang, R. Kanai, V. Lamme, C. Paffen, and M. Snodgrass for discussions. We thank the participants of our tutorial at ASSC10 in Oxford and at ASSC11 in Las Vegas for feedback. This research was supported by the NIMH, the NSF, the Keck Foundation, the Moore Foundation, and the Tom Slick Research Awards from the Mind Science Foundation.

References

1. Crick, F. and Koch, C. (2003) A framework for consciousness. *Nat Neurosci* 6:119–126.
2. Koch, C. (2004) *The Quest for Consciousness: A Neurobiological Approach*, Englewood, CO: Roberts and Publishers.
3. O'Regan, J.K. and Noe, A. (2001) A sensorimotor account of vision and visual consciousness. *Behav Brain Sci* 24:939–973. discussion 973–1031.
4. Posner, M.I. (1994) Attention: The mechanisms of consciousness. *Proc Natl Acad Sci USA* 91:7398–7403.
5. Velmans, M. (1996) *The Science of Consciousness*, London: Routledge.
6. Merikle, P.M. and Joordens, S. (1997) Parallels between perception without attention and perception without awareness. *Conscious Cogn* 6:219–236.
7. Jackendoff, R. (1996) How language helps us think. *Pragmatics Cogn* 4:1–34.

8. Prinz, J. (2004) *Gut Reactions*, New York: Oxford University Press.
9. Chun, M.M. and Wolfe, J.M. (2000). Visual attention. In Goldstein, E.B. (ed.) *Blackwell's Handbook of Perception* (Bla), pp. 272–310.
10. Wundt, W. (1874) *Grundzüge der physiologischen Psychologie*, Leipzig: Engelmann.
11. Iwasaki, S. (1993) Spatial attention and two modes of visual consciousness. *Cognition* 49:211–233.
12. Hardcastle, V.G. (1997) Attention versus consciousness: A distinction with a difference. *Cogn Stud Bull Japanese Cogn Sci Soc* 4:56–66.
13. Naccache, L., Blandin, E. and Dehaene, S. (2002) Unconscious masked priming depends on temporal attention. *Psychol Sci* 13:416–424.
14. Lamme, V.A. (2003) Why visual attention and awareness are different. *Trends Cogn Sci* 7:12–18.
15. Woodman, G.F. and Luck, S.J. (2003) Dissociations among attention, perception, and awareness during object-substitution masking. *Psychol Sci* 14:605–611.
16. Kentridge, R.W., Heywood, C.A. and Weiskrantz, L. (2004) Spatial attention speeds discrimination without awareness in blindsight. *Neuropsychologia* 42:831–835.
17. Baars, B.J. (2005) Global workspace theory of consciousness: Toward a cognitive neuroscience of human experience. *Prog Brain Res* 150:45–53.
18. Block, N. (2005) Two neural correlates of consciousness. *Trends Cogn Sci* 9:46–52.
19. Dehaene, S., Changeux, J.P., Naccache, L., Sackur, J. and Sergent, C. (2006) Conscious, preconscious, and subliminal processing: A testable taxonomy. *Trends Cogn Sci* 10:204–211.
20. Bachmann, T. (2006) A single metatheoretical framework for a number of conscious-vision phenomena. In Jing, Q. (ed.) *Psychological Science Around the World*, Vol. 1, pp. 229–242. Sussex: Psychology Press.
21. Baars, B.J. (1997) Some essential differences between consciousness and attention, perception, and working memory. *Conscious Cogn* 6:363–371.
22. Block, N. (1996) How can we find the neural correlate of consciousness? *Trends Neurosci* 19:456–459.
23. Chalmers, D.J. (1996) *The conscious mind: In search of a fundamental theory*, New York: Oxford University Press.
24. Tulving, E. (1993) Varieties of consciousness and levels of awareness in memory. In Baddeley, A. and Weiskrantz, L. (eds.) *Attention: Selection, Awareness and Control. A Tribute to Donald Broadbent*, pp. 283–299. Oxford: Oxford University Press.
25. Posner, M.I. and Petersen, S.E. (1990) The attention system of the human brain. *Annu Rev Neurosci* 13:25–42.
26. Bahrami, B., Lavie, N. and Rees, G. (2007) Attentional load modulates responses of human primary visual cortex to invisible stimuli. *Curr Biol* 17:509–513.
27. Tsushima, Y., Sasaki, Y. and Watanabe, T. (2006) Greater disruption due to failure of inhibitory control on an ambiguous distractor. *Science* 314:1786–1788.
28. Kunimoto, C., Miller, J. and Pashler, H. (2001) Confidence and accuracy of near-threshold discrimination responses. *Conscious Cogn* 10:294–340.
29. Persaud, N., McLeod, O. and Cowey, A. (2007) Post-decision wagering objectively measures awareness. *Nat Neurosci* 10:257–261.
30. James, W. (1890) *Principles of psychology*, London: MacMillan.
31. Braun, J. and Julesz, B. (1998) Withdrawing attention at little or no cost: Detection and discrimination tasks. *Percept Psychophys* 60:1–23.
32. Duncan, J. (1998) Converging levels of analysis in the cognitive neuroscience of visual attention. *Philos Trans R Soc Lond B Biol Sci* 353:1307–1317.

33. Itti, L. and Koch, C. (2001) Computational modelling of visual attention. *Nat Rev Neurosci* 2:194–203.
34. Parkhurst, D., Law, K. and Niebur, E. (2002) Modeling the role of salience in the allocation of overt visual attention. *Vis Res* 42:107–123.
35. Peters, R.J., Iyer, A., Itti, L. and Koch, C. (2005) Components of bottom-up gaze allocation in natural images. *Vis Res* 45:2397–2416.
36. Constantinidis, C. and Steinmetz, M.A. (2005) Posterior parietal cortex automatically encodes the location of salient stimuli. *J Neurosci* 25:233–238.
37. Thompson, K.G. and Bichot, N.P. (2005) A visual salience map in the primate frontal eye field. *Prog Brain Res* 147:251–262.
38. Henderson, J.M., Brockmole, J.R., Castelhano, M.S. and Mack, M. (2006). Visual Saliency does not account for Eye-Movements during Visual Search in Real-World Scenes. In Van Gompel, R., Fischer, M., Murray, W. and Hill, R. (eds.) *Eye Movement Research: Insights into Mind and Brain*. Elsevier.
39. Sperling, G. and Dosher, B. (1986) Strategy and optimization in human information processing. In Boff, K.R. Kaufman, L. and Thomas, J.P. (eds.) *Handbook of Perception and Human Performance* New York: pp. 1–65. Wiley.
40. VanRullen, R., Reddy, L. and Koch, C. (2004) Visual search and dual tasks reveal two distinct attentional resources. *J Cogn Neurosci* 16:4–14.
41. Posner, M.I., Snyder, C.R. and Davidson, B.J. (1980) Attention and the detection of signals. *J Exp Psychol* 109:160–174.
42. Jiang, Y., Costello, P., Fang, F., Huang, M. and He, S. (2006) A gender- and sexual orientation-dependent spatial attentional effect of invisible images. *Proc Natl Acad Sci USA* 103: 17048–17052.
43. McCormick, P.A. (1997) Orienting attention without awareness. *J Exp Psychol Hum* 23:168–180.
44. Rajimehr, R. (2004) Unconscious orientation processing. *Neuron* 41:663–673.
45. Sumner, P., Tsai, P.C., Yu, K. and Nachev, P. (2006) Attentional modulation of sensorimotor processes in the absence of perceptual awareness. *Proc Natl Acad Sci USA* 103:10520–10525.
46. Braun, J. and Sagi, D. (1990) Vision outside the focus of attention. *Percept Psychophys* 48:45–58.
47. Sato, W., Okada, T. and Toichi, M. (2007) Attentional shift by gaze is triggered without awareness. *Exp Brain Res* 183:87–94.
48. Li, F.E., VanRullen, R., Koch, C. and Perona, P. (2002) Rapid natural scene categorization in the near absence of attention. *Proc Natl Acad Sci USA* 99:9596–9601.
49. Reddy, L., Reddy, L. and Koch, C. (2006) Face identification in the near-absence of focal attention. *Vis Res* 46:2336–2343.
50. Reddy, L., Wilken, P. and Koch, C. (2004) Face-gender discrimination is possible in the near-absence of attention. *J Vis* 4:106–117.
51. Braun, J. (1998) Vision and attention: The role of training. *Nature* 393:424–425.
52. Joseph, J.S., Chun, M.M. and Nakayama, K. (1997) Attentional requirements in a 'preattentive' feature search task. *Nature* 387:805–807.
53. Driver, J. and Mattingley, J.B. (1998) Parietal neglect and visual awareness. *Nat Neurosci* 1:17–22.
54. Raymond, J.E., Shapiro, K.L. and Arnell, K.M. (1992) Temporary suppression of visual processing in an RSVP task: An attentional blink? *J Exp Psychol Hum Percept Perform* 18:849–860.
55. Chun, M.M. and Potter, M.C. (1995) A two-stage model for multiple target detection in rapid serial visual presentation. *J Exp Psychol Hum Percept Perform* 21:109–127.
56. Mack, A. and Rock, I. (1998) *Inattentional blindness*, Cambridge, MA: MIT Press.

57. Simons, D.J. and Rensink, R.A. (2005) Change blindness: Past, present, and future. *Trends Cogn Sci* 9:16–20.

58. Anderson, A.K. and Phelps, E.A. (2001) Lesions of the human amygdala impair enhanced perception of emotionally salient events. *Nature* 411:305–309.

59. Pastukhov, A. and Braun, J. (2007) Perceptual reversals need no prompting by attention. *J Vis* .

60. Paffen, C.L., Alais, D. and Verstraten, F.A. (2006) Attention speeds binocular rivalry. *Psychol Sci* 17:752–756.

61. Koch, C. and Tsuchiya, N. (2007) Attention and consciousness: Two distinct brain processes. *Trends Cogn Sci* 11:16–22.

62. Hofstoetter, C., Koch, C. and Kiper, D.C. (2004) Motion-induced blindness does not affect the formation of negative afterimages. *Conscious Cogn* 13:691–708.

63. Tsuchiya, N. and Koch, C. (2005) Continuous flash suppression reduces negative afterimages. *Nat Neurosci* 8:1096–1101.

64. Gilroy, L.A. and Blake, R. (2005) The interaction between binocular rivalry and negative afterimages. *Curr Biol* 15:1740–1744.

65. Macknik, S.L. and Livingstone, M.S. (1998) Neuronal correlates of visibility and invisibility in the primate visual system. *Nat Neurosci* 1:144–149.

66. Tsuchiya, N., Koch, C., Gilroy, L.A. and Blake, R. (2006) Depth of interocular suppression associated with continuous flash suppression, flash suppression, and binocular rivalry. *J Vis* 6:1068–1078.

67. Kim, C.Y. and Blake, R. (2005) Psychophysical magic: Rendering the visible 'invisible'. *Trends Cogn Sci* 9:381–388.

68. Sperling, G. (1960) The information available in brief visual presentations. *Psychol Monogr* 74:1–29.

69. Landman, R., Spekreijse, H. and Lamme, V.A. (2003) Large capacity storage of integrated objects before change blindness. *Vis Res* 43:149–164.

70. Wolfe, J.M. (1999) Inattentional amnesia. In Coltheart, V. (eds.) *Fleeting Memories* Cambridge, MA: pp. 71–94. MIT Press.

71. Galvin, S.J., Podd, J.V., Drga, V. and Whitmore, J. (2003) Type 2 tasks in the theory of signal detectability: Discrimination between correct and incorrect decisions. *Psychon Bull Rev* 10:843–876.

72. Kolb, F.C. and Braun, J. (1995) Blindsight in normal observers. *Nature* 377:336–338.

73. Wilimzig, C., Tsuchiya, N., Fahle, M., Einhäuser, W. and Koch, C. (2008) Spatial attention increases performance but not subjective confidence in a discrimination task. *J Vis* 8.5:1–10.

74. Szczepanowski, R. and Pessoa, L. (2007) Fear perception: can objective and subjective awareness measures be dissociated? *J Vis* 7:10.

75. Maia, T.V. and McClelland, J.L. (2004) A reexamination of the evidence for the somatic marker hypothesis: What participants really know in the Iowa gambling task. *Proc Natl Acad Sci USA* 101:16075–16080.

76. Clifford, C.W., Arabzadeh, E. and Harris, J.A. (2008) Getting technical about awareness. *Trends Cogn Sci* 12:54–58.

77. Schurger, A. and Sher, S. (2008) Awareness, loss aversion, and post-decision wagering. *Trends Cogn Sci* 12:209–210.

78. He, S., Cavanagh, P. and Intriligator, J. (1996) Attentional resolution and the locus of visual awareness. *Nature* 383:334–337.

79. Montaser-Kouhsari, L. and Rajimehr, R. (2004) Attentional modulation of adaptation to illusory lines. *J Vis* 4:434–444.

80. Kentridge, R.W., Nijboer, T.C. and Heywood, C.A. (2008) Attended but unseen: visual attention is not sufficient for visual awareness. *Neuropsychologia* 46:864–869.

81. Bahrami, B., Carmel, D. Walsh, V., Rees, G. and Lavie, N. (2008) Unconscious orientation processing depends on perceptual load. *J. Vis* 8 12:10–1.

82. Kentridge, R.W., Heywood, C.A. and Weiskrantz, L. (1999) Attention without awareness in blindsight. *Proc R Soc Lond B Biol Sci* 266:1805–1811.

83. Kentridge, R.W., Heywood, C.A. and Weiskrantz, L. (1999) Effects of temporal cueing on residual visual discrimination in blindsight. *Neuropsychologia* 37:479–483.

84. Melcher, D., Papathomas, T.V. and Vidnyanszky, Z. (2005) Implicit attentional selection of bound visual features. *Neuron* 46:723–729.

85. Kanai, R., Tsuchiya, N. and Verstraten, F.A. (2006) The scope and limits of top-down attention in unconscious visual processing. *Curr Biol*.

86. Biederman, I. (1972) Perceiving real-world scenes. Science 177:77–80.

87. Fei-Fei, L., Iyer, A., Koch, C. and Perona, P. (2007) What do we perceive in a glance of a real-world scene? *J Vis* 7:10.

88. Desimone, R. and Duncan, J. (1995) Neural mechanisms of selective visual attention. *Annu Rev Neurosci* 18:193–222.

89. Thorpe, S., Fize, D. and Marlot, C. (1996) Speed of processing in the human visual system. *Nature* 381:520–522.

90. Kirchner, H. and Thorpe, S.J. (2006) Ultra-rapid object detection with saccadic eye movements: Visual processing speed revisited. *Vis Res* 46:1762–1776.

91. VanRullen, R., Delorme, A. and Thorpe, S.J. (2001) Feed-forward contour integration in primary visual cortex based on asynchronous spike propagation. *Neurocomputing* 38:1003–1009.

92. VanRullen, R. and Koch, C. (2003) Visual selective behavior can be triggered by a feed-forward process. *J Cogn Neurosci* 15:209–217.

93. Rousselet, G.A., Fabre-Thorpe, M. and Thorpe, S.J. (2002) Parallel processing in high-level categorization of natural images. *Nat Neurosci* 5:629–630.

94. Einhauser, W., Mundhenk, T.N., Baldi, P., Koch, C. and Itti, L. (2007) A bottom-up model of spatial attention predicts human error patterns in rapid scene recognition. *J Vis* 7:1–13.

95. Serre, T., Oliva, A. and Poggio, T. (2007) A feedforward architecture accounts for rapid categorization. *Proc Natl Acad Sci USA* 104:6424–6429.

96. Olivers, C.N. and Nieuwenhuis, S. (2005) The beneficial effect of concurrent task-irrelevant mental activity on temporal attention. *Psychol Sci* 16:265–269.

97. Wong, E. and Weisstein, N. (1982) A new perceptual context-superiority effect: Line segments are more visible against a figure than against a ground. *Science* 218:587–589.

98. Wong, E. and Weisstein, N. (1983) Sharp targets are detected better against a figure, and blurred targets are detected better against a background. *J Exp Psychol Hum Percept Perform* 9:194–201.

99. Yeshurun, Y. and Carrasco, M. (1998) Attention improves or impairs visual performance by enhancing spatial resolution. *Nature* 396:72–75.

100. Reber, (1976) Implicit learning of synthetic languages: The role of instructional set. *J Exp Psych Hum Lean Mem* 2:88–94.

101. Luck, S.J., Vogel, E.K. and Shapiro, K.L. (1996) Word meanings can be accessed but not reported during the attentional blink. *Nature* 383:616–618.

102. Vogel, E.K., Luck, S.J. and Shapiro, K.L. (1998) Electrophysiological evidence for a postperceptual locus of suppression during the attentional blink. *J Exp Psychol Hum Percept Perform* 24:1656–1674.

103. Dehaene, S., Naccache, L., Le Clec, H.G., Koechlin, E., Mueller, M., Dehaene-Lambertz, G., van de Moortele, P.F. and Le Bihan, D. (1998) Imaging unconscious semantic priming. *Nature* 395:597–600.

104. Jiang, Y., Zhou, K. and He, S. (2007) Human visual cortex responds to invisible chromatic flicker. *Nat Neurosci* 10:657–662.

105. Wyart, V. and Tallon-Baudry, C. (2008) Neural dissociation between visual awareness and spatial attention. *J Neurosci* 28:2667–2679.

106. Schurger, A., Cowey, A., Cohen, J.D., Treisman, A. and Tallon-Baudry, C. (2008) Distinct and independent correlates of attention and awareness in a hemianopic patient. *Neuropsychologia* 46:2189–2197.

107. Koivisto, M., Revonsuo, A. and Lehtonen, M. (2005) Independence of visual awareness from the scope of attention: An Electrophysiological study. *Cereb Cortex* .

108. Koivisto, M., Revonsuo, A. and Salminen, N. (2005) Independence of visual awareness from attention at early processing stages. *Neuroreport* 16:817–821.

109. Lee, S.H., Blake, R. and Heeger, D.J. (2007) Hierarchy of cortical responses underlying binocular rivalry. *Nat Neurosci* 10:1048–1054.

110. Enns, J.T. and Di Lollo, V. (2000) What's new in visual masking? *Trends Cogn Sci* 4:345–352.

111. Lee, D.K., Itti, L., Koch, C. and Braun, J. (1999) Attention activates winner-take-all competition among visual filters. *Nat Neurosci* 2:375–381.

112. Beilock, S.L., Carr, T.H., MacMahon, C. and Starkes, J.L. (2002) When paying attention becomes counterproductive: Impact of divided versus skill-focused attention on novice and experienced performance of sensorimotor skills. *J Exp Psychol Appl* 8:6–16.

113. Lou, L. (2001) Effects of voluntary attention on structured afterimages. *Perception* 30:1439–1448.

114. Suzuki, S. and Grabowecky, M. (2003) Attention during adaptation weakens negative afterimages. *J Exp Psychol Hum Percept Perform* 29:793–807.

115. Wede, J. and Francis, G. (2007) Attentional effects on afterimages: Theory and data. *Vis Res* 47:2249–2258.

116. Orbach, J., Ehrlich, D. and Heath, H.A. (1963) Reversibility of the Necker cube. I. An examination of the concept of 'satiation of orientation'. *Percept Mot Skills* 17:439–458.

117. Leopold, D.A., Wilke, M., Maier, A. and Logothetis, N.K. (2002) Stable perception of visually ambiguous patterns. *Nat Neurosci* 5:605–609.

118. Kanai, R. and Verstraten, F.A. (2006) Attentional modulation of perceptual stabilization. *Proc Biol Sci* 273:1217–1222.

119. Dijksterhuis, A., Bos, M.W., Nordgren, L.F. and van Baaren, R.B. (2006) On making the right choice: The deliberation-without-attention effect. *Science* 311:1005–1007.

120. Berlin H. A. (in press) Neurobiological explanations of the dynamic unconscious. *Impuls – Journal of Pychology*.

121. Block, N. (2007) Consciousness, accessibility, and the mesh between psychology and neuroscience. *Behav Brain Sci* .

122. Crick, F. and Koch, C. (1998) Consciousness and neuroscience. *Cereb Cortex* 8:97–107.

123. Koch, C. and Tsuchiya, N. (2007) Phenomenology without conscious access is a form of consciousness without top-down attention. *Behavioral and Brain Sciences* 30:509–510.

124. Dehaene, S., Sergent, C. and Changeux, J.P. (2003) A neuronal network model linking subjective reports and objective physiological data during conscious perception. *Proc Natl Acad Sci USA* 100:8520–8525.

125. Tononi, G. and Edelman, G.M. (1998) Consciousness and complexity. *Science* 282:1846–1851.

126. Lamme, V.A. and Roelfsema, P.R. (2000) The distinct modes of vision offered by feedforward and recurrent processing. *Trends Neurosci* 23:571–579.

127. Haynes, J.D. and Rees, G. (2005) Predicting the orientation of invisible stimuli from activity in human primary visual cortex. *Nat Neurosci* 8:686–691.

128. Crick, F. and Koch, C. (1995) Are we aware of neural activity in primary visual cortex? *Nature* 375:121–123.

129. Braun, J., Koch, C. and Davis, J.L. (2001) *Visual attention and cortical circuits*, MIT press.

130. Crick, F. and Koch, C. (1998) Constraints on cortical and thalamic projections: The no-strong-loops hypothesis. *Nature* 391:245–250.

131. Crick, F.C. and Koch, C. (2005) What is the function of the claustrum? *Philos Trans R Soc Lond B Biol Sci* 360:1271–1279.

132. Lamme, V.A. (2006) Towards a true neural stance on consciousness. *Trends Cogn Sci* 10:494–501.

133. Goodale, M.A. and Milner, D.A. (2004) *Sight Unseen: An Exploration of Conscious and Unconscious Vision*, Oxford, UK: Oxford University Press.

134. Koch, C. and Crick, F. (2001) The zombie within. *Nature* 411:893.

135. Macknik, S.L. and Martinez-Conde, S. (2007). Neurophysiology of visual awareness. *New Encyclopedia of Neuroscience*.

136. Macknik, S.L. and Martinez-Conde, S. (2007) The role of feedback in visual masking and visual processing. *Adv Cogn Psychol*.

137. Huk, A.C., Ress, D. and Heeger, D.J. (2001) Neuronal basis of the motion aftereffect reconsidered. *Neuron* 32:161–172.

138. Tse, P.U., Martinez-Conde, S., Schlegel, A.A. and Macknik, S.L. (2005) Visibility, visual awareness, and visual masking of simple unattended targets are confined to areas in the occipital cortex beyond human V1/V2. *Proc Natl Acad Sci USA* 102:17178–17183.

139. Treisman, A.M. and Gelade, G. (1980) A feature-integration theory of attention. *Cogn Psychol* 12:97–136.

140. Wojciulik, E. and Kanwisher, N. (1998) Implicit visual attribute binding following bilateral parietal damage. *Vis Cogn* 5:157–181.

WAKING, SLEEP AND ANAESTHESIA

Intrinsic Brain Activity and Consciousness

Marcus E. Raichle, Abraham Z. Snyder

ABSTRACT

Two perspectives on brain function exist. One posits that the brain is primarily reflexive, with its activity evoked by demands of the environment. The other view is that the brain's operations are mainly intrinsic involving the maintenance of information for interpreting, responding to and predicting environmental demands. The former has motivated most neuroscience research including that with functional neuroimaging. Yet, when examined in terms of the brain's enormous energy budget, 60–80% of which is devoted to function, evoked activity including conscious perception makes a very small contribution (<5%). Given the complexity attributed to realization of consciousness it seems reasonable to ask whether the brain's intrinsic activity might serve to enable conscious perception and account for the complexity attributed to it. We approach this question from the perspective of functional neuroimaging.

BACKGROUND

The human brain is approximately 2% of the weight of the body and yet accounts for 20% of its energy consumption (for a review of this and other features of the cost of brain function see [1]). It has been estimated that upwards of 80% of this energy consumption is used to support neuronal signalling, implying that most of the energy consumed is used for functional activities. Stimulus and performance-evoked changes in brain energy consumption are surprisingly small by comparison (typically <5%) and rarely change overall brain energy consumption significantly. It is reasonable to assume that changes in brain energy consumption associated with stimulus independent thoughts (e.g., day dreaming) likewise would be small.

Because the vast majority of studies designed to study brain function have focused on stimulus or task-related changes it follows that most of our knowledge of brain function comes from studying a minor component of functional brain activity. It seems reasonable to ask how consciousness might relate to this apparent dichotomy between processes of which we are aware, provoked either by internal or external events, vs. the largely unaccounted, for functional activities of the brain. Thus, we here use 'consciousness' in the sense of subjective awareness.

Two points seem relevant to such a discussion. First, early attempts to estimate the 'bandwidth' of conscious perception arrived at surprisingly small values [2]. The numbers obtained were on the order of 10^2 bits per second or less. For comparison, incoming sensory information can be as high as 10^7 bits per second. On this view, consciousness would seem to demand a share of the brain's energy budget that is approximately equivalent to that of any type of spontaneous or evoked functional activity and, therefore, a relatively modest component of brain function from a cost perspective. However, there is another important factor to be considered.

Second, theories of consciousness have posited that realizing a conscious state depends on the existence of an organized repertoire of potential conscious states [3]. Consciousness may be viewed as a trajectory through this rich repertoire driven by changing environmental contingencies as well as internal brain states. Thus, while conscious awareness is a low bandwidth phenomenon and therefore energetically inexpensive, it is dependent upon a very complex, dynamically organized, non-conscious state of the brain that is achieved at great expense. Here we provide a view of the brain's intrinsic functional activity from the perspective of functional brain imaging studies in humans that we believe may provide some insight into this possibility.

BRAIN IMAGING

Brain imaging research, first with positron emission tomography (PET) and later with functional magnetic resonance imaging (fMRI) was provoked to focus on intrinsic activity when activity decreases (deactivations) were serendipitously noticed during task performance even when the control state was resting quietly with eyes closed [4]. This observation led to the conceptualization of a physiological baseline and the identification of a default mode of brain function [5, 6]. More recently attention has turned to an intense scrutiny of spontaneous fluctuations (noise) in the fMRI blood oxygen level dependent (BOLD) signal [7]. The result of all this work has revealed a remarkable systems level *functional* organization of the brain that transcends levels of consciousness. We posit that this represents the functional connectome of the brain and, as such, the backbone of consciousness. We view this as an extension of the concept of a 'Human Connectome' as proposed by Sporns, Tononi and Kötter [8]. Whereas the originally proposed connectome was an anatomical concept, we suggest that consciousness arises out of and is dependent on relationships among brain areas within networks defined on functional criteria.

We begin with a discussion of activity decreases as they first appeared in early functional brain imaging studies.

ACTIVITY DECREASES

Functional neuroimaging began with studies of the brain's responses to carefully controlled sensory, cognitive and motor events [9]. Such experiments fit well with the view of the brain as driven by the momentary environmental demands. The study of human cognition with neuroimaging was aided greatly by the involvement of cognitive psychologists in the 1980s whose experimental strategies for dissecting human behaviours fit well with the emerging capabilities of functional brain imaging [9]. Subtracting functional images acquired in a task state from ones acquired in a control state was a natural extension of mental chronometry [10] in which one measures the time required to complete specific mental operations isolated by the careful selection of task and control states. This approach, in various forms, has dominated the cognitive neuroscience agenda ever since with remarkably productive results.

For the better part of a decade following the introduction of subtractive methodology to neuroimaging, the vast majority of changes reported in the literature were activity increases or *activations* as they were almost universally called. Activity increases but not decreases are expected in subtractions of a control condition from a task condition as long as the *assumption of pure insertion* is valid. To illustrate, using an example based on mental chronometry, say that one's control task requires a key press to a simple stimulus such as the appearance of a point of light in the visual field, whereas the task state of interest requires a decision about the colour of the light prior to the key press. Assuming pure insertion, the response latency difference between conditions is interpretable as the time needed to perform a colour discrimination. However, the time needed to press a key might be affected by the nature of the decision process itself, violating the assumption of pure insertion. More generally, the brain state underlying any action could have been altered by the introduction of an additional process. Interestingly, functional neuroimaging helped address the question of pure insertion by employing the device of *reverse subtraction*. Thus, in certain circumstances subtracting task-state data from control-state data revealed negative responses, or *task-specific deactivations* (for examples and further discussion of this interesting issue see [11–13]). It was clearly shown, just as psychologists had suspected, that processes active in a control state could be modified when paired with a particular task.

The notion of a default mode of brain function originated from the persistent observation of activity decreases in subtraction images even when the control state was either visual fixation or eyes closed rest. What particularly caught our attention was the fact that, regardless of the task under investigation, the activity decreases almost always included the posterior cingulate and adjacent precuneus as well as dorsal and ventral medial prefrontal cortex [4].

The first formal characterization of task-induced activity decreases from our laboratory [4] generated a set of iconic images (Figure 7.1A) whose unique identity was subsequently replicated in later meta-analyses by Jeffery Binder and colleagues at the Medical College of Wisconsin [14] and Bernard Mazoyer and his colleagues [15] in France. Similar observations are now an everyday occurrence in laboratories throughout the world leaving little doubt that a specific set of brain areas decrease their activity across a remarkably wide array of task conditions when compared to a passive control condition such as visual fixation.

The finding of a network of brain areas that consistently decreased its activity during task performance (Figure 7.1A) was both surprising and challenging. Surprising because the areas involved had not previously been recognized as a system in the same way we might think of the motor or visual system. And, challenging because initially it was unclear what cognitive significance should be assigned to activity in a passive or resting condition. A prevailing sentiment was that it likely represented unconstrained cognition of a type that should be minimized by using a proper control condition for the task of interest. One would anticipate, however, if that were the case such activity would vary randomly across individuals, a hypothesis at odds with the spatial consistency of the activity decreases (Figure 7.1A). The work of Nancy

Andreasen and colleagues [16] presciently characterized this 'uncensored thinking' as random episodic memory that reflected both the active retrieval of past experiences and planning of future experiences necessary for one to experience personal identity, consciousness and self-awareness. Interestingly they associated these unconstrained processes with what later turned out to be the default network (Figure 7.1A).

The necessity of determining whether or not these task-induced activity decreases were simply 'activations' present in the resting state or something more fundamental in terms of brain organization remained for us an important and challenging question. In wrestling with this difficult issue two things came to mind that, together, we felt offered us an opportunity to move forward.

First, quantitative circulatory and metabolic PET studies demonstrated that during task-induced activity increases above a resting state, blood flow increased more than oxygen consumption [17, 18]. As a result the amount of oxygen in blood increased locally as the ratio of oxygen consumed to oxygen delivered falls. This ratio is known as the oxygen extraction fraction or the *OEF*. Activation then can be physiologically defined as a transient local decrease in the oxygen extraction or, equivalently, a transient increase in oxygen availability. The practical consequence of this observation was to lay the *physiological* groundwork for fMRI using BOLD contrast (i.e., MRI is sensitive to the level of blood oxygenation [19–22]). Using this quantitative definition of activation we were in a position to ask whether 'activations' were present in a passive state such as visual fixation or eyes closed rest. However, activation must be defined relative to something. How was that to be accomplished if there was no 'control' state for eyes closed rest or visual fixation?

The definition of a control state for eyes closed rest or visual fixation arose from a *second* critical piece of physiological information. Researchers using PET for the quantitative measurement of brain oxygen consumption and blood flow had long appreciated the fact that, across the entire brain, blood flow and oxygen consumption are closely matched at rest (see [23] for one of the earliest references; also [5]). This match is observed throughout the brain despite a nearly four-fold difference in oxygen consumption and blood flow between grey and white matter and variations in both measurements of greater than 30% within grey matter itself. As a result of this close matching of blood flow and oxygen consumption at rest, the OEF is uniform throughout the brain with the exception (modest) of the visual cortex [5]. This well-established observation led us to the hypothesis that if this observation (a uniform

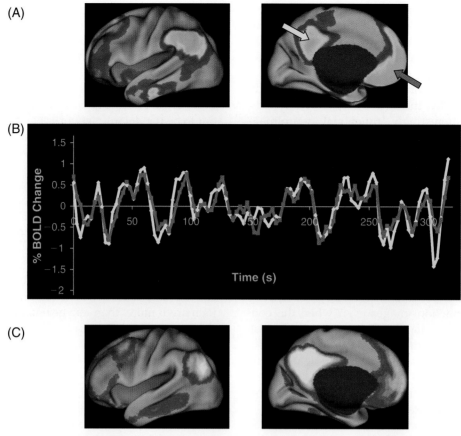

FIGURE 7.1   Brain areas consistently exhibiting activity decreases during task performance also exhibit coherent spontaneous activity in the resting state. Performance of a wide variety of tasks has called attention to a group of brain areas (A) that decrease their activity during task performance (data adapted from [4]). This particular group of brain areas has come to be known as the 'default network' and serves as an exemplar of all areas of the cerebral cortex which exhibit a systems level organization in the resting (default) state [7]. If one records the spontaneous fMRI BOLD signal activity in these areas (arrows, A) in the resting state what emerges is a remarkable correlation in the spontaneous fluctuations of the fMRI BOLD signals obtained from the two areas (B). Using these fluctuations to analyse the network as a whole [7] reveals a level of functional organization (C) that parallels that seen in the task-related activity decreases (A). These data provide a dramatic demonstration of the intrinsic organization of the human brain which likely provides a critical context for all human behaviours including conscious awareness. These data were adapted from our earlier published work [4–6, 24].

OEF at rest) was correct then activations, as defined above, were likely absent in the resting state [5]. We decided to test this hypothesis.

Using PET to quantitatively assess regional OEF, we examined two groups of normal subjects in the resting state and initially confined our analysis to those areas of the brain frequently exhibiting the aforementioned imaging signal decreases (Figure 7.1A). In this analysis we found no evidence that these areas were activated in the resting state; that is, the *average* OEF in these areas did not differ significantly from other areas of the brain. We concluded that the regional decreases, observed commonly during task performance, represented the presence of functionality that was ongoing (i.e., sustained as contrasted to transiently activated) in the resting state and attenuated only when resources were temporarily reallocated

during goal-directed behaviours; hence our original designation of them as *default functions* [5]. Thus, from a metabolic/physiologic perspective, these areas (Figure 7.1A) could not be distinguished from other areas of the brain in the resting state.

While the notion of default functionality first arose in connection with a specific set of cortical regions, now widely referred to as the default system or network (Figure 7.1A), it has since become clear that organized functional activity is a ubiquitous property of neural tissue throughout the brain at all times. Task-specific decreases from a resting state occur in many areas of the brain [25–30]. Importantly, recent work has provided direct evidence that these activity decreases represent decreases in neuronal activity [31].

Having arrived at the view that the brain has an organized default mode of function through our analysis of activity decreases, we began to take seriously claims that there was likely much more to brain function than that revealed by momentary demands of the environment. Two bodies of information have been especially persuasive.

First was the cost of intrinsic functional activity which far exceeds that of evoked activity and dominates the overall cost of brain function (see 'Background'; also [1]). Second was the remarkable degree of functional organization exhibited by intrinsic activity. For us this organization was first revealed in the activity decreases we have been discussing (Figure 7.1A). Reinforcing this view of a default mode of brain function have been the dramatic patterns of activity revealed in the analysis of the 'noise' in the fMRI BOLD signal.

'NOISE' IN THE FMRI BOLD SIGNAL

A prominent feature of fMRI is that the unaveraged signal is quite noisy (Figure 7.1B) prompting researchers to average their data to increase the signal to noise ratio in task-related fMRI responses. As it turns out, a considerable fraction of the variance in the BOLD signal in the frequency range below 0.1 Hz appears to reflect spontaneous fluctuating neural activity that exhibits striking patterns of coherence within known brain systems (Figure 7.1C) even in the absence of observable behaviours associated with those systems.

While spatial patterns of coherence in resting-state fluctuations of the fMRI BOLD signal were first noted by Biswal and colleagues in 1995 in their studies of the somatomotor cortex of humans [32], it was for us the observation of Greicius and colleagues of resting-state coherence in the default network [33] that ignited our interest. As can be seen in Figure 7.1C, the pattern of resting-state coherence in the fMRI BOLD signal faithfully recapitulates a pattern introduced to us as activity decreases during goal-directed behaviours, the so-called default network (Figure 7.1A).

Since these early observations, there has been an exponential increase in the number of studies of resting-state functional connectivity based on spontaneous fluctuations of the fMRI BOLD signal. A recent comprehensive review summarizes much of this work [7] which includes descriptions of coherent patterns of activity within most major cortical systems in the human brain. Several features of this activity deserve special mention in the present context.

While the major focus of work in this area has been on patterns of coherence within the elements of a system (e.g., the default network; Figure 7.1C) it is also

the case that anticorrelations between systems have also been noted. A dramatic representation of example was observed between the default network and what we dubbed the 'task-positive' network [24] consisting of elements of the dorsal attention system [34] and a control system used in establishing task set [35, 36]. Recall that decreases in the activity of the default network regularly occur during task performance when the dorsal attention system and associated control systems are engaged in task performance. What this observation suggests is that relationships between brain systems observed during task performance are, at least in this instance, reflected in the relationship of their spontaneous activity in the absence of a task, an observation that underscores the integrative nature of the underlying process. Interestingly, using a computational/simulation approach to understanding the neuronal dynamics of interregional connections in the monkey cortex, Honey and colleagues [37] demonstrate two anticorrelated clusters linked by prefrontal and parietal regions that are hub nodes in the underlying structural networks.

Several observations (e.g., see [38–40]) have now confirmed that the spontaneous activity reflected in the fMRI BOLD signal persists during task performance albeit modified in some cases [38]. More surprising, however, is that the spatially coherent spontaneous activity of the fMRI BOLD signal persists despite major changes in levels of consciousness. For example, in the anaesthetized monkey [41] spatially coherent spontaneous activity can be demonstrated in the oculomotor (Figure 7.2), somatomotor and visual systems as well as in elements of the default network. These observations are complimented by recent work in humans during sleep [42] where, again, patterns of spatial coherence in the fMRI BOLD signal are seen.

The persistence of this spatially coherent activity during task performance as well as across widely differing brain states seems to set it apart from much work in neurophysiology [43] where patterns of coherence typically appear in the context of a task. These task-induced patterns appear to represent the emergence of a '… unified cognitive moment' [44]. From a neurophysiologic perspective these 'cognitive moments' arise in the context of highly complex, ongoing (i.e., spontaneous) neural activity representing an ever changing balance between excitation and inhibition [45]. While much work remains to be done one is left with the impression presently that coherent, spontaneous fluctuations in the fMRI BOLD (Figure 7.1B) as well as infra-slow cortical activity observed with direct current (DC) electroencephalography [46] exhibit a temporal stationarity that distinguishes it

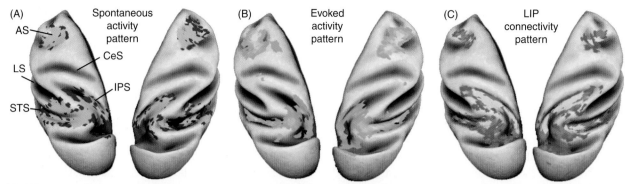

FIGURE 7.2   Cortical patterns of coherent spontaneous BOLD fluctuations are similar to those of task-evoked responses and anatomical connectivity. (A) Conjunction map of BOLD correlations within the oculomotor system on dorsal views of the monkey atlas left and right hemisphere surfaces. Voxels significantly correlated with three (dark blue) or four (light blue) oculomotor ROIs are shown. (B) Activation pattern evoked by performance of a saccadic eye movement task (average of two monkeys; adapted from [47]). (C) Density of cells labelled by retrograde tracer injections in right LIP (average of three monkeys; adapted from [48]). *Source*: This figure is from [49] with permission.

from the state-dependent, non-stationarity of most other recordings of coherent brain activity [44, 50].

A question that has arisen regarding these spontaneous fluctuations in the fMRI BOLD signal is their relationship to anatomical connectivity. At present we have only a partial answer to this question. Our studies in the anaesthetized monkey indicate quite clearly that mono-synaptic connectivity is not required (see Figures 3 and S7 in [49]). Additionally, it should be noted that development of these patterns of coherence in the human brain continues from childhood through young adulthood [51, 52] despite the fact that connections within the brain are stable during this time. Experience-induced changes in the efficacy of synapses within and among brain networks could well play an important role in sculpting lines of communication within elements of a network of functionally related brain areas.

Another factor in sculpting the patterns of spatially coherent activity exhibited by spontaneous fluctuations in the fMRI BOLD signal could be the ongoing input received by neurons. Neurons continuously receive both excitatory and inhibitory inputs [53]. The 'balance' of these stimuli determines the responsiveness (or gain) of neurons to correlated inputs and, in so doing, routes information flow in the brain [54–57]. Balance is also observed at a large systems level. For example, neurologists know that strokes damaging cortical centres controlling eye movements lead to deviation of the eyes toward the side of the lesion implying the pre-existing presence of 'balance'. Another well-known example first demonstrated in the visual system of the cat is the Sprague effect [58].

Thus, it may be that in the normal brain our genetically endowed anatomical connectivity is sculpted into a 'functional connectome' by processes of a type posited by Hebb many years ago [59] involving an interaction between spontaneous and evoked activity that begins in the embryo and extends into adulthood.

A CONCEPTUAL FRAMEWORK

At the present time it is not possible to formulate a comprehensive theory of the role of the spatially coherent brain activity reflected in the spontaneous fluctuations of the fMRI BOLD signal. Because it transcend levels of consciousness it must represent a fundamental level of brain functional organization and, if cost estimates are correct (see 'Background'), one that is of vital importance to the operation of the system. It seems to us reasonable to posit that it provides a backbone upon which the 'cognitive moments' of our conscious awareness are realized. We find an example from some of our recent work instructive in this regard.

FUTURE QUESTIONS

Many questions remain to be answered as we pursue an understanding of the brain's intrinsic activity which we view as one of the great challenges of neuroscience. We enumerate a few of them from the perspective of the work we have presented in this chapter.

What is the nature of the electrical activity associated with the spontaneous fluctuations in the fMRI BOLD signal? Our understanding of these patterns of brain activity is critically dependent on elucidating the underlying neurophysiology. Do they represent, for example, spontaneous variations in cortical excitability equivalent in some way to so-called up and down states [60–62].

Why do we see spatially coherent fluctuations in the fMRI BOLD signal? This is a question that for us goes to the heart of our understanding of the BOLD signal. Most see the BOLD signal as arising from a discrepancy between changes in blood flow and oxygen consumption with the former being greater than the latter. Often overlooked is the fact that the blood flow changes are accompanied by changes in glucose utilization independent of oxygen consumption [18]. This excess glycolysis is usually attributed to the energy needed to remove glutamate into astrocytes from synapses (for a recent review see [1]). However, it has been pointed out that glycolysis may also be playing an important role at the synapse [63]. In this regard it should be recalled that glycolysis not only provides substrate for oxidative phosphorylation but also carbon fragments for the synthesis of proteins and lipids. As Eve Marder has pointed out [64] 'the ion channels and receptors that underlie electrical signalling and synaptic transmission turn over in the membrane in minutes, hours, days and weeks'. That being the case, glycolysis may be playing a critical role in providing the metabolic precursors for this process. The 'glycolytic window' through which we view the brain with neuroimaging may well be providing a unique view of the brain's functional backbone, how it is instantiated, maintained and modified. We believe that such information will be critical to an understanding of how the brain instantiates consciousness.

Finally, how might we use information on the brain's functional connectome to evaluate altered states of consciousness? One of the practical consequences of being able to interrogate the brain's activity in the manner presented herein is that it does not require a task to be performed. The information arises out of the brain's spontaneous activity. Elimination of the need for a task makes comparisons between patients and controls as well as individual patients in different states of alertness feasible. We are optimistic that using this approach will add a new dimension to the study of consciousness in patients.

References

1. Raichle, M.E. and Mintun, M.A. (2006) Brain work and brain imaging. *Annu Rev Neurosci* 29:449–476.
2. Norretranders, T. (1998) *The User Illusion*, New York: Viking.
3. Tononi, G. and Edelman, G.M. (1998) Consciousness and complexity. *Science* 282 (5395):1846–1851.
4. Shulman, G.L., *et al.* (1997) Common blood flow changes across visual tasks: II. Decreases in cerebral cortex. *J Cogn Neurosci* 9 (5):648–663.
5. Raichle, M.E., *et al.* (2001) A default mode of brain function. *Proc Natl Acad Sci USA* 98 (2):676–682.
6. Gusnard, D.A. and Raichle, M.E. (2001) Searching for a baseline: Functional imaging and the resting human brain. *Nat Rev Neurosci* 2 (10):685–694.
7. Fox, M.D. and Raichle, M. (2007) Spontaneous fluctuations in brain activity observed with functional magnetic resonance imaging. *Nat Rev Neurosci* 8:700–711.
8. Sporns, O. and Honey, C.J. (2006) Small worlds inside big brains. *Proc Natl Acad Sci USA* 103 (51):19219–19220.
9. Posner, M. and Raichle, M. (1994) *Images of Mind*, New York: W. H. Freeman and Company, Scientific American Library.
10. Posner, M. (1986) *Chronometric Explorations of Mind*, New York: Oxford University Press.
11. Raichle, M.E. (1998) Behind the scenes of functional brain imaging: A historical and physiological perspective. *Proc Natl Acad Sci USA* 95 (3):765–772.
12. Petersen, S.E., *et al.* (1998) The effects of practice on the functional anatomy of task performance. *Proc Natl Acad Sci USA* 95 (3):853–860.
13. Raichle, M.E., *et al.* (1994) Practice-related changes in human brain functional anatomy during nonmotor learning. *Cereb Cortex* 4 (1):8–26.
14. Binder, J.R., *et al.* (1999) Conceptual processing during the conscious resting state. A functional MRI study. *J Cogn Neurosci* 11 (1):80–95.
15. Mazoyer, B., *et al.* (2001) Cortical networks for working memory and executive functions sustain the conscious resting state in man. *Brain Res Bull* 54 (3):287–298.
16. Andreasen, N.C., *et al.* (1995) Remembering the past: Two facets of episodic memory explored with positron emission tomography. *Am J Psychiatr* 152 (11):1576–1585.
17. Fox, P.T. and Raichle, M.E. (1986) Focal physiological uncoupling of cerebral blood flow and oxidative metabolism during somatosensory stimulation in human subjects. *Proc Natl Acad Sci USA* 83 (4):1140–1144.
18. Fox, P.T., *et al.* (1988) Nonoxidative glucose consumption during focal physiologic neural activity. *Science* 241 (4864): 462–464.
19. Thulborn, K.R., *et al.* (1982) Oxygenation dependence of the transverse relaxation time of water protons in whole blood at high field. *Biochim Biophys Acta* 714 (2):265–270.
20. Ogawa, S., *et al.* (1990) Brain magnetic resonance imaging with contrast dependent on blood oxygenation. *Proc Natl Acad Sci USA* 87 (24):9868–9872.
21. Ogawa, S., *et al.* (1992) Intrinsic signal changes accompanying sensory stimulation: Functional brain mapping with magnetic resonance imaging. *Proc Natl Acad Sci USA* 89 (13):5951–5955.
22. Kwong, K.K., *et al.* (1992) Dynamic magnetic resonance imaging of human brain activity during primary sensory stimulation. *Proc Natl Acad Sci USA* 89 (12):5675–5679.
23. Lebrun-Grandie, P., *et al.* (1983) Coupling between regional blood flow and oxygen utilization in the normal human brain. A study with positron tomography and oxygen 15. *Arch Neurol* 40 (4):230–236.
24. Fox, M.D., *et al.* (2005) The human brain is intrinsically organized into dynamic, anticorrelated functional networks. *Proc Natl Acad Sci USA* 102 (27):9673–9678.
25. Drevets, W.C., *et al.* (1995) Blood flow changes in human somatosensory cortex during anticipated stimulation. *Nature* 373 (6511):249–252.
26. Kawashima, R., O'Sullivan, B.T. and Roland, P.E. (1995) Positron-emission tomography studies of cross-modality inhibition in selective attentional tasks: Closing the 'mind's eye'. *Proc Natl Acad Sci USA* 92 (13):5969–5972.

27. Ghatan, P.H., *et al.* (1998) Coexistence of attention-based facilitation and inhibition in the human cortex. *Neuroimage* 7 (1):23–29.

28. Somers, D.C., *et al.* (1999) Functional MRI reveals spatially specific attentional modulation in human primary visual cortex. *Proc Natl Acad Sci USA* 96 (4):1663–1668.

29. Smith, A.T., Singh, K.D. and Greenlee, M.W. (2000) Attentional suppression of activity in the human visual cortex. *Neuroreport* 11 (2):271–277.

30. Amedi, A., Malach, R. and Pascual-Leone, A. (2005) Negative BOLD differentiates visual imagery and perception. *Neuron* 48 (5):859–872.

31. Shmuel, A., *et al.* (2006) Negative functional MRI response correlates with decreases in neuronal activity in monkey visual area V1. *Nat Neurosci* 9 (4):569–577.

32. Biswal, B., *et al.* (1995) Functional connectivity in the motor cortex of resting human brain using echo-planar MRI. *Magn Reson Med* 34 (4):537–541.

33. Greicius, M.D., *et al.* (2003) Functional connectivity in the resting brain: A network analysis of the default mode hypothesis. *Proc Natl Acad Sci USA* 100 (1):253–258.

34. Corbetta, M. and Shulman, G.L. (2002) Control of goal-directed and stimulus-driven attention in the brain. *Nat Rev Neurosci* 3 (3):201–215.

35. Dosenbach, N.U., *et al.* (2007) Distinct brain networks for adaptive and stable task control in human. *Proc Natl Acad Sci USA* 104 (26):11073–11078.

36. Dosenbach, N.U., *et al.* (2006) A core system for the implementation of task sets. *Neuron* 50 (5):799–812.

37. Honey, C.J., *et al.* (2007) Network structure of cerebral cortex shapes functional connectivity on multiple time scales. *Proc Natl Acad Sci USA* 104 (24):10240–10245.

38. Fransson, P. (2006) How default is the default mode of brain function? Further evidence from intrinsic BOLD signal fluctuations. *Neuropsychologia* 44 (14):2836–2845.

39. Fox, M.D., *et al.* (2006) Coherent spontaneous activity accounts for trial-to-trial variability in human evoked brain responses. *Nat Neurosci* 9 (1):23–25.

40. Fox, M.D., *et al.* (2007) Intrinsic fluctuations within cortical systems account for intertrial variability in human behavior. *Neuron* 56 (1):171–184.

41. Vincent, J.L., *et al.* (2007) Intrinsic function architecture in the anesthetized monkey brain. *Nature* (in press).

42. Czisch, M., *et al.* (2004) Functional MRI during sleep: BOLD signal decreases and their electrophysiological correlates. *Eur J Neurosci* 20 (2):566–574.

43. Buzsaki, G. (2006) *Rhythms of the Brain*, 5th Edition New York: Oxford University Press,

44. Varela, F., *et al.* (2001) The brainweb: Phase synchronization and large-scale integration. *Nat Rev Neurosci* 2 (4):229–239.

45. Buzsaki, G. (2007) The structure of consciousness. *Nature* 446:267.

46. Vanhatalo, S., *et al.* (2004) Infraslow oscillations modulate excitability and interictal epileptic activity in the human cortex during sleep. *Proc Natl Acad Sci USA* 101 (14):5053–5057.

47. Baker, J.T., *et al.* (2006) Distribution of activity across the monkey cerebral cortical surface, thalamus and midbrain during rapid, visually guided saccades. *Cereb Cortex* 16 (4):447–459.

48. Lewis, J.W. and Van Essen, D.C. (2000) Corticocortical connections of visual, sensorimotor, and multimodal processing areas in the parietal lobe of the macaque monkey. *J Comp Neurol* 428 (1):112–137.

49. Vincent, J.L., *et al.* (2007) Intrinsic functional architecture in the anaesthetized monkey brain. *Nature* 447 (7140):83–86.

50. Buzsaki, G. and Draguhn, A. (2004) Neuronal oscillations in cortical networks. *Science* 304 (5679):1926–1929.

51. Fair, D.A., *et al.* (2008) The maturing architecture of the brain's default network. *Proc Natl Acad Sci USA* (in press).

52. Fair, D.A., *et al.* (2007) Development of distinct control networks through segregation and integration. *Proc Natl Acad Sci USA* 104 (33):13507–13512.

53. Buzsaki, G., Kaila, K. and Raichle, M. (2007) Inhibition and brain work. *Neuron* 56 (5):771–783.

54. Laughlin, S.B. and Sejnowski, T.J. (2003) Communication in neuronal networks. *Science* 301 (5641):1870–1874.

55. Abbott, L.F. and Chance, F.S. (2005) Drivers and modulators from push-pull and balanced synaptic input. *Prog Brain Res* 149:147–155.

56. Salinas, E. and Sejnowski, T.J. (2001) Correlated neuronal activity and the flow of neural information. *Nat Rev Neurosci* 2 (8):539–550.

57. Haider, B., *et al.* (2006) Neocortical network activity *in vivo* is generated through a dynamic balance of excitation and inhibition. *J Neurosci* 26 (17):4535–4545.

58. Sprague, J.M. (1966) Interaction of cortex and superior colliculus in mediation of visually guided behavior in the cat. *Science* 153 (743):1544–1547.

59. Hebb, D.O. (1949) *The Organization of Behavior. A Neurophysiological Theory*, New York: John Wiley and Sons, Inc.

60. Petersen, C.C., *et al.* (2003) Interaction of sensory responses with spontaneous depolarization in layer 2/3 barrel cortex. *Proc Natl Acad Sci USA* 100 (23):13638–13643.

61. Hahn, T.T., Sakmann, B. and Mehta, M.R. (2006) Phase-locking of hippocampal interneurons' membrane potential to neocortical up-down states. *Nat Neurosci* 9 (11):1359–1361.

62. Compte, A., *et al.* (2003) Cellular and network mechanisms of slow oscillatory activity (<1 Hz) and wave propagations in a cortical network model. *J Neurophysiol* 89 (5):2707–2725.

63. Wu, K., *et al.* (1997) The synthesis of ATP by glycolytic enzymes in the postsynaptic density and the effect of endogenously generated nitric oxide. *Proc Natl Acad Sci USA* 94 (24):13273–13278.

64. Marder, E. and Prinz, A.A. (2004) Modeling stability in neuron and network function: The role of activity in homeostasis. *Bioessays* 24 (12):1145–1154.

Sleep and Dreaming

Giulio Tononi

ABSTRACT

Sleep brings about the most dramatic change in consciousness we are all familiar with. Consciousness nearly fades during deep sleep early in the night, and returns later on in the form of dreams despite our virtual disconnections from the outside world. Meanwhile, the brain goes through an orderly progression of changes in neural activity, epitomized by the occurrence of slow oscillations and spindles. There are also local changes in the activation of many brain regions, as indicated by imaging studies. This chapter considers sleep stages and cycles, brain centers regulating wakefulness and sleep, the neural correlates of wakefulness and sleep including changes in spontaneous neural activity and in metabolism, as well as changes in responsiveness to stimuli. Next, it reviews changes in the level of consciousness during sleep, and considers recent findings concerning the underlying mechanisms. Finally, the chapter examines how consciousness changes during dreaming and discusses the underlying neuropsychology, possible neurocognitive models, as well as the development of dreams. This overview ends with a consideration of dissociated states such as daydreaming, lucid dreaming, sleepwalking, REM sleep behavioral disorders and narcolepsy.

Studying mental activity during sleep offers a unique opportunity to find out how changes in consciousness are associated with changes in brain activity. Indeed, sleep brings about at once the most common and the most dramatic change in consciousness that healthy subjects are likely to witness – from the near-fading of all experience to the bizarre hallucinations of dreams. At the same time, the brain goes through an orderly progression of sleep stages, which can be identified by recording the electroencephalogram (EEG), eye movements (EOG, electroculogram), and muscle tone (EMG, electromyogram), and which indicate that major changes in brain activity are taking place. Within each sleep stage, there are frequent, short-lasting EEG phenomena, such as slow oscillations and spindles, which indicate precise times at which brain activity undergoes important fluctuations. There are also orderly spatial changes in the activation of many brain regions, as indicated by imaging studies. All of this happens spontaneously and reliably every night. Moreover, similar changes occur in animals, which have spearheaded detailed studies of the underlying neural mechanisms.

This chapter will first examine how sleep is traditionally subdivided into different stages that alternate in the course of the night, and consider the brain centres that determine whether we are asleep or awake. The chapter will then discuss how brain activity changes between sleep and wakefulness, and consider how this leads to the characteristic modifications of consciousness.

SLEEP STAGES AND CYCLES

In the course of the night, the EEG, EOG, and EMG patterns undergo coordinated changes that are used to distinguish among different sleep stages (Figure 8.1).

Wakefulness. During wakefulness, the EEG is characterized by waves of low amplitude and high frequency. This kind of EEG pattern is known as *low-voltage fast-activity* or *activated*. When eyes close in preparation for sleep, EEG alpha activity (8–13 Hz) becomes prominent, particularly in occipital regions. Such alpha activity is thought to correspond to an 'idling' rhythm in visual areas. The waking EOG reveals frequent voluntary eye movements and eye blinks. The EMG reveals tonic muscle activity with additional phasic activity related to voluntary movements.

Falling asleep: Stage N1. Falling asleep is a gradual phenomenon of progressive disconnection from the environment. Sleep is usually entered through a transitional state, stage 1, characterized by loss of alpha activity and the appearance of a low-voltage mixed-frequency EEG pattern with prominent theta activity (3–7 Hz). Eye movements become slow and rolling, and muscle tone relaxes. Although there is decreased awareness of sensory stimuli, a subject in stage N1 may deny that he was asleep. Motor activity may persist for a number of seconds during stage N1. Occasionally individuals experience sudden muscle contractions (hypnic jerks), sometimes accompanied by a sense of

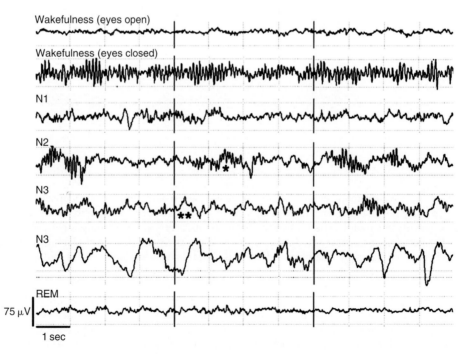

FIGURE 8.1　The human EEG during wakefulness and the different stages of sleep (*, sleep spindles; **, slow wave).

falling and dream-like imagery. Individuals deprived of sleep often have 'microsleep' episodes that consist of brief (5–10 seconds) bouts of stage 1 sleep; these episodes can have serious consequences in situations that demand constant attention, such as driving a car.

Sleep is traditionally categorized into non-rapid eye movement (NREM) sleep and REM sleep. Human NREM sleep, in turn, is divided into stages N2 and N3.

NREM sleep: Stage N2. After a few minutes in stage N1, people usually progress to stage N2 sleep. Stage N2 is heralded in the EEG by the appearance of K-complexes and sleep spindles, which are especially evident over central regions. K-complexes are made up of a high-amplitude negative sharp wave followed by a positive slow wave, and are often triggered by external stimuli. Sleep spindles are waxing and waning oscillations at around 12–15 Hz that last about 1 second and occur 5–10 times a minute. Eye movements and muscle tone are much reduced. Stage N2 qualifies fully as sleep because people are partially disconnected from the environment, meaning that they do not respond to the events around them – their *arousal threshold* is increased. If stimuli are strong enough to wake them up, people in stage N2 will confirm that they were asleep.

NREM sleep: Stage N3. Stage N2 is followed, especially at the beginning of the night, by a period called stage N3, during which the EEG shows prominent slow waves in the delta range (<2 Hz, >75 μV in humans). Eye movements cease during stage N3 and EMG activity decreases further. Stage N3 is also referred to as *slow wave sleep*, *delta sleep*, or *deep sleep*, since the threshold for arousal is higher than in stage N2. The process of awakening from slow wave sleep is drawn out, and subjects often remain confused for some time.

REM sleep. After deepening through stages N2 to N3, NREM sleep lightens and returns to stage N2, after which the sleeper enters REM sleep [1, 2] also referred to as *paradoxical sleep* [3–5] because the EEG during REM sleep is similar to the activated EEG of

waking or of stage N1. Indeed, the EEG of REM sleep is characterized by low-voltage fast-activity, often with increased power in the theta band (3–7 Hz). REM sleep is not subdivided into stages, but is rather described in terms of tonic and phasic components. Tonic aspects of REM sleep include the activated EEG and a generalized loss of muscle tone, except for the extraocular muscles and the diaphragm. REM sleep is also accompanied by penile erections. Phasic features of REM include irregular bursts of REM and muscle twitches. Behaviourally, REM sleep is deep sleep, with an arousal threshold that is as high as in slow wave sleep.

The sleep cycle. The succession of NREM sleep stages followed by an episode of REM sleep is called a sleep cycle, and lasts approximately 90–110 minutes in humans. As shown in Figure 8.2, there are a total of 4–5 cycles every night. Slow wave sleep is prominent early in the night, especially during the first sleep cycle, and diminishes as the night progresses. As slow wave sleep wanes, periods of REM sleep lengthen and show greater phasic activity. The proportion of time spent in each stage and the pattern of stages across the night is fairly consistent in normal adults. A healthy young adult will typically spend about 5% of the sleep period in stage N1, about 50% in stage N2, 20–25% in stage N3 (slow wave sleep), and 20–25% in REM sleep.

Sleep during the lifespan. Sleep patterns change markedly across the lifespan [6–10]. Newborn infants spend 16–18 hours per day sleeping, with an early version of REM sleep, called active sleep, occupying about half of their sleep time. At approximately 3–4 months of age, when sleep starts to become consolidated during the night, the sleep EEG shows more mature waveforms characteristic of NREM and REM sleep. During early childhood, total sleep time decreases and REM sleep proportion drops to adult levels. The proportion of NREM sleep spent in slow wave sleep increases during the first year of life, reaches a peak, declines during adolescence and adulthood and may disappear entirely by age 60.

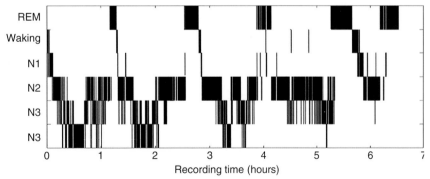

FIGURE 8.2 Hypnogram for an all-night recording in a young man. Note the occurrence of five sleep cycles, the predominance of slow wave sleep (stage N3 – the two of N3 rows correspond to stages 3 and 4 of the previous staging convention) early in the night and the increasing length of REM sleep episodes later in the night.

BRAIN CENTRES REGULATING WAKEFULNESS AND SLEEP

Wakefulness system. Maintenance of wakefulness is dependent on several heterogeneous cell groups extending from the upper pons and midbrain (the so-called *reticular activating system*, RAS [11, 12]), to the posterior hypothalamus and basal forebrain. These cell groups are strategically placed so that they can release, over wide regions of the brain, neuromodulators and neurotransmitters that produce EEG activation, such as acetylcholine, histamine, norepinephrine, glutamate, and hypocretin (Figure 8.3, red). Cholinergic cells are located in the basal forebrain and in two small nuclei in the pons: the *pedunculopontine tegmental* and *lateral dorsal tegmental* nuclei (*PPT/LDT*). Both basal forebrain and pontine cholinergic cells fire at high rates in wakefulness and REM sleep, and decrease or stop firing during NREM sleep [13–15]. Pontine cholinergic cells project to the thalamus, where they help depolarize specific and intralaminar thalamic nuclei. The latter, which are dispersed throughout the thalamus and project diffusely to the cortex, fire at very high frequencies during both wakefulness and REM sleep and help to synchronize cortical firing in the gamma (>28 Hz) range [16–18]. Cholinergic cells in the dorsal brainstem and nearby non-cholinergic cells also project to other cholinergic and non-cholinergic cells (many of them glutamatergic) in the basal forebrain, which in turn provide an excitatory input to the entire cortex [18–20].

Cholinergic neurons in the pons also project to the posterior hypothalamus, where histaminergic neurons are located in the *tuberomammillary nucleus* [21]. Histaminergic neurons, which project throughout the cortex, fire at the highest rates during wakefulness and are inhibited during both NREM and REM sleep [22]. Probably the largest contingent of the wakefulness-promoting system is made up by cells dispersed throughout the brainstem reticular formation and the basal forebrain that do not release conventional neuromodulators, but rather the ubiquitous neurotransmitter glutamate. By binding to metabotropic receptors, glutamate can act as a neuromodulator and influence the excitability of target cells. The firing patterns of these glutamatergic cells are not well characterized [18–20]. Noradrenergic cells are concentrated in the *locus coeruleus* in the upper pons, from where they project throughout the brain [23–27]. They fire tonically during wakefulness, and emit short, phasic bursts of activity during behavioural choices or salient events [13, 23–27]. By contrast, locus coeruleus neurons decrease their firing during NREM sleep, and cease firing altogether during REM sleep. Serotoninergic cells from the *dorsal raphe* nucleus also project widely throughout the brain and, like noradrenergic neurons, fire at higher levels in waking, lower levels in NREM sleep, and fall silent during REM sleep. However, in contrast to noradrenergic neurons, serotoninergic neurons are inactivated when animals make behavioural choices or orient to salient stimuli, and are activated instead during repetitive motor activity such as locomoting, grooming, or feeding [28, 29]. Dopamine-containing neurons located in the substantia nigra and ventral tegmental area, which innervate the frontal cortex, basal forebrain, and limbic structures [30], do not appear to change their firing rate depending on behavioural state, though blocking dopamine reuptake is known to promote arousal [30]. Finally, the peptide hypocretin (also known as orexin) is produced by cells in the posterior hypothalamus that provide excitatory input to all components of the waking system [31, 32]. These cells, too, are most active during waking, especially in relation to motor activity and exploratory behaviour, and almost stop firing during both NREM and REM sleep [33, 34].

Altogether, the main mechanism by which these neuromodulators and neurotransmitters produce cortical activation is by closing leakage potassium channels on the cell membrane of cortical and thalamic neurons, thus keeping cells depolarized and ready to fire.

Sleep system. At sleep onset, wakefulness-promoting neuronal groups are actively inhibited by antagonistic neuronal populations located in the hypothalamus and basal forebrain (Figure 8.3, green). Decreasing levels of acetylcholine and other waking-promoting neuromodulators and neurotransmitters lead to the opening of leak potassium channels in cortical and thalamic neurons, which become hyperpolarized

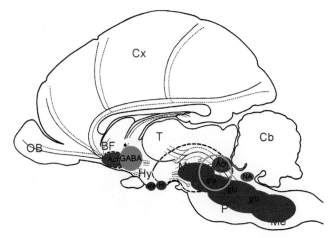

FIGURE 8.3　The major brain areas involved in initiating and maintaining wakefulness (red), NREM sleep (green), and REM sleep (orange). OB, olfactory bulb; Cx, cerebral cortex; Cb, cerebellum; T, thalamus; BF, basal forebrain; Hy, hypothalamus; Mi, midbrain; P, pons; Me, medulla oblongata; Ach, acetylcholine; glu, glutamate; NA, norepinephrine; H, histamine; ore, orexin/hypocretin.

and begin oscillating at low frequencies. Cell groups scattered within the anterior hypothalamus, including the ventrolateral preoptic area (VLPO [35, 36]) and the median preoptic nucleus [37], as well as in the basal forebrain, are involved in the initiation and maintenance of sleep. These neurons tend to fire during sleep and stop firing during wakefulness. When they are active, many of them release GABA and the peptide galanin, and inhibit most waking-promoting areas, including cholinergic, noradrenergic, histaminergic, hypocretinergic, and serotonergic cells. In turn, the latter inhibit several sleep-promoting neuronal groups [38–41]. This reciprocal inhibition provides state stability, in that each state reinforces itself as well as inhibits the opponent state.

REM sleep generator. This consists of pontine cholinergic cell groups (LDT and PPT) that are part of the wakefulness system, and nearby cell groups in the medial pontine reticular formation and medulla [3, 13, 42, 43]. Lesions in these areas eliminate REM sleep without significantly disrupting NREM sleep. Pontine cholinergic neurons produce EEG activation by releasing acetylcholine to the thalamus and to cholinergic and glutamatergic basal forebrain neurons that in turn activate the limbic system and cortex. However, while during wakefulness other waking-promoting neuronal groups, such as noradrenergic, histaminergic, hypocretinergic, and serotonergic neurons, are also active, they are inhibited during REM sleep. Other REM active neurons in the dorsal pons are responsible for the tonic inhibition of muscle tone during REM sleep. Finally, neurons in the medial pontine reticular formation fire in bursts and produce phasic events of REM sleep, such as REM and muscle twitches.

NEURAL CORRELATES OF WAKEFULNESS AND SLEEP

Wakefulness, NREM and REM sleep are accompanied by changes in spontaneous neural activity, metabolism, and responsiveness to stimuli.

Spontaneous Neural Activity

Wakefulness. The waking EEG, characterized by the presence of low-voltage fast-activity, is known as *activated* because most cortical neurons are steadily depolarized close to their firing threshold (Figure 8.4, left), and are thus ready to respond to the slightest change in their inputs. The readiness to respond of cortical and thalamic neurons enables fast and effective interactions among distributed regions of the thalamocortical system, resulting in a continuously changing sequence of specific firing patterns. Superimposed on the low-voltage fast-activity background of wakefulness one frequently observes rhythmic oscillatory episodes within the alpha (8–13 Hz), beta (14–28 Hz), and gamma (>28 Hz) range, which are usually localized to specific cortical areas. These waking rhythms are due to the activation of oscillatory mechanisms intrinsic to each cell as well as to the entrainment of oscillatory circuits among excitatory and inhibitory neurons.

NREM sleep. The EEG of NREM sleep differs markedly from that of wakefulness because of the occurrence of slow waves (<2 Hz in humans), K-complexes, and sleep spindles. The opening of leakage potassium channels due to the reduced levels of acetylcholine and other neuromodulators draws cortical and thalamic cells towards hyperpolarization and triggers a series of membrane currents that produce the *slow oscillation* (Figure 8.4, centre) [45]. As shown by intracellular recordings, the slow oscillation is made up of a hyperpolarization phase or *down-state*, which lasts a few hundreds of milliseconds, and a slightly longer depolarization phase or *up-state*. The down-state is associated with the virtual absence of synaptic activity within cortical networks. During the up-state, by contrast, cortical cells fire at rates that are as high or even higher than those seen in waking, and may even show periods of fast oscillatory activity in the gamma range.

The slow oscillation is found in virtually every cortical neuron, and is synchronized across much of the cortical mantle by cortico-cortical and thalamo-cortical

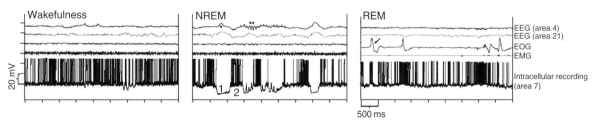

FIGURE 8.4 Simultaneous EEG, EOG, EMG, and intracellular cortical recording in a cat. During NREM sleep, the EEG trace shows slow waves (*) and sleep spindles (**), while the intracellular trace reveals the occurrence of slow oscillations in membrane potential (1 and 2 indicate down-state and up-state, respectively). During REM sleep note the absence of muscle tone and the presence of REM (arrow). *Source*: Modified from [44].

connections, which is why the EEG records high-voltage, low-frequency waves. Human EEG recordings using 256 channels have revealed that EEG slow waves behave as travelling waves that sweep across a large portion of the cerebral cortex [46]. Most of the time, the sweep starts in the very front of the brain and propagates front to back. These sweeps occur very infrequently during stage N1, around 5 times a minute during stage N2, more than 10 times a minute in stage N3. Thus, a wave of depolarization and intense synaptic activity, followed by a wave of hyperpolarization and synaptic silence, sweeps across the brain more and more frequently just as NREM sleep becomes deeper. Slow waves can originate at short intervals at multiple cortical sites, in which case they superimpose or interfere, leading to EEG waves that are shorter and more fractured. Topographically, slow waves are especially prominent over dorsolateral prefrontal cortex. *K-complexes*, which are usually triggered by external stimuli and appear particularly prominent because they are not immediately preceded or followed by other slow waves, are most likely the EEG correlate of global slow oscillations due to the near-synchronous activation of the cortical mantle by the RAS (as opposed to a single cortical source).

Sleep spindles occur during the depolarized phase of the slow oscillation and are generated in thalamic circuits as a consequence of cortical firing. When the cortex enters an up-state, strong cortical firing excites GABAergic neurons in the reticular nucleus of the thalamus. These in turn strongly inhibit thalamocortical neurons, triggering intrinsic currents that produce a rebound burst of action potentials. These bursts percolate within local thalamoreticular circuits and produce oscillatory firing at around 12–15 Hz. Thalamic spindle sequences reach back to the cortex and are globally synchronized by corticothalamic circuits, where they appear in the EEG as sleep spindles.

REM sleep. During REM sleep, the EEG returns to an activated, low-voltage fast-activity pattern that is similar to that of quiet wakefulness or stage 1 (Figure 8.4, right). As in wakefulness, the tonic depolarization of cortical and thalamic neurons is caused by the closure of leakage potassium channels. In fact, during REM sleep acetylcholine and other neuromodulators are released again at high levels, just as in wakefulness, and neuronal firing rates in several brain areas tend to be higher.

Metabolism and Blood Flow

Recently, the data obtained by recording the activity of individual neurons have been complemented by imaging studies that provide a simultaneous picture of synaptic activity over the entire brain, although at much lower resolution.

NREM sleep. Positron emission tomography (PET) studies show that metabolic activity and blood flow are globally reduced in NREM sleep compared to resting wakefulness [47, 48]. During slow wave sleep metabolic activity can be reduced by as much as 40%. Metabolic activity is mostly due to the energetic requirements of synaptic transmission, and its reduction during NREM sleep is thus most likely due the hyperpolarized phase of the slow oscillation, during which synaptic activity is essentially abolished. At a regional level, activation is especially reduced in the thalamus, due to its profound hyperpolarization during NREM sleep. In the cerebral cortex, activation is reduced in dorsolateral prefrontal cortex, orbitofrontal and anterior cingulate cortex. This deactivation is to be expected given that slow waves are especially prominent in these areas. Parietal cortex, precuneus and posterior cingulate cortex, as well as medial temporal cortex also show relative deactivations. As discussed in other chapters, the deactivation of thalamus and associated frontoparietal networks is seen in other conditions characterized by reduced consciousness, such as coma, vegetative states, and anaesthesia. By contrast, primary sensory cortices are not deactivated compared to resting wakefulness. Basal ganglia and cerebellum are also deactivated, probably because of the reduced inflow from cortical areas.

REM sleep. During REM sleep absolute levels of blood flow and metabolic activity are high, reaching levels similar to those seen during wakefulness, as would be expected based on the tonic depolarization and high firing rates of neurons. There are, however, interesting regional differences [48, 49]. Some brain areas are more active in REM sleep than in wakefulness. For example, there is a strong activation of limbic areas, including the amygdala and the parahippocampal cortex. Cerebral cortical areas that receive strong inputs from the amygdala, such as the anterior cingulate and the parietal lobule, are also activated, as are extrastriate areas. By contrast, the rest of parietal cortex, precuneus and posterior cingulate, and dorsolateral prefrontal cortex are relatively deactivated. As will be mentioned below, these regional activations and inactivations are consistent with the differences in mental state between sleep and wakefulness.

Upon awakening, blood flow is rapidly re-established in brainstem and thalamus, as well as in the anterior cingulate cortex [50]. However, it can take up to 20 minutes for blood flow to be fully re-established in other brain areas, notably dorsolateral prefrontal cortex. It is likely that this sluggish reactivation is responsible for the phenomenon of *sleep inertia* – a post-awakening deficit in alertness and performance that can last for tens of minutes.

Responsiveness to Stimuli

The most striking behavioural consequence of falling asleep is a progressive disconnection from the environment: the threshold for responding to peripheral stimuli gradually increases with the succession of NREM sleep stages N1 to N3, and remains high during REM sleep. Since cortical neurons continue to fire actively during sleep, how does this disconnection come about?

NREM sleep. Due to the progressive, intermittent hyperpolarization of thalamocortical neurons, sensory stimuli that normally would be relayed to the cortex often fail to do so because they do not manage to fire thalamocortical cells. In addition, the rhythmic hyperpolarization during sleep spindles is especially effective in blocking incoming stimuli, since it imposes an intrinsic oscillatory rhythm that effectively decouples inputs from outputs. Thus, the 'thalamic gate' to the cerebral cortex is partially closed [51]. However, sensory stimuli in various modalities can still elicit evoked potentials from the cerebral cortex, and neuroimaging studies show that primary cortical areas are still being activated [52]. As suggested by studies using transcranial magnetic stimulation (TMS) in conjunction with high-density EEG [53], it is likely that during NREM sleep the activation of primary sensory areas is not followed by the activation of higher-order areas because of a breakdown in cortical effective connectivity.

REM sleep. With the transition from NREM to REM sleep, neurons return to be steadily depolarized much as they are during quiet wakefulness, yet sensory stimuli are still ignored, as if the brain were focusing on its internal activities rather than on the environment [54], not unlike states of intense absorption. While the underlying mechanisms are not clear, the prefrontal and parietal cortical areas that are deactivated in REM sleep are important for directing and sustaining attention to sensory cortices. Sensory inputs reaching primary cortices would then find themselves to be systematically unattended. It is likely that the reduced activity in these cortical regions is a direct consequence of changes in the neuromodulatory milieu during REM sleep. Specifically, the reduction of serotonin release during REM sleep may favour a dissociative–hallucinogenic state, as seen with certain psychoactive compounds. Nevertheless, in contrast to a person in a coma or a vegetative state, a sleeping person can always be awakened if stimuli are strong enough, or especially meaningful. For example, it is well known that the sound of one's name, or the wailing of a baby, is among the most effective signals for awakening.

CONSCIOUSNESS IN SLEEP

There are two main lessons to be learned from the study of consciousness in sleep. The first is that, during certain phases of sleep, the level of consciousness can decrease and at times nearly vanish, despite the fact that neural activity in the thalamocortical system is relatively stable. The second is that, during other phases of sleep, vivid conscious experience is possible despite the sensory and motor disconnection from the environment and the loss of self-reflective thought.

Changes in the Level of Consciousness

Studying mental activity during sleep offers a unique opportunity to find out how changes in brain activity are associated with changes in consciousness [55]. When REM sleep was discovered, it was immediately noticed that, if subjects were awakened from that stage of sleep and asked whether they had a dream, they would say so at least 80% of the time. Subjects invariably reported dreams that were vivid, with characteristically intricate plots and changes of scene. Awakenings from NREM sleep, instead, yielded dreams 20% of the time or less. These findings led to the approximate equation of a physiological state, REM sleep, with a cognitive state, dreams. This equation was encouraged by the remarkable similarity between the EEG of REM sleep with that of wakefulness, as opposed to that of NREM sleep. It seemed natural to infer that the activated (low voltage, fast activity) EEG of waking and REM sleep would support vivid conscious experience, while the deactivated (high voltage, slow activity) EEG of NREM sleep would not.

However, later studies have shown that the relationship between consciousness and sleep stages is more complicated. By just changing the question from 'tell me if you had a dream' to 'tell me anything that was going through your mind just before you woke up', the percentages of recalls from NREM sleep reaches as high as 60%. It is now clear that reports indicative of conscious experience, including dream-like experiences, can be elicited during any stage of sleep [56, 57].

Sleep onset. Reports from sleep stage 1 are very frequent (80–90% of the time) but also very short. Usually people report hallucinatory experiences, so-called *hypnagogic hallucinations* (Greek for 'leading into sleep'). In contrast to typical dreams, hypnagogic hallucinations are often static, similar to single snapshots or a short sequence of still frames. For instance a subject may report: '… *I could feel myself moving just the way the sea moves our boat when I was out fishing today*'. This and the following examples are taken from [56, 58].

NREM sleep. A substantial number of awakenings from NREM sleep yield no report whatsoever, especially early in the night when stage N3 is prevalent. Thus, early slow wave sleep is the only phase of adult life during which healthy human subjects may deny that they were experiencing anything at all. On the other hand, between 60% and 80% of the time, awakenings from NREM sleep yield reports with experiential content. The length of NREM reports is widely distributed. Their median length is similar to that of reports from sleep onset. However, there are many very short reports early in the night and much longer reports later in the night [59], considerably longer than those typically obtained at sleep onset or even during quiet wakefulness. Reports from NREM sleep, especially early in the night, are often thought-like, for example: '*I kept thinking about my upcoming exam and about the subject matter that it will contain…*' Later in the night, they can be much more hallucinatory and, generally speaking, more dream-like.

REM sleep. Awakenings from REM sleep yield reports 80–90% of the time, a percentage similar to that obtained at sleep onset. Especially in the morning hours, the percentage is close to 100%, which is of course the report rate for wakefulness. Most REM reports have the characteristics of typical dreams: complex, temporally unfolding hallucinatory episodes that can be as vivid as waking experience. For example, as reported by Allan Hobson [58]: '*As the climbing party rounds the trail to the right, I am suddenly on a bicycle, which I steer through the group of climbers. It becomes clear that I make a complete circuit of the peak (at this level) by staying on the grass. There is, in fact, a manicured lawn surface continuing between the rocks and the crags … Then the scene changes to Martha's Vineyard Island (though I was still on the same bicycle) … and then to a shopping centre, a restaurant, a dance, and a meeting of faculty colleagues … one of my colleague's wives is seen as a blonde when, in reality, she is a brunette. The sense of movement, which is continuous, becomes particularly delightful when I become practically weightless and glide along a golf fairway. At the dance there is a Baltic group wearing embroidered peasant garb and stamping the floor to a loud band (I can hear the drums especially)*'. Remarkably, the median word count of REM sleep reports is even higher than that of wakefulness reports, whether quiet or active. This finding seems to fit with the notion that dreams

are single-minded, and thus less frequently interrupted by extraneous thoughts, than waking consciousness. Also, the average length of REM reports increases with the duration of the REM sleep episode. By contrast, there is no such relationship for NREM sleep reports [59].

What are the processes underlying the systematic changes in the level of consciousness during different phases of sleep? At first, it was assumed that the fading of consciousness during certain phases of sleep was due to the brain shutting down. However, while metabolism is reduced, the thalamocortical system remains active also during stage N3, with mean firing rates during the up-state of the slow oscillation that are comparable to those of quiet wakefulness [51]. Indeed, most other aspects of neural activity during the up-state of the sleep slow oscillation, including gamma activity, resemble those observed during wakefulness [60]. Why, then, does consciousness fade during certain phases of sleep and return during others?

An intriguing possibility is that the level of consciousness during sleep may be related to the degree of bistability of thalamocortical networks. Even though the level of activation of cortical neurons during the up-state of NREM slow oscillations is as high as in wakefulness and REM sleep, the up-state of NREM sleep is intrinsically unstable, in that it is inexorably terminated by the occurrence of a down-state – a generalized, stereotypical cessation of activity that can last for a tenth of a second or more. The transition from up- to down-states appears to be due to depolarization-dependent potassium currents and to short-term synaptic depression, both of which increase with the amount of prior activation [51]. Indeed, during NREM sleep the stimulation of cortical neurons typically precipitates a down-state, and even spontaneous activity cannot last for long before a down-state is triggered.

From this perspective, the incidence of spontaneous slow waves can provide a telling indicator of the degree of bistability in thalamocortical networks. Thus, during stage N1, at the transition between wakefulness and sleep, the cortex enjoys periods of activation that can last up to a minute before a large slow wave sweeps through, which is consistent with reports of short, hallucinatory sequences upon awakening. In stage N2 early in the night, the EEG is similar to that of stage N1, but the intervals between large slow waves are much shorter, on average 12 seconds. Accordingly, reports are not only short, but also thought-like in character. In stage N2 later in the morning, the intervals between large slow waves are longer, and reports are correspondingly longer and more dream-like. The hallmark of slow wave sleep, which is prevalent early in the night, are the large slow

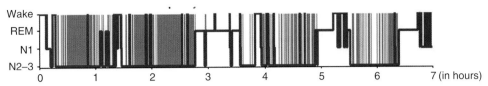

FIGURE 8.5   Incidence of large slow waves depending on sleep stage and time of night.

waves that sweep through the cortex more than 10 times a minute in stage N3 (Figure 8.5), suggesting an extreme degree of bistability. Correspondingly, reports are usually of short duration and often thought-like; at times, no experiential content is reported. In stark contrast, during REM sleep, which predominates later in the night, the EEG is tonically activated and there are no slow waves sweeping the cortex. Accordingly, REM reports are on average much longer, 2–7 times more than in NREM sleep, and usually yield vivid, prototypical dreams.

Why would the level of consciousness reflect the degree of bistability of thalamocortical networks? A possible answer is offered by the integrated information theory of consciousness [61], which states that the level or quantity of consciousness is given by a system's capacity to generate integrated information. According to the theory, the brain substrate of consciousness is a complex of neural elements within the thalamocortical system that has a large repertoire of available states (information), yet cannot be decomposed into a collection of causally independent subsystems (integration). In this view, integrated information would be high during wakefulness because thalamocortical networks have a large repertoire of global firing patterns that are continuously available on a background of tonic depolarization. During early NREM sleep, by contrast, the ensuing bistability would reduce this global repertoire through two mechanisms. First, a local activation would cause a local down-state preventing effective interactions with other brain areas. As a consequence, the main thalamocortical complex would break down into causally independent modules (loss of integration). Second, to the extent that global activation patterns can still occur, they too would be rapidly followed by a global, stereotypical down-state, thereby greatly reducing the repertoire of available states (loss of information).

To test these predictions, it is not sufficient to observe activity levels or patterns of temporal correlations among distant brain regions (functional connectivity), but it is crucial to employ a perturbational or causal approach (effective connectivity). For this purpose, TMS-evoked brain responses were recorded using a high-density EEG system to investigate to what extent cortical regions can interact causally (integration) and produce differentiated responses (information) [53]. As shown in Figure 8.6A, TMS applied to various cortical regions during wakefulness induced a sustained response made of changing patterns of activity. Specifically, a sequence of time-locked, high-frequency (20–35 Hz) oscillations occurred in the first 100 ms and was followed by a few slower (8–12 Hz) components that persisted until 300 ms. Source modelling revealed that the initial response to TMS was followed by spatially and temporally differentiated patterns of activation presumably mediated by long-range ipsilateral and transcallosal connections.

As soon as the subjects transitioned into stage N1, the TMS-evoked response grew stronger at early latencies but became shorter in duration due to dampening of later fast waves. With the onset of NREM sleep, the brain response to TMS changed markedly. The initial wave doubled in amplitude and became slower. Following this large wave, no further TMS-locked activity could be detected, except for a negative rebound between 80 and 140 ms. Specifically, fast waves, still visible during stage N1, were completely obliterated, and all TMS-evoked activity had ceased by 150 ms. Moreover, as shown in Figure 8.6B left, the activity evoked by TMS remained localized to the site of stimulation and did not propagate to connected brain regions, presumably because of the induction of a local down-state. This finding indicates that during early NREM sleep, when the level of consciousness is reduced, effective connectivity among cortical regions breaks down, implying a corresponding breakdown of cortical integration.

In subsequent experiments, it was found that, when applied to a median centroparietal region, each TMS pulse would trigger a full-fledged, high-amplitude slow wave that closely resembled spontaneous ones and that travelled through much of the cortex [62]. Spatially, the TMS-evoked slow wave was associated with a broad and stereotypical response: cortical currents spread, like an oil-spot, from the stimulated site to the rest of the brain. The large negative peak evoked by the TMS pulse, corresponding to a global cortical down-state, demonstrates that during early NREM sleep activation is inevitably followed by deactivation, suggesting that the repertoire of possible firing patterns (information) is drastically reduced

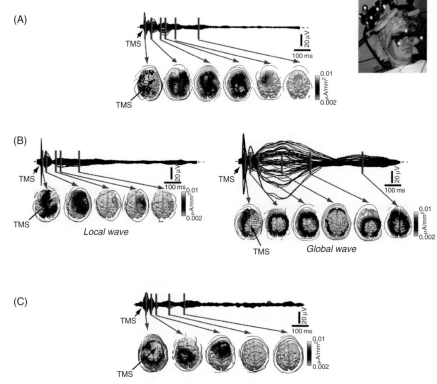

FIGURE 8.6 Spatiotemporal cortical current maps of TMS-induced activity during (A) wakefulness, (B) NREM, and (C) REM sleep. On the top right is the setup for TMS/EEG. From the EEG data, current sources corresponding to periods of significant activations were plotted on the subject's MRI. Note for TMS during wakefulness the rapidly changing patterns of activation, lasting up to 300 ms and involving several different areas (right premotor cortex stimulation is shown, but similar results are observed for other stimulation sites, including midline centroparietal regions); for TMS during NREM sleep either a brief activation that remains localized to the area of stimulation (right premotor cortex stimulation) or a global wave of activation that affects indiscriminately and stereotypically the entire cortex (midline centroparietal stimulation); and for TMS during REM sleep, an intermediate pattern of activation. *Source*: From [53, 62] and Tononi and Massimini, unpublished data).

(Figure 8.6B, right). Importantly, such stereotypical responses could be induced even when, for the preceding seconds, there were no slow waves in the spontaneous EEG, indicating that perturbations can reveal the potential bistability of a system irrespective of its observed state.

By contrast, during REM sleep late in the night, when dreams become long and vivid and the level of consciousness returns to levels close to those of wakefulness, the responses to TMS also recovers and comes to resemble more closely those observed during wakefulness: as shown in Figure 8.6C, evoked patterns of activity become more complex and spatially differentiated, although some late components are still missing. Altogether, these TMS–EEG measurements suggest that the sleeping brain, despite being active and reactive, changes dramatically in its capacity to generate integrated information: it either breaks down in causally independent modules, or it bursts into a global, stereotypical response, in line with the predictions of the integrated information theory [61].

Importantly, the use of a perturbational approach (TMS–EEG) reveals that during NREM sleep cortical circuits may be intrinsic bistable even during periods of stable ongoing EEG with no overt slow waves.

Dreams: Consciousness in the Absence of Sensory Inputs and Self-reflection

Just as striking as the near-loss of consciousness during certain phases of sleep is its remarkable preservation during other phases. This is especially true of REM sleep awakenings, which yield almost without exception reports of vivid dreams. Perhaps the most remarkable property of dreams is how similar they can be to waking consciousness, to the point that the dreamer may be uncertain whether he is awake or asleep. This means that the sleeping brain, disconnected from the real world, is capable of generating an imagined world, a virtual reality, which is fairly similar to the real one and is indeed experienced as real (Box 8.1).

BOX 8.1

NEUROCOGNITIVE MODELS OF DREAMING

Building on the cognitive model of Foulkes [63] and on the work of Hall on content analysis of dreams [64], William Domhoff has recently attempted a synthesis that he calls the neurocognitive model of dreaming [65, 66]. Domhoff proposes that dreaming is what the mature brain does when (1) primary sensory cortices are relatively inactivated, thus enforcing a partial disconnection from the external world; (2) dorsolateral prefrontal cortices are relatively inactivated, thus reducing our ability to exercise reflection and decision making; and (3) a subsystem of brain regions, comprising limbic and paralimbic structures as well as several association areas at the temporo-parieto-occipital junction, is at a sufficient level of activation. According to Domhoff's model, dream-like experiences can occur not only in NREM sleep, but also during wakefulness, provided sensory and prefrontal cortices are sufficiently quiet.

Like Foulkes, Domhoff emphasizes that the dreaming subsystem, when activated, is drawing on memory schemas and general knowledge to produce a kind of dramatized version of the world, and that these dramatizations are an active act of imagination, rather than a mere reaction to random activation. More specifically, Domhoff argues that the system of scripts and schemas activated in dreams is nothing else but the organizational basis for all human knowledge and beliefs. Basic-level categories, which can be represented by a single image, reflect distinctions among types of animals, such as cats and dogs, types of social interactions, such as friendly and aggressive, or types of actions, such as walking and running. Spatial relations categories are, for example, 'up', 'down', 'in front of', and 'in back of'. Finally, sensorimotor categories are based on experiences related to temperature, motion, and touch. The systematic occurrence of basic experiential categories in dreams is confirmed by the analysis of thousands of dreams from all over the world according to the Hall/van de Castle system [64].

Dreams may also build upon figurative thinking: conceptual metaphors, metonymies, ironies, and conceptual blends. As pointed out by Lakoff and Johnson [67], hundreds of primary conceptual metaphors actually map common experiential categories. For example, basic experiences like warmth and motion are used to understand more difficult concepts like friendship (they have a warm relationship) and time (time flies by). Just as in waking thought, figurative thinking may be used in dreams when it expresses a conception better and more succinctly than an experiential concept does. To this extent, some dreams may indeed be symbolic.

Finally, based on content analysis, Domhoff concludes that most dreams deal with personal concerns – typical ones are being inappropriately dressed, being lost, or being late for an examination. Personal concerns are very stable over the years, as well as across cultures, which may explain why dreams themes are stable across life across individuals, and around the world. Such personal concerns are also the subject of recurrent dreams, and of the repetitive nightmares experienced by people suffering from post-traumatic stress disorder (generally in stage N2). Curiously, personal concerns in dreams are often stuck in the past, in a way that fits with the persistence of negative memories stored in the amygdala and other limbic circuits that are part of the brain's fear system.

Perceptual modalities and submodalities that are experienced in wakefulness are represented in dreams: dreams are highly visual, in full colour, rich of different shapes and movements, but they also have sound, tactile feelings, smells, and tastes, as well as pleasure and pain [56]. The categories that are the stuff of dreams are the same as those that constitute the fabric of wakefulness – objects, animals, people, faces, places, and so on. Dream experiences are not necessarily all vivid and perceptual – there are also faint ideas, just as in wakefulness, and various kinds of thoughts. Dreams are also rich in emotion: in fact, emotions are often very intense, especially fear and anxiety. Hearing speech or conversation is also extremely frequent, and speech patterns are as grammatically correct as in waking life. Finally, there is a good correlation between our waking and dreaming selves with respect to mood, imaginativeness, and predominant concerns. For example, people dream most often about the individuals and interests that preoccupy them in waking life, and they show aggression in dreams towards the same people with whom they are in conflict in waking life.

Despite the remarkable similarities between waking and dreaming consciousness, dreaming consciousness often presents some distinctive features. These include: (1) disconnection from the environment; (2) internal generation of a world-analogue; (3) reduction of voluntary control and reflective thought; (4) amnesia; and (5) high emotional involvement.

Disconnection. The most obvious difference between dreaming and waking consciousness is the profound disconnection of the dreamer from his current environment. Only occasionally do external stimuli manage to be incorporated in dreams, the most effective being a spray of water or pressure on the limbs. The disconnection is so effective that even the regular erections occurring during REM sleep dreams almost never make it into the dream's content. It is also difficult to influence dream content with pre-sleep stimuli, even strong ones such as viewing a horror movie just before going to bed. Instead, all sensory experiences in dreams are generated internally: they are, strictly speaking, hallucinations. The disconnection is also evident on the motor side. For example, a feeling of weightlessness is commonplace in dreams, as are the experience of floating or flying. It is possible that the peculiar, effortless nature of motor activities in dreams has something to do with the activation of motor programmes in the absence of proprioceptive feedback signalling. As would be expected, the sensory and motor disconnection of dreams are neatly reflected in the reduced activation of primary sensory and motor areas in PET studies of REM sleep [68].

Internal generation of a world-analogue. Given the sleeper's disconnection from the external world, all dream consciousness is generated internally. Dreams, rather than being at the mercy of bottom-up signals and events from the environment, take a top-down approach by following a narrative script and using a set of well-rehearsed formulas: if waking consciousness is like watching a news broadcast, dreaming is more like watching a movie produced by an imaginative director (rather than by a camera bouncing around at random). In selecting scenes, the dream director is not particularly choosey: any actor, dress, means of transportation, or food item that is readily available will do. Indeed, as in some B-movies, characters and objects seem to be chosen for their role in each scene, with little regard for factual truth or plausibility, and without caring about the mixing of incongruent characteristics, or inconsistencies between one scene and the other. Thus, chimerical creatures, sudden transformations, and physically impossible objects are not infrequent. While the ability to dream requires the ability to imagine, dream images are generally

more vivid, presumably because they do not have to compete with external signals. Also, in dreams there is a strong tendency for a single train of related thoughts and images to persist for extended periods without disruption or competition from other thoughts or images ('*single-mindedness*' [69]). From a neuroimaging perspective, the internal generation of a world-analogue is consistent with the strong activation of temporo-occipital and parahippocampal association areas that is observed in REM sleep [48, 49].

Reduced voluntary control and reflective thought. During dreaming there is a prominent reduction of voluntary control, whether of action, thought, or attention. With the exception of lucid dreaming (see below), the dreamer has no control on what he is going to dream, and is largely a passive spectator. Reflective thought processes are also impaired in characteristic ways. Again with exception of lucid dreams, dreaming is almost always delusional, in the sense that events and characters in the dream are taken for real. While the dreamer experiences thoughts, there is a severe impairment of the ability to pursue goals effectively, to analyse situations intelligently, to question assumptions, to reason properly, and to make appropriate decisions. For example, holding contradictory beliefs is quite common in dreams, and a dreamer easily accepts impossible events or situations, such as flying. There is often uncertainty about orientation in space (where one is in the dream), about time (when the dream is taking place in personal history), and person (confusion about the gender, age, and identity of dream characters). When dreaming, one cannot stop and reflect rationally on what one should be doing, nor imagine other scenarios (after all, one is already imagining the dream). Once again, these characteristics of dreaming consciousness are consistent with neuroimaging findings: dorsolateral prefrontal cortex, which is involved in volitional control and self-monitoring, is especially deactivated during REM sleep [48, 49].

Amnesia. Memory is drastically impaired both within the dream and for the dream. Working memory is not working well, as it is extremely difficult to hold anything in mind during a dream. Episodic memory is also not functioning properly. Remarkably little makes it into dreams of recent episodes of the dreamer's life. While individual items from waking experience sometimes are incorporated into a dream, they do so in new and unrelated contexts, and true declarative memories for wakening episodes are found in a very small percentage of dreams. For example, in a study where subjects had intensively played the computer game Tetris, there was no episodic memory in subsequent dreams that the subject had indeed played Tetris. In fact, dreams of healthy subjects were indistinguishable from those of profoundly amnesic subjects, who could not remember having played Tetris whether they were dreaming or awake. In contrast, both normal and amnesic subjects often reported perceptual fragments, such as falling blocks on a computer screen, especially at sleep onset, but there were no episodic memories associated with these fragments [70]. Even previous events within a dream are soon forgotten and do not appear to influence the subsequent evolution of dream experiences. Instead, dreams are characterized by what has been called 'hyperassociativity', as if the network of association were much wider and less constricted than in wakefulness. Finally, dreams themselves are extremely fleeting: if the dreamer does not wake up, they are forever lost, and even upon awakening they vanish extremely rapidly unless they are written down or recorded. This is true even of the most intense dreams, even if they are accompanied by great emotion. It is not clear why the dreaming brain is so profoundly amnesic since, for example, parahippocampal and limbic circuits are highly active during REM sleep ([48, 49], although prefrontal cortex, which also plays a role in episodic memory, is deactivated). As is the case with daydreaming (see below), the source and structure of experienced events (external, highly constrained, vs. internal, less constrained) is a crucial determinant of recall. Perhaps changes in neuromodulators also play a role, specifically the silence of noradrenergic neurons whose activity is involved in the conversion of neural activity into neural plasticity [71].

Hyperemotionality. Many dreams are characterized by a high degree of emotional involvement, especially fear and anxiety, to a degree rare in waking life. This has led to the suggestion that the initial impetus for constructing dream narratives may originate in perceived threats or conflicts. Whether or not this interpretation has merits, REM sleep is in fact associated with a marked activation of limbic and paralimbic structures such as the amygdala, the anterior cingulate cortex, the insula, and medial orbitofrontal cortex.

In summary, there are many aspects of dreaming consciousness that can be found in textbooks of psychopathology, including hallucinations, delusions, reduced orientation and attention, impaired memory, loss of voluntary control and reflective thought. Since hallucinations and delusions are the hallmark of psychosis, it is not surprising that a connection between dreams and madness has often been suggested. However, the closest psychiatric conditions are not the major psychoses, but the so-called acute confusional state or delirium, which is often due to withdrawal from alcohol and drugs and is characterized by many

of the same symptoms as dreams – hallucinations and delusions, impaired orientation and attention, intense emotions, loss of directed thought and self-reflection, frequent confabulations, as well as by a reduced responsiveness to the external world [72]. The remarkable regional differences in activation during REM sleep are probably responsible for many of the differences between waking and dreaming consciousness [56]. It is still unclear what is responsible in turn for these regional differences, although once again it is likely that neuromodulatory systems may be involved. For example, since monoaminergic systems are silent during REM sleep, acetylcholine is alone in maintaining brain activation. Consistent with imaging results, cholinergic innervation is especially strong in limbic and paralimbic areas and much weaker in dorsolateral prefrontal cortex.

Neuropsychology of Dreaming

The analysis of patients with brain lesions indicates that the ability to dream depends on specific forebrain regions rather than on the brainstem REM sleep generator [73, 74]. In most cases of global cessation of dreaming, there is damage to the parieto-temporo-occipital junction (uni- or bilaterally), while the brainstem and the polygraphic features of REM sleep are preserved. The parieto-temporo-occipital junction is important for mental imagery, for spatial cognition (on the right side) and for symbolic cognition (on the left side), all central features of dreaming. More restricted lesions produce the cessation of visual dreaming. In all these patients, these functions were at least partially impaired during wakefulness. Thus, the ability to dream seems to go hand in hand with the ability to imagine and with visuospatial skills. Indeed, these areas are among those that are most activated during REM sleep, although it is unknown to what extent they may be activated during NREM dreaming.

The close relationship between dream generation and waking imagery is borne out by longitudinal studies of dreaming in children, which show that dreaming progresses in parallel with the child's waking ability to imagine and his visuospatial skills (Box 8.2). Thus, children of age 2–3, although they obviously can see and even speak of everyday people, objects, and events, cannot imagine them, nor can they dream of them. Similarly, if people are blind from birth, they cannot construct visual images during wakefulness, nor can they dream visually (dreams of blind people are otherwise just as vivid as those of sighted subjects). However, if people become blind after the age of

BOX 8.2

THE DEVELOPMENT OF DREAMS

When do children start dreaming, and what kind of dreams do they have? These questions have been addressed in a series of studies by David Foulkes in children between the ages of 3 and 15 years [77]. Foulkes's laboratory studies showed that children under the age of 7 awakened from REM sleep recall dreaming only 20% of the time, compared with 80–90% in adults. NREM sleep awakenings before age 7 produced some recall only 6% of the time. For both REM and NREM sleep awakenings, recall came first from awakenings late in the night.

Preschoolers' dreams are often static and plain, such as seeing an animal, thinking about eating or sleeping – 'they are more like a slide than a movie'. There are no characters that move, no social interactions, very little feeling of any sort, and they do not include the dreamer as an active character. There are also no autobiographic, episodic memories, and Foulkes suggests that the paucity of childrens' dreams is closely related to infantile amnesia: both would be due to the inability of preschoolers to exercise conscious episodic recollection. Children's dreams are more positive than adult dreams: preschoolers never reported fear in dreams, and there are few aggressions, misfortunes, and negative emotions. Note that children who have *night terrors*, in which they awaken early in the night from slow wave sleep and display intense fear and agitation, are terrorized not by any dream, but by disorientation due to incomplete awakening.

Between ages 5 and 7 dream reports become longer, although still infrequent. Dreams may contain short sequences of events in which characters move about and interact, but the dream narratives are not very well developed. At around age 7, dream reports become longer and more frequent, the child's self becomes an actual participant in the dream, with thoughts and even feelings, and dreams begin to acquire a narrative structure and to reflect autobiographic, episodic memories.

Foulkes also found that recall frequency was best correlated with the ability to produce waking mental imagery, and not with language ability. If childrens' dreams seem rare and not well developed, then, it is not because of an inability to report dreams. Instead, the frequency of dream reporting in young children is correlated with their visuospatial skills. Visuospatial skills are known to depend on the parietal lobes, which are not fully myelinated until age 7. Recall that blind adults have visual imagination and dreaming only if they lost their sight after age 7. These data suggest that dreaming is a gradual cognitive development that is tightly linked to the development of visual imagination. According to Foulkes, studying the development of dreams is tantamount to studying the development of consciousness.

---

seven, they generally can still construct visual images, and they do have visual dreams [75, 76].

Global cessation of dreaming can also be produced by bilateral lesions of white matter tracts underlying ventromedial prefrontal cortex [74]. White matter tracts in this region are the ones that used to be severed in prefrontal leucotomy, once performed on many schizophrenic patients. Most leucotomized patients complained of global cessation of dreaming as well as of lack in initiative, curiosity, and fantasy in waking life. Many of the nerve fibers travelling in the ventromedial white matter originate or end in limbic areas. In addition, the ventromedial white matter contains dopaminergic projections to the frontal lobe. Once again, these lesion data are consistent with imaging results since limbic areas are highly active during REM sleep. By contrast, lesions of forebrain areas that are deactivated during REM sleep, such as the dorsolateral prefrontal cortex, sensorimotor cortex, and primary visual cortex, do not affect the ability to dream. Also, many patients with brainstem lesions are able to dream, though it is unclear whether REM sleep was preserved. However, it is well known that certain antidepressant treatments that suppress REM sleep do not eliminate dreaming.

DISSOCIATED STATES

This last section will consider a series of conditions that lie as it were in between waking and sleep: they partake of some features typical of waking consciousness as well as of some characteristics of consciousness in sleep – that is, they represent dissociated states [78]. Some of these conditions, such as daydreaming and lucid dreaming, are perfectly normal, and can even be learned; others occur in the context of certain sleep disorders. Other conditions, known as *parasomnias*, include some of the most remarkable examples of pathological dissociation between consciousness, awareness of the environment, reflective consciousness, and behaviour.

Daydreaming

A common definition of daydreaming is 'a dream-like musing or fantasy while awake, especially of the fulfilment of wishes or hopes'. For experimental purposes, daydreaming can be defined as 'stimulus-independent mentation', that is, as waking images and thoughts that are independent of the task at hand [79]. Daydreaming is extremely common. Indeed, no matter how hard one concentrates on the task at hand, a surprising amount of time is spent drifting off into fantasies and interior monologues of one kind or another. If subjects are periodically interrupted for thought sampling during a signal-detection task, they report stimulus independent mentation at least 35% of the time, even under heavy processing loads. Their reports also indicate discontinuities and scene changes that are more frequent that in REM sleep. There have been attempts at further categorizing waking mental activities and validating such categories using questionnaires and factor analysis. Relevant dimensions are (1) directed or operant vs. non-directed or respondent thought (the former voluntarily directed towards accomplishing a task); (2) stimulus bound vs. stimulus independent; (3) realistic vs. fanciful; (4) well-integrated (orderly, connected, coherent) vs. degenerated; and (5) vivid vs. non-vivid. A prototypical daydream would be non-directed, stimulus-independent, fanciful, and non-integrated. Recall of waking images and thoughts experienced while daydreaming can be as poor as dream recall, possibly because, just as dream images, daydreaming images cannot be referenced by external events.

The neural circuits involved in daydreaming are beginning to be studied. For instance, using both thought sampling and brain imaging [80], a recent study showed that mind wandering is associated with activity in the same default network of cortical regions that are active when the brain is not actively engaged in a task [81]. Regions of the default network that exhibited greater activity during mind wandering included bilateral medial prefrontal cortex, anterior cingulate, posterior cingulate, precuneus, insula, left angular gyrus, as well as superior temporal cortex. In addition, individuals' reports of the tendency of their minds to wander were correlated with activity in this network [80]. Based on these results, however, it would seem that the circuits activated during daydreaming may actually be different from those involved in dreaming, given that, for instance, posterior cingulate, precuneus, and lateral parietal cortex are relatively deactivated during REM sleep [48, 49, 82].

Lucid Dreaming

Dreams usually involve loss of self-reflection and of reality testing. Hallucinations and delusions in dreams are typically thought to be real rather than dreamt up. Sometimes, however, a dreamer can become aware that he is dreaming [83–86]. Under such circumstances, the dreamer is able to remember the circumstances of waking life, to think clearly, and to act deliberately upon reflection, all while experiencing a dream world that seems vividly real. Lucid dreaming can be cultivated, typically by a pre-sleep autosuggestion procedure: the key is to remember that, if one is experiencing something bizarre, such as floating in space, it must be a dream rather than a waking experience. In fact, lucid dreamers often attempt to fly: if they succeed, they know they are probably dreaming. Lucid dreaming has been extensively studied in the laboratory by asking trained subjects to carry out distinctive patterns of voluntary eye movements when they realize they are dreaming. The prearranged eye movement signals appear on the polygraph records during REM sleep, proving that the subjects had indeed been lucid during uninterrupted REM sleep. This strategy has been used to demonstrate that time intervals estimated in lucid dreams are very close to actual clock time, that dreamed breathing corresponds to actual respiration, and that dreamed movements result in corresponding patterns of muscle twitching. Stable lucid dreams apparently only occur during REM sleep, especially in the early morning, when REM sleep is accompanied by intense phasic phenomena. It is plausible, but not proven, that the deactivation of dorsolateral prefrontal cortex that is generally observed during REM sleep may not occur during lucid dreams.

Sleepwalking

Sleepwalking refers to various complex motor behaviours, including walking, that are initiated during deep NREM sleep, typically during stage N3 (see also Chapter 9). Some episodes may be limited to sitting up, fumbling, picking at bedclothes, and mumbling. Patients usually stand up and walk around quietly and aimlessly.

Sleepwalkers walk around with open eyes and some-times speak, though slowly and often inarticulately. They behave as if they were wide awake though their awareness of their actions is very restricted. Occasionally, sleepwalkers become agitated, with thrashing about, screaming, running, and aggressive behaviour. A highly publicized case is that of Ken Parks, a sleepwalker who, after falling asleep at home, arose to drive to his in-laws, strangled his father-in-law into unconsciousness, and stabbed his mother-in-law to her death.

Sleepwalking is frequent in children, but it can per-sist in up to 1% of adults. In predisposed individu-als, attacks can be precipitated by forced arousals, for example by placing the subject afoot. Sleepwalking is regarded as a disorder of arousal with frequent but incomplete awakening from slow wave sleep. If awakened during an episode, sleepwalkers typically do not report any dream-like mental activity, although in a few cases hallucinations have been reported. There is almost never any memory of the behaviours carried out while sleepwalking. The episodes begin while the EEG shows high-amplitude slow waves. During the episodes, the EEG decreases in ampli-tude and increases in frequency, usually leading to the appearance of mixed-frequency patterns typical of stage N1. There may also be rhythms resembling the alpha rhythm of waking, but slower by 1–2 Hz and not abolished by eye opening or visual stimula-tion. During short episodes of sitting up with eyes open and moving around, the EEG may show slow waves throughout – providing a clear-cut dissocia-tion between observable behaviour, brain activity and consciousness.

A recent study has succeeded in performing neu-roimaging during a sleepwalking episode using sin-gle photon emission computed tomography, a variant of PET [87] (Chapter 9). The patient, a 16-year-old man, stood up with his eyes open and a scared facial expression. After a few seconds, he sat down, pulled on the EEG leads and spoke a few unintelligible words. The EEG showed diffuse, high-voltage rhyth-mic slow wave activity. Compared to waking, regional cerebral blood flow was decreased during sleepwalk-ing in frontoparietal associative cortices, just as it is in slow wave sleep. This deactivation of prefrontal corti-ces during normal sleep and sleepwalking is consist-ent with the lack of self-reflective consciousness and recall that characterize both conditions. However, blood flow was higher during sleepwalking than in slow wave sleep in the posterior cingulate cortex and anterior cerebellum, and the thalamus was not deac-tivated as it is during normal slow wave sleep. Thus, at least in this patient, sleepwalking seems to arise

from the selective activation of thalamo-cingulate circuits and the persisting deactivation of other tha-lamocortical systems. Normally, the entire forebrain is either awake or asleep. Sleepwalking thus appears to constitute a dissociated state where some brain areas are 'awake' while others are 'asleep'. It is likely that, in different patients or at different times in the same patient, different areas may be awake or asleep.

Sleeptalking is a more frequent occurrence than sleepwalking, and it can occur both in NREM and REM sleep. The majority of sleep speeches contain at least a few words, but they range from a single, mum-bled utterance to several minutes of perfectly intelli-gible talk, the latter more frequently associated with REM sleep. Sometimes sleeptalk is clearly a soliloquy, at other times it may resemble telephone conversa-tion. While there is some correspondence between sleeptalking and dream content, more often one has the impression of multiple, concurrent stream of men-tal activity that occur independently and in parallel. Such instances suggest that the speech-production system may be active in relative isolation from dream consciousness, thereby constituting another example of dissociation.

REM Sleep Behaviour Disorder

This disorder, which affects mostly elderly males, is characterized by vigorous, often violent episodes of dream enactment, with punching, kicking, and leaping from bed [78]. Patients often injure them-selves or their spouses. For example, a male subject would dream of defending his wife, but in enacting his dream he would actually forcefully strike her in bed. In rare cases there can be well-articulated speech. Polysomnographic recordings demonstrate that such episodes occur during REM sleep. Unlike sleepwalk-ers, who usually have no recollection of what they were thinking or dreaming at the time of their actions, people with REM sleep behaviour disorder can usu-ally recall their dreams in detail. Conscious experi-ence during an episode is extremely vivid, as in the most animated dreams, and is fully consistent with the motor activity displayed.

Much before the clinical syndrome was recognized in humans, sleep researchers had observed that, if cer-tain regions of the pons that are normally responsible for inhibiting muscle tone and motor programmes during REM sleep are lesioned, cats seem to 'enact their dreams' of raging, attacking, fleeing, or eating while not responding to external stimuli [88–90]. In humans, the disorder most often occurs without an obvious cause, but it is sometimes associated with neurological conditions. It may indeed result from minute lesions in the pons, it may anticipate the development of Parkinson's disorder, and it may be triggered acutely by certain drugs (certain antidepressants) or by withdrawal (ethanol).

Narcolepsy and Cataplexy

Narcolepsy is characterized by daytime sleepiness (sleep attacks), cataplexy (muscle weakness attacks), hypnagogic hallucinations and sleep paralysis [78]. Narcolepsy usually begins with excessive sleepiness and unintentional naps in the teens and twenties. Sleepiness is especially strong during periods of inactivity and may be relieved by short naps. When narcoleptics fall asleep, they usually go straight into REM sleep. Not surprisingly, patients complain that they have a short attention span, have poor memory, and sometimes behave in an automatic, uncontrolled way. The sleepiness seems to be due to a problem staying awake rather than to an increased need for sleep, since narcoleptics generally get enough sleep at night. In more than half of the cases, narcolepsy is accompanied by cataplexy. This is a sudden loss of muscle tone, typically brought on by strong emotions such as laughter or anger. The sudden weakness may be generalized and force the patient to collapse to the ground, or it may be localized to the voice, the chin, or a limb. Each episode generally lasts only a few minutes. Consciousness and awareness of the environment are preserved during cataplectic attacks, unless sleep intervenes. Hypnagogic hallucinations are dream-like hallucinations, mostly visual, that occur at sleep onset or when drowsy. Sleep paralysis is a frightening feeling of being fully conscious but unable to move, which may occur on awakening or falling asleep, like a temporary version of the locked-in syndrome (see Chapter 15). Healthy individuals can experience hypnagogic hallucinations, especially when sleep deprived, and may also experience sleep paralysis. However, while laughter and other emotional stimuli can produce muscle relaxation in normals, cataplexy is definitely an abnormal phenomenon. Sleep paralysis and cataplexy are probably due to the inappropriate activation of the brainstem mechanisms responsible for abolishing muscle tone during REM sleep. Narcolepsy–cataplexy are known to be associated with a defect in the hypocretin–orexin system [91]. Narcoleptic dogs and mice have a mutation in the gene for hypocretin or its receptors and, in the brain of narcoleptic patients, there is a loss of hypocretin cell groups in the posterior hypothalamus.

References

1. Aserinsky, E. and Kleitman, N. (1953) Regularly occurring periods of ocular motility and concomitant phenomena during sleep. *Science* 118: 273–274.
2. Dement, W. and Kleitman, N. (1957) Cyclic variations in EEG during sleep and their relation to eye movements, body motility, and dreaming. *Electromyogr Clin Neurophysiol* 9:673–690.
3. Jouvet, M. (1962) Research on the neural structures and responsible mechanisms in different phases of physiological sleep. *Arch Ital Biol* 100:125–206.
4. Jouvet, M. (1965) Paradoxical sleep – a study of its nature and mechanisms. *Prog Brain Res* 18:20–62.
5. Jouvet, M. (1998) Paradoxical sleep as a programming system. *J Sleep Res* 7 (Suppl 1):1–5.
6. Carskadon, M.A., Harvey, K., Duke, P., Anders, T.F., Litt, I.F. and Dement, W.C. (2002) Pubertal changes in daytime sleepiness, 1980. *Sleep* 25:453–460.
7. Peirano, P., Algarin, C. and Uauy, R. (2003) Sleep–wake states and their regulatory mechanisms throughout early human development. *J Pediatr* 143:S70–S79.
8. Carskadon, M.A., Acebo, C. and Jenni, O.G. (2004) Regulation of adolescent sleep: Implications for behavior. *Ann NY Acad Sci* 1021:276–291.
9. Jenni, O.G. and Carskadon, M.A. (2004) Spectral analysis of the sleep electroencephalogram during adolescence. *Sleep* 27:774–783.
10. Ohayon, M.M., Carskadon, M.A., Guilleminault, C. and Vitiello, M.V. (2004) Meta-analysis of quantitative sleep parameters from childhood to old age in healthy individuals: Developing normative sleep values across the human lifespan. *Sleep* 27:1255–1273.
11. Moruzzi, G. and Magoun, H.W. (1949) Brainstem reticular formation and activation of the EEG. *Electroencephalogr Clin Neurophysiol* 1:455–473.
12. Lindsley, D.B., Bowden, J.W. and Magoun, H.W. (1949) Effect upon the EEG of acute injury to the brainstem activating system. *Electroencephalogr Clin Neurophysiol* 1:475–486.
13. Hobson, J.A., McCarley, R.W. and Wyzinski, P.W. (1975) Sleep cycle oscillation: Reciprocal discharge by two brainstem neuronal groups. *Science* 189:55–58.
14. el Mansari, M., Sakai, K. and Jouvet, M. (1989) Unitary characteristics of presumptive cholinergic tegmental neurons during the sleep–waking cycle in freely moving cats. *Exp Brain Res* 76:519–529.
15. Lee, M.G., Hassani, O.K., Alonso, A. and Jones, B.E. (2005b) Cholinergic basal forebrain neurons burst with theta during waking and paradoxical sleep. *J Neurosci* 25:4365–4369.
16. McCormick, D.A. (1989) Cholinergic and noradrenergic modulation of thalamocortical processing. *Trends Neurosci* 12:215–221.
17. Steriade, M. (2004) Acetylcholine systems and rhythmic activities during the waking–sleep cycle. *Prog Brain Res* 145:179–196.
18. Jones, B.E. (2005a) Basic mechanisms of sleep–wake states. In Kryger, M.H. Roth, T. and Dement, W.C. (eds.) *Principles and Practice of Sleep Medicine*, 4th Edition, pp. 136–153. Philadelphia, PA: Elsevier Saunders.
19. Jones, B.E. (2003) Arousal systems. *Front Biosci* 8:s438–s451.
20. Jones, B.E. (2005b) From waking to sleeping: Neuronal and chemical substrates. *Trends Pharmacol Sci* 26:578–586.
21. Brown, R.E., Stevens, D.R. and Haas, H.L. (2001) The physiology of brain histamine. *Prog Neurobiol* 63:637–672.
22. Takahashi, K., Lin, J.S. and Sakai, K. (2006) Neuronal activity of histaminergic tuberomammillary neurons during wake–sleep states in the mouse. *J Neurosci* 26:10292–10298.

23. Foote, S.L., Aston-Jones, G. and Bloom, F.E. (1980) Impulse activity of locus coeruleus neurons in awake rats and monkeys is a function of sensory stimulation and arousal. *Proc Natl Acad Sci USA* 77:3033–3037.

24. Aston-Jones, G. and Bloom, F.E. (1981a) Activity of norepinephrine-containing locus coeruleus neurons in behaving rats anticipates fluctuations in the sleep–waking cycle. *J Neurosci* 1:876–886.

25. Aston-Jones, G. and Bloom, F.E. (1981b) Nonrepinephrine-containing locus coeruleus neurons in behaving rats exhibit pronounced responses to non-noxious environmental stimuli. *J Neurosci* 1:887–900.

26. Berridge, C.W. and Abercrombie, E.D. (1999) Relationship between locus coeruleus discharge rates and rates of norepinephrine release within neocortex as assessed by *in vivo* microdialysis. *Neuroscience* 93:1263–1270.

27. Aston-Jones, G. and Cohen, J.D. (2005) An integrative theory of locus coeruleus-norepinephrine function: Adaptive gain and optimal performance. *Annu Rev Neurosci* 28:403–450.

28. McGinty, D.J. and Harper, R.M. (1976) Dorsal raphe neurons: Depression of firing during sleep in cats. *Brain Res* 101:569–575.

29. Jacobs, B.L., Martin-Cora, F.J. and Fornal, C.A. (2002) Activity of medullary serotonergic neurons in freely moving animals. *Brain Res Rev* 40:45–52.

30. Monti, J.M. and Monti, D. (2007) The involvement of dopamine in the modulation of sleep and waking. *Sleep Med Rev* 11:113–133.

31. Peyron, C., Wurts, S., Srere, H., Heller, H. and Edgar, D.T.K. (1998) mRNA level of brain-derived neurotrophic factor (BDNF) increases in several brain regions after sleep deprivation. *Soc Neurosci Abstr* 24:1430.

32. Sakurai, T. (2007) The neural circuit of orexin (hypocretin): Maintaining sleep and wakefulness. *Nat Rev Neurosci* 8:171–181.

33. Lee, M.G., Hassani, O.K. and Jones, B.E. (2005a) Discharge of identified orexin/hypocretin neurons across the sleep–waking cycle. *J Neurosci* 25:6716–6720.

34. Mileykovskiy, B.Y., Kiyashchenko, L.I. and Siegel, J.M. (2005) Behavioral correlates of activity in identified hypocretin/orexin neurons. *Neuron* 46:787–798.

35. Sherin, J.E., Shiromani, P.J., McCarley, R.W. and Saper, C.B. (1996) Activation of ventrolateral preoptic neurons during sleep. *Science* 271:216–219.

36. Szymusiak, R., Alam, N., Steininger, T.L. and McGinty, D. (1998) Sleep–waking discharge patterns of ventrolateral preoptic/anterior hypothalamic neurons in rats. *Brain Res* 803:178–188.

37. Suntsova, N., Szymusiak, R., Alam, M.N., Guzman-Marin, R. and McGinty, D. (2002) Sleep–waking discharge patterns of median preoptic nucleus neurons in rats. *J Physiol* 543:665–677.

38. Szymusiak, R., Steininger, T., Alam, N. and McGinty, D. (2001) Preoptic area sleep-regulating mechanisms. *Arch Ital Biol* 139:77–92.

39. McGinty, D. and Szymusiak, R. (2003) Hypothalamic regulation of sleep and arousal. *Front Biosci* 8:s1074–s1083.

40. McGinty, D., Gong, H., Suntsova, N., Alam, M.N., Methippara, M., Guzman-Marin, R. and Szymusiak, R. (2004) Sleep-promoting functions of the hypothalamic median preoptic nucleus: Inhibition of arousal systems. *Arch Ital Biol* 142:501–509.

41. Saper, C.B., Scammell, T.E. and Lu, J. (2005) Hypothalamic regulation of sleep and circadian rhythms. *Nature* 437:1257–1263.

42. McCarley, R.W. (2004) Mechanisms and models of REM sleep control. *Arch Ital Biol* 142:429–467.

43. Siegel, J.M. (2005) REM sleep. In Kryger, M.H., Roth, T. and Dement, W.C. (eds.) *Principles and Practice of Sleep Medicine*, 4th Edition. Philadelphia, PA: pp. 120–135. Elsevier Saunders.

44. Steriade, M., Timofeev, I. and Grenier, F. (2001a) Natural waking and sleep states, a view from inside neocortical neurons. *J Neurophysiol* 85:1969–1985.

45. Steriade, M., Timofeev, I. and Grenier, F. (2001b) Natural waking and sleep states: A view from inside neocortical neurons. *J Neurophysiol* 85:1969–1985.

46. Massimini, M., Huber, R., Ferrarelli, F., Hill, S. and Tononi, G. (2004) The sleep slow oscillation as a traveling wave. *J Neurosci* 24:6862–6870.

47. Maquet, P., Degueldre, C., Delfiore, G., Aerts, J., Péters, J.M., Luxen, A. and Franck, G. (1997) Functional neuroanatomy of human slow wave sleep. *J Neurosci* 17:2807–2812.

48. Braun, A.R., Balkin, T.J., Wesenten, N.J., Carson, R.E., Varga, M., Baldwin, P., Selbie, S., Belenky, G. and Herscovitch, P. (1997) Regional cerebral blood flow throughout the sleep–wake cycle. An H2(15)O PET study. *Brain* 120:1173–1197.

49. Maquet, P., Peters, J., Aerts, J., Delfiore, G., Degueldre, C., Luxen, A. and Franck, G. (1996) Functional neuroanatomy of human rapid-eye-movement sleep and dreaming. *Nature* 383:163–166.

50. Balkin, T.J., Braun, A.R., Wesensten, N.J., Jeffries, K., Varga, M., Baldwin, P., Belenky, G. and Herscovitch, P. (2002) The process of awakening: A PET study of regional brain activity patterns mediating the re-establishment of alertness and consciousness. *Brain* 125:2308–2319.

51. Steriade, M. (2003) The corticothalamic system in sleep. *Front Biosci* 8:D878–D899.

52. Portas, C.M., Krakow, K., Allen, P., Josephs, O., Armony, J.L. and Frith, C.D. (2000) Auditory processing across the sleep–wake cycle: Simultaneous EEG and fMRI monitoring in humans. *Neuron* 28:991–999.

53. Massimini, M., Ferrarelli, F., Huber, R., Esser, S.K., Singh, H. and Tononi, G. (2005) Breakdown of cortical effective connectivity during sleep. *Science* 309:2228–2232.

54. Llinas, R.R. and Pare, D. (1991) Of dreaming and wakefulness. *Neuroscience* 44:521–535.

55. Hobson, J.A. (1988) *The Dreaming Brain*, New York: Basic Books.

56. Hobson, J.A., Pace-Schott, E.F. and Stickgold, R. (2000) Dreaming and the brain: Toward a cognitive neuroscience of conscious states. *Behav Brain Sci* 23:793–842. Discussion 904–1121.

57. Hobson, J.A. and Pace-Schott, E.F. (2002) The cognitive neuroscience of sleep: Neuronal systems, consciousness and learning. *Nat Rev Neurosci* 3:679–693.

58. Hobson, J.A. (2002) *Dreaming: An introduction to the science of sleep*, Oxford, New York: Oxford University Press.

59. Stickgold, R., Malia, A., Fosse, R., Propper, R. and Hobson, J.A. (2001) Brain-mind states: I. Longitudinal field study of sleep/wake factors influencing mentation report length. *Sleep* 24:171–179.

60. Sejnowski, T.J. and Destexhe, A. (2000) Why do we sleep? *Brain Res* 886:208–223.

61. Tononi, G. (2004) An information integration theory of consciousness. *BMC Neurosci* 5:42.

62. Massimini, M., Ferrarelli, F., Esser, S.K., Riedner, B.A., Huber, R., Murphy, M., Peterson, M.J. and Tononi, G. (2007) Triggering sleep slow waves by transcranial magnetic stimulation. *Proc Natl Acad Sci USA* 104:8496–8501.

63. Foulkes, D. (1985) *Dreaming: A Cognitive-Psychological Analysis*, Hillsdale, NJ: L. Erlbaum Associates.

64. Hall, C.S. and Van de Castle, R.L. (1966) *The content analysis of dreams*, New York: Appleton-Century-Crofts.

65. Domhoff, G.W. and Hall, C.S. (1996) *Finding meaning in dreams: A quantitative approach*, New York: Plenum Press.

66. Domhoff, G.W. (2003) *The scientific study of dreams: Neural networks, cognitive development, and content analysis*, 1st Edition Washington, DC: American Psychological Association.

67. Lakoff, G. and Johnson, M. (2003) *Metaphors we live by*, Chicago, IL: University of Chicago Press.

68. Braun, A.R., Balkin, T.J., Wesensten, N.J., Gwadry, F., Carson, R.E., Varga, M., Baldwin, P., Belenky, G. and Herscovitch, P. (1998) Dissociated pattern of activity in visual cortices and their projections during human rapid eye movement sleep. *Science* 279:91–95.

69. Rechtschaffen, A. (1978) The single-mindedness and isolation of dreams. *Sleep* 1:97–109.

70. Stickgold, R., Malia, A., Maguire, D., Roddenberry, D. and O'Connor, M. (2000) Replaying the game: Hypnagogic images in normals and amnesics. *Science* 290:350–353.

71. Cirelli, C., Pompeiano, M. and Tononi, G. (1996) Neuronal gene expression in the waking state: A role for the locus coeruleus. *Science* 274:1211–1215.

72. Hobson, J.A. (1997) Dreaming as delirium: A mental status analysis of our nightly madness. *Semin Neurol* 17:121–128.

73. Bischof, M. and Bassetti, C.L. (2004) Total dream loss: A distinct neuropsychological dysfunction after bilateral PCA stroke. *Ann Neurol* 56:583–586.

74. Solms, M. (1997) *The Neuropsychology of Dreams: A Clinico-Anatomical Study*, Mahwah, NJ: L. Erlbaum Associates.

75. Hollins, M. (1985) Styles of mental imagery in blind adults. *Neuropsychologia* 23:561–566.

76. Buchel, C., Price, C., Frackowiak, R.S. and Friston, K. (1998) Different activation patterns in the visual cortex of late and congenitally blind subjects. *Brain* 121 (Pt 3):409–419.

77. Foulkes, D. (1999) *Children's dreaming and the development of consciousness*, Cambridge, MA: Harvard University Press.

78. Mahowald, M.W. and Schenck, C.H. (2005) REM sleep parasomnias. In Kryger, M.H., Roth, T. and Dement, W. (eds.) *Principles and Practice of Sleep Medicine*, 4th Edition. Philadelphia, PA: pp. 897–916. Elsevier Saunders.

79. Singer, J.L. (1993) Experimental studies of ongoing conscious experience. *Ciba Found Symp* 174:100–116. discussion 116–122.

80. Mason, M.F., Norton, M.I., Van Horn, J.D., Wegner, D.M., Grafton, S.T. and Macrae, C.N. (2007) Wandering minds: The default network and stimulus-independent thought. *Science* 315:393–395.

81. Raichle, M.E., MacLeod, A.M., Snyder, A.Z., Powers, W.J., Gusnard, D.A. and Shulman, G.L. (2001) A default mode of brain function. *Proc Natl Acad Sci USA* 98:676–682.

82. Schwartz, S. and Maquet, P. (2002) Sleep imaging and the neuropsychological assessment of dreams. *Trends Cogn Sci* 6:23–30.

83. LaBerge, S.P. (1980) Lucid dreaming: An exploratory study of consciousness during sleep. In *Dissertation Abstracts International*, pp 1966–1966. US: ProQuest Information & Learning.

84. LaBerge, S., Levitan, L. and Dement, W.C. (1986) Lucid dreaming: Physiological correlates of consciousness during REM sleep. *J Mind Behav* 7:251–258.

85. LaBerge, S., Bootzin, R.R., Kihlstrom, J.F. and Schacter, D.L. (1990) Lucid dreaming: Psychophysiological studies of consciousness during REM sleep. In *Sleep and Cognition*, pp 109–126. Washington, DC, US: American Psychological Association.

86. LaBerge, S. (2000) Lucid dreaming: Evidence and methodology. *Behav Brain Sci* 23:962.

87. Bassetti, C., Vella, S., Donati, F., Wielepp, P. and Weder, B. (2000) SPECT during sleepwalking. *Lancet* 356:484–485.

88. Jouvet, M. (1979) What does a cat dream about? *Trends Neurosci* 2:280–282.

89. Sastre, J.P. and Jouvet, M. (1979) Oneiric behavior in cats. *Physiol Behav* 22:979–989.

90. Morrison, A.R. (1988) Paradoxical sleep without atonia. *Arch Ital Biol* 126:275–289.

91. Dauvilliers, Y., Arnulf, I., and Mignot, E. (2007) Narcolepsy with Cataplexy, *Lancet* 369(9560):499–511.

Sleepwalking (Somnambulism)
Dissociation Between 'Body Sleep' and 'Mind Sleep'
Claudio L. Bassetti

ABSTRACT

Sleepwalking (SW) consists of a deambulatory activity with reduced levels of consciousness which occurs during incomplete arousals from slow wave sleep. Patients behave semi-purposefully, but cannot be awakened and have no recall of the episodes. SW is common ($\approx$10%) in schoolchildren and uncommon ($\approx$2–4%) in adults. Eating, sexual behaviour, injuries and violence can complicate SW. Pathophysiologically, the dissociation between 'body and mind sleep' of SW is thought to arise from the isolated hyper-arousability of specific (striato-limbic?) neuronal networks. Etiologically, SW is determined by genetic, neurological, psychiatric and triggering (e.g., fever, drugs, alcohol, stress,...) factors. Diagnosis relies on history. Video-polysomnography may be needed to rule out other conditions. Treatment of SW includes the identification of involved etiological factors, measures to make the sleep environment safe and the use of benzodiazepines or antidepressants.

DEFINITION

Sleepwalking (SW, syn. somnambulism) consists of complex motor behaviours that interrupt night sleep. It is initiated during sudden arousals from slow wave sleep and culminates in a deambulatory activity with an altered state of consciousness and judgement [1].

HISTORICAL REMARKS

Sleepwalking (SW) is known since ancient times (Galen and Socrates may have been somnambulic) [2]. Homer described in 'Odyssey' a youth named Elpenor who after awakening from deep sleep run off a roof injuring himself. Dante described in 'La Divina Commedia' the SW of the Purgatory's souls, and Shakespeare the SW of 'Macbeth'. In his book *Dracula* Bram Stoker described hereditary SW in the Westerna family.

Violence and injuries related to SW and their forensic implications have been discussed in the medical literature since the 19th century [3, 4]. Neurologists at the turn to the 20th century (including Charcot, Dejerine and Oppenheim) discussed the existence of epileptic, psychogenic (hysterical, hypnosis-induced), toxic (alcoholic), post-traumatic and sleep-related deambulatory episodes (poriomania, dromomania) [4–7].

In his classical book *Sleep and Wakefulness* (first edition in 1939) Nathaniel Kleitman pointed out that the term SW, if used to denote walking while asleep, represents a misnomer since it corresponds rather to 'walking in the course of an interruption of night's sleep'[8]. First systematic clinical studies on SW were performed in the 1940s and 1950s in the US army [9]. Systematic polysomnographic studies of SW were performed first in the 1960s [10–12].

Pathophysiologically, De Morsier suggested in the 1930s an analogy between SW and daytime states with impaired consciousness such as confusional states and epileptic automatisms [13]. Kleitman underlined the difference between wakefulness and consciousness in the context of SW [8]. Broughton expanded these concepts proposing SW as a disorder of arousal (with increased but incomplete arousability from slow wave sleep) because of the co-existence in SW of mental confusion, automatic behaviour, non-reactivity to external stimuli, retrograde amnesia and decreased amplitude/increased latencies of visual evoked potentials [14].

EPIDEMIOLOGY

The frequency of SW is age-dependent [15]. The peak frequency of about 10–15% is observed in children around the age of 8–12 years [1, 15, 16]. In one out of four cases SW persists beyond the age of 10 years [15].

In adults the frequency of SW has been estimated to be around 2–4%, although less than 1% present SW at least weekly [17, 18]. SW affects both genders equally [1, 15, 18]. A positive family history of SW is frequent (see below).

CLINICAL FEATURES

During SW patients wake up suddenly, sit up, look around with a confused stare, leave the bed and deambulate. Movements are typically slow and clumsy at the beginning, more coordinated and physiologic later (patients often can avoid obstacles while walking). Movements can be repetitive and purposeless, on other occasions they appear complex and meaningful (eating, drinking, cooking, driving a car) [19]. Occasionally, movements are rapid (Figure 9.1). The patient suddenly jumps out of bed, appears agitated and belligerent and may even run (a situation for which the term 'somnomania' was suggested [3]).

During SW the eyes are open and staring. Patients can speak and answer to questions, usually however in an incomprehensible manner. Shouting can accompany agitated SW episodes. Autonomic activation (sweating, tachycardia, tachypnea) is more common in confusional arousals and sleep terrors than in SW.

Patients are difficult to awaken, and when awakened appear confused. They may return spontaneously to bed and lie down. There is usually no recall of SW episodes. Dream-like experiences are however occasionally reported particularly in adult SW [20]. Occasionally SW appears to respond to a perceived threat (fire, earthquake, bomb) [3, 21].

Complications

Self-injuries are possible, more frequently in adult SW. This may occur during such acts as jumping out of the window or walking on a roof [22].

Violence during SW occurs mainly in adult and male patients (in 30% of 74 adult sleepwalkers in an own series [20]). Reports of homicidal, filicidal and suicidal SW are known since the 19th century [3, 22–27]. In a systematic review of 32 cases drawn from medical and forensic literature physical contact and

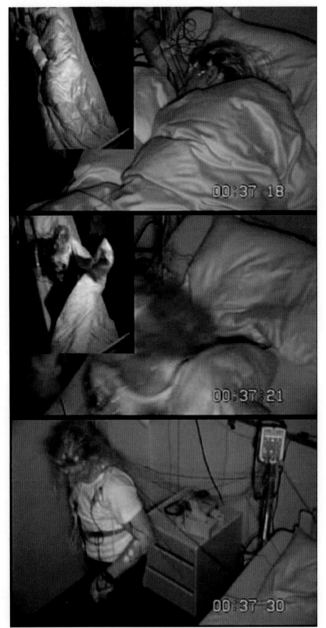

FIGURE 9.1 30-year old man (B.S.) with SW. Three pictures (12 seconds separate the first from the last picture) taken from a nocturnal videography documents the abrupt beginning of a SW episode.

proximity were found to be often involved in violent behaviour associated with SW/sleep terrors [28].

Nocturnal eating (somnophagia), often rapid and compulsory, can appear in association with SW, in females more than males [29]. In a series of 74 adults sleepwalkers nocturnal eating was reported by 34% of patients [20].

Abnormal sexual behaviour during sleep (sleep sex, sexsomnia) in form of indecent exposure, sexual intercourse, sexual assault, moaning and masturbation has

also been reported in association with SW, in males more then females [30].

Onset/Course

More often, SW appears between the age of 5 and 15 years, with a peak around 8–12 years. Earlier and later onsets (including 'de novo' in adulthood) are possible [21]. Childhood SW usually disappears around puberty.

Typically, SW occurs once per night and in the first third of the night (about 1 hour after sleep onset). The frequency of SW is however very variable and can range from few episodes in a lifetime up to several [5, 6] episodes per night [21]. In addition, SW can occur also in the latter two-thirds of the night and even during daytime naps [21]. The duration of SW ranges from 1–3 to 7–10 minutes, rarely longer. Patients are typically difficult to be awaken during an SW episode. Episodes of SW often end with the patient returning to his bed.

Associated Features

Patients with SW have a higher frequency of sleep terrors (pavor nocturnus), confusional arousals, enuresis and sleep talking [3, 14, 18]. In some but not all studies an association with bruxism and sleep starts was observed [18]. An association with complex nocturnal hallucinations has also been reported [31, 32].

Migraine and psychiatric symptoms/disturbances have also been linked with SW [18, 33, 34].

NEUROPHYSIOLOGICAL FEATURES

Neurophysiologically it is known since the 1960s that SW occurs during sudden but in complete arousals (Figure 9.2) from slow wave sleep [11, 14]. Less commonly SW, particularly in adults, may occur out of other sleep stages [21, 35].

SW episodes are rarely recorded in the sleep laboratory [11, 14]. An episode of SW is typically preceded by high amounts of slow wave activity occasionally in form of high-voltage, rhythmic slow delta waves which are typically accentuated over the frontal and central derivations (hypersynchronous delta waves, HSD [11, 36]). Occasionally runs of alpha waves can appear diffusely or focally (e.g., over the central regions) in the delta wave sleep preceding a SW episode [37]. The heart rate accelerates abruptly during but not before the sudden arousal.

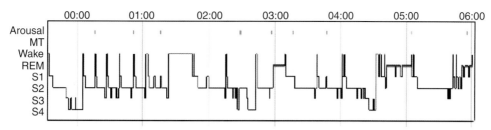

FIGURE 9.2   32-year old man (T.K.) with SW. About 1 hour after sleep onset six recurrent episodes of sudden arousal from slow wave sleep.

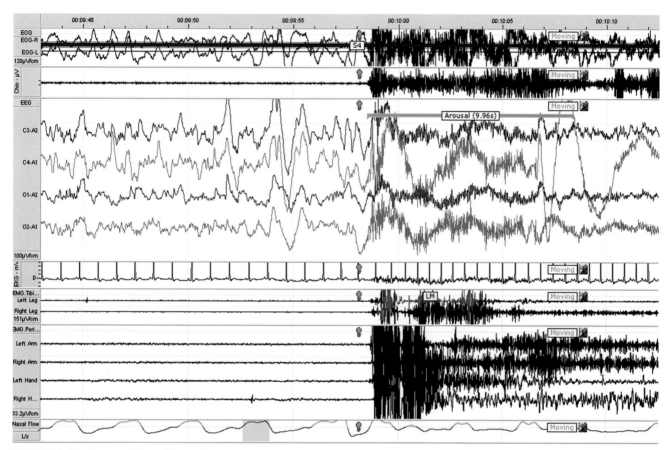

FIGURE 9.3   27-year old man (S.B.) with SW. About 1 hour after sleep onset sudden arousal from slow wave sleep.

The post-arousal electroencephalography (EEG) demonstrates variable patterns including rhythmic, high-voltage frontally accentuated delta activity (which seems to be associated with rather simple behavioural episodes [38]); diffuse delta–theta activity; mixed delta–theta–alpha–beta activity (Figure 9.3); alpha or beta activity [38, 39].

The polysomnography of patients with SW is characterized by an increased fragmentation of slow wave sleep (particularly during the first non-rapid eye movement (NREM) episode) and by the recurrent appearance of HSD [11, 36]. The number of arousals from slow wave sleep (SWS) is increased [40] whereas the amounts of SWS are decreased [41, 42]. An abnormal CAP (cyclic alternating pattern) with a decrease in phase 1 and increase in phase 2 was observed in chronic sleepwalkers [43].

Sleep deprivation may increase the diagnostic yield of sleep studies in SW [35]. It is noteworthy, that sleep deprivation leads also to an increase of HSD [36].

Occasionally, particularly in adult SW, phasic muscle activity during rapid eye movement (REM) sleep is increased (in 20% of 74 patients with adult sleep-walker in an own study [20]). Some series noted an increased frequency of sleep disordered breathing and periodic limb movements in sleep in patients with SW (see 'Triggering Factors').

The EEG is typically normal in sleepwalkers [20, 44]. During sleep as well as wakefulness focal epileptiform activities have been however sporadically observed.

ETIOLOGY

SW arises from genetic, developmental, somatic and psychological factors. Predisposing, priming and precipitating factors have been identified.

Predisposing Factors: Genetic Influences

The familial occurrence of SW was first documented in 1942 [45]. The frequency of SW in first-degree relatives is at least 10 times greater than in the general population [46]. In a twin study monozygotic twins were found to be concordant for the symptom SW six times more than dizygotic twins [47]. In the Finnish Twin Cohort the frequency of SW was similar in monyzygotic and dizygotic twins, however the concordance rate was also higher for monozygotic twins (0.55 vs. 0.32) [17]. The phenotypic variance related to genetic factors has been estimated to be about 57–66% in childhood SW and 36–80% in adult SW [17].

The HLA marker DQB1*05 may represent a susceptibility marker for SW [48]. In a study of 60 sleepwalkers this marker was found in 35% of patients (vs. 15% of matched controls).

Priming Factors: Psychiatric and Neurological Influences

Current or past mental disorders are more common in patients with SW than in patients without SW [18]. Schizoid, obsessive, compulsive, anxious, phobic, depressive symptoms or profiles have been found in patients with SW [24, 26, 49]. Overall the link between psychopathology and SW is considered however to be weak [1]. Furthermore, a history of major psychological trauma appears to be rare in SW [50].

Several disorders of the central nervous system including stroke, head trauma, encephalitis, Tourette's syndrome and migraine have been linked with (often adult) SW [51, 52]. In the absence of a specific correlation between SW and the topographical, pathological

or neurochemical characteristics of these brain disorders the nature of the link between SW and neurological conditions (as this is the case also for psychiatric disorders) appears to be non-specific one.

Triggering Factors: Precipitating Influences

Several triggering factors are known from clinical experience. However, only a few systematic studies have been performed. The pertinent literature was reviewed recently [53].

Sleep fragmentation: This may be related to sleep disordered breathing [54, 55], restless legs/periodic limb movements in sleep, internal stimuli (e.g., bladder distension) or external stimuli (light, noise) [1]. This may play a role in the observed association between SW and thyrotoxicosis [52]. In a series of 74 adult sleepwalkers sleep disordered breathing was found 'only' in 25% of patients and periodic limb movements in 12% of patients [20].

Slow wave sleep rebound: This can be observed for example after sleep deprivation and at the beginning of CPAP treatment for sleep apnea [56]. Experimentally a sleep deprivation of 36 hours has led to an increase in frequency and complexity of episodes during the recovery night compared with baseline in patients with SW [35].

Fever is often reported to trigger episodes of SW [1].

Alcohol, often in combination of other factors, is not infrequently involved [22, 24]. Up to 10% of adult patients with SW consume alcohol at bedtime [18]. Direct experimental evidence that alcohol may trigger or worsen SW is however lacking [57].

Several *medications* including zolpidem/benzodiazepines [58, 59], thioridazine/neuroleptics [49, 60], stimulants/aminergic (dopaminergic) drugs [26, 61], antidepressants/serotonin reuptake inhibitors (e.g., paroxetin) [60], antihistaminics [60] and lithium [62] may trigger SW episodes also in the absence of a positive history of SW [60]. Nevertheless, only 4% of adult patients with SW consume psychotropic drugs [18].

Mental stress is often reported by patients as triggers of SW or as involved in increasing its frequency [18].

Pregnancy usually leads to a decrease of SW [52].

PATHOPHYSIOLOGY

Any pathophysiological model of SW must explain the simultaneous appearance of (1) complex motor behaviours (including deambulation) out of deep sleep in and (2) an impaired state of consciousness. The co-existence of complex motor behaviours and impaired consciousness corresponds to a state dissociation (between 'body and mind sleep'), the neurophysiological, anatomical and chemical nature and origin of which remains speculative [63].

Animal and human data suggests that the variety of complex motor behaviours associated with SW could arise from the activation of neuronal networks in subcortical and brainstem regions responsible for the generation of (innate, archaic) emotional and motor behaviours. The activation of such 'central pattern generators' during SW, epileptic or psychogenic spells could explain the similar phenomenology of complex motor behaviours (including deambulation, eating, sexual activity, violent acts) seen with such different underlying conditions [64–66]. If this hypothesis is correct, SW could be viewed as a disorder characterized by the 'hyper-arousability' of specific (striato-limbic?) neuronal networks.

The impaired state of consciousness typical of SW implies on the other hand an insufficient activation of prefrontal cortical areas necessary for purposeful behaviour/planning, insight/judgement and inhibition of emotional responses. These areas have been shown by neuroimaging studies to be inactivated during physiological sleep.[1] The incomplete/difficult awakening of sleepwalkers from deep sleep could therefore correspond to a 'hypo-arousability' of (prefrontal?) cortical areas. This hypothesis could explain why factors that increase slow wave sleep (which exhibits maximal power over the prefrontal areas [67]) trigger SW as well as the similarities between the mental state of sleepwalkers and that of normal subjects with protracted/difficult awakening from sleep (sleep inertia, sleep drunkenness).

One SPECT (single photon emission computed tomography) study supports the concept of state dissociation underlying SW. Compared to cerebral blood flow (CBF) data obtained in 24 subjects during wakefulness the CBF of a single patient during SW was found to be increased in the posterior cingulate cortex and cerebellar vermis and decreased in frontal and parietal association cortices (Figure 9.4) [68]. This observation, in line with Broughton's original suggestion of SW as an arousal disorder, suggests the presence of a specific activation of thalamo-cingulo-cortical pathways (implicated in the control of complex motor and emotional behaviour) while other thalamocortical pathways (including those projecting to the frontal lobes) remain inhibited. The appearance at the different ages and during different nights in the same patient of SW,

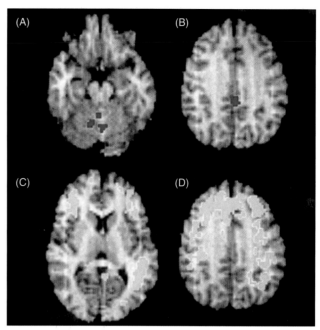

FIGURE 9.4   SPECT findings in a 22-year old man with familial SW (with permission from Bassetti et al. (2000). The highest increases of regional cerebral blood flow (>25%) during SW compared with quiet stage 3 to 4 NREM sleep are found in the anterior cerebellum – i.e. vermis (A), and in the posterior cingulate cortex (Brodmann area 23 [Tailarach coordinate $x = -4, y = -40, z = 31$], B). However, in relation to data from normal volunteers during wakefulness ($n = 24$), large areas of frontal and parietal association cortices remain deactivated during SW, as shown in the corresponding parametric maps (z-threshold $= -3$). Note the inclusion of the dorsolateral prefrontal cortex (C), mesial frontal cortex (D) and left angular gyrus (C) within these areas.

sleep terrors, confusional arousals could be explained by the recruitment of distinct although partially overlapping thalamo-cingulo-cortical pathways.

The fundamental cause of state dissociation in SW remains unknown. The existence of different predisposing, priming and triggering factors of SW (see 'Etiology') as well as of different forms of SW (see 'Differential Diagnosis') prove that the dynamic physiological reorganization that the brain undergoes at the transition from one state to another (in the case of SW from deep sleep to lighter sleep/wakefulness) represents a complex and fragile process that undergoes developmental maturation and can be impaired by different (neurological, psychological, pharmacological…) factors.

Although SW may represent a behavioural disorder unique to the human species [70], dissociated states of being are known also in the animal kingdom (e.g., unihemispheric sleep in dolphins, flight during sleep in birds) [65]. This offers the opportunity for an experimental approach to the study of the above

---

[1]This explains the neuropsychological characteristics of mental activities in sleep including dreams [69].

mentioned 'dynamical reorganizational brain processes' and its dysfunctions.

The association of SW with migraine suggests the possible involvement of the serotonin system in both [33, 34]. This hypothesis is further supported by the observation that several factors known to trigger SW (including fever, lithium and antidepressants) activate the serotoninergic system [71]. The involvement of cholinergic and GABA(A) pathways has been proposed based on theoretical speculations and the result of transcranial magnetic stimulation studies in awake sleepwalkers [72]. Considering the essential physiological role of the hypocretin (orexin) system in state stabilization [73] and the fact that narcolepsy represents the dissociated disorder 'par excellence'[74], an involvement of this hypothalamic system – possibly with the dopamin system (which is known to interact with the hypocretin system [75]) – appears also to be possible.

DIAGNOSIS

The diagnosis is usually based on typical history. Videography done at home can be of diagnostic help. Sleep studies in the sleep laboratory rarely documents episodes of SW but can show the typical polysomnographical/EEG findings of patients with SW. Furthermore, they can help to rule our disorders that may erroneously be diagnosed as SW (e.g., sleep epilepsy). Finally, sleep tests can rule out the co-existence of sleep disorders that may trigger SW episodes (sleep disordered breathing, periodic limb movements in sleep).

DIFFERENTIAL DIAGNOSIS

Is It SW?

In otherwise healthy subjects SW must be differentiated mainly from REM sleep behaviour disorder and other parasomnias, nocturnal (morpheic) seizures, dissociative spells, toxic encephalopathies (secondary to drug/alcohol intake and leading to incomplete/confusional arousals and sleep drunkenness, 'syndrome d'Elpénor'[26]), metabolic encephalopathies (e.g., hypoglycemia secondary to insulinoma [76]) and nocturnal volitional (waking) behaviour/malingering (see Table 9.1).

In elderly patients with cognitive impairment sensory deprivation in the night may lead to episodes of nocturnal confusion (sundowning phenomena).

TABLE 9.1 Diagnostic Approach and Differential Diagnosis of SW

a. *Is it SW or another nocturnal motor 'spell'?*
History/videography/video-polysomnography are decisive

SW 'sensu strictu'
REM sleep behaviour disorder (without SW)
Nocturnal epilepsy (without SW)
Confusional arousals/sleep drunkenness
    Idiopathic
    Secondary to sleep apnea or other sleep disorders
    Secondary to toxic/metabolic encephalopathy
Nocturnal wandering/sundowning in demented
(Alzheimer's) patients
Dissociative 'spells'
Volitional (waking) behaviour

b. *It is SW, which form/cause?*
History, clinical context/examination and ancillary tests (e.g. brain MRI, EEG…) are decisive

In the context of:
    NREM parasomnia
    Overlap parasomnia or REM sleep behaviour disorder
    Neurological disorders (including Parkinson)
    Nocturnal epilepsy (epileptic wandering)
    Psychiatric disorders

In patients with neurological and psychiatric disorders deambulatory activity (pacing), if appearing at night, may also be mistaken for SW. Wandering behaviour is in fact quite common in Alzheimer's disease. It is typically associated with severe dementia, disturbed sleep, delusions, injuries and caregiver distress [77]. Its pathophysiology remains obscure.

Diagnostic Work-up: Which Form/Cause of SW?

See Table 9.1.

1. SW in the context of arousal disorders (NREM parasomnias)
   This is certainly the most common and best known form of SW.
2. SW in the context of parasomnia overlap syndrome
   These patients exhibit both SW and REM sleep behaviour disorder [78].
   The existence of SW in the context of REM sleep behaviour remains controversial/poorly known [79, 80].
3. SW in the context of nocturnal epilepsy (epileptic wandering)
   Nocturnal seizures of temporal and frontal lobe have been reported to manifest with somnambulism

(usually called in this context 'epileptic nocturnal wandering') [81–83]. This existence of epileptic wandering was known already by Charcot [2, 84]. Patients may exhibit during such episodes dystonic postures and violent behaviours. The EEG displays an epileptiform activity.

4. SW in the context of psychogenic disorders

Psychogenic dissociative states, as discussed already by Charcot, can present with SW [4, 85].

5. SW in neurological disorders

This is a yet poorly known context for SW.

Besides the association of SW with migraine, stroke, head trauma and encephalitis [33, 34], SW was linked more recently with neurodegenerative disorders such as Machado-Joseph and Parkinson's disease [86, 87].

TREATMENT

Triggering factors and predisposition situations should be avoided.

The patients' sleep environment should be made safe (sleeping on the first floor, securing doors/windows, removing potentially dangerous objects,…).

Stress-reducing treatments (including hypnosis) can be of help in selected patients [88].

Clonazepam (0.5 mg at bedtime, to be increased up to 2–3 mg) is the drug of first choice for SW [89].

Other benzodiazepines (including flurazepam, triazolam and diazepam), antiepileptics (including carbamazepine, phenytoin and gabapentin), antidepressants (including imipramine, trazodone and paroxetin) and melatonin have been reported to be effective in both childhood and adult SW, although only in single cases or very small series [21, 52, 90–93].

Treatment of sleep disordered breathing can improve the control of SW [92].

FORENSIC ASPECTS

Already Charcot – in the late 19th century – was involved in a medico-legal expertise of a patient accused of attempted murder and pleading innocence because he was a somnambulist. In a famous case published in 1878 the patient, asked to plead, said 'I am guilty in my sleep, but not guilty in my senses'[3]. Seven criteria have been suggested by Mahowald for the evaluation of sleep-related violence cases: (1) presence of sleep disorder by history/sleep tests?; (2) duration of 'spells'; (3) character of behaviour (senseless?)?; (4) behaviour after the 'spell' (perplexity,

horror?)?; (5) amnesia?; (6) timing of 'spell' after sleep onset and (7) prior sleep deprivation? [94].

CONCLUSION

The complex, semi-purposeful behaviour observed during sleepwalking can be viewed as the result of a specific and isolated activation of specific (striato-limbic?) neuronal networks during slow wave sleep. This state dissociation results from a wide range of genetic, neurological, psychiatric and triggering influences.

Clinically, SW is relevant because of the associated risk of injuries and violence and the fact that, particularly in adults, a variety of disorders (including epilepsy) may lead to an automatic deambulatory activity during sleep.

Scientifically, the study of SW offers a unique perspective on the control mechanisms of complex emotional behaviors and more generally on dissociated states of being.

Overall, SW – while raising fundamental questions about the biological bases of consciousness, behaviour and free will – represents a fascinating challenge for modern neurosciences.

References

1. American Academy of Sleep Medicine (2005). *The International Classification of Sleep Disorders*, 2nd Edition. American Academy of Sleep Medicine, Rochester.
2. Goetz, C.G. (1987) *Charcot the Clinician. The Tuesday Lessons*, New York: Raven Press.
3. Yellowlees, D. (1878) Homicide by a Somnambulist. *J Ment Sci* 24:451–458.
4. Charcot, J.M. (1892) Le somnambulisme hytérique spontané considéré au point de vue nosographique et médico-légal. *Gaz hebd de méd et de chirurgie* 2–3.
5. Charcot, J.M. (1887–1888) *Leçons du mardi à la Salpêtrière, Policlinique, I et II*, Paris: A. Delahaye.
6. Dejerine, J. (1914) *Sémiologie des affections du système nerveux*, Paris: Masson.
7. Oppenheim, H. (1913) *Lehrbuch der Nervenkrankheiten*, Berlin: S. Karger.
8. Kleitman, N. (1939) *Sleep and Wakefulness*, Chicago: University of Chicago Press.
9. Sandler, S.A. (1945) Somnambulism in the armed forces. *Mental Hygiene* 29:236–247.
10. Gastaut, H. and Brougton, R. (1965) A clinical and polygraphic study of episodic phenomena during sleep. In J. Wortis, (ed.) *Recent Advances in Biological Psychiatry*, New York: Plenum Press. pp. 197–221.
11. Jacobson, A., Kales, A., Lehmann, D. and Zweizig, J.R. (1965) Somnambulism: All-night electroencephalographic studies. *Science* 148:975–977.
12. Kales, A., Jacobson, A., Paulson, M.J., Kales, J.D. and Walter, R.D. (1966) Somnambulism: Psychophysiological correlates. *Arch Gen Psychiatr* 14:386–394.

13. De Morsier, G. (1931) Les amnésie transitoires. Conception neurologique des états dits: somnambulisme naturel, état second, automatisme comitial ambulatoire. *Encéphale* 26:18–41.

14. Broughton, R.J. (1968) Sleep disorders: Disorders of arousal? *Science* 159:1070–1078.

15. Laberge, L., Trembley, R.E., Vitaro, F. and Montplaisir, J. (2000) Development of parasomnias from childhood to early adolescence. *Pediatrics* 106:67–73.

16. Petit, D., Touchette, E., Trembley, R.E., Boivin, M. and Montplaisir, J. (2007) Dyssomnias and parasomnias in early childhood. *Pediatrics* 119:1016–1025.

17. Hublin, C., Kaprio, J., Partinen, M., Heikkilä, K. and Koskenvuo, M. (1997) Prevalence and genetics of sleepwalking. A population-base twin study. *Neurology* 48:177–181.

18. Ohayon, M.M., Guilleminault, C. and Priest, R.G. (1999) Night terrors, sleepwalking, and confusional arousals in the general population. Their relationship to other sleep and mental disorders. *J Clin Psychiatr* 60:268–274.

19. Schenck, C.H. and Mahowald, M.W. (1995) A polysomnographically documented case of adult somnambulism with long-distance automobile driving and frequent nocturnal violence: Parasomnia with continuing danger as a noninsane automatism. *Sleep* 18:765–772.

20. Bassetti, C. and Vadilonga, D. (2000) Adult sleepwalking: Clinical, neurophysiological, and neuroimaging findings. *J Sleep Res* 9 (Suppl 1):13.

21. Kavey, N.B., Whyte, J., Resor, S.R. and Gidro-Frank, S. (1990) Somnambulism in adults. *Neurology* 40:749–752.

22. Broughton, R., Billings, R., Cartwright, R., *et al.* (1994) Homicidal somnambulism: A case report. *Sleep* 17:253–264.

23. Brouardel, P., Motet, D. and Garnier, P. (1893) Affaire Valrof: double tentative du neurtre-somnabulisme allégué. *Ann Hyyg Pub Méd Lég* 29:497–524.

24. Hartmann, E. (1983) Two cases reports: night terrors with sleepwalking a potentially lethal disorder. *J Nerv Ment Dis* 171:503–505.

25. Gottlieb, P., Christensen, O. and Kramp, P. (1986) On serious violence during sleepwalking. *Br J Psychiatr* 149:120–121.

26. Bornstein, S., Guegen, B. and Hache, E. (1995) Syndrome d'Elpénor ou meurtre somnambulique. *Ann Méd-Psychol* 154:195–201.

27. Cartwright, R. (2004) Sleepwalking violence: A sleep disorder, a legal dilemma, and a psychological challenge. *Am J Psychiatr* 161:1149–1158.

28. Pressmann, M.R. (2007) Disorders of arousal from sleep and violent behavior: The role of physical contact and proximity. *Sleep* 30:1039–1047.

29. Vetrugno, R., Manconi, M., Ferini-Strambi, L., Provini, E., Plazzi, G. and Montagna, P. (2006) Nocturnal eating: Sleep-related eating disorder or night eating syndrome? A videopolysomnographic study. *Sleep* 29:949–954.

30. Andersen, M.L., Poyares, D., Alves, R.S.C., Skomro, R. and Tufik, S. (2007) Sexsomnia: Abnormal sexual behavior during sleep. *Brain Res Rev* 56:271–282.

31. Kavey, N.B. and Whyte, J. (1993) Somnambulism associated with hallucinations. *Psychosomatics* 34:86–90.

32. Silber, M.H., Hansen, M.R. and Girish, M. (2005) Complex nocturnal visual hallucinations. *Sleep Med* 6:363–366.

33. Barabas, G., Ferrari, M. and Matthews, W.S. (1983) Childhood migraine and somnambulism. *Neurology* 33:948–949.

34. Casez, O., Dananchet, Y. and Besson, G. (2005) Migraine and somnambulism. *Neurology* 65:1334–1335.

35. Joncas, S., Zadra, A., Paquet, J. and Montplaisir, J. (2002) The value of sleep deprivation as a diagnostic tool in adult sleepwalkers. *Neurology* 58:936–940.

36. Pilon, M., Zadra, A., Joncas, S. and Montplaisir, J. (2006) Hypersynchronous delta waves and somnambulism: Brain topography and effect of sleep deprivation. *Sleep* 29:77–84.

37. Guilleminault, C., Poyares, D., Aftab, F.A. and Palombini, L. (2001) Sleep and wakefulness in somnambulism: A special analysis study. *J Psychosom Res* 51:411–416.

38. Zadra, A., Pilon, M., Joncas, S., Rompré, S. and Montplaisir, J. (2004) Analysis of postarousal EEG activity during somnambulistic episodes. *J Sleep Res* 13:279–284.

39. Schenck, C.H., Parejy, J.A., Patterson, A.L. and Mahowald, M.W. (1998) Analysis of polysomnographic events surrounding 252 slow-wave sleep arousals in thirty-eight adults with injurious sleep walking and terrors. *J Clin Neurophysiol* 15:159–166.

40. Blatt, I., Peled, R., Gadoth, N. and Lavie, P. (1991) The value of sleep recording in evaluating somnambulism in young adults. *Electroencephalogr Clin Neurophysiol* 78:407–412.

41. Gaudreau, H., Joncas, S., Zadra, A. and Montplaisir, J. (2000) Dynamics of slow-wave activity during the NREM sleep of sleepwalkers and control subjects. *Sleep* 23:755–762.

42. Espa, F., Ondzé, B., Deglise, P., Billiard, M. and Besset, A. (2000) Sleep architecture, slow wave activity, and sleep spindles in adult patients with sleepwalking and sleep terrors. *Clin Neurophysiol* 78:407–412.

43. Guilleminault, C., Kirisoglu, C., da Rosa, A.C., Lopes, C. and Chan, A. (2006) Sleepwalking, a disorder of NREM sleep instability. *Sleep Med* 7:163–170.

44. Soldatos, C.R., Vela-Bueno, A., Bixler, E.O., Schweitzer, P.K. and Kales, A. (1980) Sleepwalking and night terrors in adulthood. Clinical EEG findings. *Clin Electroencephalogr* 11:136–139.

45. Davis, E., Hayes, M. and Kirman, B.H. (1942) Somnambulism. *Lancet* 1:186, .

46. Kales, A., Soldatos, C.R., Bixler, E.O., *et al.* (1980) Hereditary factors in sleepwalking and night terrors. *Br J Psychiatr* 137:111–118.

47. Bakwin, H.I. (1970) Sleepwalking in twins. *Lancet* 2 (7670):446–447.

48. Lecendraux, M., Mayer, G., Bassetti, C., Neidhart, E., Chappuis, R. and Tafti, M. (2003) HLA and genetic susceptibility to sleepwalking. *Mol Psychiatr* 8:114–117.

49. Scott, A.I.F. (1988) Attempted strangulation during phenothiazine-induced sleep-walking and night terrors. *Br J Psychiatr* 153:692–694.

50. Hartman, D., Crisp, A.H., Sedgwick, P. and Borrow, S. (2001) Is there a dissociative process in sleepwalking and night terrors. *Postgrad Med J* 77:244–249.

51. Mori, T., Suzuki, T., Terashima, Y., Kawai, N., Shiraishi, H. and Koizumi, J. (1990) Chronic herpes simplex encephalitis with somnambulism: CT, MR and SPECT findings. *Jpn J Psychiatr Neurol* 44:735–739.

52. Hughes, J.R. (2007) A review of sleepwalking (somnambulism): The enigma of neurophysiology and polysomnography with differential diagnosis of complex partial seizures. *Epilepsy Behav* 11:483–491.

53. Pressmann, M.R. (2007) Factors that predispose, prime and precipitate NREM parasomnias in adults: Clinical and forensic implications. *Sleep Med Rev* 11:5–30.

54. Espa, F., Dauvilliers, Y., Ondze, B., Billiard, M. and Besset, A. (2002) Arousal reactions in sleepwalking and night terrors in adults: The role of respiratory events. *Sleep* 25:871–875.

55. Guilleminault, C., Palombini, L., Pelayo, R. and Chervin, R. (2003) Sleepwalking and sleep terrors in prepubertal children: What triggers them? *Pediatrics* 111:17–25.

56. Millman, R.P., Kipp, G.J. and Carskadon, M.A. (1991) Sleepwalking precipitated by treatment of sleep apnea with nasal CPAP. *Chest* 99:750–751.

57. Pressmann, M.R., Mahowald, M.W., Schenck, C.H. and Bornemann, M.C. (2007) Alcohol-induced sleepwalking or confusional arousal as a defense to criminal behavior: A review of scientific evidence, methods and forensic implications. *J Sleep Res* 16:198–212.

58. Sansone, R. and Sansone, L.A. (2008) Zolpidem, somnambulism and nocturnal eating. *Gen Hosp Psychiatr* 30:90–91.

59. Lauerma, H. (1991) Nocturnal wandering caused by restless legs and short-acting benzodiazepines. *Acta Psychiatr Scand* 83:492–493.

60. Huapaya, L.V.M. (1979) Seven cases of somnambulism induced by drugs. *Am J Psychiatr* 136:985–986.

61. Khazaal, Y., Krenz, Z. and Zullino, D.F. (2003) Buproprion induced somnambulism. *Addict Biol* 8:1429–1433.

62. Charney, D.S., Kales, A., Soldatos, C.R. and Nelson, J.C. (1979) Somnambulistic-like episodes secondary to combined lithium-narcoleptics treatment. *Br J Psychiatr* 135:418–424.

63. Mahowald, M.K. and Schenck, C.H. (1992) Dissociated states of wakefulness and sleep. *Neurology* 42 (Suppl 6):44–52.

64. Berntson, G.G. and Micco, D.J. (1976) Organization of brainstem behavioral systems. *Brain Res Bull* 1:471–483.

65. Mahowald, M. and Schenck, C.H. (2000) Parasomnias: Sleepwalking and the law. *Sleep Med Rev* 4:321–339.

66. Tassinari, C.A., Rubboli, G., Gardella, E., et al. (2005) Central pattern generators for a common semiology in fronto-limbic seizures and in parasomnias. A neurotologic approach. *Neurol Sci* 26:225–232.

67. Werth, E., Achermann, P. and Borbély, A. (1997) Fronto-occipital EEG power gradients in human sleep. *J Sleep Res* 6:102–112.

68. Bassetti, C., Vella, S., Donati, F., Wielepp, P. and Weder, B. (1999) SPECT during sleepwalking. *Lancet* 356:484–485.

69. Schwartz, S. and Maquet, P. (2002) Sleep imaging and the neuropsychological assessment of dreams. *Trends Cogn Sci* 6:23–30.

70. Kantha, S.S. (2003) Is somnambulism a distinct disorder of humans and not seen in non-human primates? *Med Hypotheses* 61:5–6.

71. Juszczack, G.R. and Swiergiel, A.H. (2005) Serotoninergic hypothesis of sleepwalking. *Med Hypotheses* 64:28–32.

72. Oliviero, A., Della Marca, G., Tonali, P.A., Pilato, F., Saturno, E., et al. (2005) Functional involvement of cerebral cortex in human narcolepsy. *J Neurol* 252:56–61.

73. Saper, C.B., Chou, T.C. and Scammell, T.E. (2001) The sleep switch: Hypothalamic control of sleep and wakefulness. *Trends Neurosci* 24:726–731.

74. Baumann, C. and Bassetti, C.L. (2005) Hypocretin and narcolepsy. *Lancet Neurol* 10:673–682.

75. Harris, G.C. and Aston-Jones, G. (2006) Arousal and reward: A dichotomy in orexin function. *Trends Neurosci* 29:571–577.

76. Suzuki, K., Miyamoto, M., Miyamato, T. and Hirata, K. (2007) Insulinoma with early-morning abnormal behavior. *Intern Med* 46:405–408.

77. Rolland, Y., Payoux, P., Lauwers-Cances, V., et al. (2005) A SPECT study of wandering behavior in Alzheimer's disease. *Int J Geriatr Psychiatr* 20:816–820.

78. Schenck, C.H., Boyd, J.L. and Mahowald, M.W. (1997) A parasomnia overlap syndrome involving sleepwalking, sleep terrors, and REM sleep behaviour disorder in 33 polysomnographically confirmed cases. *Sleep* 20:972–981.

79. Tachibana, N., Sugita, Y., Trashima, K., Teshima, Y., Shimizu, T. and Hishikawa, Y. (1991) Polysomnographic characteristics of healthy elderly subjects with somnambulism-like behaviors. *Biol Psychiatr* 30:4–14.

80. De Cock Cochen, V.C., Vidaihlet, M., Leu, S., et al. (2007) Restoration of normal motor control in Parkinson's disease during REM sleep. *Brain* 130:450–456.

81. Pedley, T.A. and Guilleminault, C. (1977) Episodic nocturnal wanderings responsive to anticonvulsant drug therapy. *Ann Neurol* 2:30–35.

82. Plazzi, G., Tinuper, P., Montagna, P., provini, F. and Lugaresi, E. (1995) Epileptic nocturnal wanderings. *Sleep* 18:749–756.

83. Nobili, L., Francione, S., Cardinale, F. and Lo Russo, G. (2002) Epileptic nocturnal wanderings with a temporal lobe origin: A stereo-electroencephalographic study. *Sleep* 25:669–671.

84. Goetz, C.G. (2004) Medical-legal issues in Charcot's neurologic career. *Neurology* 62:1827–1833.

85. Schenck, C.H., Milner, D.M., Hurwitz, T.D., et al. (1989) Dissociative disorders presenting as somnambulism: Polysomnographic, video and clinical documentation. *Dissociation* 2:194–204.

86. Kushida, C.A., Clerk, A.A., Kirsch, C.M., Hotson, J.R. and Guilleminault, C. (1995) Prolonged confusion with nocturnal wandering arising from NREM and REM sleep: A case report. *Sleep* 18:757–764.

87. Poryazova, R., Waldvogel, D. and Bassetti, C.L. (2007) Sleepwalking in patients with Parkinson disease. *Arch Neurol* 64:1–4.

88. Reid, W.H. (1975) Treatment of sleepwalking in military trainees. *Am J Psychother* 35:27–37.

89. Schenck, C.H. and Mahowald, M. (1996) Long-term, nightly benzodiazepine treatment of injurious parasomnias and other disorders of disrupted nocturnal sleep in 170 adults. *Am J Med* 100:333–337.

90. Wilson, S.J., Lillywhite, A.R., Potokar, J.P., Bell, C.J. and Nutt, D.J. (1997) Adult night terrors and paroxetine. *Lancet* 350:185.

91. Liliwhite, A.R., Wilson, S.J. and Nutt, D.J. (1994) Successful treatment of night terrors and somnambulism with paroxetine. *Br J Psychiatr* 164:551–554.

92. Guilleminault, C., Kirisoglu, C., Bao, G., Arias, V., Chan, A. and Li, K.K. (2005) Adult chronic sleepwalking and its treatment based on polysomnography. *Brain* 128:1062–1068.

93. Cooper, A.J. (1987) Treatment of coexistent night-terrors and somnambulism in adults with imipramine and diazepam. *J Clin Psychiatr* 48:209–210.

94. Mahowald, M.W., Bundlie, S.R., Hurwitz, T.D. and Schenck, C.H. (1990) Sleep violence – forensic science implications: Polygraphic and video documentation. *J Forensic Sci* 35:413–432.

General Anaesthesia and Consciousness

Michael T. Alkire

ANAESTHETIC AWAKENINGS

Consciousness is widely held to be a neurobiological property of the brain [1]. Without a brain, there is no consciousness. Anaesthesiologists are in a particularly useful position to help with the modern scientific study of consciousness because it is part and parcel of the profession to chemically induce a temporary reversible state of unconsciousness for surgery. We are the experts at manipulating levels of consciousness. Embarrassingly, however, we do not always get it right.

On rare occasions, patients having general anaesthesia for surgery will remain conscious and aware during their operation, while appearing to be completely anaesthetized. This complication, known as intraoperative awareness, may occur as often as once in every 1000–2000 general anaesthetic cases [2]. This complication highlights the fact that the scientific understanding of consciousness is imperfect. Yet, progress in anaesthesia research towards understanding the neurobiology of consciousness is being made. Within the last decade, a focus on the neurobiology of consciousness from the anaesthesia research community has generated a number of theories [3–7] and reviews about anaesthesia and consciousness [8–11]. This chapter will offer a systems level perspective of current thinking regarding how anaesthesia affects consciousness.

TO STUDY CONSCIOUSNESS, MAKE CONSCIOUSNESS THE DEPENDENT VARIABLE

Using anaesthesia, we are in an excellent position to proceed with the study of consciousness as a dependent variable [12]. This is not a new concept, as the proposal of using anaesthetics as tools for investigating the mind was stated most eloquently by Henry K. Beecher in 1947, 'Experimental reproducibility of clinical states is a first requisite in the study of many problems of medicine. With anaesthetic agents we seem to have a tool for producing and holding at will, and at little risk, different levels of consciousness – a tool that promises to be of great help in studies of mental phenomena. Thus, anaesthesia, in presenting a reversible depression, enables the study of the life process itself. The potentialities for future discoveries in this field seem scarcely to have been tapped' [13].

Anaesthetics can be used as tools in the study of consciousness because they provide a stable reproducible temporary reduction or elimination of consciousness from which comparisons in brain functioning can be made throughout transitions between the conscious and unconscious state and vice versa. The 'depth' of a person's unconsciousness can be directly controlled by the amount of anaesthesia that is given. When anaesthetic dose manipulation is thus coupled with a number of modern neuroscience techniques, such as electrophysiology or functional brain imaging, a powerful methodology emerges for localizing brain regions whose activity might represent specific neural correlates of consciousness.

The ability of anaesthetics to cause a loss of consciousness is dose dependent. There is a minimal dose that must be given in order for a person to become unconscious. This dose varies slightly from person to person. In the operating room, a loss of consciousness is defined as a loss of the ability of a patient to respond to a verbal request to move, or failure of the patient to move to a rousing shake. This clinically useful definition offers a rough guidepost for knowing when something rather drastic has changed in the functioning of a patient's brain, but its ultimate utility for understanding the neurobiology of consciousness may be limited.

THE ANAESTHETIC TOOLBOX

Anaesthetics are broadly classified into two primary categories depending on their route of administration, either intravenous or inhalational. The intravenous agents are generally used for rapid induction of anaesthesia, though they can also be used as a continuous infusion to provide maintenance of anaesthesia. Commonly used modern intravenous (induction) agents include the barbiturates: *sodium thiopental* and *methohexital*; the carboxylated imidazole derivative, *etomidate*; 2,6-diisopropylphenol or *propofol*; and the dissociative agent, *ketamine*. Sedative agents are also given through the intravenous route. These include the benzodiazepines: now most commonly *midazolam*; the alpha-2 agonists, *clonidine* and *dexmedetomidine*; and the opiate analgesics.

Inhaled agents are either gases at room temperature, such as *nitrous oxide* or *xenon*, or they are vapours of volatile liquids, such as the commonly used modern anaesthetic agents: *isoflurane*, *sevoflurane* and *desflurane*. These agents are given to patients to maintain anaesthesia over longer periods of time using calibrated vaporizers, which mix a small controlled portion of the agent's vapour (usually only around 1–5%) with a carrier gas (usually oxygen or an oxygen in air mixture). By turning the calibrated dosage knob on the vaporizer to a particular set point, an anaesthesiologist can give an exact desired amount of a particular agent. The concept of the vaporizer was a great advance in anaesthesia delivery as it allowed for the rapid titration of the agents to match the momentary needs of a particular operation [14].

The doses of inhaled anaesthetics are discussed in terms of their relative potency by referring to the amount needed to prevent movement to a surgical stimulation. The minimum alveolar (i.e., lung) concentration (MAC) of an inhaled agent needed to prevent movement in 50% of subjects in response to a painful surgical stimulation is defined as 1 MAC [15]. To prevent movement during surgery, anaesthetics are given at a cumulative dose that adds up to a value slightly above 1 MAC. MAC-awake is the point at which response to verbal command is lost in 50% of patients. This is typically considered the point at which consciousness is lost and occurs at 0.3–0.4 MAC in younger, healthy individuals [16].

CELLULAR MECHANISM(S) OF ANAESTHESIA

In 1901 two German scientists (working independently) discovered that the amount an anaesthetic molecule dissolved in olive oil correlated with its ability to block the swimming of tadpoles [17, 18]. This observation became known as the Meyer–Overton correlation. It suggested that lipids may be a site of anaesthetic action and it dominated thinking about the mechanism of anaesthesia for nearly a century. In 1984, Nicholas P. Franks and William R. Lieb demonstrated that there was a correlation between anaesthetic potency and the ability of anaesthetics to competitively inhibit firefly luciferase, a pure soluble protein (i.e., no lipids involved) [19]. This seminal observation suggested anaesthetics might work through a different mechanism than a nonspecific interaction with lipid membranes. Instead, anaesthetics might work by specific interactions with cellular protein channels. These are the types of channels that control synaptic transmission. A plethora of studies now detail how anaesthetics interact with numerous ligand-gated ion channels [20, 21].

The cellular targets most closely linked with anaesthetic action involve anaesthetic-induced enhancement of inhibitory currents mediated by gamma-amino butyric acid (GABA) and glycine protein channels, reductions of excitatory currents mediated by glutamate and acetylcholine protein channels, and most recently enhancement of background potassium leak currents (causing intracellular hyperpolarization, an effect which reduces a cell's chances of firing an action potential) [20, 21]. These are generally considered the most plausible cellular targets accounting for anaesthetic action, however, alternative hypotheses still exist [22–26].

Yet once the principle cellular target of anaesthetic action is identified, questions still remain. Why should anaesthetic interactions with that cellular target cause a loss of consciousness? More importantly, what shuts down in the brain at the precise moment consciousness is lost? Does the whole brain shut down and take consciousness away? Or, is there a special network of consciousness neurons that must be affected? What if we could watch the brain turning on and off with anaesthesia, would we find where the consciousness neurons are? To begin addressing these questions, we first turn towards brain imaging.

INTRODUCTION TO FUNCTIONAL BRAIN IMAGING

Functional brain imaging is distinct from structural brain imaging in that a functional brain imaging scan reveals what parts of the brain are functioning over a specific time window in relation to a specific task or a specific cognitive state of the brain. Structural brain imaging simply reveals the structural form of brain tissue. Two commonly used functional imaging methods with positron emission tomography (PET) are measures of either regional cerebral blood flow (rCBF) or cerebral metabolic rate of glucose utilization (rCMRglu). Both measures serve as an indirect correlate for the regional changes in underlying functional neuronal activity [27, 28]. Functional magnetic resonance imaging (fMRI) is another blood flow based technique that has a fast imaging window, on the order of seconds, which measures regional changes in the blood oxygen level-dependent (BOLD) signal as a correlate for neuronal activity [29]. Functional brain imaging works because brain areas that are more active, such as when thinking, require more metabolic support and consequently a regional increase in blood flow occurs to support the increased metabolic demands.

A basic understanding of how anaesthesia affects cerebral blood flow (CBF) and cerebral metabolism is now available as common textbook material [30, 31]. In general, essentially all anaesthetic agents decrease global cerebral metabolism in a dose-dependent manner with variable effects on global CBF [32]. The exception to this generality is the dissociative anaesthetic agent ketamine. Recent human neuroimaging data show that ketamine has a heterogeneous effect on cerebral metabolism with an overall net effect of increasing global cerebral metabolism [33].

More representative of the anaesthetic state is the fact that anaesthetics cause a rather large decrease in cerebral metabolism that is dose dependent. A qualitative example of the magnitude of this cerebral metabolic reduction is illustrated in Figure 10.1. The figure shows high-resolution PET scans of cerebral glucose metabolism in a single subject studied on three different occasions under two different increasing doses of desflurane anaesthesia, compared with no anaesthesia. The amount of glucose metabolism occurring in any particular brain area can be quantified by comparing the colour within the brain region of interest to the scale bar of glucose utilization. Brighter colours indicate more activity. Thus, a glance at Figure 10.1 reveals what anaesthesia does to functional neuronal activity in the living human brain; anaesthesia decreases global rCMRglu. Essentially, anaesthesia seems to work everywhere in the brain to 'turn off' all the neurons at once. The magnitude of the global decrease is generally proportional to the dose of the anaesthesia delivered [31]. It can be seen that sedation with desflurane to the point where the subject was sleepy, yet still readily responsive to a request to move, was associated with a fairly limited decrease in global cerebral metabolism for this subject of around 5–10% from baseline. For this subject, consciousness was lost at a

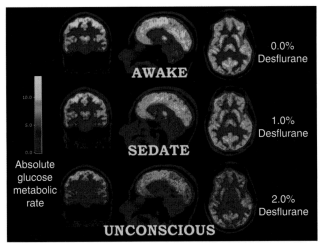

FIGURE 10.1   High-resolution PET images of absolute regional cerebral glucose metabolism from one subject studied on three different occasions. The subject was studied in the awake condition without any anaesthesia and then again on a separate occasion while breathing 1.0% desflurane, which made the subject feel slightly sedated. The subject was then studied a third time while breathing 2.0% desflurane, which made the subject unconscious. The figure illustrates how anaesthesia causes a global metabolic suppression. The blue ghosting around the brain shows the background radiation emanating from the subject's soft tissues. This is not normally seen with lower-resolution PET cameras.

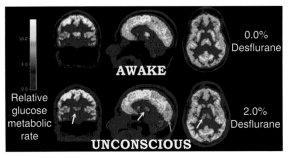

FIGURE 10.2   High-resolution PET images are shown of relative regional cerebral glucose metabolism from the same subject as displayed in Figure 10.1. The scans are identical, except that the unconscious scan has now been placed on a relative colour scale that equalizes the relative metabolic rate occurring in the frontal lobe region. This allows one to see with the naked eye that regional relative metabolic activity within the thalamus is more suppressed than is the activity in the frontal lobe. Examining relative glucose metabolic rates allows the lack of thalamic activity during the unconsciousness produced by desflurane anaesthesia to be more readily appreciated (white arrows). This relative scale also reveals that the primary visual cortex is also regionally suppressed with desflurane anaesthesia (green arrow).

desflurane dose of 2% when the global cerebral metabolic reduction was about 30%.

One could end the examination at this point and be left with the firm conclusion that anaesthesia seems to work everywhere in the brain. However, there is more information that can be obtained. Additional questions can be asked. Which, if any, brain regions were 'turned off' relatively more than others? By understanding if certain anaesthetics had specific regional effects it might be possible to link specific actions of specific anaesthetics to their regional effects in the brain. For instance, if one agent turns off the visual cortex more so than any other agent, then it might be the most interesting to study as a probe of visual consciousness. Might some anaesthetic have a greater tendency to 'turn off' say the cortex more so than the subcortical structures [34]? If so, then the anaesthetic's site of action might be more specifically localized to the cortex and it might be an interesting probe to investigate the relative contributions of cortical vs. subcortical functioning in generating consciousness.

To investigate questions about regional selectivity of anaesthetic effects the metabolic rates in a reference brain region can be equilibrated and the rest of the brain proportionally scaled to show where regional differences might have occurred in comparison with other brain regions. This procedure is shown in Figure

10.2. The same awake and unconscious desflurane scans that were used in Figure 10.1 are again used, except this time the colour scale has been adjusted to match intensity between conditions in the frontal lobe and mid-cingulate regions. Scaling the colour of the unconscious scan to match that of the awake scan reveals two brain regions that have a relative suppression effect. The thalamus (white arrows in Figure 10.2) and the posterior occipital lobe encompassing the primary visual cortical region (green arrow in Figure 10.2) are relatively more suppressed than other brain regions during desflurane-induced unconsciousness for this subject. Thus, desflurane might be an interesting probe for studying both visual consciousness and the relative contribution played by thalamic activity in maintaining consciousness.

NEUROIMAGING STUDIES OF ANAESTHESIA IN HUMANS

The regional effects of most anaesthetic agents have been studied with neuroimaging in humans at doses near to, or just more than, those required to produce unconsciousness. A case has been made for a common effect of most, if not all, agents involving thalamic metabolism/blood flow and thalamocortical–corticothalamic connectivity [3, 35]. This observation, that relative thalamic suppression is a common effect amongst a number of anaesthetics, led to the development of the 'thalamic consciousness switch' hypothesis of anaesthetic-induced unconsciousness [3]. This hypothesis proposed that anaesthetic suppression of activity within the thalamocortical system (as defined by thalamocortical, thalamoreticulocortical and corticothalamic network interactions) could occur through a multitude of anaesthetic interactions at various brain sites which all ultimately converged to hyperpolarize network neurons in the thalamocortical system. The fact that anaesthetics have an ability to affect thalamocortical signalling is well recognized from *in vivo* electrophysiological work in animals [36, 37]. Figure 10.3 illustrates the relative regional effects of anaesthetics found to date.

The figure shows the thalamus is a common site of effect for all agents and sleep. The figure also reveals that a common effect is present for a number of the agents involving the posterior cingulate and medial parietal cortical areas. Another common effect between a few of the agents is seen in the medial basal forebrain areas. Each of these other common regional effects may also have some importance for the neural correlates of consciousness [38]. The studies differ in the anaesthetic endpoints examined. An unconsciousness endpoint was used for the non-REM sleep image, the propofol correlation image, the propofol rCBF image, the sevoflurane rCBF image, the xenon rCMRglu image and the halothane and isoflurane conjunction image. Heavy sedation, where one or a few of the study subjects may have lost consciousness at some point was the behavioural endpoint for each of the other studies.

When the idea of a thalamic consciousness switch was originally developed in relation to human neuroimaging [3], it took into account rCMRglu or rCBF effects involving the thalamus that were observed in humans as a site of a common overlapping regional effect between: the benzodiazepines – lorazepam [39] and midazolam [40]; the intravenous anaesthetic agent propofol [41]; and the inhalational agents isoflurane and halothane [3]. Further additional empirical study over the intervening years has remained consistent with the thalamic overlap effect and has shown replications of propofol's thalamic effects [42, 43], along with an overlapping thalamic effect for the additional inhalational anaesthetic agent sevoflurane [44]. Additionally, recent studies with another newer class of sedative anaesthetics, the alpha-2 adrenoreceptor agonists, dexmedetomidine [45] and clonidine [46] have also shown a consistent overlapping regional suppression effect involving the thalamus at doses that cause heavy sedation or at doses that are just beyond a loss of consciousness endpoint. Furthermore, two recent replication studies of the lorazepam [47] and sevoflurane [48] regional results have strengthened support for the hypothesis of a common regional suppressive effect of anaesthetics involving the thalamus. Pain and vibrotactile sensory processing were also previously examined during increasing doses of isoflurane [49] and propofol [50] anaesthesia, respectively. Both agents cause signal suppression at the level of the thalamus during anaesthetic-induced unconsciousness. If one considers the relative thalamic

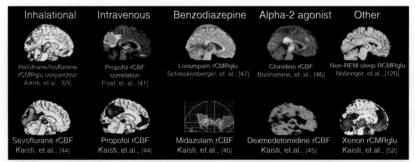

FIGURE 10.3   The regional effects of anaesthetics on brain function are shown in humans that were given various anaesthetic agents at doses which caused, or nearly caused a loss of consciousness. The data are from nine different groups of investigators and encompass the study of nine different agents. The particular agent results are displayed under each drugs category. The inhalational agents examined are halothane and isoflurane [3], sevoflurane [44] and xenon (located under other as an inert noble gas) [51]. The intravenous general anaesthetic agent examined was propofol [41, 44]. The intravenous sedative agents examined were the benzodiazepines, lorazepam [47] and midazolam [40], as well as the alpha-2 agonists, clonidine [46] and dexmedetomidine [45]. Also shown are the results from non-REM sleep [52]. The regional effects were measured using either blood flow or glucose metabolism based techniques. The images were reoriented, and resized to allow the direct overlapping effects between studies to be visually compared. The original colour scales were used. Nevertheless, all images show regional decreases of activity caused by anaesthesia compared to the awake state, except the propofol correlation image and the clonidine correlation image, which shows whereincreasing anaesthetic dose correlates with decreasing blood flow. The figure identifies that the regional suppressive effects of anaesthetics involving the thalamus is a common finding associated with anaesthetic-induced unconsciousness.

suppression of desflurane, as seen in Figure 10.2, then desflurane can be added to this list. However, a full study of desflurane awaits completion.

Most recently, the effects of xenon anaesthesia were imaged [51, 53]. Xenon is an inert noble gas that causes full anaesthesia when inhaled at doses of around 65–75%. It is thought to have minimal to no effect on the GABA ligand channels, yet it does have effects on the *N*-methyl-*D*-Aspartate (NMDA) receptors. However, more recent findings suggest xenon also has important effects on 2-pore background potassium channels [51]. Most interestingly, whatever xenon's cellular mechanisms of action might turn out to be, it too demonstrates a regionally specific effect involving the thalamus when humans are rendered unconscious.

Despite the often dramatic technical differences between studies, the one finding that emerges as potentially robust for anaesthetic effects on consciousness is that when consciousness goes away, or nearly goes away with any number of different anaesthetics, a relative decrease in thalamic activity occurs. This relative effect always has to be interpreted in the broader context of the rather large 30–60% decrease in global metabolism. Nevertheless, the thalamic effect implies that there is a minimal amount of regional thalamic activity that may be necessary to maintain consciousness. Therefore, thalamocortical network interactions emerge as potentially important component of the neural correlate of consciousness.

Common regional effects between agents may suggest a shared underlying mechanism of action. Ori and colleagues noted early on that one of the only common regional metabolic effects seen across a multitude of animal studies was that they all caused metabolic suppression of the somatosensory cortex [54]. Given that the majority of the regional metabolic PET signal originates from synaptic activity and that the thalamus receives a large afferent input from the cerebral cortex, the actual site of mechanistic overlap among agents might be displaced from the thalamus and may actually reside in the cerebral cortex [54]. Such an idea fits well with electrophysiologic studies of anaesthesia [37], and with one study on the regional cerebral metabolic effects of enflurane in the rat, where enflurane's metabolic effects involving the thalamus were unilaterally prevented with an ipsilateral cortical ablation [55].

SITE OF ACTION: THALAMUS?

The regional interaction between the thalamus and anaesthetics supports the proposed localized thalamic consciousness switch [3], such a switch mechanism

may be a central component of a broader dose-related anaesthetic cascade of effects [6]. At the cellular level, anaesthetic agents compromise the natural firing patterns of thalamic network neurons (i.e., thalamocortical, corticothalamic and reticulothalamic cells) by hyperpolarizing their resting membrane potentials [56–58]. As a result, and in a manner that parallels the mechanisms underlying physiologic sleep, a greater proportion of these network cells experience bursting rather than tonic activity [59]. This, in effect, blocks or diminishes synaptic transmission of sensory information through the thalamus and diminishes the high frequency rhythms that characterize the spontaneous activity associated with the awake state and dreaming mentation [60–64].

An example of the dose-dependent ability of isoflurane to reduce the reliability of sensory transmission through the sensory thalamus is shown in Figure 10.4. The figure shows the electrophysiology work of Detsch *et al.* who recorded thalamic unit activity in the rat following a temporary 100 Hz stimulation of mechanoreceptors [65]. The thalamic units tonically

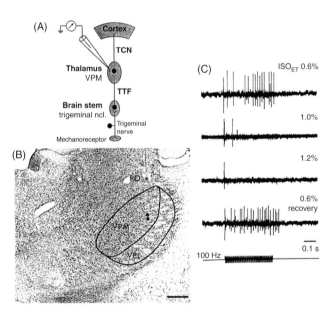

FIGURE 10.4 Isoflurane reduces thalamic neuron responsiveness to somatosensory stimulation in a dose-dependent manner. (A) The experimental setup showing recording of thalamocortical neurons with stimulation of mechanoreceptor. (B) Histology image showing location of the recording electrodes in somatosensory thalamus (VPM). (C) Thalamic neuron fires in a tonic manner to 100 Hz stimulation at 0.6% isoflurane. Increasing the isoflurane dose to 1.0% causes the neuron to fire primarily only to the onset of the stimulation. Increasing the isoflurane dose to 1.2% causes the neuron to fire essentially only an initial burst of activity with the simulation onset. Recovery of the tonic firing ability occurs when the isoflurane dose is once again set to 0.6%. Thus, somatosensory throughput through the thalamus is reduced with increasing dose of isoflurane in a repeatable and reversible manner.

followed the stimulation at low isoflurane levels, but would show only an initial burst to the stimulation when the isoflurane levels were higher. This finding is consistent with the thalamic consciousness switch hypothesis as it shows that thalamic unit activity switches its firing pattern in a reversible manner with increasing anaesthesia dose. Interestingly, further work by this group suggests that the decrease in thalamic firing rates that occur at higher anaesthetic doses is likely due to a decrease in excitatory cortico-thalamic feedback, mediated by both glutamatergic and GABAergic effects [66]. This suggests that the switch in thalamic unit activity is driven primarily through a reduction in afferent corticothalamic feedback and is not necessarily a direct effect of anaesthesia on the thalamic neurons themselves.

The cellular mechanism or mechanisms through which a thalamic consciousness switch might work remain unknown. Nevertheless, two facts converge to suggest that neuronal nicotinic acetylcholine receptors (nAChRs) are a plausible anaesthetic target. First, neuronal nAChRs are potently inhibited by many anaesthetics at subanaesthetic doses [67, 68]. This fact suggests that nAChRs are inhibited in significant proportions at the concentration of anaesthesia associated with a loss of consciousness. Second, the $\alpha4\beta2$ subtype of the nAChR has its highest density of expression in the thalamus [69], suggesting that the localized decrease in regional thalamic activity seen in anaesthesia brain imaging studies might be due to a regionally localized antagonism of nAChRs and might really be a reflection of a localized direct action of anaesthetics on the thalamus and not just a secondary reduction caused by decreased corticothalamic activity.

Alkire *et al.* directly investigated whether thalamic nicotinic mechanisms might play a role in mediating the unconsciousness component of inhalational anaesthesia [70]. This idea was tested in sevoflurane anaesthetized rats that were given enough sevoflurane to induce a loss of the righting reflex (LORR – a correlate for unconsciousness). With rats rendered unconscious, minuscule amounts of nicotine were microinfused into the thalamus of each rat through a previously implanted cannula that was aimed at the central medial (CM) nucleus of the thalamus. The CM is an important component of the intralaminar (ILN) thalamic nuclei and it represents the rostral extension of the ascending reticular activating system (ARAS). Previous work by Miller and coworkers had discovered that the CM thalamus plays a role in arousal and seizure propagation [71, 72]. Miller found that microinfusions of GABA agonists into the CM thalamus would cause a rat to lose consciousness, often within 90 seconds. As shown in Box 10.1, when Alkire *et al.* [70] gave nicotine microinfusions localized to the

CM thalamus, rats awoke from anaesthesia, despite still being in the middle of a chamber filled with anaesthesia.

The case for the thalamic consciousness switch would seem to be strongly supported by the nicotine reversal of unconsciousness experiment. Importantly, however, Alkire and colleagues also tried to induce unconsciousness with intrathalamic microinfusions of mecamylamine a nicotinic antagonist. If thalamic nicotinic mechanisms were causal to anaesthetic-induced unconsciousness and the thalamus was a switch site mediating the 'consciousness off' component of anaesthesia, then intrathalamic mecamylamine should rapidly induce a loss of consciousness. This would be a similar experiment to that reported by Miller and colleagues with their GABAergic agonists [71]. Interestingly, mecamylamine did not induce a loss of consciousness. In fact, it did not even appear to change the dose of sevoflurane that was required to cause a loss of the righting reflex. The overall pattern of results, where the agonist reversed the unconsciousness producing effect of anaesthesia and the antagonist failed to cause a loss of consciousness, suggests that the ILN thalamus may act more as a consciousness 'on' switch, than as a consciousness 'off' switch. Yet, further work is needed to clarify why GABAergic agonists into the ILN could produce unconsciousness, yet a nicotinic antagonist could not.

SITE OF ACTION: CORTEX?

The brain imaging studies do not provide a definitive answer as to where anaesthetics first work to cause unconsciousness. Brain scans of anaesthesia are obtained at steady state doses of anaesthesia and offer no temporal dynamics regarding the process of becoming unconscious. Even if rapid imaging is attempted, the temporal dynamics are likely far too slow to clarify which region (i.e., thalamus or cortex) is affected first by anaesthesia and thus could be considered the primary cause of anaesthetic-induced unconsciousness. This is not just a chicken-or-the-egg phenomenon. If it is the thalamus which is shutting down first and then dragging the cortex down with it, then this suggests one might be able to selectively interact with the thalamus to change one's state of consciousness. Alternatively, if it is the cortex which is shutting down first and then dragging down the thalamus, then the thalamic effect seen in the brain imaging studies may be epiphenomenal to the loss of consciousness.

A number of empirical findings support the hypothesis that the main effect of anaesthesia occurs in the cortex. In human neuroimaging data, Alkire

BOX 10.1

NICOTINIC REVERSAL OF ANAESTHETIC-INDUCED UNCONSCIOUSNESS

The sequential pictures are from a representative video that shows an anaesthetized unconscious rat lying on its back (Figure 10.5A). Shortly after a microinfusion of nicotine into its central medial thalamus the rat begins to arouse (Figure 10.5B–D). He turns over and begins to

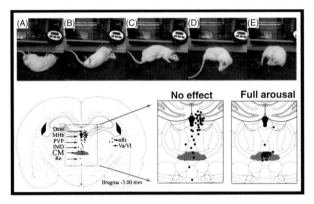

FIGURE 10.5 How to reverse anaesthetic-induced unconsciousness.

ambulate, as if immune to the consciousness suppressing action of anaesthesia (Figure 10.5E). This dramatic reversal of the unconsciousness component of anaesthesia lasts only a few minutes, a time consistent with the pharmacology of nicotine. The arousal response generally did not occur if the microinfusion of nicotine did not involve the CM thalamus (the grey shaded region of the lower rat brain anatomy pictures). The histology schematics show the locations of infusions and their corresponding behavioural responses. The reversal of unconsciousness is a site-specific effect that depends upon changing the activity of neurons within the intralaminar CM thalamus. Abbreviations: CM: central medial thalamus, Dent: dentate gyrus of the hippocampus, IMD: intermediodorsal nucleus, MHb: medial habenular nucleus, nRt: thalamic reticular nucleus, Re:reuniens thalamic nucleus, PVP: paraventricular thalamic nucleus (posterior), Va/Vl: ventral anterior and ventral lateral thalamic nucleus. Rat atlas image from Paxino's and Watson [73] (with permission).

and Haier found that the amount of global metabolic suppression that occurs in each various brain region during propofol anaesthesia (a presumed GABA agonist) was highly correlated with the known regional densities of the GABAergic receptors [74]. Brain regions with more GABA receptors had a larger decrease in regional glucose metabolism, a potential straightforward explanation for the global metabolic decrease seen with anaesthesia. Lukatch and MacIver found *in vitro* evidence that anaesthetics slow cortical oscillatory activity independent of subcortical structures [75]. Antkowiak tested the ability of most anaesthetics to suppress firing rates in cultured slice preparations of neocortical neurons and whether the depression of such firing rates involved GABAergic mechanisms [76]. All anaesthetics at clinically relevant doses decreased spontaneous firing rates of cortical cells and for most agents tested this was a GABAergic effect that could be blocked with the GABAergic antagonist bicuculline. Hentschke *et al.* recently measured the change in cortical firing rates that occurred as rats were exposed to increasing doses of inhaled anaesthetics [77]. They then correlated the changes in firing rates with the concentrations of anaesthetics that increase GABAergic currents *in vitro*. They found

a reasonable correlation between the *in vivo* suppression of cortical firing rates and the *in vitro* effects of anaesthetics on GABA currents. Taken together these studies offer strong support for the idea that anaesthetics have their primary site of action in the cortex.

The most compelling evidence that anaesthetics first work in the cortex to cause a loss of consciousness, and then affect the thalamus, comes from a recent study by Velly *et al.* [78]. These investigators studied human Parkinson's patients who had previously had chronic stimulating electrodes placed into their subthalamic nucleus. The patients were undergoing general anaesthesia to have the pacemaker portion of the stimulator implanted. During a slow careful induction of anaesthesia with either propofol or sevoflurane the investigators monitored cortical electroencephalography (EEG) and subcortical EEG through the stimulator electrode using the electrical contact points that passed through the thalamus. As shown in Box 10.2, when the patient's lost consciousness, a clear change in the cortical EEG occurred first and then the thalamus EEG changed, but not until approximately 10 minutes later.

The findings from Velly and colleagues indicate that anaesthetics first 'turn off' the cortex well before

BOX 10.2

The box summarizes the findings from Velly et al. [78]. During a slow titrated induction of anaesthesia, cortical surface EEG (F3–C3) and subcortical (ESCoG) electrogenesis (i.e., essentially thalamic EEG) was recorded from Parkinson's patients through their deep-brain stimulator electrode (p0–p3) (Figure 10.6). At the point of the loss of consciousness with either propofol (n = 13) or sevoflurane (n = 12) a large change in the cortical EEG pattern of activity occurred, as shown in the raw EEG epochs from a representative subject. A large increase in delta wave activity occurred, as shown in the power spectral analysis. At the same time, the thalamic EEG signal did not change with loss of consciousness, though a slight increase in theta activity seems apparent. The thalamus did not show EEG slowing similar to that found in the cortex at loss of consciousness until 5 minute after the patients were intubated. The middle graph, from a representative subject, shows (in red)

a time–trend plot for a dimensional activation (DA) parameter (an estimate for EEG signal complexity) and (in green) power spectra for the cortical and thalamic EEG signals. A dramatic decrease in cortical DA occurs with the loss of consciousness. The thalamic DA does decrease with anaesthesia, but only slowly over several minutes. The lower graph shows group data regarding the value of the DA parameter determined from either the cortical or the thalamic EEG to discriminate consciousness from unconsciousness. Also shown is the value of the DA parameter identifying patients who were likely to move during laryngoscopy (i.e., during the placement of the endotracheal tube) from those who were not. Put simply, the effect of the anaesthetic on the cortex determined whether patients were conscious or not and the effect of the anaesthetic on the thalamus determined whether patients would move with intense somatosensory stimulation or not.

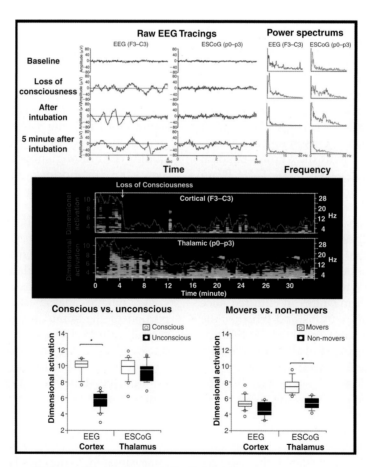

FIGURE 10.6   Chicken or egg? Who is off first, the cortex or the thalamus?

'turning off' the thalamus. The findings temporally localize the loss of consciousness with anaesthesia to an effect on the cerebral cortex. This result offers strong support to those who would wish to place the neural correlates of consciousness in the cerebral cortex. The data also strongly suggest that the decrease in relative thalamic activity found in the brain imaging studies of anaesthesia occurs as a direct result of a decreased corticothalamic feedback to the thalamus. An interpretation consistent with the modelling results of Destexhe [79].

SITE OF ACTION: OTHER SPECIFIC AREAS?

Many other components of the brain's arousal systems will also be affected by anaesthesia. A number of hypothalamic systems may have relevance for interactions with anaesthesia. The orexin system has been implicated in mediating a state-related 'flip-flop' switching mechanism that stabilizes the brain in either a state of consciousness or a state of sleep [80, 81]. The tuberomammillary nucleus (TMN) has been implicated in mediating a component of the sedative nature of GABAergic anaesthetics [82]. More recent work provides evidence that the limbic system participates in regulating the arousal suppressing aspects of anaesthesia [83]. Most recently, an area in the midbrain has been identified and named the mesopontine tegmental anaesthesia area (MPTA) because microinjections of barbiturates into this area cause a rapid apparent loss of consciousness [84]. The overlapping regional effect of anaesthetics involving the thalamus may involve at some level the effects anaesthetics have on normal sleep pathways [3, 82, 85]. However, the results from Velly et al. [78] make this possibility much less likely. Nonetheless, anaesthetic interactions with sleep pathways may be more of a factor for sedative agents or when anaesthetics are only given at sedative doses. Together these studies reveal that the process by which anaesthetics suppress arousal and cause unconsciousness likely involves a complex network of interacting components of the brain's arousal systems, for which the thalamus is but one (perhaps central) component.

IS CONSCIOUSNESS IN THE PARIETAL CORTEX?

The second most consistent anaesthetic-related regional overlap in the brain imaging studies involves the posterior cingulate and medial parietal cortical areas. These posterior areas are of some interest as potential neural correlates of consciousness for five primary reasons. First, as noted above, and as seen in Figure 10.3, a number of these anaesthetic agents suppress activity in these posterior brain regions. Second, these posterior parietal regions have been noted to show a relative decrease in functioning during other altered states of consciousness, such as during the persistent vegetative state [86] and sleep [87]. Laureys noted further that a functional disconnection of this region with frontal brain regions appeared associated with the unconsciousness of the persistent vegetative state [88] and restoration of connectivity between this brain region and frontal brain regions was associated with the return to consciousness [89]. Third, these regions, especially the posterior cingulate area, are involved in memory retrieval [90, 91]. This retrieval effect has recently been shown to be multimodal and independent of response contingency; prompting Shannon and Buckner [92] to 'suggest that conceptions of posterior parietal cortical function should expand beyond attention to external stimuli and motor planning to incorporate higher-order cognitive functions'. Fourth, some evidence links activity in these regions, especially the medial parietal lobes, to the first person perspective of consciousness. A line of research enquiry has developed in which the neural correlates of consciousness are sought using a technique in which experimental subjects manipulate their intra-personal perspective of an external situation [93–95]. Such studies have identified that the medial parietal areas are involved in generating the first person perspective. Such localization would seem to fit well with the long established link between neglect syndromes and parietal damage. Fifth and finally, recent work has shown that the posterior cingulate and medial posterior parietal areas seem to be involved in the generation of the baseline functional state of the human brain [96]. One interpretation of this baseline concept is that these brain regions are active as a reflection of ones self-conscious state when the brain is not involved in any specific cognitive task.

Recent evidence indicates that baseline activity in these posterior brain regions is probably not a correlate for baseline conscious brain activity. Vincent et al. studied the pattern of how spontaneous fluctuation in baseline functional magnetic resonance imaging (fMRI) signals share a temporal coherence within widely distributed cortical systems, including the 'default' system for both humans and monkeys [97]. They found that coherent system fluctuations were still present within the 'default' system of completely unconscious anaesthetized monkeys. A finding that indicates this system is not in general a primary neural correlate of baseline consciousness; nor is it specifically a unique correlate of human consciousness.

SITE OF ACTION: NETWORK INTERACTIONS

As stated by Tononi and Edelman [98], 'Activation and deactivation of distributed neural populations in the thalamocortical system are not sufficient bases for conscious experience unless the activity of the neuronal groups involved is integrated rapidly and effectively'. Following this logic, it is unlikely that a full characterization of the effects of anaesthetic agents can be made by observing only the regionally specific and global suppressive effects of these agents. A more comprehensive assessment would seem to require an additional understanding of how these agents affect functional integration across neural systems [99]. Tononi has further theorized that consciousness depends on a process of information integration within the thalamocortical system [100]. Thus, anaesthetics can be seen as substances that cause unconsciousness because they prevent the ability of information to be integrated in a timely manner across widely dispersed areas of the thalamocortical system [3, 7, 37, 101, 102]. Evidence that anaesthetics block functional connectivity, a finding that would support a loss of the ability to integrate information, has been found in animal models of anaesthesia, with human PET imaging, and in one recent human fMRI study of sevoflurane anaesthesia [35, 103, 104].

The disconnection of thalamocortical connectivity idea as a basis for anaesthetic-induced unconsciousness was supported by a recent functional and effective connectivity analysis of inhalational anaesthesia [35]. Using a path analysis approach it was determined that anaesthetic-induced unconsciousness in humans is associated with a change in effective thalamocortical and corticocortical connectivity, such that the thalamus and cortex no longer effectively interact with one another at the point of anaesthetic-induced unresponsiveness (see Figure 10.7). The data-driven approach to the network modelling procedure used in the connectivity analysis directed attention towards the lateral cerebello-thalamo-cortical system. The presumed primary role of the cerebello-thalamo-cortical system is in motor control. The cerebellar inputs to the cortex travelling through the thalamus are thought to represent excitatory influences on motor output regions (M1) after substantial sampling of incoming sensory and motor information [105, 106]. Disruption of cerebello-thalamo-cortical signalling during anaesthesia is thus an interesting empirical finding that may fit well with Cotterill's idea that consciousness is a controller of motor output [107].

A DETAILED LOOK AT THE DOSE-DEPENDENT PHENOMENOLOGY OF ANAESTHESIA

The effects of anaesthetics on consciousness do not represent an all-or-nothing process. They are dose dependent. To provide the non-clinician with a proper frame of reference, a detailed overview of the dose-related effects anaesthetics have on brain functioning is offered. In terms of consciousness, there is an important relationship between the dose of anaesthesia and the 'depth' of a person's unconsciousness. What becomes apparent from the phenomenology of clinical anaesthesia is that a primary capacity of anaesthesia to cause unconsciousness is a dose-related function of its ability to prevent an active process of arousal from occurring in the brain. Much confusion about this point arises for non-clinicians because, in the operating room, anaesthesia is delivered in a rapid manner to allow the clinician to swiftly take control of the patient's airway. Thus, for most people who experience anaesthesia for an operation, all they remember is 'being there' and then 'not being there' and then 'being there' again in the recovery room, with surgery having ended usually about an hour previously.

In a research setting, if one were to be exposed to a low dose of an inhalational anaesthetic agent at a dose of 0.1 MAC (or about 1/10th of that needed for surgery) for about a half-hour, one would not automatically become unconscious. One would certainly smell the odour of the drug and have the feeling that they were being affected to some extent by the drug. One might experience a paradoxical hyperalgesic response such that a painful stimulation will feel more painful because of the exposure to the low dose of anaesthetic [108]. This hyperalgesic effect peaks at doses around 0.1 MAC and then it is rapidly replaced by sensations of analgesia at doses around 0.2 MAC. Next, and still at these relatively low doses of 0.1–0.3 MAC, memory will start to become significantly impaired [109], with explicit-conscious memory failing before implicit-unconscious memory [110, 111]. Implicit memory remains somewhat intact at levels up to about 0.6 MAC [112].

If the dose was then increased to 0.2 MAC and held steady for about a half-hour, most of the above effects would likely intensify and four additional

(A)   (B)

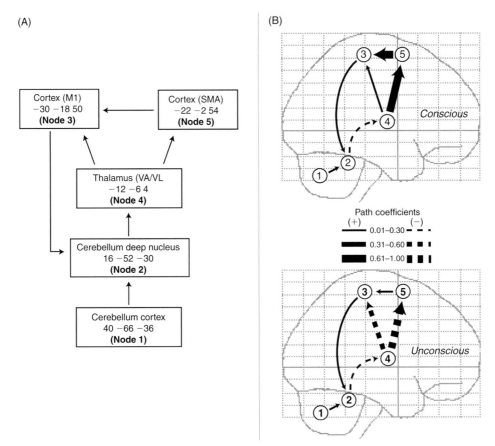

FIGURE 10.7 Effective connectivity changes with anaesthetic-induced unconsciousness in the human lateral cerebello-thalamo-cortical network [35]. Part (A) of the figure shows the network nodes, with their Talariach coordinates, and their modelled interactions. Structural equation modelling of this limited corticothalamic network (B) reveals that effective connectivity dramatically changes within this network, especially involving the thalamocortical and corticocortical interactions depending on the presence or absence of consciousness. Such a connectivity analysis approach can reveal network interactions and regional effects that might otherwise be missed with more traditional analysis techniques.

effects would start to appear. (1) An intoxicated feeling would become evident and a person might then have the sense that time itself was slowing down. One's perception of the visual world might take on a rather strange disconnection in how the microseconds of consciousness flow together. This would be experienced similar to frames in a movie that were being shown too slowly, so that the action occurred in a jerky manner from one frame to the next. (2) A feeling of a disconnection from the environment or a sense of being more focused would likely occur and this might prompt one to laugh about this or feel giddy. (3) A feeling of numbness or tingling in the hands and feet would appear. This feeling is similar to when an arm or leg is 'waking up' after having 'fallen asleep'. (4) Most importantly, an unmistakable feeling of tiredness and drowsiness would become noticeable. Indeed, if a person was left without being stimulated, even a well-rested person would soon close their eyes and

fall asleep. At this point, if the person was allowed to sleep, then they could easily be aroused by common sensory stimulation such as a verbal request to move their hand or by a light touch.

If the dose were increased slightly further to 0.3 MAC and held steady, essentially no new sensations would appear, but each of the above effects would intensify. As the time slowing effect intensifies, reaction times would now become noticeably and measurably slower. Yet a person's sense of time would become so distorted that 10 minutes might pass by during the time the person subjectively feels that only a single minute has passed. Perhaps even more intriguing is that the person might feel that certain timed events, which took a known amount of time to experience and complete when they were not exposed to any anaesthesia, were now going by much faster. Analgesia would intensify and an individual might not feel the poke of a pin. A person's attention might become fixated on a single aspect of something in the environment. A person's eyelids would soon become too heavy to keep open and the feeling of drowsiness would be replaced by a strong desire to be asleep. If allowed to fall asleep, it would now be more difficult to awaken the person. At the 0.3 MAC dose, it might take yelling the person's name or physically shaking them to cause them to arouse. When they did awaken, they would move and speak slowly in a drunk-like uncoordinated manner. Movements would be predominately gross motor movements with an apparent lack of fine motor control. If the person was then again left without stimulation, they would quickly fall back to sleep. At the exact same time that a person would transition to unconsciousness, if they were holding something in their hand, they would drop it. Thus, at the point of unconsciousness, a distinct decrease in somatic muscle tone occurs. Also, not long after 'falling asleep' most people will snore, as the anaesthesia drug relaxes the muscles of the tongue and upper airway. Indeed, the snoring reflects the fact that anaesthetics take away one's ability to keep their own airway open and this is why anaesthesia care is required when an anaesthetic is given.

The switch from conscious/responsive to unconscious/unresponsive occurs in a fraction of a second. We have all experienced the rapidity of this state transition. When one falls asleep in an upright position, such as on an aeroplane or in a car, one's head often falls forward with a sudden collapse. When the head hits the chest, the sudden jolt often arouses the person from their slumber and they often think something like, 'Oh, I just fell asleep'. In that brief instant, both a transition to sleep and a transition back to wakefulness occur. It appears from the phenomenology of low-dose anaesthesia exposure that the transition to anaesthetic-induced unconsciousness during exposure to low-dose anaesthesia probably occurs through a similar, if not identical mechanism as that which mediates the transition to a state of sleep-induced unconsciousness. This assumption is made because subjects exposed to a low dose of anaesthesia will readily fall asleep and can readily be aroused over and over again every few minutes. However, at deeper levels of anaesthesia, as found in the study of the Parkinson's patients, a different type of unconsciousness appears to occur because subjects can no longer transition rapidly between states of consciousness. This deeper level of unconsciousness, likely driven by anaesthetic effects on the cortex, would probably not share much of the neurobiology associated with sleep physiology.

Once at an anaesthetic dose level above that which causes unconsciousness, a person would not be able to respond to a specific command to move, but they would still be able to make an apparent purposeful movement if they received a painful enough stimulation. Thus, for example, if a surgeon cuts the abdomen of an appendectomy patient who appears unconscious at a 0.7 MAC dose of an inhaled anaesthetic agent, the surgeon might be surprised to find the patient's hand reaching up to stop the cutting. The patient would not be able to express a coherent thought or memory about this situation, but they may arouse enough to grimace and utter an audible groan. Suppression of all movement occurs at still deeper levels of anaesthesia, with levels above 1 MAC usually considered sufficient for surgical anaesthesia. Thereafter, increasing anaesthetic doses lead to decreased cardiovascular stability and, with some agents, an isoelectric EEG. Deeper anaesthesia than that is potentially lethal from cardiovascular collapse.

From the phenomenology of clinical anaesthesia it can be seen that the anaesthetic state arises through a sequential dose-dependent progressive suppression of the brain's ability to arouse itself into a conscious state. At low anaesthetic doses people want to be asleep, but they can wilfully keep themselves awake. This is analogous to driving home extremely tired and fighting to stay awake. At slightly higher doses of anaesthesia it takes a more robust external stimulation to fight the drug effects on the arousal system and bring the brain back to consciousness. At even slightly higher doses the intensity of the stimulus needed to generate an arousal response increases further. Finally, even the most painful stimulation cannot generate enough of an arousal influence to awaken the brain. This process of anaesthetic blockade of arousal is illustrated in Box 10.3.

The box summarizes much of the work of Antognini and colleagues who have investigated anaesthetic effects on cortical EEG arousal in a goat model of anaesthesia [113, 114]. Their goat model was developed to allow for the differential delivery of anaesthetics either to the head or to the body of a goat and they have been able to determine the relative contributions made by either the brain or the spinal cord to the actions of anaesthetics at preventing movement to painful stimulation [115]. An emerging conclusion from this line of work is that the spinal cord is now thought to be a major site of action for mediating the MAC response of anaesthesia [116, 117]. However, the brain is still thought to play a role in mediating the MAC response for certain anaesthetics [118, 119]. Most importantly, regardless of where an anaesthetic is acting to prevent movement to a painful stimulation, as Box 10.3 shows, a primary effect of surgical doses of anaesthesia is to block the process of cortical arousal and prevent the transition to a conscious state in response to an external painful stimulation.

BOX 10.3

The box illustrates how either painful somatic stimulation or direct electrical stimulation to components of the ARAS will generate a cortical EEG arousal response, but only when the dose of anaesthesia is below the 1 MAC surgical level. The pink highlighted areas show the changes in the EEG pattern from one of high voltage slow activity (usually associated with deep sleep or unconsciousness) to one of low voltage fast activity (usually associated with wakefulness or consciousness) (Figure 10.8). For the somatic stimulation, a clamp was placed on the foot of an anaesthetized goat at various increasing doses of isoflurane anaesthesia. Note that arousal does not occur at the 1.1 MAC dose or the 1.4 MAC dose and a burst-suppression pattern (i.e., temporary isoelectric EEG) occurs at the 1.4 MAC dose. The effect of direct brain electrical stimulation is shown in the lower portion of the box. The black dots on the axial brain drawings show stimulation sites. Stimulation intensity is shown at the arrows. The highlighted pink areas again show a transition from high voltage slow activity to low voltage fast activity following the stimulation. This EEG change implies a transition towards a more conscious state. When compared to the stimulation that caused arousal, even greater stimulation intensities fail to cause arousal when the dose of anaesthesia is greater than 1 MAC. *Source*: Modified from [113, 114], with permission.

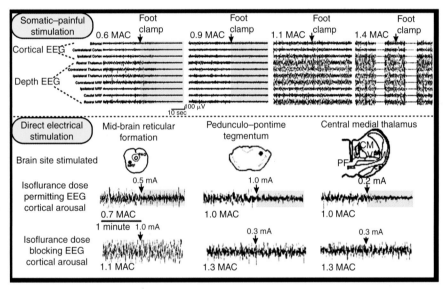

FIGURE 10.8 Anaesthesia maintains unconsciousness by blocking arousal.

CONCLUSIONS

The notion that anaesthetics might offer novel experimental insights into the functioning of the human mind is not a new one. In fact, it has been around for nearly as long as anaesthesia itself. As reported by H.K. Beecher [13], the English chemist Sir Humphry Davy experimented on himself on the day after Christmas in the year 1799 regarding the nature of the newly discovered gas nitrous oxide. As a consequence of breathing the gas, he made a remarkable discovery concerning the nature of human consciousness. Following his experiment Davy reported, 'As I recovered my former state of mind, I felt an inclination to communicate the discoveries I had made during the experiment. I endeavored to recall the ideas, they were feeble and indistinct; one collection of terms, however, presented itself: and with the most intense belief and prophetic manner, I exclaimed…, Nothing exists but thoughts! The universe is composed of impressions, ideas, pleasures and pains!' Davy's anaesthetic-induced awakening about the nature of the universe and where his mind fit into the cosmic scheme of things is a powerful testament to the ability of anaesthetics to help unravel the puzzle of human consciousness. Two centuries later, the scientific study of consciousness has risen to the forefront of neuroscience enquiry and Davy's insight that 'Nothing exists but thoughts!' is now one popular contemporary view regarding the neurobiology of consciousness [1, 120].

It appears that a convergence of evidence points towards the cortex and its interactions as part of the thalamocortical system, as being critically involved with mediating not only anaesthetic-induced unconsciousness, but also with mediating other forms of altered states of consciousness [38]. It appears that anaesthetics cause unconsciousness because they suppress cortical functioning, block arousal through the thalamus and stop the process of information integration within the thalamocortical system on which consciousness depends.

References

1. Crick, F. (1994) *The Astonishing Hypothesis*, Scribner.
2. Sebel, P.S., *et al.* (2004) The incidence of awareness during anesthesia: A multicenter United States study. *Anesth Analg* 99 (3):833–839. table of contents.
3. Alkire, M.T., *et al.* (2000) Toward a unified theory of narcosis: Brain imaging evidence for a thalamocortical switch as the neurophysiologic basis of anesthetic-induced unconsciousness. *Conscious Cogn* 9 (3):370–386.
4. Flohr, H. (1995) An information processing theory of anaesthesia. *Neuropsychologia* 33 (9):1169–1180.
5. Hameroff, S. (1998) Anesthesia, consciousness and hydrophobic pockets – a unitary quantum hypothesis of anesthetic action. *Toxicol Lett* 100–101:31–39.
6. John, E.R. and Prichep, L.S. (2005) The anesthetic cascade: A theory of how anesthesia suppresses consciousness. *Anesthesiology* 102 (2):447–471.
7. Mashour, G.A. (2004) Consciousness unbound: Toward a paradigm of general anesthesia. *Anesthesiology* 100 (2):428–433.
8. Alkire, M.T. and Miller, J. (2005) General anesthesia and the neural correlates of consciousness. *Prog Brain Res* 150:229–244.
9. Hameroff, S.R. (2006) The entwined mysteries of anesthesia and consciousness: Is there a common underlying mechanism? *Anesthesiology* 105 (2):400–412.
10. Hudetz, A.G. (2006) Suppressing consciousness: Mechanisms of general anesthesia. *Semin Anesth Perioperat Med Pain* 25:196–204.
11. Mashour, G.A. (2006) Integrating the science of consciousness and anesthesia. *Anesth Analg* 103 (4):975–982.
12. Alkire, M.T., *et al.* (1998) Towards the neurobiology of consciousness: Using brain imaging and anesthesia to investigate the anatomy of consciousness. In *Toward a Science of Consciousness II* S.R. Hameroff, *et al.* (eds.). MIT Press. pp. 255–268.
13. Beecher, H.K. (1947) Anesthesia's second power: Probing the mind. *Science* 105:164–166.
14. Morris, L.E. (1952) A new vaporizer for liquid anesthetic agents. *Anesthesiology* 13 (6):587–593.
15. Eger II, E.I., *et al.* (1965) Minimum alveolar anesthetic concentration: A standard of anesthetic potency. *Anesthesiology* 26 (6):756–763.
16. Newton, D.E., *et al.* (1990) Levels of consciousness in volunteers breathing sub-MAC concentrations of isoflurane. *Br J Anaesth* 65 (5):609–615.
17. Meyer, H.H. (1901) Zur theorie der alkoholnarkose. Der einfluss wechselnder temperature auf wirkungsstärke und theilungscoefficient der narcotica. *Arch Exp Pathol Pharmakol* 46:338–346.
18. Overton, C.E. (1901) *Studien uber die narkose zugleich ein beitrag zur allgemeinen pharmakologie*, Gustav Fischer.
19. Franks, N.P. and Lieb, W.R. (2004) Seeing the light: Protein theories of general anesthesia, 1984. *Anesthesiology* 101 (1):235–237.
20. Campagna, J.A., *et al.* (2003) Mechanisms of actions of inhaled anesthetics. *New Engl J Med* 348 (21):2110–2124.
21. Franks, N.P. (2006) Molecular targets underlying general anaesthesia. *Br J Pharmacol* 147 (Suppl 1):S72–S81.
22. Eckenhoff, R.G. (2001) Promiscuous ligands and attractive cavities: How do the inhaled anesthetics work? *Mol Interv* 1 (5):258–268.
23. Eckenhoff, R.G. and Shuman, H. (1991) Localization of volatile anesthetic molecules at the subcellular and molecular level. *Ann NY Acad Sci* 625:755–756.
24. Ishizawa, Y., *et al.* (2002) G protein-coupled receptors as direct targets of inhaled anesthetics. *Mol Pharmacol* 61 (5):945–952.
25. Kaech, S., *et al.* (1999) Volatile anesthetics block actin-based motility in dendritic spines. *Proc Natl Acad Sci USA* 96 (18):10433–10437.
26. Tsuchiya, M., *et al.* (1990) Halothane enhances the phosphorylation of H1 histone and rat brain cytoplasmic proteins by protein kinase C. *Life Sci* 46 (11):819–825.
27. Phelps, M.E., *et al.* (1977) Positron tomography: 'In vivo' autoradiographic approach to measurement of cerebral hemodynamics and metabolism. *Acta Neurol Scand Suppl* 64:446–447.
28. Raichle, M.E., *et al.* (1984) Dynamic measurements of local blood flow and metabolism in the study of higher cortical function in humans with positron emission tomography. *Ann Neurol* 15 (Suppl):S48–S49.
29. Ogawa, S., *et al.* (1990) Brain magnetic resonance imaging with contrast dependent on blood oxygenation. *Proc Natl Acad Sci USA* 87 (24):9868–9872.
30. Drummond, J.C. and Patel, P. (2000) Cerebral blood flow and metabolism. In *Anesthesia* R.D. Miller (eds.) Churchill-Livingstone. pp. 1203–1256.
31. Michenfelder, J.D. (1988) *Anesthesia and the Brain*, New York: Churchill-Livingstone,
32. Heinke, W. and Schwarzbauer, C. (2002) *In vivo* imaging of anaesthetic action in humans: Approaches with positron emission tomography (PET) and functional magnetic resonance imaging (fMRI). *Br J Anaesth* 89 (1):112–122.
33. Langsjo, J.W., *et al.* (2004) Effects of subanesthetic ketamine on regional cerebral glucose metabolism in humans. *Anesthesiology* 100 (5):1065–1071.
34. Alkire, M.T., *et al.* (1995) Cerebral metabolism during propofol anesthesia in humans studied with positron emission tomography. *Anesthesiology* 82 (2):393–403.
35. White, N.S. and Alkire, M.T. (2003) Impaired thalamocortical connectivity in humans during general-anesthetic-induced unconsciousness. *Neuroimage* 19 (2 Pt 1):402–411.
36. Steriade, M. (2001) Impact of network activities on neuronal properties in corticothalamic systems. *J Neurophysiol* 86 (1):1–39.
37. Angel, A. (1993) Central neuronal pathways and the process of anaesthesia. *Br J Anaesth* 71 (1):148–163.
38. Baars, B.J., *et al.* (2003) Brain, conscious experience and the observing self. *Trends Neurosci* 26 (12):671–675.

39. Volkow, N.D., *et al.* (1995) Depression of thalamic metabolism by lorazepam is associated with sleepiness. *Neuropsychopharmacology* 12 (2):123–132.

40. Veselis, R.A., *et al.* (1997) Midazolam changes cerebral blood flow in discrete brain regions: An H2(15)O positron emission tomography study. *Anesthesiology* 87 (5):1106–1117.

41. Fiset, P., *et al.* (1999) Brain mechanisms of propofol-induced loss of consciousness in humans: A positron emission tomographic study. *J Neurosci* 19 (13):5506–5513.

42. Veselis, R.A., *et al.* (2004) Thiopental and propofol affect different regions of the brain at similar pharmacologic effects. *Anesth Analg* 99 (2):399–408.

43. Kaisti, K.K., *et al.* (2003) Effects of sevoflurane, propofol, and adjunct nitrous oxide on regional cerebral blood flow, oxygen consumption, and blood volume in humans. *Anesthesiology* 99 (3):603–613.

44. Kaisti, K.K., *et al.* (2002) Effects of surgical levels of propofol and sevoflurane anesthesia on cerebral blood flow in healthy subjects studied with positron emission tomography. *Anesthesiology* 96 (6):1358–1370.

45. Prielipp, R.C., *et al.* (2002) Dexmedetomidine-induced sedation in volunteers decreases regional and global cerebral blood flow. *Anesth Analg* 95 (4):1052–1059.

46. Bonhomme, V., *et al.* (2008) Effect of clonidine infusion on distribution of regional cerebral blood flow in volunteers. *Anesth Analg* 106:899–909.

47. Schreckenberger, M., *et al.* (2004) The thalamus as the generator and modulator of EEG alpha rhythm: A combined PET/EEG study with lorazepam challenge in humans. *Neuroimage* 22 (2):637–644.

48. Schlunzen, L., *et al.* (2004) Effects of subanaesthetic and anaesthetic doses of sevoflurane on regional cerebral blood flow in healthy volunteers. A positron emission tomographic study. *Acta Anaesthesiol Scand* 48 (10):1268–1276.

49. Antognini, J.F., *et al.* (1997) Isoflurane anesthesia blunts cerebral responses to noxious and innocuous stimuli: A fMRI study. *Life Sci* 61 (24):L349–L354.

50. Bonhomme, V., *et al.* (2001) Propofol anesthesia and cerebral blood flow changes elicited by vibrotactile stimulation: A positron emission tomography study. *J Neurophysiol* 85 (3):1299–1308.

51. Rex, S., *et al.* (2006) Positron emission tomography study of regional cerebral metabolism during general anesthesia with xenon in humans. *Anesthesiology* 105 (5):936–943.

52. Nofzinger, E.A., *et al.* (2002) Human regional cerebral glucose metabolism during non-rapid eye movement sleep in relation to waking. *Brain* 125 (Pt 5):1105–1115.

53. Laitio, R.M., *et al.* (2007) Effects of xenon anesthesia on cerebral blood flow in humans: A positron emission tomography study. *Anesthesiology* 106 (6):1128–1133.

54. Ori, C., *et al.* (1986) Effects of isoflurane anesthesia on local cerebral glucose utilization in the rat. *Anesthesiology* 65 (2):152–156.

55. Nakakimura, K., *et al.* (1988) Metabolic activation of intercortical and corticothalamic pathways during enflurane anesthesia in rats. *Anesthesiology* 68 (5):777–782.

56. Steriade, M., *et al.* (2001) Natural waking and sleep states: A view from inside neocortical neurons. *J Neurophysiol* 85 (5):1969–1985.

57. Nicoll, R.A. and Madison, D.V. (1982) General anesthetics hyperpolarize neurons in the vertebrate central nervous system. *Science* 217 (4564):1055–1057.

58. Berg-Johnsen, J. and Langmoen, I.A. (1987) Isoflurane hyperpolarizes neurones in rat and human cerebral cortex. *Acta Physiol Scand* 130 (4):679–685.

59. Steriade, M. (1994) Sleep oscillations and their blockage by activating systems. *J Psychiatr Neurosci* 19 (5):354–358.

60. Steriade, M. (2000) Corticothalamic resonance states of vigilance and mentation. *Neuroscience* 101 (2):243–276.

61. Angel, A. (1991) The G. L. Brown lecture. Adventures in anaesthesia. *Exp Physiol* 76 (1):1–38.

62. Llinas, R.R. and Pare, D. (1991) Of dreaming and wakefulness. *Neuroscience* 44 (3):521–535.

63. Lytton, W.W. and Sejnowski, T.J. (1991) Simulations of cortical pyramidal neurons synchronized by inhibitory interneurons. *J Neurophysiol* 66 (3):1059–1079.

64. Buzsáki, G. and Chrobak, J.J. (1995) Temporal structure in spatially organized neuronal ensembles: A role for interneuronal networks. *Curr Opin Neurobiol* 5 (4):504–510.

65. Detsch, O., *et al.* (1999) Isoflurane induces dose-dependent changes of thalamic somatosensory information transfer. *Brain Res* 829 (1–2):77–89.

66. Vahle-Hinz, C., *et al.* (2007) Contributions of GABAergic and glutamatergic mechanisms to isoflurane-induced suppression of thalamic somatosensory information transfer. *Exp Brain Res* 176 (1):159–172.

67. Flood, P., *et al.* (1997) Alpha 4 beta 2 neuronal nicotinic acetylcholine receptors in the central nervous system are inhibited by isoflurane and propofol, but alpha 7-type nicotinic acetylcholine receptors are unaffected. *Anesthesiology* 86 (4):859–865.

68. Violet, J.M., *et al.* (1997) Differential sensitivities of mammalian neuronal and muscle nicotinic acetylcholine receptors to general anesthetics. *Anesthesiology* 86 (4):866–874.

69. Gallezot, J.D., *et al.* (2005) *In vivo* imaging of human cerebral nicotinic acetylcholine receptors with 2-18F-fluoro-A-85380 and PET. *J Nucl Med* 46 (2):240–247.

70. Alkire, M.T., *et al.* (2007) Thalamic microinjection of nicotine reverses sevoflurane-induced loss of righting reflex in the rat. *Anesthesiology* 107:264–272.

71. Miller, J.W. and Ferrendelli, J.A. (1990) Characterization of GABAergic seizure regulation in the midline thalamus. *Neuropharmacology* 29 (7):649–655.

72. Miller, J.W., *et al.* (1989) Identification of a median thalamic system regulating seizures and arousal. *Epilepsia* 30 (4):493–500.

73. Paxino, G. and Watson, C. (2004) *The rat brain in stereotaxic coordinates*, 5th Edition. Elsevier Academic Press.

74. Alkire, M.T. and Haier, R.J. (2001) Correlating *in vivo* anaesthetic effects with *ex vivo* receptor density data supports a GABAergic mechanism of action for propofol, but not for isoflurane. *Br J Anaesth* 86 (5):618–626.

75. Lukatch, H.S. and MacIver, M.B. (1996) Synaptic mechanisms of thiopental-induced alterations in synchronized cortical activity. *Anesthesiology* 84 (6):1425–1434.

76. Antkowiak, B. (1999) Different actions of general anesthetics on the firing patterns of neocortical neurons mediated by the GABA(A) receptor. *Anesthesiology* 91 (2):500–511.

77. Hentschke, H., *et al.* (2005) Neocortex is the major target of sedative concentrations of volatile anaesthetics: Strong depression of firing rates and increase of GABAA receptor-mediated inhibition. *Eur J Neurosci* 21 (1):93–102.

78. Velly, L.J., *et al.* (2007) Differential dynamic of action on cortical and subcortical structures of anesthetic agents during induction of anesthesia. *Anesthesiology* 107:(in press).

79. Destexhe, A. (2000) Modelling corticothalamic feedback and the gating of the thalamus by the cerebral cortex. *J Physiol Paris* 94 (5–6):391–410.

80. Sakurai, T. (2007) The neural circuit of orexin (hypocretin): Maintaining sleep and wakefulness. *Nat Rev Neurosci* 8 (3):171–181.

81. Saper, C.B., *et al.* (2005) Hypothalamic regulation of sleep and circadian rhythms. *Nature* 437 (7063):1257–1263.

82. Nelson, L.E., *et al.* (2002) The sedative component of anesthesia is mediated by GABA(A) receptors in an endogenous sleep pathway. *Nat Neurosci* 5 (10):979–984.

83. Ma, J. and Leung, L.S. (2006) Limbic system participates in mediating the effects of general anesthetics. *Neuropsychopharmacology* 31 (6):1177–1192.

84. Sukhotinsky, I., *et al.* (2007) Neural pathways associated with loss of consciousness caused by intracerebral microinjection of GABA A-active anesthetics. *Eur J Neurosci* 25 (5):1417–1436.

85. Lydic, R. and Biebuyck, J.F. (1994) Sleep neurobiology: Relevance for mechanistic studies of anaesthesia [editorial]. *Br J Anaesth* 72 (5):506–508.

86. Laureys, S., *et al.* (2004) Brain function in coma, vegetative state, and related disorders. *Lancet Neurol* 3 (9):537–546.

87. Maquet, P. (2000) Functional neuroimaging of normal human sleep by positron emission tomography. *J Sleep Res* 9 (3):207–231.

88. Laureys, S., *et al.* (1999) Impaired effective cortical connectivity in vegetative state: Preliminary investigation using PET. *Neuroimage* 9 (4):377–382.

89. Laureys, S., *et al.* (2000) Restoration of thalamocortical connectivity after recovery from persistent vegetative state. *Lancet* 355 (9217):1790–1791.

90. Rugg, M.D. and Wilding, E.L. (2000) Retrieval processing and episodic memory. *Trends Cogn Sci* 4 (3):108–115.

91. Rugg, M.D., *et al.* (2002) The neural basis of episodic memory: Evidence from functional neuroimaging. *Philos Trans R Soc Lond B Biol Sci* 357 (1424):1097–1110.

92. Shannon, B.J. and Buckner, R.L. (2004) Functional-anatomic correlates of memory retrieval that suggest nontraditional processing roles for multiple distinct regions within posterior parietal cortex. *J Neurosci* 24 (45):10084–10092.

93. Zeman, A. (2001) Consciousness. *Brain* 124 (Pt 7):1263–1289.

94. Kircher, T.T. and Leube, D.T. (2003) Self-consciousness, self-agency, and schizophrenia. *Conscious Cogn* 12 (4):656–669.

95. Vogeley, K., *et al.* (2004) Neural correlates of first-person perspective as one constituent of human self-consciousness. *J Cogn Neurosci* 16 (5):817–827.

96. Burton, H., *et al.* (2004) Default brain functionality in blind people. *Proc Natl Acad Sci USA* 101 (43):15500–15505.

97. Vincent, J.L., *et al.* (2007) Intrinsic functional architecture in the anaesthetized monkey brain. *Nature* 447 (7140):83–86.

98. Tononi, G. and Edelman, G.M. (1998) Consciousness and complexity. *Science* 282 (5395):1846–1851.

99. Cariani, P. (2000) Anesthesia, neural information processing, and conscious awareness. *Conscious Cogn* 9 (3):387–395.

100. Tononi, G. (2004) An information integration theory of consciousness. *BMC Neurosci* 5 (1):42.

101. Sugiyama, K., *et al.* (1992) Halothane-induced hyperpolarization and depression of postsynaptic potentials of guinea pig thalamic neurons *in vitro*. *Brain Res* 576 (1):97–103.

102. Ries, C.R. and Puil, E. (1999) Mechanism of anesthesia revealed by shunting actions of isoflurane on thalamocortical neurons. *J Neurophysiol* 81 (4):1795–1801.

103. Imas, O.A., *et al.* (2005) Volatile anesthetics disrupt frontal-posterior recurrent information transfer at gamma frequencies in rat. *Neurosci Lett* 387 (3):145–150.

104. Peltier, S.J., *et al.* (2005) Functional connectivity changes with concentration of sevoflurane anesthesia. *Neuroreport* 16 (3):285–288.

105. Jueptner, M., *et al.* (1997) The relevance of sensory input for the cerebellar control of movements. *Neuroimage* 5 (1):41–48.

106. Gross, J., *et al.* (2002) The neural basis of intermittent motor control in humans. *Proc Natl Acad Sci USA* 99 (4):2299–2302.

107. Cotterill, R.M. (2001) Cooperation of the basal ganglia, cerebellum, sensory cerebrum and hippocampus: Possible implications for cognition, consciousness, intelligence and creativity. *Prog Neurobiol* 64 (1):1–33.

108. Zhang, Y., *et al.* (2000) Inhaled anesthetics have hyperalgesic effects at 0.1 minimum alveolar anesthetic concentration. *Anesth Analg* 91 (2):462–466.

109. Alkire, M.T. and Gorski, L.A. (2004) Relative amnesic potency of five inhalational anesthetics follows the Meyer–Overton rule. *Anesthesiology* 101 (2):417–429.

110. Ghoneim, M.M. (2004) Drugs and human memory (part 1): Clinical, theoretical, and methodologic issues. *Anesthesiology* 100 (4):987–1002.

111. Ghoneim, M.M. (2004) Drugs and human memory (part 2). Clinical, theoretical, and methodologic issues. *Anesthesiology* 100 (5):1277–1297.

112. Renna, M., *et al.* (2000) The effect of sevoflurane on implicit memory: A double-blind, randomised study. *Anaesthesia* 55 (7):634–640.

113. Antognini, J.F. and Carstens, E. (1999) Isoflurane blunts electroencephalographic and thalamic-reticular formation responses to noxious stimulation in goats. *Anesthesiology* 91 (6):1770–1779.

114. Carstens, E. and Antognini, J.F. (2005) Anesthetic effects on the thalamus, reticular formation and related systems. *Thalamus relat syst* 3 (1):1–7.

115. Antognini, J.F. and Kien, N.D. (1994) A method for preferential delivery of volatile anesthetics to the *in situ* goat brain. *Anesthesiology* 80 (5):1148–1154.

116. Rampil, I.J. (1994) Anesthetic potency is not altered after hypothermic spinal cord transection in rats. *Anesthesiology* 80 (3):606–610.

117. Rampil, I.J., *et al.* (1993) Anesthetic potency (MAC) is independent of forebrain structures in the rat. *Anesthesiology* 78 (4):707–712.

118. Antognini, J.F., *et al.* (2007) Hexafluorobenzene acts in the spinal cord, whereas o-difluorobenzene acts in both brain and spinal cord, to produce immobility. *Anesth Analg* 104 (4):822–828.

119. Antognini, J.F., *et al.* (2002) Does the immobilizing effect of thiopental in brain exceed that of halothane? *Anesthesiology* 96 (4):980–986.

120. Edelman, G.M. and Tononi, G. (2000) *A Universe of Consciousness*, Basic Books.

COMA AND RELATED CONDITIONS

Coma

G. Bryan Young

ABSTRACT

Coma is a state of unarousable unconsciousness due to dysfunction of the brain's ascending reticular activating system (ARAS), which is responsible for arousal and the maintenance of wakefulness. Anatomically and physiologically the ARAS has a redundancy of pathways and neurotransmitters; this may explain why coma is usually transient (seldom lasting more than 3 weeks). Emergence from coma is succeeded by outcomes ranging from the vegetative state to complete recovery, depending on the severity of damage to the cerebral cortex, the thalamus or their integrated function. The clinical and laboratory assessments of the comatose patient are reviewed, along with an analysis of how various conditions (structural brain lesions, metabolic and toxic disorders, trauma, infections, seizures, hypothermia and hyperthermia) produce coma. Management issues include the determination of the cause and reversibility (prognosis) of neurological impairment, support of the patient, definitive treatment when possible and then ethical considerations for those situations where marked disability is predicted with certainty.

In this review the definition and pathophysiology of coma are discussed. Then the major conditions that produce coma are reviewed from the aspect of how they induce a comatose state. Practical issues for diagnosis and initial management are discussed along with the differential diagnosis of coma mimics. Finally, the issues of prognosis and ethical management of the patient with coma are addressed.

WHAT IS COMA?

Coma is a state of unarousable unconsciousness, characterized by a failure of the arousal/alerting system of the brain (ascending reticular activating system or ARAS). For practical purposes this includes failure of eye opening to stimulation, a motor response no better than simple withdrawal type movements and a verbal response no better than simple vocalization of nonword sounds. This presupposes that the motor pathways and systems that would allow the person to respond if he/she were conscious are intact.

PATHOPHYSIOLOGY OF COMA

Alerting or arousal is a function of the ARAS. Arousal to wakefulness is a prerequisite for awareness (see preceding chapters). This arousal system is anatomically represented by a number of structures in the rostral brainstem tegmentum, the diencephalon and projections to the cerebral cortex [1]. Principal among these are acetyl choline-producing neurons in the peribrachial nuclei, made up of the pedunculopontine tegmental and lateral dorsal tegmental nuclei. These project rostrally in two major pathways: (1) a dorsal pathway that synapses with the midline and nonspecific thalamic nuclei, which then send a glutaminergic projection to large areas of the cerebral cortex and (2) a ventral pathway from the rostral brainstem tegmentum that reaches the basal forebrain, especially the posterior hypothalamus, where axon terminals act on neurons that synthesize histamine and others synthesizing hypocretin or orexin (see Figure 11.1) [1]. These also contribute to cortical arousal. Thus the ARAS is a complex system with some redundancy of pathways that are involved in arousal and maintenance of wakefulness. This may explain the recovery of the arousal system after initial coma, almost always within 3 weeks from coma onset in most patients.

The reversible unconsciousness of sleep relates to dynamic inhibition of the above-mentioned neurotransmitter systems involved in arousal [2]. Centres

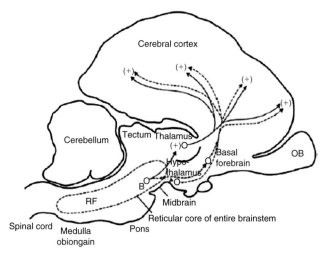

FIGURE 11.1   The nuclei and pathways of the dorsal and ventral components of the ARAS that originate in the cholinergic cells of the reticular formation. The dorsal pathway, represented by solid lines, activates the cerebral cortex via the thalamus. The ventral pathway (dashed lines) involves the hypothalamus and basal forebrain in cortical activation. OB: olfactory bulb, OC: optic chiasm, RF: reticular formation. *Source*: Taken from Jones (2000) with permission from W.B. Saunders, publisher.

for sleep are mainly in the preoptic region of the hypothalamus and use gamma-amino butyric acid (GABA), an inhibitory neurontransmitter. Adenosine, a neuromodulator, provides feedback inhibition of the arousal system as well. Hypothetically, a marked physiological imbalance of the sleep over arousal centres could also produce coma.

HOW DO VARIOUS DISORDERS PRODUCE COMA?

The following disorders may produce at least transient coma:

1. Structural brain lesions
2. Metabolic and nutritional disorders
3. Exogenous toxins
4. CNS infections and septic illness
5. Seizures
6. Temperature-related: hypothermia and hyperthermia
7. Trauma

It seems axiomatic that to do so these conditions must interfere with the ARAS, either diffusely or at strategic sites. The various clinical entities/disorders will be briefly discussed in turn.

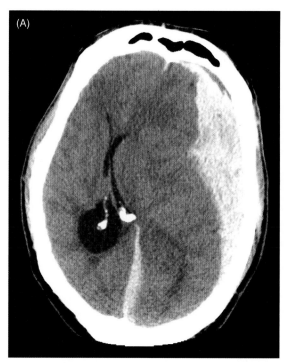
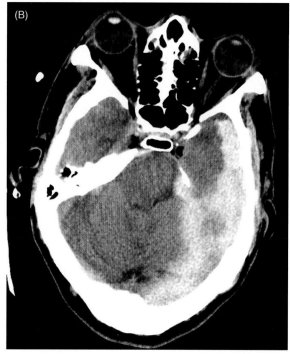

FIGURE 11.2   An example of horizontal shift of supratentorial structures with coma. (A) and (B) show an acute left subdural haematoma in a deeply unconscious 25 years old man who lost consciousness after a brief lucid interval following a motor vehicle accident. He was deeply comatose with a left oculomotor nerve palsy at the time of the CT scan. There is a massive shift of the midline from left to right in (A), yet in (B), there is minimal displacement or compression of the brainstem.

Structural Brain Lesions

Structural lesions are those that directly destroy or compress brain tissue. In the case of coma, this must include ARAS structures or acutely render the cerebral cortex diffusely dysfunctional. Single destructive lesions, for example ischaemic stroke, haemorrhage, inflammatory lesions or tumours, that involve the rostral ARAS, diencephalons, cerebral cortex (usually bilaterally but occasionally just the left cerebral hemisphere) or their interconnections acutely can produce coma. With more rostral lesions, the arousal system reactivates itself and awakening and sleep and wake cycles return within 2–3 weeks [3].

Single supratentorial mass lesions can produce coma by causing 'herniation', a shift of brain structures from one intracranial compartment into another. Plum and Posner [3] held that these lesions produced coma through downward displacement and compression of the diencephalon or mesial temporal lobe structures through the tentorial opening, 'central' and 'uncal' herniations, respectively. However, an alternative view is that the initial impairment of consciousness more commonly relates to *lateral* rather than downward herniation. This concept was initially proposed by Hasenjäger and Spatz [4] and by Miller Fisher in 1984 [5]. More recently Ropper [6–8]

has provided convincing evidence for subfalcial herniation with modern neuroimaging and careful postmortem examinations (see Figure 11.2). Indeed, there is a direct correlation of the shift of midline supratentorial structures (septum pellucidum or pineal gland) in millimetres (mm) and the depth of impairment of consciousness. Most cases of coma show a 9mm or greater lateral shift. The initial oculomotor nerve palsy attributed to uncal herniation is more likely related to stretching of the third cranial nerve over the clivus, as part of the lateral supratentorial displacement [8]. Transtentorial herniation does occur, but it is a relatively late event, often terminal, and is associated with brainstem damage. The loss of reactivity of the contralateral pupil, oculomotor palsy on the side opposite the mass lesion, is usually due to intrinsic brainstem damage from compression [9]. Such patients with intrinsic brainstem haemorrhages from compression are usually unsalvageable.

Metabolic, Nutritional and Toxic Encephalopathies

There are numerous encephalopathies due to organ failure (hepatic, renal, pulmonary, cardiovascular, adrenal), electrolyte disturbances (hyponatremia,

TABLE 11.1   Toxidromes

Syndrome	Drug examples	Features
Sympathomimetic	Cocaine, amphetamines, lysergic acid diethylamide, ephedrine and pseudoephedrine	Increased heart rate and blood pressure; pupils are dilated but reactive, sweating, agitation, hallucinations, seizures
Sympatholytic	Opiates, alpha-2 agonists, sedatives and ethanol	Small but reactive pupils, hypotension, bradycardia, respiratory depression
Cholinergic syndrome	Organophosphates, carbamate insecticides	Increased sweating, small pupils, increased sweating, salivation, bronchial secretions and gastrointestinal activity, confusion, seizures, coma, respiratory failure
Anticholinergic syndrome	First generation antihistamines, tricyclic antidepressants, benztropine, jimson weed, deadly nightshade	Pupils dilated and often unreactive, tachycardia, decreased sweating, ileus, fever, urinary retention

hypernatremia, hypocalcemia, hypercalcemia, hypomagnesemia, hypermagnesemia, hypophosphatemia), hypoglycaemia, hyperglycaemia, disturbances in thyroid function, inborn errors of metabolism (e.g., porphyria, mitochondrial disorders). Most of these cause reversible, functional dysfunction of the ARAS and cause a more diffuse disturbance without localizing signs (e.g., hemiplegia or pupillary unreactivity). Some may be associated with multifocal myoclonus, which is not epileptic in nature and probably arises from the nucleus gigantocellularis in the medulla. It seems likely that these disorders impair the polysynaptic function of the ARAS. There are some caveats to this over-simplified statement, however. Furthermore, there are clinical and laboratory differences that help to distinguish these disorders. Based on the history, past history of underlying illnesses and the context of the coma, the clinician will usually have some clues to the nature of the underlying cause or general class of illness.

Table 11.1 lists the principal toxidromes, a constellation of features peculiar to certain classes of drugs. Knowledge of these can be of considerable help to the clinician in raising suspicions of specific drug intoxications.

Similarly, observing the pattern of respirations combined with a simple blood gas analysis can narrow the possible causes of metabolic and toxic causes of coma (see Table 11.2).

Some helpful aspects of the clinical examination:

(A) Pupillary reflexes can be affected with drugs that have anticholinergic properties, for example pupils may be unreactive with massive overdoses of tricyclic antidepressants. Also, with massive overdoses of barbiturates, all brainstem reflexes, including pupillary responses, may be reversibly abolished. This can also occur in profound hypoglycaemia or anoxic–ischaemic encephalopathy, with variable degrees of reversibility of lost brain functions (in that these conditions can cause neuronal death if the insult is severe and prolonged). Pupils can be small but reactive in opiate intoxication.

(B) The vestibular-ocular reflex (VOR), tested with oculocephalic or oculovestibular procedures, can be selectively impaired, without affecting pupillary or other cranial nerve reflexes in Wernicke's encephalopathy. This happens because there is a selective involvement of grey matter structures adjacent to the ventricles and cerebral aqueduct in Wernicke's encephalopathy; this includes the vestibular nuclei involved in the VOR. We have also found that large or cumulative doses of sedative drugs can selectively and transiently abolish the VOR [10].

(C) Profound neuromuscular weakness, similar to Guillain-Barré syndrome: Hypophosphatemia, when acute and profound, can be seen in the 'refeeding syndrome' in which phosphate is driven intracellularly after a glucose load in severely malnourished individuals [11]. Flaccid quadriplegia is also sometimes a feature of acute, severe hypokalemia or hypomagnesemia.

(D) Seizures, most commonly myoclonic (with bilaterally synchronous jerks, distinct from multifocal myoclonus described above), can occur in number of metabolic encephalopathies including: hyponatremia, hyperosmolar states (especially in nonketotic hyperglycaemia, where

TABLE 11.2 Classification of Ventilatory Patterns

Breathing pattern	Metabolic pattern	pH, PaCO$_2$, HCO$_3$	Specific conditions
Hyperventilation	Metabolic acidosis	pH <7.3, PaCO$_2$ <30 mmHg, HCO$_3$ <17 mmol/L	Uremia, diabetic ketoacidosis, lactic acidosis, salicylates, methanol, ethylene glycol
Hyperventilation	Respiratory alkalosis	pH >7.45, PaCO$_2$ <30 mm, HCO$_3$ > 17 mmol/L	Hepatic failure, acute sepsis, acute salicylate intoxication, cardiopulmonary states with hypoxaemia, psychogenic causes
Hypoventilation	Respiratory acidosis	pH <7.35 (if acute), PaCO$_2$ >90 mmHg, HCO$_3$ >17 mmol/L	Respiratory failure from central (e.g., brain or spinal cord) or peripheral nervous system disease, chest conditions or deformities. Coma only with severe hypercarbia
Hypoventilation	Metabolic alkalosis	pH >7.45, PaCO$_2$ > 45 mmHg, HCO$_3$ >30 mmol/L	Vomiting, alkali ingestion. Usually no impairment of consciousness; if so, suspect psychogenic unresponsiveness or additional cause

seizures can be misleadingly focal), hypocalcemia, extreme hypercalcemia, uraemia, advanced hepatic encephalopathy, hypoglycaemia and in post-resuscitation encephalopathy after cardiac arrest. In the latter situation, myoclonic status epilepticus is almost always fatal, without recovery of awareness. We have found this is due to widespread neuronal death in a pattern that is very distinct from the pattern of neuronal loss after status epilepticus [12].

Systemic and CNS Infections

Systemic infections, or, more precisely, systemic inflammation (including pancreatitis, trauma and burns), can cause an encephalopathy that is usually reversible and resembles metabolic encephalopathies in general [13]. Proposed mechanisms include impaired microcirculation (similar to that found in other organs in sepsis), alternations in the brain's neurotransmitters from plasma amino acid imbalance, direct and indirect effects of cytokines, generation of free radicals and secondary effects from the failure of other organs [13]. Electroencephalographs (EEGs) show a graded pattern of severity ranging from mild slowing to a burst-suppression pattern [13]. Mortality is 70% with the latter category, but patients die from multiorgan failure rather than nervous system complications. There are multiple potential mechanisms that are not mutually exclusive [13].

Bacterial meningitis begins as an acute purulent infection within the subarachnoid space. The multiplication and lysis of bacteria with the subsequent release of bacterial cell wall components in the subarachnoid space is the initial step in the induction of an inflammatory response. It is probable that the encephalopathy that accompanies purulent meningitis shares some of the mechanisms found in sepsis-associated encephalopathy.

The multiplication and lysis of bacteria in the subarachnoid space leads to the release of bacterial cell wall components. Lipopolysaccharide molecules (endotoxins), a cell wall component of gram-negative bacteria, and teichoic acid and peptidoglycan, cell wall components of the pneumococcus, induce meningeal inflammation by stimulating the production of inflammatory cytokines and chemokines by microglia, astrocytes, monocytes, microvascular endothelial cells and white blood cells in the cerebrospinal fluid (CSF) space. A large number of cytokines and chemokines (cytokines that induce chemotactic migration in leukocytes) are present in meningeal inflammation; the most thoroughly understood cytokines are tumour necrosis factor (TNF) and interleukin-1 (IL-1). A number of pathophysiologic consequences result from the presence of the inflammatory cytokines in CSF. TNF and IL-1 act synergistically to alter the permeability of the blood–brain barrier. The alteration in blood–brain barrier permeability during bacterial meningitis results in vasogenic cerebral oedema and allows leakage of serum proteins and other molecules into the CSF, contributing to the formation of a purulent exudate in the subarachnoid space. The purulent exudate obstructs the flow of CSF through the ventricular system and diminishes the resorptive capacity of the arachnoid granulations in the dural sinuses.

This leads to obstructive and communicating hydrocephalus and interstitial oedema. The exudate also surrounds and narrows the diameter of the lumen of the large arteries at the base of the brain, and inflammatory cells infiltrate the arterial wall (vasculitis). This in combination with the alterations in cerebral blood flow (CBF) that occur in this infection results in cerebral ischaemia, focal neurological deficits and stroke. The inflammatory cytokines recruit polymorphonuclear leukocytes from the bloodstream and upregulate the expression of selectins on cerebral capillary endothelial cells and leukocytes, which allows leukocytes to adhere to vascular endothelial cells and subsequently migrate into the CSF. Neutrophils degranulate and release toxic metabolites that contribute to cytotoxic oedema, cell injury and death. The adherence of leukocytes to capillary endothelial cells increases the permeability of blood vessels allowing leakage of plasma proteins into the CSF, further contributing to the inflammatory exudate in the subarachnoid space. The degranulation of leukocytes and cerebral ischaemia resulting from alterations in CBF causes cytotoxic oedema. The combination of interstitial, vasogenic and cytotoxic oedema leads to raised intracranial pressure (ICP) and coma. In addition, bacteria and the inflammatory cytokines induce the production of excitatory amino acids, reactive oxygen and nitrogen species (free oxygen radicals, nitric oxide and peroxynitrite), and other mediators that induce massive apoptosis of brain cells.

Thus coma in purulent meningitis can result initially from the toxic effects of inflammatory mediations and then secondary complications: cerebral oedema, obstructive and communicating hydrocephalus, seizure activity, and the cerebrovascular complications of arteritis, ischaemic and haemorrhagic infarctions and septic venous sinus thrombosis.

Fungal meningitis and meningitis due to parasites (e.g., toxoplasmosis) probably share some of these mechanisms.

Encephalitis, either from direct infection of the brain by viruses or due to an immune-mediated, post-infectious mechanism, alters blood–brain barrier permeability and the extracellular milieu of the brain in addition to causing other inflammatory changes described above. Direct tissue destruction is often diffuse or multifocal, although the encephalitides of herpes simplex virus and rabies are more regionally specific.

The diagnosis of purulent, bacterial or fungal meningitis and some encephalitides, especially herpes simplex encephalitis, is largely dependent on lumbar puncture and CSF analysis (see below), but neuroimaging often of considerable assistance in encephalitis.

Specific therapy is available for the purulent, tuberculous, fungal and parasitic infections and for herpes simplex encephalitis.

Hyperthermia and Hypothermia

Hypothermia is defined as a core body temperature below 35°C, but as a primary cause of coma the temperature is usually below 28°C. Coma is preceded by delirium and then stupor, almost in a dose dependent manner. At temperatures less than 28°C, the pupillary light reflex is lost and the patient may appear to be brain dead. There is also a risk of ventricular fibrillation and cardiac arrest.

The EEG shows evolutionary changes with slowing at 30°C and changes to a burst-suppression pattern between 20°C and 22°C and becomes isoelectric at 20°C. This presumably reflects a progressive failure of synaptic transmission in the brain. There is also a progressive decrease in CBF by 6% for each 1°C drop in body temperature. At <25°C CBF becomes pressure passive with loss of autoregulation.

Hypothermia may be accidental, primary (usually due to a hypothalamic disorder) or secondary to loss of autonomic function, as in high spinal cord injuries, hypothyroidism, adrenal failure, Wernicke's encephalopathy, advanced sepsis or sedative drug intoxication. In the last five conditions of the secondary group the coma is usually due to the underlying condition rather than the hypothermia itself.

Hyperthermia or fever is defined as a body temperature of >38.5°C. Temperatures of >42°C directly produce encephalopathy, with slowing of EEG rhythms and often seizures. The latter probably relate to an increase in extracellular glutamate, an excitatory neurotransmitter as well as impaired functioning of the sodium–potassium pump in neuronal and glial cell membranes. Elevated temperature can arise as a result of disorders of heat production, diminished heat dissipation or hypothalamic dysfunction. Causes of increased heat production include malignant hyperthermia (a disorder of the sarcoplasmic reticulum in muscle, causing a release of ionized calcium into the muscle cytoplasm, causing action–contraction coupling of actin and myosin filaments), thyrotoxicosis, neuroleptic malignant syndrome (a central nervous system (CNS) dysfunction with increased muscle tone, often due to drugs that block dopamine receptors), cocaine or amphetamine abuse, salicylate intoxication or convulsive status epilepticus. Impaired heat dissipation can be due to heatstroke, autonomic dysfunction, use of anticholinergic medications and a hot environment. Hypothalamic and brainstem disorders include strokes, trauma or encephalitis affecting temperature-regulating centres.

Trauma

Coma that occurs immediately following trauma can range from primary injury, including concussion and diffuse axonal injury (DAI) to brain death. Secondary brain injury can cause coma that onsets after a lucid interval or complicates concussion or DAI without such a lucid period. Occasionally status epilepticus can be responsible (see Chapter 19).

Concussion

Concussion is the transient loss of consciousness after a blow to the head [14]. More recently a transient, post-traumatic dazed state has also been included in the definition [14]. Concussion is often accompanied by an anterograde post-traumatic amnesia (the inability to lay down new memories for a variable period (minutes to days) after the injury) plus or minus a shorter period of retrograde amnesia that precedes the injury. In animal models of concussion and in limited human studies there is often a transient impairment of brainstem function, including loss of pupillary and corneal reflexes and apnoea. The subject may or may not have a few generalized clonic movements similar to a convulsive seizure, but is more often flaccidly immobile.

There is no consistent neuropathology in animal models of concussion. Variable degrees of diffuse or regional axonal injury have been described; occasionally petechial or more macroscopic haemorrhages or contusions are encountered. However, brains are often morphologically normal. Since structural lesions are not essential, concussion appears to be more a disturbance of function than of structure [15].

The types of injuries that produce concussion are usually associated with acceleration/deceleration of the head, most often with a rotational component in the antero-posterior or lateral plane (i.e., angular acceleration). This has been confirmed in animal models. If the skull is fixed consciousness is not impaired unless the skull is greatly deformed. Thus, it has been proposed that there is a dynamic physical and functional distortion of the ARAS, especially the rostral brainstem tegmentum, the projection to the thalamus, the thalamus itself or to the rostral thalamic projection to the cortex [14]. Holbourn [16] using a gelatin model, showed that most of the distortion and shearing forces occurred in the cerebral subcortical region. However, the anatomy of the human brain allows for considerable rotational stress to occur at or near the union of the cerebral hemispheres and the brainstem.

The skull deformation and fluid percussion theories for concussion do not have as much credulity as the above mechanisms, as evidence for sufficiently raised ICP is lacking [14, 15].

Beyond the biomechanical insights that have been fairly well established, there is still considerable controversy about the fundamental mechanisms for the loss of consciousness and impairment of memory [15]. Several hypotheses have been proposed, but none has been established or accepted [14, 15]. The vascular theory, one of reduced blood flow to all or parts of the brain, would not account for the very abrupt loss of consciousness and is contradicted by metabolic studies that show an initial hypermetabolic state. Other theories have somewhat better support and are not mutually exclusive. A convulsive theory could explain the abrupt loss of consciousness, the initial hypermetabolic state of the cortex and the post-traumatic amnesia [14, 15]. It also could be incorporated into the cholinergic (in which there is a massive release of acetylcholine) and the centripetal theory, in which the more rostral parts of the ARAS, especially the cerebral cortex is especially dysfunctional. The reticular theory localizes dysfunction to the reticular formation but does not provide a mechanism. Other variants include the concept of deformation of neuronal membranes, which can open certain ion channels, and the release of other neurotransmitters, including glutamate, an excitotoxic neurotransmitter that could cause seizures [15].

Diffuse Axonal Injury

DAI is characterized by loss of consciousness at the time of the trauma, but the duration of coma is much longer than with concussion. Patients usually regain eye opening within 2–3 weeks, related to recovery of function of the subcortical arousal systems mentioned above. The recovery of awareness is variable, ranging from mild impairment, through mild disability, severe disability and the minimally conscious state to the persistent/permanent vegetative state.

DAI produced the same types of mechanical stresses that produce concussion, only the forces are greater, causing shearing injuries to the cerebral white matter. In severe cases the brainstem is also involved. Pathological studies in humans usually involved patients who died days or weeks after the injury. The characteristic lesions were 'axon retraction balls', the retracted ends of severed axons. These were interpreted as occurring at the time of injury with physical disruption of the axons coursing through the white matter. Subsequent studies of animal models showed that the axons are usually intact after the injury and that damage to the cytoskeleton, possibly due to an influx of calcium into the axon, leads to disruption and fragmentation of the axon [17].

Neuroradiological confirmation of DAI is problematic, in that the axons cannot be visualized. Magnetic resonance imaging (MRI) scans can detect petechial haemorrhages, which serve as an imperfect surrogate marker for DAI. Haemorrhages in the corpus callosum and the dorsolateral rostral brainstem usually indicate severe DAI. Newer techniques including tensor tract imaging and a protocol that magnifies the susceptibility artifact from blood or iron in the brain parenchyma will likely prove to be more sensitive than older techniques [18] (Figure 11.2). Somatosensory evoked response testing, although it utilizes a single sensory pathway, has proven to be sensitive and specific for severe DAI [17]. Magnetic transcranial cortical motor stimulation could also be used to assess the corticospinal motor integrity (Figure 11.3).

Secondary Brain Injury

'Secondary brain injury' refers to insults to the injured brain evolve subsequent to the initial injury. They are important in that they are often detectable, preventable and treatable. These are mainly:

1. *Intracranial haemorrhage*: Bleeding can occur into the brain parenchyma or the extracerebral space,

either as subarachnoid, subdural or epidural haemorrhage(s). The incidence of haemorrhages in hospital admissions for traumatic head injury is about 25%, but this increases to over 50% when such patients are admitted in coma [18]. The mechanisms by which haemorrhages produce coma by their mass effect are discussed above under 'Structural Brain Lesions'. Haematomas also produce both local and remote effects on the brain. With parenchymal haemorrhages there is disruption of focal structures by the bleeding. Intraparenchymal and extracerebral haematomas can produce regional ischaemia by pressure on capillaries in the underlying tissue; the release of vasoactive substances; and simply by mechanical pressure and distortion of brain tissue [18]. Remote effects relate to raised ICP (see below).

2. *Raised ICP*: The intracranial compartment is fixed and any increase in mass, for example by blood or oedema of tissues, is accommodated by changes in other compartments (CSF, intravascular or brain) to prevent a rise in ICP up to a point, at which ICP rises exponentially. Destructive effects occur by brain herniation (see above) or by reduced perfusion pressure. Perfusion pressure is equal to the ICP minus mean arterial blood pressure (BP). Autoregulation, related to dilatation or constriction of brain arteries and arterioles, allows for a constant total brain perfusion until a critical point, usually at a mean arterial pressure of about

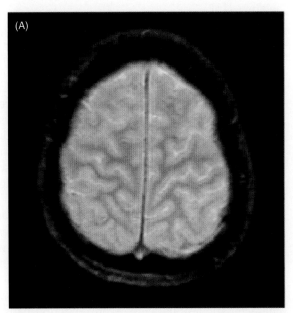
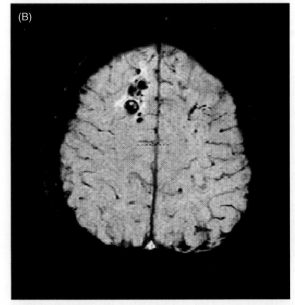

FIGURE 11.3   (A) Conventional GRE (fast imaging with steady-state precession, 500/18, 15° flip angle, 78 Hz per pixel, two signals acquired, 4 mm thick sections) and (B) Susceptibility weighted imaging (SWI) (three-dimensional fast low-angle shot, 57/40, 20° flip angle, 78 Hz per pixel, 64 partitions, one signal acquired, 2-mm thick sections reconstructed over 4 mm) MR images from the same brain region in a child with traumatic brain injury illustrating the increased ability of SWI to detect haemorrhagic DAI lesions. *Source*: Reproduced from [18].

60 mmHg, after which perfusion follows the mean arterial BP in a pressure-passive manner. With markedly raised ICP this can produce ischaemic damage or even brain death if the ICP exceeds the mean BP.

3. *Other*: Secondary insults to the brain may result from prolonged seizures, sepsis or profound electrolyte disturbances. We [19]have found that at least 8% of patients comatose from brain injury are in nonconvulsive status epilepticus (NCSE). Most often this is undetectable unless an EEG is done. Since status epilepticus can damage the brain, it is important the seizures be detected early and are treated promptly and effectively. The liberal use of EEG in the ICU is helpful; continuous monitoring for at least 48 hours increases the yield of detection of NCSE and, in patients with seizures, provides feedback that the seizures are controlled and that the sedation/anaesthesia is not excessive.

DIFFERENTIAL DIAGNOSIS

Coma can be mimicked by the locked-in state and by psychogenic unresponsiveness.

Locked-in Syndrome

In the locked-in syndrome (see the more complete discussion in Chapter 15), the patients are conscious and have wake–sleep cycles. They are, however, unable to express themselves in the usual manner due to profound paralysis of the limbs and lower brainstem-innervated musculature. Most often this is due to a lesion in the basis pontis, as might be caused by an occlusion of the basilar artery or central pontine myelinolysis. This produces an upper-motor neuron palsy of all four limbs, the lower cranial nerves, including the tongue, palate, jam and lower facial muscles (pseudobulbar palsy). The patient has vertical eye movements and can often open and close the eyes voluntarily. In this way such patients can give motor feedback and communication can be established. The most famous example of this is that of Jean-Dominique Bauby, who, while locked in from a basis pontis stroke, 'wrote' the book *The Diving Bell and the Butterfly* (1995) [20] by communicating with coded eye blinks. Other causes of a de-efferented state include severe neuromuscular paralysis from polyneuropathy or a failure of neuromuscular transmission, as might be caused by the prolonged action of a neuromuscular blocking agent. In these situations the patient does not usually have the vertical eye movements and may even lose the pupillary reflexes in severe Guillain-Barré

syndrome with autonomic involvement. This condition can even mimic brain death [21].

Psychogenic Unresponsiveness

In psychogenic unresponsiveness, as in the locked-in syndrome, the patient is awake and aware, but does not communicate or give an outward expression that he/she is conscious. This can be a 'pseudocoma' like state, in which the patient is immobile, or more commonly as pseudoseizures or nonepileptic seizures. In this situation the unresponsiveness is psychogenic in origin. A clue that the patient is conscious is the presence of nystagmus with caloric testing. In coma with intact brainstem reflexes the eyes show tonic deviation towards the ear injected with cold water; nystagmus with caloric testing implies preserved consciousness.

Patients may display a variety of behaviours or be motionless. Behaviours that should raise the suspicion of pseudoseizures include: having eyes closed during a seizure (video recording of patients having seizures have almost always observed that the eyes are open during genuine seizures but closed during pseudoseizures). Other clues are that the eyes may face the floor, regardless of how the patient is positioned. The patient may avoid being tickled by rolling over. Unusual movements, such as holding onto and shaking the siderails of the bed, asynchronous movements in what otherwise resembles a convulsive seizure (epileptic jerks are typically synchronous) and susceptibility to suggestion, are often found in pseudoseizures, but are rare in genuine seizures.

Confirmatory tests are occasionally helpful but are often unnecessary. EEGs show a normal awake pattern with blocking of the alpha rhythm with passive eye opening. Capillary or arterial blood gas testing in pseudoseizures are usually normal or may show a respiratory alkalosis from hyperventilation, as opposed to the profound, mixed metabolic-respiratory acidosis of a convulsive seizure. Serum prolactin is elevated following genuine convulsive or complex seizures, but not with pseudoseizures or most simple partial seizures. This test lacks sensitivity and it takes days/weeks for the laboratory testing to be reported.

MANAGEMENT OF THE COMATOSE PATIENT

Diagnostic and therapeutic steps should be taken virtually simultaneously. This usually requires a team of physicians and nurses. These steps will be discussed separately for clarity.

Diagnostic Steps

1. *Obtain a history and do a general examination*: Just
as with awake and communicative patients,
the history is vital. Of course, with comatose
patients the history is obtained from relatives,
friends and eye witnesses, by phone if necessary.
How the patient took ill/collapsed can give
important clues. Did the patient have a seizure?
Was trauma involved? Had the patient lost
consciousness gradually or was there fluctuation,
as might be seen in metabolic disorders or
subdural haematoma? Was the patient febrile
or having chills (suggesting a CNS or systemic
infection)? The patient's background can be
important. Did the patient have cancer, profound
depression (raising the possibility of drug
overdose), or a history of drug or alcohol abuse?
Is there an underlying illness, such as diabetes
mellitus, adrenal, hepatic or renal failure,
immunosuppression (either drug-induced or
acquired)? What drugs was the patient taking?

Hospital records can be helpful, as can medical
alert bracelets or other medical information on
his/her person.

The general, in addition to a focused neurological,
examination can give important clues. The vital
signs are helpful, for example the presence of
fever, hypothermia, shock and the respiratory
pattern. Skin color: jaundice, pallor, cyanosis,
cherry red discolouration of the lips (carbon
monoxide poisoning), petechial bleeding
(raising the possibility of a seizure, thrombotic
thrombocytopenic purpura, meningococcemia,
Rocky mountain spotted fever, vasculitis or
septic emboli) is worth noting. Are there needle
marks, suggestive of drug abuse? Are there signs
of chronic liver failure, for example distended
veins around the umbilicus or spider nevi? Is
there evidence of organ failure? Is there evidence
of trauma, especially head injury (e.g., signs of a
basal skull fracture with hemotympanium, Battle's
sign (bruising over the mastoids), raccoon eyes
(indicating a fracture of the orbital roof))? A bitten
tongue is presumptive evidence of a convulsive
seizure. A preretinal haemorrhage should raise
suspicion of a ruptured intracranial aneurysm.
Roth spots in the retinal may signify endocarditis,
leukaemia or septic emboli. Buccal pigmentation
could indicate underlying adrenal insufficiency.

2. *Is the patient truly in coma?* See the 'Differential
Diagnosis' section above.

3. *Localize the anatomical–physiological site of the
coma* (see Chapter 19): Usually if the brainstem
functions are preserved the site is more rostral or
the brain has been affected in a diffuse manner
that relatively spares the more resistant cranial
nerve nuclei. There are some caveats, however
(see 'Metabolic and Toxic' sections above).
The Glasgow Coma Scale (GCS) is commonly
used to grade the severity of the impairment of
consciousness. It was initially designed for the
assessment of trauma victims in the emergency
room, but it is commonly employed to track the
progress or worsening of ICU patients (Table 11.3).
Although there are better scales for ICU patients,
for example the Reaction Level Scale – 85 [22] and
the FOUR scoring system [23], the GCS will likely
remain.

4. *Request blood work*: As mentioned above, arterial
or capillary blood gas determination can be very
helpful in the presence of hyperventilation and
occasionally in hypoventilation and for some
toxidromes. In addition, it is always wise to check
the serum glucose, calcium, sodium, potassium,
magnesium, phosphate, urea and creatinine.
Liver function tests should be done if there is
suspicion of hepatic failure. The international
normalized ratio (INR) is sensitive to acute
hepatocellular failure. A 'drug screen' is rarely
comprehensive but can be specified to include
alcohol, benzodiazepines, barbiturates, opiates,
cocaine, amphetamines, tricyclic antidepressants,
salicylates, acetaminophen and other agents. Some
drugs, for example antihistamines may not have
an available assay and one must go on clinical
suspicions. A blood culture should be done in the
presence of fever or hypothermia.

5. *Neuroimaging*: A CT scan is most commonly
used as it is quick, available and requires less
preparation than an MRI scan. Imaging is
essential when there is a strong possibility of a
structural brain lesion or for diagnosing specific
disorders. Focal signs, such as a hemiparesis or
an oculomotor palsy in a comatose patient should
prompt a scan. However, coma may precede
such focal signs in patients with supratentorial
lesions, even mimicking a coma (see herniations
above). Thus, neuroimaging is also indicated when
structural lesions are possible or of the diagnosis
is uncertain. The CT is sensitive to intracranial
haemorrhages, major shifts of midline structures
and mass effect. The MRI is superior in showing
the early signs of herpes simplex encephalitis and
for brainstem lesions (CT often shows bone artifact
obscuring posterior fossa structures). MRI can be

TABLE 11.3   The Glasgow Coma Scale

Item	Factor	Score
Best motor response	Obeys	6
	Localizes	5
	Withdraws (flexion)	4
	Abnormal flexion	3
	Extensor response	2
	Nil	1
Verbal response	Oriented	5
	Confused conversation	4
	Inappropriate words	3
	Incomprehensible sounds	2
	Nil	1
Eye opening	Spontaneous	4
	To speech	3
	To pain	2
	Nil	1

combined with imaging of arteries and veins, for example for venous thrombosis. CT angiography is somewhat better than magnetic resonance (MR) angiography for aneurysms or vasculitis.

6. *Lumbar puncture*: This is indicated if there is suspicion of meningitis, especially bacterial, fungal or tuberculous and also for the detection of meningeal cancer. Lumbar puncture can also confirm subarachnoid haemorrhage from a ruptured aneurysm. The CT scan picks up about 95% of these acutely and would be expected to be positive in patients in coma from an aneurysm that ruptured the same day. Its sensitivity declines to less than 50% after a few days, however. Xanthochromia or a yellow staining of the CSF from haemoglobin breakdown products can be suspected clinically and confirmed by spectrophotometry. More specific diagnostic testing, apart from culture, stains, cytology and flow cytometry include polymerase chain reaction (PCR) for herpes simplex virus 1 and 2, broad range bacterial PCR, specific meningeal pathogen PCR, PCR for *M. tuberculosis*, reverse transcriptase PCR for enteroviruses, PCR for West Nile virus, PCR for Epstein Barr virus, PCR for varicella zoster virus, PCR for cytomegalovirus DNA, PCR for HIV RNA and RT-PCR for rabies virus. Antigen screening can be done for cryptococcal and histoplasma polysaccharide antigens. Antibody screens in the CSF are available for herpes simplex virus (serum:CSF antibody ratio of <20:1), arthropod-borne viruses, *Borrelia burgdorferi* (for suspected Lyme disease) and rabies virus; complement fixation antibody testing for *C. immitis* can also be performed.

7. *EEG*: This can be of great help in detecting seizures; it seems appropriate to request one, even in the emergency room when the cause of coma is not apparent and brainstem reflexes are intact. DeLorenzo and colleagues [24] have shown that least 14% of patients who failed to waken after a convulsive seizure were in NCSE. As mentioned above, seizures may be acquired in the ICU; those at highest risk are those with structural brain lesions. Monitoring for 48 hours is optimal for seizure detection.

CARE OF THE COMATOSE PATIENT

The comatose patient requires the care of the intensive care unit, unless only palliation is intended. Airway management, to prevent aspiration or asphyxiation and to provide adequate ventilation, is of prime importance and the patient should have an endotracheal tube in place. Most patients require assisted ventilation to assure adequate oxygenation and carbon dioxide clearance. Vascular support to maintain adequate cerebral and renal perfusion may require volume expansion and/or inotropic agents or vaso-pressors. Intensivists are skilled in such management, along with line insertion and monitoring of vital signs and ventilation.

Special steps such as the insertion of ICP monitor-ing devices are indicated when ICP is high or likely to become elevated, for example, in traumatic brain injury with an abnormal CT scan and a GCS of 8 or less.

Continuous EEG monitoring should be considered for patients in status epilepticus receiving anaesthetic agents, those who have not regained consciousness after witnessed seizures or those with a high risk of seizures. Intermittent monitoring of somatosensory evoked potentials is used in some centres to monitor head injured patients; changes can indicate the devel-opment or growth of an intracerebral haematoma. Specialized monitoring with microdialysis catheters, special probes for regional blood flow, serial transcra-nial Doppler each have their place in special units where there is expertise in using these techniques. Further research is needed to establish their practical value.

PROGNOSIS AND ETHICAL MANAGEMENT OF THE COMATOSE PATIENT

The neurologist is often asked to provide a progno-sis for patients in coma. This has obvious implications for decision making for further management. It is not always possible to provide an accurate prognosis; in some conditions the main determinant of outcome is not neurological. The neurologist should not be placed in a position as the major prognosticator when the nervous system is affected in a potentially reversible manner. For example, in sepsis and multiorgan failure, the encephalopathy is usually secondary to systemic disease and can recover if the systemic inflammatory state resolves and other organs recover. When judging whether or not the prognosis is poor, the neurologist is best to address only those conditions that are capa-ble of causing neuronal death.

Brain Death

Most industrialized countries have developed guide-lines for declaration of 'brain death' and have equated this with death of the individual [25]. The essential clinical elements are: (1) an identified aetiology that is capable of causing neuronal death; (2) the patient is in coma and is on a ventilator; (3) cranial nerve reflexes (pupillary, corneal, vestibular-ocular, pharyngeal and laryngeal) are absent; (4) there are no movements aris-ing from the brain and no response to stimulation; and (5) the patient is apneic. When the clinical criteria can-not be applied, the absence of intracranial perfusion is necessary for the declaration of brain death. Some countries require ancillary testing as part of the proto-col, even when the clinical criteria are met [25].

Anoxic–Ischaemic Encephalopathy After Cardiac Arrest (Post-resuscitation Encephalopathy)

Prognostic guidelines have been developed by a Quality Subcommittee of the American Academy of Neurology [26]. These were result of an evidence-based review of articles published before the advent of hypothermic treatment of such patients. The fol-lowing were deemed reliable predictors of an outcome that was no better than institutionalized dependency and marked disability (no false positives): myoclonus status epilepticus; by day 3 post-resuscitation the loss of pupillary light or corneal reflexes or a motor response no better than extensor posturing. The only ancillary tests that also had 0% false positives for this outcome were bilateral loss of the N20 response with somatosensory stimulation of the median nerve at the wrist or a serum neuronal specific enolase concentra-tion $>33\,\mu g/L$. A subsequent small prospective study performed on initially comatose patients after resus-citation identified two of nine patients with motor responses no better than extension by day 3 who recovered awareness (their motor responses recovered by days 5 and 6, respectively) [27]. The other clinical features were validated. The guidelines will likely require revision after further study, to accommodate the patients treated with hypothermia.

We [28] have also studied later somatosensory steady-state evoked potentials (SSEP) responses and found the preservation of the N70 to be reliably asso-ciated with recovery of awareness. It is likely that event-related responses (e.g., mismatch negativity, the P300 and N400 responses) will also be helpful in pre-dicting a more favourable prognosis [29]. Functional MRI also holds promise both for favourable and unfa-vourable outcomes after cardiac arrest [30].

Traumatic Brain Injury

In estimating prognosis, traumatic brain injury is more difficult than anoxic–ischaemic encephalopathy unless the patient is brain dead. There are no widely accepted guidelines. Decisions are made on a case-by-case basis. The outcome is primarily dependent on the level of consciousness at the time of the injury and the age of the patient (older patients fare much worse than younger individuals). Bilaterally, unreactive pupils as a sign indicate a poor prognosis and imminent death. Evoked potentials hold great promise, as they test sensory pathways running through the brainstem and ultimately to the cerebral cortex. Bilateral loss of the intracranial component of SSEPs is associated with a mortality or outcome no better than vegetative state in at least 95% of cases [31]. Refinements in MRI imaging (mentioned above) should prove to be prognostically valuable. As with anoxic–ischaemic encephalopathy, the preservation of later components of SSEPs or the presence of event-related potentials is suggestive of a favourable outcome.

Other Conditions

Severe hypoglycaemia can cause neuronal death. It is likely that similar criteria used for anoxic–ischaemic encephalopathy would apply to these patients, but it seems unlikely that a large series will be studied.

Acute/fulminant hepatic failure can be associated with severe cerebral oedema and even brain death. However, we caution clinicians to be careful in making definitive prognostic statements on these patients, as some will recover awareness even with clinical and MRI findings that would have a poor prognosis if the cause for the coma was cardiac arrest. Encephalitides, whether viral or immune-mediated, ischaemic or haemorrhagic strokes cause structural brain damage that is highly variable. Examination and neuroimaging will usually allow for a reasonable determination of the projected deficits.

ETHICAL MANAGEMENT OF THE COMATOSE PATIENT

The practice of medicine is fundamentally one of practical morality/ethics. As physicians we are to do our best for the patient. Most ethicists hold with the four principles of biomedical ethics proposed by Beauchamp and Childress [32]: autonomy, nonmalficence, beneficence and justice. Autonomy prevails among these; the patient's wishes for self-determination are to be respected and honoured. Of course, the patient in coma cannot speak for himself/herself and a determination or estimate his/her preferences

is gleaned from substitute decision makers or written advance directives.

Nonmalficence is the duty of the physician not to do harm to the patient; beneficence involves doing what is best for the patient and justice concerns the just use of public resources in the health care system, with fair treatment and even distribution.

Applying ethical principles helps to avoid medical paternalism and opens a dialogue between health care professionals and the patient's substitute decision maker(s). It is the physician's responsibility to explain to the substitute decision maker the medical issues, including the prognosis, and to indicate the responsibilities of the substitute decision maker, along with the guiding principles mentioned above. If the patient's wishes are not known, an attempt should be made to use the best collective judgement of loved ones and the health care professionals, in a patient-centred approach, to arrive at a decision. Occasionally a hospital ethicist or ethics committee can be used to provide objective advice, but not to make decisions. Rarely is it necessary to refer to the courts to make such decisions.

The decision to remove life-supporting therapy is always difficult, but the above steps (establishing the prognosis, respecting the autonomy of the patient and discussing the options and appropriate level of care) are necessary to make appropriate, patient-centred conclusions. The help of the intensive care team in describing the staged withdrawal of life supports and administration of medications to remove the appearance of distress of the dying patient is the final step in explaining the process.

FUTURE DIRECTIONS

Improvements in the management of comatose patients await dissemination of knowledge regarding appropriate investigation and prognostication and the development of evidence-based guidelines. Further research is needed to validate newer innovations. It is important to 'stay tuned' to the evolving discipline of neurocritical care.

References

1. Vincent, S.R. (2000) The ascending reticular activating system – from aminergic neurons to nitric oxide. *J Chem Neuroanat* 18:23–30.
2. Evans, B.M. (2003) Sleep, consciousness and the spontaneous and evoked electrical activity of the brain. Is there a cortical integrating mechanism? *Clin Neurophysiol* 33:1–10.
3. Plum, F. and Posner, J.B. (1980) *The Diagnosis of Stupor and Coma*, 3rd Edition. Philadelphia, PA: F.A. Davis.

4. Hasenjäger, T. and Spatz, H. (1937) Über örtliche Veränderungern der Konfiguration des Gehrins beim Hindruk. *Arch Psychiat Nervenk* 107:193–222.

5. Fisher, C.M. (1984) Acute brain herniation: A revised concept. *Semin Neurol* 4:417–421.

6. Ropper, A.H. (1986) Lateral displacement of the brain and level of consciousness in patients with an acute hemispheric mass. *New Engl J Med* 314:953–958.

7. Ropper, A.H. (1989) A preliminary MRI study of the geometry of brain displacement and level of consciousness with acute intracranial masses. *Neurology* 39:622–627.

8. Ropper, A.H., *et al.* (1991) Clinicopathological correlation in a case of pupillary dilation from cerebral hemorrhage. *Arch Neurol* 48:1166–1169.

9. Ropper, A.H. (1990) The opposite pupil in herniation. *Neurology* 40:1707–1710.

10. Morrow, S.A. and Young, G.B. (2007) Selective abolition of the vestibular-ocular reflex by sedative drugs. *Neurocrit Care* 6:45–48.

11. Kraft, M.D., *et al.* (2005) Review of the refeeding syndrome. *Nutr Clin Pract* 20:625–633.

12. Young, G.B., *et al.* (1990) The significance of myoclonic status epilepticus in post-anoxic coma. *Neurology* 40:1843–1848.

13. Wilson, J.X. and Young, G.B. (2003) Sepsis-associated encephalopathy: Evolving concepts. *Can J Neurol Sci* 30:98–105.

14. Ropper, A.H. and Gorson, K.C. (2007) Concussion. *New Engl J Med* 356:166–172.

15. Shaw, N.A. (2002) The neurophysiology of concussion. *Prog Neurobiol* 67:281–344.

16. Povlishok, J.T. (1993) Pathobiology of traumatically induced axonal injury in animals and man. *Ann Emerg Med* 22:980.

17. Ashwal, S., *et al.* (2006) Susceptibility-weighted imaging and proton magnetic resonance spectroscopy in assessment of outcome after pediatric traumatic brain injury. *Arch Phys Med Rehabil* 87 (Suppl 2):S50–S58.

18. Moulton, R. (1998) Head injury. In *Coma and Impaired Consciousness: A Clinical Perspective* G.B. Young, A.H. Ropper, and C.F. Bolton, (eds.) New York: McGraw-Hill. pp. 149–181.

19. Young, G.B. and Doig, G.S. (2005) Continuous EEG monitoring in intensive care unit patients: Epileptiform activity in etiologically distinct groups. *Neurocrit Care* 2:5–10.

20. Bauby, J.-D. (1997) *The Diving Bell and the Butterfly*, New York: Kropf.

21. Freedman, Y., *et al.* (2003) Simulation of brain death from fulminant deefferentation. *Can J Neurol Sci* 30:397–404.

22. Starmark, J.-E., Holmgren, E., *et al.* (1988) Current reporting of responsiveness in acute cerebral disorders. *J Neurosurg* 69:692.

23. Wijdicks, E.F., *et al.* (2005) Validation of a new coma scale: The FOUR score. *Ann Neurol* 58:585–593.

24. Delorenzo, R.J., *et al.* (1998) Persistent non-convulsive status epilepticus following the control of convulsive status epilepticus. *Epilepsia* 39:833–840.

25. Wijdicks, E.F., *et al.* (2002) Brain death worldwide: Accepted fact but no global consensus on diagnostic criteria. *Neurology* 58:20–25.

26. Wijdicks, E.F.M., *et al.* (2006) Practice parameter: Prediction of outcome in comatose survivors after cardiopulmonary resuscitation (an evidence-based review). Report of the Quality Standards Subcommittee of the American Academy of Neurology. *Neurology* 67:203–210.

27. Al Thenayan, E.A., *et al.* (2007) The validity of predictors of poor neurological outcome following therapeutic hypothermia for cardiac arrest. *Can J Neurol Sci* 34 (Suppl 2): S38.

28. Young, G.B., *et al.* (2005) Anoxic-ischemic encephalopathy: Clinical and electrophysiological associations with outcome. *Neurocrit Care* 2:159–164.

29. Wang, J.T., *et al.* (2004) Prognostic value of evoked responses and event-related brain potentials in coma. *Can J Neurol Sci* 31:438–450.

30. Gofton, T.E., *et al.* (2007) Functional MRI and EEG in the comatose survivor of cardiac arrest. *Can J Neurol Sci* 34 (Suppl 2):S37.

31. Firsching, R. and Frowein, R.A. (1990) Multimodality evoked potentials and early prognosis in comatose patients. *Neurosurg Rev* 13:141–146.

32. Beauchamp, T.L. and Childress, J.F. (2001) *Principles of Biomedical Ethics*, 5th Edition. Oxford: University Press.

Brain Death

James L. Bernat

ABSTRACT

Brain death is the determination of human death by showing the irreversible cessation of the clinical functions of the brain. Whole-brain death is human death because of the loss of the organism as a whole. Brain death is primarily a clinical diagnosis but laboratory tests showing the cessation of intracranial blood flow can be used to confirm it in cases in which the clinical tests cannot be fully performed or correctly interpreted, or to expedite organ donation. The world's principal religions accept brain death with few exceptions. Despite a few residual areas of controversy, brain death is a durable concept that has been accepted well and has formed the basis of successful public policy in diverse societies throughout the world.

Brain death is the common, colloquial term for the determination of human death by showing the irreversible cessation of the clinical functions of the brain. Although the term *brain death* is hallowed by history and accepted in common usage, it is a misleading and unfortunate term. It promotes confusion by wrongly implying that there are different kinds of death or that it is only the brain that dies in such cases. Notwithstanding these shortcomings, I use the term but only in the manner I define here. The terms *cerebral death* and *neocortical death* should be abandoned because they incorrectly suggest that destruction of the cerebral hemispheres is sufficient for death. *Death determined by brain criteria* is a more accurate term than *brain death.*

HISTORY

Brain death is an artifact of modern medical technology. Beginning with the development of positive-pressure ventilators in the 1950s, patients with complete apnoea and paralysis could be successfully ventilated permitting the temporary continuation of heartbeat and circulation that otherwise would have ceased rapidly. By the late 1950s, several patients who developed apnoea resulting from complete destruction of the brain had their ventilation and, hence, circulation supported temporarily. Mollaret and Goulon called this state *coma dépassé* (beyond coma) because affected patients had a depth of unresponsiveness unlike that of any previously recorded [1]. They expressed uncertainty whether patients with *coma dépassé* were alive or dead. These patients had some features usually associated with being alive (e.g., heartbeat, circulation, digestion, and excretion) but other features associated with being dead (e.g., no breathing, no movement, and no reflex responses). It became clear that physicians could not state confidently whether patients with *coma dépassé* were alive or dead until first there was agreement on what it meant for humans to be dead in a technological era.

In 1968, the Harvard Medical School Ad Hoc Committee first provided criteria to substantiate the claim that patients with permanent cessation of neurological function were not simply irreversibly comatose but were in fact dead, and therefore could serve as organ donors without organ procurement causing their death [2]. Over the past four decades, the concept of brain death has become nearly universally accepted and enshrined in laws and practice guidelines throughout the developed world and in many parts of the undeveloped world. Brain death determination is currently practiced in at least 80 countries [3]. While a few areas of persisting controversy remain, brain death is the one bioethical issue that has achieved the highest level of consensus and acceptance, permitting the enactment of uniform laws allowing its practice [4].

THE CONCEPT OF DEATH

The practice of brain death determination is predicated upon a concept of death that affords brain functions a critical role in life. In the pre-technological era, it was unnecessary to make explicit the concept of human death because all bodily systems critical to life (the so-called vital functions of breathing, heartbeat, circulation, and brain functions) were mutually interdependent and ceased within minutes of each other whenever one ceased. But the advent of positive-pressure ventilation permitted the dissociation of vital functions: all brain functions could have ceased irreversibly yet ventilation and circulation could be continued because of mechanical support. The technologically created dissociation of vital functions created an ambiguity in death determination and raised the essential question: which vital functions are most vital to life?

In a series of articles over the past 27 years, my Dartmouth colleagues and I provided a rigorous biophilosophical argument that the human organism was dead when all clinical brain functions ceased irreversibly, irrespective of mechanical continuation of ventilation and support of circulation [5–9]. This argument, providing a conceptual basis for brain death, was cited by the (United States) President's Commission for the Study of Ethical Problems in Medicine and Biomedical and Behavioral Research in their influential book *Defining Death* [10], and has been regarded by many scholars, including opponents, as the standard conceptual defense of whole-brain death [11].

The Dartmouth analysis of death is conducted in four sequential phases: (1) agreeing upon the 'paradigm' of death – the set of preconditions that makes an analysis possible; (2) the philosophical task of determining the definition of death by making explicit the consensual concept of death that has been confounded by technology; (3) the philosophical and medical task of determining the best criterion of death – that measurable condition that shows that the definition has been fulfilled by being both necessary and sufficient for death; and (4) the medical–scientific task of determining the tests of death for physicians to employ at the patient's bedside to demonstrate that the criterion of death has been fulfilled with no false positive and minimal false negative determinations [8].

The paradigm of death comprises seven conditions: (1) *death* is a non-technical word thus defining it should make explicit its ordinary, consensual meaning and not contrive to redefine death; (2) death, like life, is fundamentally a biological (not a social) phenomenon, thus its definition must conform to the empirical facts of biological reality; (3) the definitional domain should be restricted to the death of *homo sapiens* and related higher vertebrates for whom death is a univocal phenomenon; (4) the term *death* can be applied directly and categorically only to organisms, other uses are metaphorical; (5) all higher organisms must be either dead or alive, none can reside in both states or in neither; (6) death is an event and not a process: it is the event separating the processes of dying and bodily disintegration; and (7) death is irreversible. Elsewhere I have explained and defended these conditions in detail [8].

There are three competing criteria of brain death, popularly known as whole-brain death, brain stem death, and the higher-brain formulation [7]. The whole-brain formulation of death is the original concept of brain death, enjoys the greatest prevalence throughout the world, by far, and is the concept my Dartmouth colleagues and I endorse and defend. Brain stem death is practiced in the United Kingdom and a few other countries. Whole-brain death and brain stem death are nearly congruent in practice and rarely produce instances of disagreement. The higher-brain formulation has been propounded by several academic scholars but has not been endorsed by any medical society, and forms the basis of no medical practice or law in any country or jurisdiction.

THE DEFINITION AND CRITERION OF DEATH

Whole-Brain Death

The whole-brain criterion of death is based on a definition of death as the irreversible cessation of the critical functions of the organism as a whole. The organism as a whole is not synonymous with the whole organism (the sum of its parts). Rather it is the set of the organism's emergent functions (properties of a whole not possessed by any of its component parts) that integrate and regulate its subsystems to create the interrelatedness and unity of the organism. The biophilosophical concept of the organism as a whole [8] embraces the concept of an organism's critical system [12]. Death is the irreversible loss of the critical functions of the organism as a whole because of the destruction of the organism's critical system.

The criterion of death satisfying this definition is the irreversible cessation of the clinical functions of the entire brain (whole brain). The critical functions of the organism as a whole include those of respiration and control of circulation executed by the brain stem, neuroendocrine control systems for homeostatic regulation executed by the diencephalon, and (the most exquisite emergent function) conscious awareness somehow executed by in the thalami, the cerebral hemispheres, and their connections. Because all these functions must be irretrievably lost for death, the clinical functions

served by each of these structures must be proved to be permanently absent.

Despite its categorical-sounding name, the whole-brain criterion does not require the irreversible cessation of functioning of every brain neuron. Rather, it requires only the irreversible cessation of all clinical functions of the brain, namely those measurable at the bedside by clinical examination. Some brain cellular activities, such as random electroencephalographic (EEG) activity, may remain recordable after brain death [13]. This electrical activity that results from isolated surviving neurons, although measurable, does not generate a clinical function of the brain or contribute to the functioning of the organism as a whole and, thus, is irrelevant to the determination of death.

The progression to whole-brain death from an initial brain injury usually requires the pathophysiological process of transtentorial brain herniation to produce widespread destruction of the neuronal systems that provide the brain's clinical functions [14]. When the brain is diffusely injured by head trauma, massive intracranial haemorrhage, hypoxic–ischaemic damage during cardiopulmonary arrest or asphyxia, or enlarging intracranial mass lesions, brain oedema within the rigidly fixed skull causes intracranial pressure to rise to levels exceeding mean arterial blood pressure, or in some cases, exceeding systolic blood pressure. At this point, intracranial circulation ceases and nearly all brain neurons that were not destroyed by the initial brain injury are secondarily destroyed by the cessation of intracranial circulation. This process culminates in the destruction of the brain stem. The whole-brain formulation thus provides a fail-safe mechanism to eliminate false positive brain death determinations and assure the loss of the critical functions of the organism as a whole. Showing the absence of all intracranial circulation is sufficient to prove widespread destruction of all critical neuronal systems.

Brain Stem Death

The brain stem criterion of death also is based on a definition of death of the cessation of the organism's integrated, unified functioning. Brain stem theorists argue, however, that the criterion on death should be simply the irreversible loss of the capacity for consciousness combined with the irreversible loss of the capacity to breathe [15, 16]. Christopher Pallis, the most eloquent proponent of the concept of brain stem death, pointed out that the brain stem is at once the through-station for nearly all hemispheric input and output, the centre generating conscious wakefulness, and the centre of breathing. Therefore, destruction of the brain stem produces loss of brain functions that is sufficient for death. He epitomized the role of the brain stem in brain death: 'the irreversible cessation of brain stem function implies death of *the brain as a whole*' [16]. Pallis also correctly observed that most of the clinical tests for whole-brain death measure the loss of brain stem functions.

There are two serious problems with the brain stem criterion. First, because it does not require cessation of the clinical functions of the diencephalon or cerebral hemispheres, it creates the possibility of misdiagnosis of death resulting from a pathological process that appears to destroy all brain stem activities but that preserves a degree of conscious awareness that cannot be clinically detected. I called such a possibility a 'super locked-in syndrome' [7]. I am unaware of the existence of such a case but it remains possible.

The second problem of the brain stem criterion is that by not requiring intracranial circulatory arrest, it eliminates the fail-safe feature of the whole-brain formulation to confidently demonstrate global neuronal destruction. As a practical matter, it also eliminates the possibility of using a confirmatory test to show cessation of intracranial circulation, thereby guaranteeing the irreversible loss of consciousness and of the brain's other clinical functions.

Higher-Brain Formulation

In the early days of the brain death debate, Robert Veatch proposed a refinement in the concept of brain death that became known as the higher-brain formulation. He argued that because it was man's cerebral cortex that defined the person, and not the primitive brain stem structures, the loss of the higher functions served by the cortex should define death. He proposed that death should be defined formally as 'the irreversible loss of that which is considered to be essentially significant to the nature of man' [17]. He rejected the idea that death should be based upon the biophilosophical concept of an organism's loss of the capacity to integrate bodily function. His definition of death thus was unique for *homo sapiens* and was centred upon the unique attribute of human conscious awareness [18]. Veatch's idea became popular, particularly among some philosophers and medical ethicists, where it remains embraced. But despite over three decades of scholarly articles endorsing the higher-brain formulation, it has failed utterly as a public policy. No lawmakers in any jurisdiction have succeeded in changing laws to incorporate it and no physicians or medical societies in any country practice or permit it.

Although Veatch did not explicitly stipulate this point, the criterion of death that satisfies his definition is the irreversible loss of consciousness and cognition. Thus, patients in persistent vegetative states (PVS) would be declared dead by this definition. But, despite their profound disability, and the tragic irony of persistently non-cognitive life, all societies, cultures, and laws throughout the world consider PVS patients as alive. Practice guidelines permit the withdrawal of life-sustaining treatment from PVS patients under certain conditions to allow them to die, but nowhere are they summarily declared dead [19]. The higher-brain formulation is an inadequate concept of death because it fails the first condition of the paradigm of death: to make explicit our underlying consensual concept of death and not to contrive a new definition of death. Rather, the higher-brain formulation is a contrived redefinition of death that neither comports with biological reality nor is consistent with prevailing societal beliefs and laws.

The Circulatory Formulation

Brain death is not accepted universally and has had opponents from the time it was first popularized in the 1960s. Early critics claimed brain death practices violated Christian religious beliefs [20]. Later critics detected inconsistencies between the definition and criterion of death of the whole-brain formulation [18, 21]. Current critics reject outright the concept of brain death and, in its place, propose the circulatory formulation of death: the organism is not dead until its systemic circulation ceases irreversibly. The circulatory idea had its conceptual birth by the philosopher Josef Seifert [22] and received its conceptual consolidation by Alan Shewmon, its most eloquent and persuasive advocate, in several influential recent articles [23, 24].

Shewmon summoned evidence that the brain performs no qualitatively different forms of bodily integration than the spinal cord and concludes that therefore it should be granted no special status above other organs in death determination. He presented a series of cases of what he infelicitously called 'chronic brain death' in which a group of brain dead patients were treated aggressively and had their circulation maintained for many months or longer [25]. He concluded that these cases proved that the concept of brain death is inherently counterintuitive, for how could a dead body continue visceral organ functioning for extended periods, gestate infants, or grow?

First I question how many of the patients in Shewmon's series were truly brain dead or might have been examined incorrectly. (However, the most extreme case cited by Shewmon – a child rendered brain dead by meningitis and ventilated with continued circulation for 16 years – was proved at autopsy to have no recognizable brain tissue and clearly had been brain dead [26].) Second, I observe that prolonged physiological maintenance of the circulation of brain dead patients represents a *tour de force* that reflects our current impressive critical care technological virtuosity. Third, on more conceptual grounds, I argue that the circulatory formulation has the inverse problem of the higher-brain formulation. While the higher-brain formulation generates a criterion that is necessary but insufficient for death, the circulatory formulation generates a criterion that is sufficient but unnecessary for death. Elsewhere I have provided arguments supporting this conclusion based on the fact that it is unnecessary for a determination of death to require the cessation of functions of any organs that do not serve the critical functions of the organism as a whole [6, 8]. Finally, although I concede that Shewmon and other critics have shown weaknesses in the coherence of the whole-brain formulation, these arguments have not swayed the majority of scholars, medical professionals, or the public who experience a conceptual and intuitive attraction to the whole-brain formulation and find it sufficiently coherent and useful to wish to preserve it as public policy [9].

THE TESTS OF DEATH

Brain death tests must be used to determine death only in the unusual death determination in which a patient's ventilation is supported. In an apnoeic patient, if positive-pressure ventilation is neither employed nor planned, the traditional tests to determine death – the prolonged absence of breathing and heartbeat – can be used confidently. These tests are completely predictive of death because the brain will be rapidly destroyed by the resultant hypoxaemia and ischaemia from apnoea and asystole, at which time death will have occurred.

Beginning with the 1968 Harvard Medical School Ad Hoc Committee report, advocates for brain death have proposed a series of bedside tests to show that the whole-brain criterion of death has been satisfied. Numerous batteries of brain death tests were published in the 1970s. In 1981, the Medical Consultants to the President's Commission published a test battery that was quickly accepted, and superseded previous batteries [27]. In 1995, following an evidence-based review of the brain death scientific literature by Eelco Wijdicks [28], the Quality Standards Subcommittee

of the American Academy of Neurology published a practice parameter for determining brain death in adults that forms the current standard for brain death determination in the United States [29]. Similar test batteries have been published in Canada [30, 31] and in the majority of European countries [32]. The individual tests have been described in detail by Wijdicks [33, 34] and are outlined in Table 12.1.

All brain death tests require satisfying preconditions of irreversibility. The cause of the loss of brain functions must be known to be structural and irreversible, and must be sufficient to account for the clinical signs. Before brain death can be declared, the clinician must scrupulously exclude potentially reversible metabolic encephalopathies, such as those from hypothermia, hypoglycemia, or organ failure, as well as toxic encephalopathies, such as those caused by depressant drug intoxication or neuromuscular blockade. To prove that the brain damage is permanent it is critical to exclude potentially reversible conditions that have been reported to mimic the clinical findings in brain death including severe de-efferentation from Guillain-Barré syndrome, hypothermia, and intoxication with drugs that depress central or peripheral nervous system function [33].

The clinical examination for brain death must demonstrate three cardinal signs: (1) profound coma with utter unresponsiveness to noxious stimuli; (2) absence

TABLE 12.1   The Clinical Determination of Brain Death

(A) Preconditions
   1. Diagnosis is considered in a diffusely brain damaged patient with coma and apnoea.
   2. A structural brain lesion is demonstrable that accounts for the clinical findings.
   3. Potentially reversible metabolic and toxic conditions have been excluded.
   4. Physicians performing the test have sufficient training.

(B) Examination elements (all must be present)
   1. Coma with utter unresponsiveness.
   2. Absence of all brain stem reflexes: pupillary, corneal, vestibulo-ocular, gag, cough.
   3. Apnoea in the presence of hypercapnea.

(C) Process
   1. Findings confirmed in at least two examinations separated by a time interval.
   2. The time interval varies as a function of the patient's age and cause of brain death.
   3. The second examination can be omitted if a confirmatory test is performed (Table 12.2).
   4. The patient is declared dead at the fulfilment of the second test.
   5. The family is offered the opportunity for organ donation.
   6. A medical record note itemizes test results and declaration.

of all brain stem-mediated reflexes, including pupillary light/dark reflexes, corneal reflexes, vestibulo-ocular reflexes, gag reflexes, and cough reflexes; and (3) complete apnoea in the face of maximal chemoreceptor stimulation by adequate hypercapnia [35]. Serial neurological examinations over a time interval (determined by the patient's age and cause of brain injury) are necessary unless a confirmatory laboratory test is also used.

Patients with brain death show the deepest coma possible with utter unresponsiveness to all stimuli. They make no movements and lie completely still when the ventilator is stopped. They are insensate to all stimuli. Deep tendon reflexes may be retained but usually are absent. Muscle tone is flaccid and 'posturing' phenomena must be absent. The 'Lazarus sign' of bilateral arm elevation and abduction is a cervical motor neuron reflex movement that is seen occasionally during apnoea testing in unequivocally brain dead patients [36]. Other reflex motor 'automatisms' also may be rarely seen [37].

True apnoea must be present in brain death. The stimulus to breathe in comatose patients usually results from the hypercapnic and not hypoxaemic effect on medullary breathing centres. Therefore, to prove true apnoea, the $PACO_2$ must be raised to levels of at least 50 torr – and preferably exceeding 60 torr – with no respiratory effort present. The technique of apnoeic oxygenation protects the PAO_2 from falling to dangerously low levels as the $PACO_2$ rises during testing. The description of techniques and problems of apnoea testing were reviewed recently by Lang and Heckman [38].

All reflexes innervated by the cranial nerves must be entirely absent in brain death including the pupillary light/dark reflexes to bright light and darkness, corneal touch reflexes, vestibulo-ocular reflexes tested with 50 mL ice water caloric irrigation of the external auditory canals, gag reflexes to tongue depressor stimulation of the throat, and pharyngeal cough reflex during endotracheal tube suctioning.

The demonstration of unresponsive coma, apnoea, and brain stem areflexia shows the absence of the clinical functions of the brain. Physicians determining brain death next must show that the absence of these functions is irreversible. Irreversibility can be demonstrated by excluding the contribution of potentially reversible metabolic or toxic factors and by showing a structural basis for the absent brain functions. Brain CT scan may be sufficient for this purpose in cases of massive traumatic brain injury or subarachnoid haemorrhage with transtentorial herniation.

In cases of hypoxic–ischaemic neuronal injury suffered during cardiopulmonary arrest, repeated examinations followed by an interval of time are necessary. The interval between examinations varies as a function of the patient's age, the nature of the condition causing brain death, and the performance of confirmatory laboratory tests. The interval between serial examinations is longer in infants or when caused by hypoxic–ischaemic neuronal injury, and shorter when accompanied by a positive confirmatory test.

The clinical tests for whole-brain death and for brain stem death are identical. There are no accepted tests for the higher-brain formulation because it has achieved no medical or legal acceptance. The principal difference between tests for whole-brain and brain stem death lies in the availability of confirmatory tests measuring cessation of intracranial blood flow to prove the whole-brain criterion.

A laboratory test to confirm the clinical determination of brain death is useful to expedite brain death determination when organ donation is planned, when facial injury or pre-existing disease preclude adequate clinical testing, or in medico-legal circumstances in which it is desirable to have objective documentation of the absence of brain functions. The available confirmatory tests are listed in Table 12.2. Showing electrocerebral silence by EEG is the oldest confirmatory test but generates too many false positive determinations to be reliable. EEG assesses only the integrity of thalamocortical reverberating circuits and does not directly inspect brain stem function. Electrocerebral silence may be seen in patients with severe vegetative states who clearly are not brain dead [39]. Linking EEG with measurements showing the absence of brain stem auditory evoked potentials or somatosensory evoked potentials improves its reliability in brain death by additionally providing a direct measurement of brain stem electrical activity [40, 41].

TABLE 12.2 Confirmatory Tests for Brain Death

(A) Indications
1. Clinical examination cannot be completed or interpreted confidently
2. Expedite determination to facilitate timely organ procurement
3. Medico-legal reasons

(B) Tests showing absent intracranial circulation (preferred)
1. Radionuclide intravenous angiography
2. Transcranial Doppler ultrasound
3. Computed tomographic angiography
4. Magnetic resonance angiography
5. Magnetic resonance diffusion/perfusion

(C) Tests showing absent neuronal electrical function (both required)
1. Electroencephalography
2. Brain stem auditory evoked responses

The most reliable confirmatory tests are those demonstrating the cessation of intracranial blood flow. Intracranial blood flow ceases once intracranial pressure exceeds mean arterial blood pressure. Two widely available and reliable tests to show cessation of intracranial circulation are intravenous cerebral isotope angiography [42] and transcranial Doppler ultrasound [43–45]. Both have been shown to have high positive and negative predictive values to confirm whole-brain death when performed and interpreted properly. They require examiner experience to detect the presence or absence of small amounts of blood flow.

There have been several reports demonstrating the absence of intracranial circulation in brain death using other techniques, including brain SPECT (Single Photon Emission Computed Tomography) scintigraphy [46, 47], magnetic resonance diffusion-weighted imaging [48], magnetic resonance angiography [49], and computed tomographic angiography (CTA) [50, 51]. Of these newer techniques, although we have only preliminary data, CTA appears to be the most useful and most widely available. Once it has been adequately validated, it will probably replace the other imaging techniques as the preferred confirmatory test for brain death. A recent survey of the confirmatory test preferences of neurointensivists disclosed that radionuclide imaging is more frequently ordered by older physicians and transcranial Doppler ultrasound by younger physicians [52]. Young and Lee compared the reported predictive values of each test [53].

In most brain death cases, rostrocaudal transtentorial herniation from transmitted supratentorial pressure waves secondarily destroys the brain stem and most other neurons by ischaemic infarction. However, in the unusual brain death case caused by a primary brain stem or cerebellar haemorrhage or other destructive lesion of the posterior fossa, intracranial pressure may not rise to levels sufficient to interfere with intracranial circulation, thereby eliminating the possibility of detecting intracranial circulatory arrest in a blood flow confirmatory test [54, 55]. In such cases, the absence of both EEG activity and brain stem auditory and somatosensory potentials can be used as a confirmatory test. The electrical tests also are useful when brain death determinations are performed several days into the course of brain death, after intracranial pressure has fallen to levels below mean arterial blood pressure.

AETIOLOGY AND PATHOGENESIS

The most common causes of brain death in adults are traumatic brain injury, massive intracranial (especially subarachnoid) haemorrhage, expanding intracranial mass lesions, and hypoxic–ischaemic neuronal damage suffered during cardiac arrest. Children become brain dead most commonly from these disorders and/or from asphyxia or meningitis [56].

The pathogenesis of brain death usually comprises three phases. The primary brain insult destroys neurons in a widespread pattern and produces diffuse cerebral oedema which increases in severity over 24–48 hours. The oedematous brain adds volume that, within the fixed skull, raises intracranial pressure. In phase two, as intracranial pressure rises and exceeds mean arterial blood pressure (in massive subarachnoid haemorrhage it often exceeds systolic blood pressure), intracranial circulation ceases because intracranial resistance to blood flow exceeds systemic blood pressure. At this time, all neurons not killed by the primary process and brain oedema become infracted secondarily by global intracranial ischaemia. Phase three occurs several days later when intracranial pressure spontaneously falls permitting renewed blood flow through the necrotic brain [57].

The extent of gross or microscopic necrosis present at autopsy is proportional to the duration of ventilator use following cessation of intracranial circulation. In the early reports on the pathology of brain death, patients' brains showed liquefactive necrosis, a condition called 'respirator brain'. These changes took a week or so to develop following brain death. In the contemporary era, evidence of frank necrosis at autopsy is seen less frequently because of more rapid brain death determination [58].

DIFFERENTIAL DIAGNOSIS

Very few clinical situations mimic brain death. Occasionally, patients with severe depressant drug intoxication, neuromuscular blockade, or hypothermia can show no evidence of clinical brain functions and be mistaken for brain death if these potentially reversible conditions have not been not excluded. Patients with severe Guillain-Barré syndrome have been mistaken for brain death [59]. The vegetative state, locked-in syndrome, coma, and other states of unresponsiveness can be excluded by careful examination [60].

A more common problem is in the differential diagnosis of individual signs of brain death. Cranial nerve reflexes may have been abolished by pre-existing disease. For example, a patient's pupillary light/dark reflexes may be absent because of severe diabetes. Or a patient's vestibulo-ocular reflexes may be absent because of prior treatment with vestibulotoxic aminoglycoside drugs. Patients with chronic obstructive pulmonary disease who chronically retain CO_2 may not breathe in response to elevations of $PACO_2$ during apnoea testing because of chronic CO_2 insensitivity. Whenever possible, it is desirable to restrict brain death determination to clinicians experienced in performing it. Clinical algorithms should be followed when less experienced clinicians perform the determination [61].

DETERMINATION IN PRACTICE

The clinical tests used to determine brain death are well known and accepted but guidelines vary somewhat among countries [3] and among hospitals within countries [62]. Of greater concern, empirical studies of the adequacy of physicians' bedside testing for brain death, including apnoea testing, have shown unfortunate and widespread variability in performing the tests properly and recording the results completely [63–65] as well as variability in the testing protocols required by hospital policies [66]. These discouraging findings suggest the disquieting implication that some physicians probably are declaring patients dead using brain death tests when the patients may not be dead. This inaccuracy suggests the need for better standardization of brain death testing and adequate training to assure that testing is performed and recorded properly.

One confounding factor is the conceptual confusion among physicians and other health professionals about brain death, irreversible coma, and the definition of death. A widely quoted older study showed an appalling misunderstanding of the definitions and boundaries of these categories by many critical care physicians and nurses, the very professionals expected to be most knowledgeable about brain death [67]. A more recent survey of medical students provided somewhat more encouraging results [68] but all experienced neurologists know that brain death is inadequately understood by fellow physicians and nurses. Laura Siminoff and colleagues showed widespread misunderstanding of brain death and related states among the public [69]. Careful explanation of the concept of brain death to family members can improve their understanding and acceptance as well as improve consent for organ donation [70]. The educational need to correct public and professional misunderstanding is obvious.

In a 2002 survey, Eelco Wijdicks found that brain death is currently practiced in at least 80 countries but the testing protocols vary somewhat among countries [3].

Brain death is practiced widely throughout the Western world but is also practiced in a growing number of countries in the non-Western world, such as in the Islamic Middle East [71] and in India [72]. Because of the variation in test batteries among countries, international standardization of brain death testing was designated as the principal project of the Ethics Committee of the World Federation of Neurology during the next decade (Prof. F. Gerstenbrand, personal communication, 25 June 2004). Simple guidelines for the determination of brain death are needed to guide inexperienced physicians in countries where neurologists may not be available [73] and in which there are no facilities for confirmatory tests. The brain death practice guidelines published by the California Medical Association are exemplary [74].

For the past several years, I have become increasingly disturbed by the continued publication of reports of improper brain death determinations and my own personal experience of witnessing errors in examinations of patients purported to be brain dead who were not. Although brain death ideally is a fundamentally a clinical determination, accurately diagnosing it requires skill, experience, and scrupulous attention to detail. I have reluctantly concluded that, as a matter of practice, and especially for those who lack the necessary skill or experience, it is desirable also to perform a test showing the absence of intracranial blood flow to confirm the clinical diagnosis [57].

CHILDREN

The Task Force for the Determination of Brain Death in Children asserted that children over 12 months of age can be tested using the same protocol as for adults. The Task Force recommended that, because younger children may be more amenable to improvement, they require a longer interval between serial examinations and always should have a confirmatory laboratory test in addition to the clinical assessment before brain death is diagnosed [75]. More recent evidence-based recommendations for protocols of brain death testing in children [76, 77] and neonates [78] are available.

RELIGIOUS VIEWS

Early commentators on brain death asserted that its concept and practice were compatible with the beliefs of the world's principal religions [79]. While that assertion was debatable in 1977, it is largely true now. Among Christian believers, Protestantism has accepted brain death without serious exception [80]. The decades-long debate in Roman Catholicism [20] that saw brain death approved by successive pontifical academies was finally settled in 2000 when Pope John Paul II, in an address to the 18th Congress of the International Transplantation Society, formally stated that brain death determination was compatible with Roman Catholic beliefs and teachings [81]. The Pope's statement was reaffirmed in a recent publication of the Pontifical Academy of Sciences [82].

A rabbinic debate on brain death persists in Judaism. Reform and Conservative rabbis accept brain death almost without exception. But the Orthodox Jewish rabbinate remains split between acceptance and rejection. Orthodox authorities such as the Talmudic scholar–physician Fred Rosner argue that brain death is compatible with traditional Jewish law because it is the modern physiological equivalent of decapitation [83]. Other Talmudic authorities, such as Rabbi David Bleich, however, reject brain death because death as understood in Jewish law requires the irreversible cessation of both cardiac and respiratory activity [84]. In general, the strictest Orthodox rabbis continue to oppose brain death on Talmudic grounds.

The former opposition of Islam to brain death was reversed in 1986 by a decree from the Council of Islamic Jurisprudence Academy. Now, religious authorities in several Islamic countries, including in conservative Whahabian Saudi Arabia, permit brain death and organ transplantation [71]. Hindu culture in India endorses brain death [72] as does Shinto-Confucian Japan following a lengthy social battle [85].

All states in the United States have enacted statutes or written administrative regulations permitting physicians to declare death by brain death determination [86]. In the 1990s, two states amended their laws to accommodate religious opposition. New Jersey enacted a religious exemption providing that any citizen who could show that brain death determination violated 'personal religious beliefs or moral convictions' could not be declared brain dead [87]. New York amended its administrative regulations on brain death declaration to provide a similar though more restricted exemption [86].

ORGAN DONATION

The principal reason for societies to allow physicians to practice brain death is to acknowledge biological reality, particularly with advances in ICU technology that permit increasingly prolonged physiological maintenance of a patient's organ subsystems after the demise of the organism as a whole. The principal current utility of brain death is to permit multiple vital organ procurement for transplantation. The desire to obtain transplantable vital organs was a motivating factor in the development of the Harvard Ad Hoc Committee's pioneering 1968 report [88, 89]. At the time of the Harvard report, there was also no legally acceptable means to discontinue life-sustaining therapy once it had been started; the adoption of brain death determination provided such a means.

Current laws and medical practice guidelines in most societies permit the withdrawal of life-sustaining therapy from living hopelessly ill patients. Robert Truog argued that brain death determination is an anachronism that should be abandoned because it has outlived its usefulness: it is no longer necessary to declare a patient dead to discontinue supportive therapy [90]. Truog further called for the dissociation of the relationship between death declaration and vital organ donation, and for the abandonment of the dead-donor rule [91]. I believe that these efforts, while understandable in intent, are misguided.

The dead-donor rule is the ethical axiom of unpaired multi-organ procurement for transplantation: the organ donor must first be dead, and it is unethical to kill even hopelessly ill donors for their organs despite the intent to save others and with the patient's consent [92]. Truog has suggested that the dead-donor rule in vital organ transplantation could be dropped if two conditions were met: (1) the donor patient was hopelessly ill and beyond being harmed because of neurological devastation or imminently dying and (2) the patient had previously consented to serve as an organ donor [90]. The problem with this idea is not that patients will be harmed because they probably would not, given Truog's two conditions. Rather, the problem is that eliminating the dead-donor rule may diminish public confidence in the organ donation enterprise. The public needs to maintain confidence that physicians will remove their vital unpaired organs only after they are dead. Public confidence is fragile and can be jeopardized by publicized claims of physician malfeasance, even when false.

The resistance to implementing protocols permitting organ donation after cardiac death (DCD) is the latest example of the fragility of public confidence in the organ transplantation enterprise. The United States National Academy of Sciences Institute of Medicine has endorsed protocols (formerly called 'non-heart-beating organ donation') that permit organ donation immediately after cardiac death with family consent. Suitable DCD candidate donors have suffered severe brain damage and are on ventilators, but are not brain dead. The patient's surrogate decision maker has ordered cessation of life-sustaining therapy to permit the patient to die because this decision is in accordance with the patient's previously stated wishes [93, 94].

DCD protocols are being implemented in ever greater numbers of hospitals throughout the developed world in response to two needs: (1) to increase the scarce supply of transplantable organs to try to meet the demand for them and (2) to respond to the desire of families to have dying relatives become organ donors. DCD now accounts for a growing number of cadaveric organ donors among organ procurement organizations [95]. Most DCD protocols follow the procedure listed in Table 12.3.

Protocols permitting DCD were introduced to try to increase the finite brain dead organ donor pool by making more efficient an organ donation scheme that was practiced prior to the era of brain death [96]. This seemingly simple scheme has met resistance from the public for two reasons: (1) uncertainty if the patient is unequivocally dead after 5 minutes of asystole and (2) the fear of a causal connection between the family's desire for organ donation and their decision to withhold life-sustaining therapy. I have argued recently that these protocols are consistent with prevailing statutes of death and do not violate the dead-donor rule [97]. The unfortunate and highly publicized 'scandal' arising when the Cleveland Clinic simply considered initiating a DCD protocol is a measure of the fragility of public confidence in death determination and organ donation. The public's tenuous confidence in the ability and impartiality of physicians to correctly diagnose death, upon which the cadaveric organ donation

enterprise rests, could be jeopardized by unnecessarily and unwisely sacrificing the dead-donor rule.

ACKNOWLEDGEMENT

Portions of this chapter were published in Bernat, J.L. (2005) The concept and practice of brain death. *Prog Brain Res* 150:369–379. Copyright Elsevier 2005 (with permission of publisher and author).

References

1. Mollaret, P. and Goulon, M. (1959) Le coma dépassé (mémoire préliminaire). *Rev Neurol* 101:3–15.
2. Ad Hoc Committee (1968) A definition of irreversible coma: Report of the Ad Hoc Committee of the Harvard Medical School to Examine the Definition of Brain Death. *JAMA* 205:337–340.
3. Wijdicks, E.F.M. (2002) Brain death worldwide: Accepted fact but no global consensus in diagnostic criteria. *Neurology* 58:20–25.
4. Capron, A.M. (2001) Brain death – well settled yet still unresolved. *N Engl J Med* 344:1244–1246.
5. Bernat, J.L., *et al.* (1981) On the definition and criterion of death. *Ann Intern Med* 94:389–394.
6. Bernat, J.L. (1998) A defense of the whole-brain concept of death. *Hastings Cent Rep* 28 (2):14–23.
7. Bernat, J.L. (1992) How much of the brain must die in brain death? *J Clin Ethics* 3:21–26.
8. Bernat, J.L. (2002) The biophilosophical basis of whole-brain death. *Soc Philos Policy* 19:324–342.
9. Bernat, J.L. (2006) The whole brain concept of death remains optimum public policy. *J Law Med Ethics* 34:35–43.
10. President's Commission for the Study of Ethical Problems in Medicine and Biomedical and Behavioral Research (1993) *Defining Death: Medical, Legal and Ethical Issues in the Determination of Death*, Washington, DC: U.S. Government Printing Office, pp. 31–43.
11. Shewmon, D.A. and Shewmon, E.S. (2004) The semiotics of death and its medical implications. *Adv Exp Med Biol* 550:89–114.
12. Korein, J. and Machado, C. (2004) Brain death: Updating a valid concept for 2004. *Adv Exp Med Biol* 550:1–14.
13. Grigg, M.M., *et al.* (1987) Electroencephalographic activity after brain death. *Arch Neurol* 44:948–954.
14. Posner, J.B., *et al.* (2007) *Plum and Posner's Diagnosis of Stupor and Coma*, 4th Edition. New York: Oxford University Press, pp. 88–118.
15. Conference of Medical Royal Colleges and Their Faculties in the United Kingdom. (1976) Diagnosis of brain death. *BMJ* 2:1187–1188.
16. Pallis, C. and Harley, D.H. (1996) *ABC of Brainstem Death*, 2nd Edition. London: British Medical Journal Publishers.
17. Veatch, R.M. (1973) The whole brain-oriented concept of death: An outmoded philosophical formulation. *J Thanatol* 3:13–30.
18. Veatch, R.M. (1993) The impending collapse of the whole-brain definition of death. *Hastings Cent Rep* 23 (4):18–24.
19. Jennett, B. (2002) *The Vegetative State: Medical Facts, Ethical and Legal Dilemmas*, Cambridge: Cambridge University Press, pp. 97–125.
20. Byrne, P.A., *et al.* (1979) Brain death – an opposing viewpoint. *JAMA* 242:1985–1990.

TABLE 12.3   Protocol for Organ DCD

1. A decision is made by a lawful surrogate decision maker to withdraw life-sustaining treatment from a hopelessly ill patient and allow the patient to die because of a poor prognosis and the patient's prior wishes to refuse life-sustaining treatment in this circumstance.
2. A lawful surrogate decision maker provides consent for organ donation from the patient once the patient is declared dead.
3. The withdrawal of life-sustaining treatment and declaration of cardiac death is planned and timed with readiness of the organ procurement team.
4. The patient is extubated and receives the same palliative care during dying as non-donors during extubation.
5. The patient's resulting apnoea or hypopnea leads to cardiac asystole.
6. Death is declared following 5 minutes of asystole.
7. Organ procurement proceeds immediately after death declaration, usually successfully procuring the kidneys and often the liver and other organs.

21. Halevy, A. and Brody, B. (1993) Brain death: Reconciling definitions, criteria, and tests. *Ann Intern Med* 119:519–525.

22. Seifert, J. (1993) Is brain death actually death? A critique of redefinition of man's death in terms of 'brain death'. *Monist* 76:175–202.

23. Shewmon, D.A. (2001) The brain and somatic integration: Insights into the standard biological rationale for equating 'brain death' with death. *J Med Philos* 26:457–478.

24. Shewmon, D.A. (2004) The 'critical organ' for the organism as a whole: Lessons from the lowly spinal cord. *Adv Exp Med Biol* 550:23–42.

25. Shewmon, D.A. (1998) Chronic 'brain death': Meta-analysis and conceptual consequences. *Neurology* 51:1538–1545.

26. Repertinger, S., *et al.* (2006) Long survival following bacterial meningitis-associated brain destruction. *J Child Neurol* 21:591–595.

27. Medical Consultants to the President's Commission (1981) Report of the medical consultants on the diagnosis of death to the President's commission for the study of ethical problems in medicine and biomedical and behavioral research. Guidelines for the determination of death. *JAMA* 246:2184–2186.

28. Wijdicks, E.F.M. (1995) Determining brain death in adults. *Neurology* 45:1003–1011.

29. American Academy of Neurology Quality Standards Subcommittee (1995) Practice parameters for determining brain death in adults [summary statement]. *Neurology* 45:1012–1014.

30. Canadian Neurocritical Care Group (1999) Guidelines for the diagnosis of brain death. *Can J Neurol Sci* 26:64–66.

31. Shemie, S.D., *et al.* (2006) Severe brain injury to neurological determination of death: Canadian forum recommendations. *CMAJ* 174:S1–S13.

32. Haupt, W.F. and Rudolf, J. (1999) European brain death codes: A comparison of national guidelines. *J Neurol* 246:432–437.

33. Wijdicks, E.F.M. (2001) The diagnosis of brain death. *N Engl J Med* 344:1215–1221.

34. Wijdicks, E.F.M. (2001) *Brain Death*, Philadelphia, PA: Lippincott Williams & Wilkins, pp. 61–90.

35. Marks, S.J. and Zisfein, J. (1990) Apneic oxygenation in apnea tests for brain death: A controlled trial. *Arch Neurol* 47:1066–1068.

36. Saposnik, G., *et al.* (2005) Spontaneous and reflex movements in 107 patients with brain death. *Am J Med* 118:311–314.

37. Jain, S. and DeGeorgia, M. (2005) Brain death-associated reflexes and automatisms. *Neurocrit Care* 3:122–126.

38. Lang, C.J. and Heckmann, J.G. (2005) Apnea testing for the diagnosis of brain death. *Acta Neurol Scand* 112:358–369.

39. Boutros, A.R. and Henry, C.E. (1982) Electrocerebral silence associated with adequate spontaneous ventilation in a case of fat embolism: A clinical and medicolegal dilemma. *Arch Neurol* 39:314–316.

40. Goldie, W.D., *et al.* (1981) Brainstem auditory and short-latency somatosensory evoked responses in brain death. *Neurology* 31:248–256.

41. Facco, E., *et al.* (2002) Role of short-latency evoked potentials in the diagnosis of brain death. *Clin Neurophysiol* 113:1855–1866.

42. Flowers, W.M.Jr. and Patel, B.R. (1997) Radionuclide angiography as a confirmatory test for brain death: A review of 229 studies in 219 patients. *South Med J* 90:1091–1096.

43. Ducrocq, X., *et al.* (1998) Brain death and transcranial Doppler: Experience in 130 cases of brain dead patients. *J Neurol Sci* 160:41–46.

44. de Freitas, G.R. and Andre, C. (2006) Sensitivity of transcranial Doppler for confirming brain death: A prospective study of 270 cases. *Acta Neurol Scand* 13:426–432.

45. Monteiro, L.M., *et al.* (2006) Transcranial Doppler ultrasonography to confirm brain death: A meta-analysis. *Intensive Care Med* 32:1937–1944.

46. Donohoe, K.J., *et al.* (2003) Procedural guidelines for brain death scintigraphy. *J Nucl Med* 44:846–851.

47. Munari, M., *et al.* (2005) Confirmatory tests in the diagnosis of brain death: Comparison between SPECT and contrast angiography. *Crit Care Med* 33:2068–2073.

48. Lovblad, K.O. and Bassetti, C. (2000) Diffusion-weighted magnetic resonance imaging in brain death. *Stroke* 31:539–542.

49. Karantanas, A.H., *et al.* (2002) Contributions of MRI and MR angiography in early diagnosis of brain death. *Eur Radiol* 12:2710–2716.

50. Qureshi, A.I., *et al.* (2004) Computed tomographic angiography for the diagnosis of brain death. *Neurology* 62:652–653.

51. Leclerc, X., *et al.* (2006) The role of spiral CT for the assessment of the intracranial circulation in suspected brain death. *J Neuroradiol* 33:90–95.

52. Boissy, A.R., *et al.* (2005) Neurointensivists' opinions about death by neurological criteria and organ donation. *Neurocrit Care* 3:115–121.

53. Young, B. and Lee, D. (2004) A critique of ancillary tests of brain death. *Neurocrit Care* 1:499–508.

54. Ferbert, A., *et al.* (1986) Isolated brainstem death. *Electroencephalogr Clin Neurophysiol* 65:157–160.

55. Kosteljanetz, M., *et al.* (1988) Clinical brain death with preserved cerebral arterial circulation. *Acta Neurol Scand* 78:418–421.

56. Staworn, D., *et al.* (1994) Brain death in pediatric intensive care unit patients: Incidence, primary diagnosis, and the clinical occurrence of Turner's triad. *Crit Care Med* 22:1301–1305.

57. Bernat, J.L. (2004) On irreversibility as a prerequisite for brain death determination. *Adv Exp Med Biol* 550:161–167.

58. Wijdicks, E.F.M. and Pfeifer, E.A. (2008) Neuropathology of brain death in modern transplant era. *Neurology* 70:1234–1237.

59. Friedman, Y., *et al.* (2003) Simulation of brain death from fulminant de-efferentation. *Can J Neurol Sci* 30:305–306.

60. Bernat, J.L. (2006) Chronic disorders of consciousness. *Lancet* 367:1181–1192.

61. Kaufman, H.H. and Lynn, J. (1986) Brain death. *Neurosurgery* 19:850–856.

62. Hornby, K., *et al.* (2006) Variability in hospital-based brain death guidelines in Canada. *Can J Anaesth* 53:613–619.

63. Earnest, M.P., *et al.* (1986) Testing for apnea in brain death: Methods used by 129 clinicians. *Neurology* 36:542–544.

64. Mejia, R.E. and Pollack, M.M. (1995) Variability in brain death determination practices in children. *JAMA* 274:550–553.

65. Wang, M.Y., *et al.* (2002) Brain death documentation: Analysis and issues. *Neurosurgery* 51:731–735.

66. Powner, D.J., *et al.* (2004) Variability among hospital policies for determining brain death in adults. *Crit Care Med* 32:1284–1288.

67. Youngner, S.J., *et al.* (1989) 'Brain death' and organ retrieval. A cross-sectional survey of knowledge and concepts among health professionals. *JAMA* 261:2205–2210.

68. Frank, J.I. (2001) Perceptions of death and brain death among fourth-year medical students: Defining our challenge as neurologists (abst). *Neurology* 56:A429.

69. Siminoff, L., *et al.* (2004) Death and organ procurement: Public beliefs and attitudes. *Kennedy Inst Ethics J* 14:217–234.

70. Ormrod, J.A., *et al.* (2005) Experiences of families when a relative is diagnosed brain stem dead: Understanding of death, observation of brain stem death testing, and attitudes to organ donation. *Anaesthesia* 60:1002–1008.

71. Yaqub, B.A. and Al-Deeb, S.M. (1996) Brain death: Current status in Saudi Arabia. *Saudi Med J* 17:5–10.

72. Jain, S. and Maheshawari, M.C. (1996) Brain death – the Indian perspective. In Machado, C. (ed.) *Brain Death*, pp. 261–263. Amsterdam: Elsevier.

73. Baumgartner, H. and Gerstenbrand, F. (2002) Diagnosing brain death without a neurologist: Simple criteria and training are needed for the non-neurologist in many countries. *BMJ* 324:1471–1472.

74. Shaner, D.M., *et al.* (2004) Really, most SINCERELY dead: Policy and procedure in the diagnosis of death by neurologic criteria. *Neurology* 62:1683–1686.

75. Task Force for the Determination of Brain Death in Children (1987) Guidelines for the determination of brain death in children. *Arch Neurol* 44:587–588.

76. Shemie, S.D., *et al.* (2007) Diagnosis of brain death in children. *Lancet Neurol* 6:87–92.

77. Banasiak, K.J. and Lister, G. (2003) Brain death in children. *Curr Opin Pediatr* 15:288–293.

78. Ashwal, S. (1997) Brain death in the newborn. Current perspectives. *Clin Perinatol* 24:859–882.

79. Veith, F.J., *et al.* (1977) Brain death: A status report of medical and ethical considerations. *JAMA* 238:1651–1655.

80. Campbell, C.S. (1999) Fundamentals of life and death: Christian fundamentalism and medical science. In Youngner, S.J. *et al.* (eds.) *The Definition of Death: Contemporary Controversies*, pp. 194–209. Baltimore: John Hopkins University Press.

81. Furton, E.J. (2002) Brain death, the soul, and organic life. *Natl Cathol Bioeth Q* 2:455–470.

82. Pontifical Academy of Sciences (2007) *The Signs of Death*. Scripta Varia 110, Vatican City: Pontifical Academy of Sciences.

83. Rosner, F. (1999) The definition of death in Jewish law. In Youngner, S.J. *et al.* (eds.) *The Definition of Death: Contemporary Controversies*, pp. 210–221. Baltimore: John Hopkins University Press.

84. Bleich, J.D. (1979) Establishing criteria of death. In Rosner, F. and Bleich, J.D. (eds.) *Jewish Bioethics*, pp. 277–295. New York: Sanhedrin Press.

85. Lock, M. (1995) Contesting the natural in Japan: Moral dilemmas and technologies of dying. *Cult Med Psychiatr* 19:1–38.

86. Beresford, H.R. (1999) Brain death. *Neurol Clin* 17:295–306.

87. Olick, R.S. (1991) Brain death, religious freedom, and public policy: New Jersey's landmark legislative initiative. *Kennedy Inst Ethics J* 4:275–288.

88. Giacomini, M. (1997) A change of heart and a change of mind? Technology and the redefinition of death in 1968. *Soc Sci Med* 44:1465–1482.

89. Belkin, G.S. (2003) Brain death and the historical understanding of bioethics. *J Hist Med Allied Sci* 58:325–361.

90. Truog, R.D. (1997) Is it time to abandon brain death? *Hastings Cent Rep* 27 (1):29–37.

91. Truog, R.D. and Robinson, W.M. (2003) Role of brain death and the dead-donor rule in the ethics of organ transplantation. *Crit Care Med* 31:2391–2396.

92. Robertson, J.A. (1999) The dead donor rule. *Hastings Cent Rep* 29 (6):6–14.

93. Institute of Medicine (1997) *Non-Heart-Beating Organ Donation: Medical and Ethical Issues in Procurement*, Washington, DC: National Academy Press.

94. Institute of Medicine (2000) *Non-Heart-Beating Organ Transplantation: Practice and Protocols*, Washington, DC: National Academy Press.

95. Bernat, J.L., *et al.* (2006) Report of a national conference on donation after cardiac death. *Am J Transplant* 6:281–291.

96. Sheehy, E., *et al.* (2003) Estimating the number of potential organ donors in the United States. *N Engl J Med* 349:667–674.

97. Bernat, J.L. (2006) Are organ donors after cardiac death really dead? *J Clin Ethics* 17:122–132.

The Assessment of Conscious Awareness in the Vegetative State

Adrian M. Owen, Nicholas D. Schiff and Steven Laureys

ABSTRACT

The assessment of patients in the vegetative state is extremely complex and depends frequently on subjective interpretations of the observed spontaneous and volitional behaviour. In recent years, a number of studies have demonstrated an important role for functional neuroimaging in the identification of residual cognitive function, and even conscious awareness, in some patients fulfilling the clinical criteria for vegetative state. Such studies, when successful, may be particularly useful where there is concern about the accuracy of the diagnosis and the possibility that residual cognitive function has remained undetected. However, use of these techniques in severely brain-injured persons is methodologically complex and requires careful quantitative analysis and interpretation. In addition, ethical frameworks to guide research in these patients urgently need to be developed to accommodate these emerging technologies.

INTRODUCTION

In recent years, improvements in intensive care have increased the number of patients who survive severe acute brain injuries. Although the majority of these patients recover from coma within the first days of the insult, others evolve to a state of 'wakeful unawareness' or vegetative state. Clinically, recognizing unambiguous signs of conscious perception of the environment and of the self in such patients can be extremely challenging. This difficulty is reflected in frequent misdiagnoses of the condition and confusion between the vegetative state and related conditions such as minimally conscious state and locked-in syndrome [1, 2]. Like all severely brain-injured patients, bedside evaluation of residual brain function in vegetative state is difficult because motor responses may be very limited or inconsistent. In addition, the clinical assessment of cognitive function relies on inferences drawn from present or absent responses to external stimuli at the time of the examination [3]. Recent advances in functional neuroimaging suggest a novel solution to this problem; in several cases, so-called activation studies have been used to identify residual cognitive function and even *conscious awareness* in patients who are assumed to be vegetative, yet retain cognitive abilities that have evaded detection using standard clinical methods. In this chapter, we first describe the major clinical characteristics of vegetative state following severe brain injury. We then discuss the contribution of neuroimaging studies to the assessment of conscious awareness in the vegetative state. Finally, we review the major methodological and ethical impediments to conducting such studies in disorders of consciousness.

CLINICAL DESCRIPTION

Patients in the vegetative state are awake, but are assumed to be entirely unaware of self and environment [4, 5]. Jennett and Plum cited the Oxford English Dictionary to clarify their choice of the term 'vegetative': to be vegetate is to 'live a merely physical life devoid of intellectual activity or social intercourse' and vegetative describes 'an organic body capable of growth and development but devoid of sensation and thought'. 'Persistent vegetative state' is a term that was chosen arbitrarily to describe a vegetative state present 1 month after acute traumatic or non-traumatic brain injury but does not imply irreversibility [6]. 'Permanent vegetative state' denotes irreversibility. The Multi-Society Task Force on vegetative state concluded that 3 months following a non-traumatic brain injury and 12 months after traumatic injury, the condition of vegetative patients may be regarded as 'permanent'. These guidelines are best applied to patients who have suffered diffuse traumatic brain injuries and post-anoxic events; other non-traumatic aetiologies may be less well predicted (see for example [7, 8]) and require further considerations of aetiology and mechanism in evaluating prognosis. Even after long and arbitrary delays, some exceptional patients may show limited recovery. This is more likely in patients with non-traumatic coma without cardiac arrest who survive in the vegetative state for more than 3 months. The diagnosis of

vegetative state should be questioned when there is any degree of sustained visual pursuit, consistent and reproducible visual fixation, or response to threatening gestures [6]. It is essential to establish the formal absence of any sign of conscious perception or deliberate action before making the diagnosis (Box 13.1).

RESTING BRAIN FUNCTION

In the vegetative state, the brainstem is relatively spared whereas the grey or white matter of both cerebral hemispheres is widely and severely injured. Overall cortical metabolism of vegetative patients is 40–50% of normal values [9–20]. Some studies however, have found normal cerebral metabolism [17] or blood flow [21] in patients in a persistent vegetative state. In *permanent* vegetative state (i.e., 12 months after a trauma or 3 months following a non-traumatic brain injury), brain metabolism values drop to 30–40% of normal values (Figure 13.1) [9]. This progressive loss of metabolic functioning over time is the result of progressive Wallerian and transsynaptic neuronal degeneration. Characteristic of vegetative patients is a relative sparing of metabolism in the brainstem (encompassing the pedunculopontine reticular formation, the hypothalamus and the basal forebrain) [22]. The functional preservation of these structures allows for the preserved arousal and autonomic functions in these patients. Another hallmark of the vegetative state is a systematic impairment of metabolism in the polymodal associative cortices (bilateral prefrontal regions, Broca's area, parieto-temporal and posterior parietal areas and precuneus) [18]. These regions are known to be important in various functions that are necessary for consciousness, such as attention, memory and language

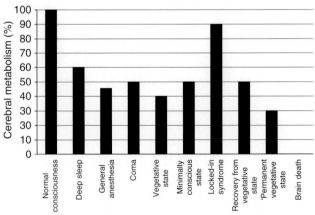

FIGURE 13.1 Cerebral metabolism in the different diagnostic groups. *Source*: Adapted from Laureys *et al.* (2004) *Lancet Neurol* 9:537–546.

BOX 13.1

VEGETATIVE PATIENTS WITH ATYPICAL BEHAVIOURAL FRAGMENTS

Stereotyped responses such as grimacing, crying or occasional vocalization are frequently observed on examination of vegetative state patients. These behaviours are assumed to arise primarily from brainstem circuits and limbic cortical regions that are preserved in the vegetative state. Rarely, however, patients meeting the diagnostic criteria for the vegetative state exhibit behavioural features that prima facie appear to contravene the diagnosis. A series of studies of chronic vegetative patients examined with multimodal imaging techniques identified three such patients with unusual behavioural fragments. Using FDG-PET (fluorodeoxyglucose-positron emission tomography), structural magnetic resonance imaging (MRI) and magnetoencephalography (MEG) preserved islands of higher resting brain metabolism measured by PET imaging and incompletely preserved evoked MEG gamma-band responses were correlated with structural imaging and behavioural fragments [17]. Among those studied was a patient who had been in a vegetative state for 20 years who infrequently expressed single words (typically epithets) in isolation of environmental stimulation [23]. MRI images demonstrated severe subcortical injuries. Resting FDG-PET measurements of the patient's brain revealed a global cerebral metabolic rate of <50% of normal across most brain regions with small regions in the left hemisphere expressing higher levels of metabolism (see Figure 13.2). MEG responses to bilateral auditory stimulation were confined to the left hemisphere and localized to primary auditory areas. Taken together, the imaging and neurophysiological data appeared to identify isolated sparing of left sided thalamo-cortical-basal ganglia loops that normally support language

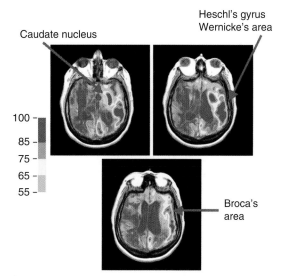

FIGURE 13.2   Preservation of regional cerebral metabolic activity in a vegetative state patient. FDG-PET data for vegetative state patient with occasional expression of isolated words is displayed co-registered with structural MRI (from Schiff *et al.* [23]). PET voxels are normalized by region and expressed on a colour scale ranging from 55% to 100% of normal.

function in Heschl's gyrus, Broca's area and Wernicke's area. Similar observations in two other vegetative state patients provide novel evidence that isolated cerebral networks may remain active in rare vegetative state patients. Importantly, the preservation of these isolated behaviours does not herald further recovery in patients in chronic vegetative states who have been repeatedly examined and carefully studied with imaging tools. Reliable observations of such unusual features should prompt further investigation in an individual patient.

[24]. It is still unknown whether the observed metabolic impairment in this large cortical network reflects an irreversible structural neuronal loss [25] or functional and potentially reversible damage. However, in those rare and fortunate cases where vegetative patients recover awareness of self and environment, positron emission tomography (PET) shows a functional recovery of metabolism in these same cortical regions [19]. Moreover, the resumption of long-range functional connectivity between these associative cortices and the intralaminar thalamic nuclei parallels the restoration of their functional integrity [26]. The cellular mechanisms

which underlie this functional normalization remain unclear: axonal sprouting, neurite outgrowth, cell division (known to occur predominantly in associative cortices in normal primates) [27] have been proposed as candidate processes.

BRAIN ACTIVATION STUDIES

While metabolic studies are useful, they can only identify functionality at the most general level; that is, mapping cortical and subcortical regions that are *potentially* recruitable, rather than relating neural activity within such regions to specific cognitive processes [13]. On the other hand, methods such as $H_2^{15}O$ PET and functional magnetic resonance imaging (fMRI) can be used to link residual neural activity to the presence of covert cognitive *function*. In short, functional neuroimaging, or so-called activation studies, have the potential to demonstrate distinct and specific physiological responses (changes in regional cerebral blood flow (rCBF) or changes in regional cerebral haemodynamics) to controlled external stimulation in the absence of any overt response (e.g., a motor action) on the part of the patient (Box 13.2). In the first of such studies, $H_2^{15}O$ PET was used to measure rCBF in a post-traumatic vegetative patient during an auditorily presented story told by his mother [28]. Compared to non-word sounds, activation was observed in the anterior cingulate and temporal cortices, possibly reflecting emotional processing of the contents, or tone, of the mother's speech. In another patient diagnosed as vegetative, Menon *et al.* [7] also used PET, but to study covert *visual* processing in response to familiar faces. During 'experimental' scans, the patient was presented with pictures of the faces of family and close friends, while during 'control' scans scrambled versions of the same images were presented which contained no meaningful visual information whatsoever. Previous imaging studies in healthy volunteers have shown that such tasks produce robust activity in the right fusiform gyrus, the so-called human 'face area' (e.g., [29, 30]). The same visual association region was activated in the vegetative patient when the familiar face stimuli were compared to the meaningless visual images [7, 31] (Figure 13.3).

In cohort studies of patients unequivocally meeting the clinical diagnosis of the vegetative state, simple noxious somatosensory [32] and auditory [20, 33] stimuli have shown systematic activation of primary sensory cortices and lack of activation in higher-order associative cortices from which they were functionally disconnected. High intensity noxious electrical stimulation activated midbrain, contralateral thalamus and primary somatosensory cortex in each and every one of the 15 vegetative patients studied, even in the absence of detectable cortical evoked potentials [32]. However, secondary somatosensory, insular, posterior parietal and anterior cingulate cortices, which were activated in all control subjects, failed to show significant activation in a single vegetative patient (Figure 13.4).

Moreover, in the vegetative state patients, the activated primary somatosensory cortex was shown to exist as an island, functionally disconnected from

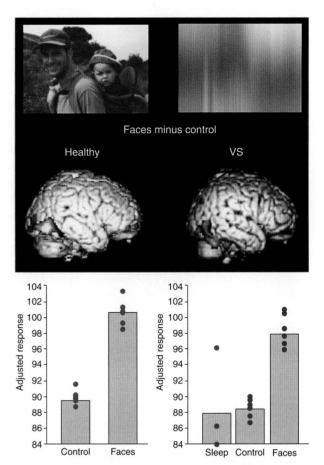

FIGURE 13.3 Example stimuli (top) from the face perception task used by Menon *et al.* [7]. Surface rendered normalized PET data from the familiar face perception task superimposed on standard 3D magnetic resonance template (middle) for a healthy control subject (left) and a patient diagnosed as vegetative state (right). Subtraction shown is faces minus control stimuli. In both cases, strong right hemisphere activation in the fusiform gyrus is clearly visible. Graphs below represent individual adjusted blood flow response for each scan (red dots) within each condition at peak coordinates within this region. The vegetative state patient fell asleep during three scans (labelled 'sleep'). *Source:* Figure adapted from Menon *et al.* [7].

higher-order associative cortices of the pain matrix. Similarly, although simple auditory click stimuli activated bilateral primary auditory cortices in vegetative patients, hierarchically higher-order multimodal association cortices were not activated. Moreover, a cascade of functional disconnections were observed along the auditory cortical pathways, from primary auditory areas to multimodal and limbic areas [33] suggesting that the observed residual cortical processing in the vegetative state does not lead to integrative processes which are thought to be necessary for awareness.

In a recent review of the relevant literature it was argued that functional neuroimaging studies in

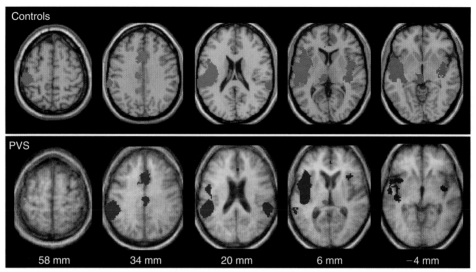

FIGURE 13.4 (Upper) Brain regions, shown in red, that activated during noxious stimulation in controls (subtraction stimulation–rest). (Lower) Brain regions that activated during stimulation in vegetative state patients, shown in red (subtraction stimulation–rest) and regions that activated less in patients than in controls (interaction (stimulation vs. rest) × (patient vs. control)), shown in blue. Projected on transverse sections of a normalized brain MRI template in controls and on the mean MRI of the patients (distances are relative to the bicommissural plane). *Source*: Adapted from Laureys *et al.* [32].

patients meeting the clinical criteria for vegetative state should be conducted hierarchically [34, see also 35]; beginning with the simplest form of processing within a particular domain (e.g., auditory) and then progressing sequentially through more complex cognitive functions. By way of example, a series of auditory paradigms was described that had all been successfully employed in functional neuroimaging studies of vegetative patients. These paradigms increased in complexity systematically from basic acoustic processing to more complex aspects of language comprehension and semantics. Indeed, in a recent study exploring the utility of this approach residual language function in a group of seven vegetative and five minimally conscious patients has been graded according to their brain activation on this hierarchical series of paradigms [36]. Three patients, diagnosed as vegetative, demonstrated some evidence of preserved speech processing, whilst the remaining four patients showed no significant activation at all, even in response to sound when compared to silence. The authors suggested that such a hierarchy of cognitive tasks provides the most valid mechanism for defining the depth and breadth of preserved cognitive function in patients meeting the clinical criteria for persistent vegetative state and discuss how such an approach might be extended to allow clear inferences about the level of 'awareness' or consciousness to be made.

A question that is often asked of such studies, however, is whether the presence of 'normal' brain activation in patients who are diagnosed as vegetative indicates a level of conscious awareness, perhaps even similar to that which exists in healthy volunteers when performing the same tasks. Many types of stimuli, including faces, speech and pain will elicit relatively 'automatic' responses from the brain; that is to say, they will occur without the need for wilful intervention on the part of the participant (e.g., you cannot choose to *not* recognize a face, or to *not* understand speech that is presented clearly in your native language). By the same argument, 'normal' neural responses in patients who are diagnosed as vegetative do not necessarily indicate that these patients have any conscious experience associated with processing those same types of stimuli. Thus, such patients *may* retain discreet islands of subconscious cognitive function, which exist in the absence of awareness.

The logic described above exposes a central conundrum in the study of conscious awareness and in particular, how it relates to the vegetative state. Deeper philosophical considerations notwithstanding, the only reliable method that we have for determining if another being is consciously aware is to ask him/her. The answer may take the form of a spoken response or a non-verbal signal (which may be as simple as the blink of an eye, as documented cases of the locked-in syndrome have demonstrated), but it is this answer that allows us to infer conscious awareness. In short, our ability to know unequivocally that another being is consciously aware is ultimately determined, not by

BOX 13.2

METHODOLOGICAL ISSUES

The acquisition, analysis and interpretation of neuroimaging data in severe brain injury are methodologically extremely complex. In quantitative PET studies, the absolute value of cerebral metabolic rates depends on many assumptions for which a consensus has not been established in cases of cerebral pathology. For example, the estimation of the cerebral metabolic rate of glucose using FDG-PET requires a correction factor, known as the lumped constant. It is generally accepted that this lumped constant is stable in normal brains. However, in traumatic brain injury, a significant global *decrease* in lumped constant has recently been reported [37] and in severe ischaemia, regional lumped constant values are known to *increase* significantly as a result of glucose transport limitation [38]. Second, cerebral glucose use as measured by FDG may not always be tightly coupled with oxygen use in patients because altered metabolic states, including anaerobic glycolysis, may occur acutely after brain injury [39–41]. Third, because PET provides measurements per unit volume of intracranial contents, they may be affected by the inclusion of metabolically inactive spaces such as cerebrospinal fluid or by brain atrophy which may artificially lower the calculated cerebral metabolism [42, 43].

As described in the main text, so-called activation studies using $H_2^{15}O$ PET or fMRI together with established sensory paradigms provide a direct method for assessing cognitive processing and even conscious awareness in severely brain-injured patients. However, like metabolic studies, these investigations are methodologically complex and the results are rarely equivocal. For example, in brain-injured patients, the coupling between neuronal activity and local haemodynamics, essential for all $H_2^{15}O$ PET and fMRI activation measurements, is likely to be different from healthy control [44–47], making interpretation of such datasets extremely difficult. Notwithstanding this basic

methodological concern, the choice of experimental paradigm is also critical. For example, abnormal brainstem auditory evoked responses may make the use of auditory stimuli inappropriate and alternative stimuli (i.e., visual) should be considered. The paradigm should also be sufficiently complex to exercise the cognitive processes of interest, preferably beyond those that are simply involved in stimulus perception, yet not so complex that they might easily overload residual cognitive capacities in a tired or inattentive patient. In addition, it is essential that the experimental paradigm chosen produces well-documented, anatomically specific, robust and reproducible activation patterns in healthy volunteers in order to facilitate interpretation of imaging data in patients. In vegetative state, episodes of low arousal and sleep are also frequently observed and close patient monitoring (preferably by means of simultaneous electroencephalographic (EEG) recording) during activation scans is essential to avoid such periods. Spontaneous movements during the scan itself may also compromise the interpretation of functional neuroimaging data, particularly scans acquired using fMRI. Data processing of functional neuroimaging data may also present challenging problems in patients with acute brain injury. For example, the presence of gross hydrocephalus or focal pathology may complicate co-registration of functional data (e.g., acquired with PET or fMRI) to anatomical data (e.g., acquired using structural MRI), and the normalization of images to a healthy reference brain. Under these circumstances statistical assessment of activation patterns is complex and interpretation of activation foci in terms of standard stereotaxic co-ordinates may be impossible. Finally, where PET methodology is employed, issues of radiation burden must also be considered and may preclude longitudinal or follow-up studies in many patients.

whether they are aware or not, but by their ability to communicate that fact through a recognized behavioural response. But what if the ability to blink an eye or move a hand is lost, yet conscious awareness remains? By definition, patients who are diagnosed as vegetative are not able to elicit such behavioural responses. Following the logic of this argument then, even if such a patient *were* consciously aware, he/she

would, by definition, have no means for conveying that information to the outside world.

A novel approach to this conundrum has recently been described, using fMRI, to demonstrate preserved conscious awareness in a patient fulfilling the criteria for a diagnosis of vegetative state [48, 49]. In mid-2005, the patient was involved in a road traffic accident. On admission to hospital she had a Glasgow

Coma Scale score of 4. A computed tomography scan revealed diffuse brain swelling, intraventricular blood in the left lateral ventricle, low attenuation in the left frontal lobe close to the corpus callosum and attenuation change in the right frontal and left posterior temporal regions. The following day she underwent a bifrontal decompressive craniectomy and a month later a ventriculoperitoneal shunt was inserted into the right lateral ventricle. Between the time of the accident and the fMRI scan in early January 2006, the patient was assessed by a multidisciplinary team employing repeated standardized assessments consistent with the procedure described by Bates [50]. Throughout this period the patient's behaviour was consistent with accepted guidelines defining the vegetative state [51]. She would open her eyes spontaneously, exhibited sleep/wake cycles and had preserved, but inconsistent, reflexive behaviour (startle, noxious, threat, tactile, olfactory). No elaborated motor behaviours (regarded as 'voluntary' or 'willed' responses), were observed from the upper or lower limbs. There was no evidence of orientation, fixation or tracking to visual or auditory stimuli. No overt motor responses to command were observed.

Prior to the fMRI scan, the patient was instructed to perform two mental imagery tasks when cued by the instructions 'imagine playing tennis' or 'imagine visiting the rooms in your home'. These instructions were elaborated outside of the scanner in an attempt to induce a rich and detailed mental picture during the scan itself. Thus, one task involved imagining playing a vigorous game of tennis, swinging for the ball with both forehand and backhand, for the entire duration of each scanning block. The other task involved imagining moving slowly from room to room in her house, visualizing the location and appearance of each item of furniture as she did so. In a third condition, the patient was asked to 'just relax'.

Importantly, these particular tasks were chosen, not because they involve a set of fundamental cognitive processes that are known to reflect conscious awareness, but because imagining playing tennis and imagining moving around the house elicit extremely reliable, robust and statistically distinguishable patterns of activation in specific regions of the brain. For example, in a series of studies in healthy volunteers [48, 52] imagining playing tennis has been shown to elicit activity in the supplementary motor area, a region known to be involved in imagining (as well as actually performing) co-ordinated movements, in each and every one of 34 participants scanned. In contrast, imagining moving from room to room in a house commonly activates the parahippocampal cortices, the posterior parietal lobe and the lateral premotor cortices,

all regions that have been shown to contribute to imaginary, or real, spatial navigation.

Given the reliability of these responses across individuals, activation in these regions can be used as a 'neural marker', confirming that the participant retains the ability to understand instructions, to carry out different mental tasks in response to those instructions and, therefore, is able to exhibit willed, voluntary *behaviour* in the absence of any overt action.

When the patient who was clinically diagnosed as vegetative was asked to imagine playing tennis, significant activity was observed in the supplementary motor area that was statistically indistinguishable from that observed in healthy awake volunteers (see Figure 13.5). In contrast, the instruction to imagine

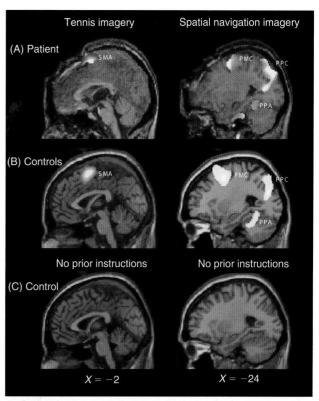

FIGURE 13.5 (A) Supplementary motor area (SMA) activity during tennis imagery and parahippocampal gyrus (PPA), posterior parietal lobe (PPC) and lateral premotor cortex (PMC) activity while imagining moving around a house in the patient described by Owen *et al.* [49]. (B) Statistically indistinguishable activity in all four brain regions in a group of 12 healthy volunteers asked to perform the same imagery tasks. (C) The result when a healthy volunteer underwent exactly the same fMRI procedure as the patient described by Owen *et al.* [50], with the exception that non-instructive sentences (e.g., 'The man played tennis', 'The man walked around his house') were used. Using an identical statistical model to that used with the patient, *no* significant sustained activity was observed in the SMA, the PPA, the PPC, the PMC, nor any other brain region. All results are similarly thresholded at a False Discovery Rate (FDR) $p < .05$, corrected for multiple comparisons.

walking through the rooms of her house elicited significant activity in the parahippocampal gyrus, the posterior parietal cortex and the lateral premotor cortex, which was again indistinguishable from that observed in healthy volunteers (Figure 13.5). It was concluded that, despite fulfilling all of the clinical criteria for a diagnosis of vegetative state, this patient retained the ability to understand spoken commands and to respond to them through her brain activity, rather than through speech or movement, confirming beyond any doubt that she was consciously aware of herself and her surroundings.

Of course, sceptics may argue that the words 'tennis' and 'house' could have automatically triggered the patterns of activation observed in the supplementary motor area, the parahippocampal gyrus, the posterior parietal lobe and the lateral premotor cortex in this patient in the absence of conscious awareness. However, no data exists supporting the inference that such stimuli can unconsciously elicit sustained haemodynamic responses in these regions of the brain. Indeed, considerable data exists to suggest such words do not elicit the responses that were observed. For example, although it is well documented that some words can, under certain circumstances, elicit wholly automatic neural responses in the absence of conscious awareness, such responses are typically transient (i.e., lasting for a few seconds) and, unsurprisingly, occur in regions of the brain that are associated with word processing. In the patient described by Owen et al. [48, 49], the observed activity was not transient, but persisted for the full 30 seconds of each imagery task, that is far longer than would be expected, even given the haemodynamics of the fMRI response. In fact, these task-specific changes persisted until the patient was cued with another stimulus indicating that she should rest. Such responses are impossible to explain in terms of automatic brain processes. In addition, the activation observed in the patient was not in brain regions that are known to be involved in word processing, but rather, in regions that are known to be involved in the two imagery tasks that she was asked to carry out. Again, sustained activity in these regions of the brain is impossible to explain in terms of unconscious responses to either single 'key' words or to short sentences containing those words. In fact, in a supplementary study [49], non-instructive sentences containing the same key words as those used with the patient (e.g., 'The man enjoyed playing tennis') were shown to produce *no* sustained activity in any of these brain regions in healthy volunteers (see Figure 13.5, lower panel).

The most parsimonious explanation is, therefore, that this patient was consciously aware and wilfully

---

BOX 13.3

ETHICAL ISSUES

Severely brain-injured, non-communicative patients raise several ethical concerns. Foremost is the concern that diagnostic and prognostic accuracy is assured, as treatment decisions typically include the possibility of withdrawal of life support. At present, although the approaches discussed above hold great promise to improve both diagnostic and prognostic accuracy, the standard approach remains the careful and repeated neurological examination by a trained examiner.

Ethical concerns are often raised concerning the participation of severely brain-injured patients in neuroimaging activation studies (especially to assess pain perception), studies that require invasive procedures (e.g., intra-arterial or jugular lines required for quantification of PET data or modelling) or the use of neuromuscular paralytics. By definition, unconscious or minimally conscious patients cannot give informed consent to participate in clinical research and written approval is typically obtained from family or legal representatives depending on governmental and hospital guidelines in each country. Nonetheless, it is not without precedent for studies in these patient populations to be refused for grants, ethics committee approval or data publication based on a view that no research study is ethical in patients who cannot provide consent. We side with a proposed ethical framework that emphasizes balancing access to research and medical advances alongside protection for vulnerable patient populations [53]. Severe brain injury represents an immense social and economic problem that warrants further research. Unconscious, minimally conscious and locked-in patients are very vulnerable and deserve special procedural protections. However, it is important to stress that they are also vulnerable to being denied potentially life-saving therapy if clinical research cannot be performed adequately.

following the instructions given to her, despite her diagnosis of vegetative state.

CONCLUSIONS

Vegetative state presents unique problems for diagnosis, prognosis, treatment and everyday management (Box 13.3). At the patient's bedside, the evaluation of possible cognitive function in these patients is difficult because voluntary movements may be very small, inconsistent and easily exhausted. Functional neuroimaging appears to offer a complimentary approach to the clinical assessment of patients with vegetative state and other altered states of consciousness and can objectively describe (using population norms) the regional distribution of cerebral activity at rest and under various conditions of stimulation. Indeed, in some rare cases, functional neuroimaging has demonstrated preserved cognitive function and even (in two cases so far) *conscious awareness* in patients who are assumed to be vegetative, yet retain cognitive abilities that have evaded detection using standard clinical methods. In our opinion, the future use of PET, MEG/EEG and especially fMRI will substantially increase our understanding of severely brain-injured patients.

ACKNOWLEDGEMENTS

Steven Laureys is Senior Research Associate at the Fonds National de la Recherche Scientifique de Belgique (FNRS) and is supported by grants from the European Commission. Nicholas Schiff is supported by NS02172, NS43451 and the Charles A. Dana Foundation. Adrian M. Owen is supported by the Medical Research Council, UK and thanks Dr. Martin Coleman and the Cambridge Impaired Consciousness Research Group and the staff of the Welcome Trust Research Facility for their major contribution to some of the work described in this chapter [48, 49]. The authors thank the James S. McDonnell Foundation for funding the present work.

References

1. Andrews, K., Murphy, L., Munday, R. and Littlewood, C. (1996) Misdiagnosis of the vegetative state: Retrospective study in a rehabilitation unit. *BMJ* 313 (7048):13–16.
2. Childs, N.L., Mercer, W.N. and Childs, H.W. (1993) Accuracy of diagnosis of persistent vegetative state. *Neurology* 43 (8):1465–1467.
3. Wade, D.T. and Johnston, C. (1999) The permanent vegetative state: Practical guidance on diagnosis and management. *BMJ* 319 (7213):841–844.
4. Jennett, B. and Plum, F. (1972) Persistent vegetative state after brain damage. A syndrome in search of a name. *Lancet* 1 (7753):734–737.
5. Jennett, B. (2002) *The Vegetative State: Medical Facts, Ethical and Legal Dilemmas*, Cambridge: Cambridge University Press.
6. The Multi-Society Task Force on PVS (1994) Medical aspects of the persistent vegetative state (1). *New Engl J Med* 330 (21):1499–1508.
7. Menon, D.K., Owen, A.M., Williams, E.J., *et al.* (1998) Cortical processing in persistent vegetative state. *Lancet* 352 (9123):200.
8. Wilson, B.A., Gracey, F. and Bainbridge, K. (2001) Cognitive recovery from 'persistent vegetative state': Psychological and Personal Perspectives. *Brain Injury* 15 (12):1083–1092.
9. Tommasino, C., Grana, C., Lucignani, G., Torri, G. and Fazio, F. (1995) Regional cerebral metabolism of glucose in comatose and vegetative state patients. *J Neurosurg Anesthesiol* 7 (2):109–116.
10. De Volder, A.G., Goffinet, A.M., Bol, A., Michel, C., de, B.T. and Laterre, C. (1990) Brain glucose metabolism in postanoxic syndrome. Positron emission tomographic study. *Arch Neurol* 47 (2):197–204.
11. Levy, D.E., Sidtis, J.J., Rottenberg, D.A., *et al.* (1987) Differences in cerebral blood flow and glucose utilization in vegetative versus locked-in patients. *Ann Neurol* 22 (6):673–682.
12. Rudolf, J., Ghaemi, M., Haupt, W.F., Szelies, B. and Heiss, W.D. (1999) Cerebral glucose metabolism in acute and persistent vegetative state. *J Neurosurg Anesthesiol* 11 (1):17–24.
13. Momose, T., Matsui, T. and Kosaka, N. (1989) Effect of cervical spinal cord stimulation (cSCS) on cerebral glucose metabolism and blood flow in a vegetative patient assessed by positron emission tomography (PET) and single photon emission computed tomography (SPECT). *Radiat Med* 7 (7):243–246.
14. Rudolf, J., Sobesky, J., Ghaemi, M. and Heiss, W.D. (2002) The correlation between cerebral glucose metabolism and benzodiazepine receptor density in the acute vegetative state. *Eur J Neurol* 9 (6):671–677.
15. Edgren, E., Enblad, P., Grenvik, A., *et al.* (2003) Cerebral blood flow and metabolism after cardiopulmonary resuscitation. A pathophysiologic and prognostic positron emission tomography pilot study. *Resuscitation* 57 (2):161–170.
16. Beuthien-Baumann, B., Handrick, W., Schmidt, T., *et al.* (2003) Persistent vegetative state: Evaluation of brain metabolism and brain perfusion with PET and SPECT. *Nucl Med Comm* 24 (6):643–649.
17. Schiff, N.D., Ribary, U., Moreno, D.R., *et al.* (2002) Residual cerebral activity and behavioural fragments can remain in the persistently vegetative brain. *Brain* 125 (Pt 6):1210–1234.
18. Laureys, S., Goldman, S., Phillips, C., *et al.* (1999) Impaired effective cortical connectivity in vegetative state: Preliminary investigation using PET. *Neuroimage* 9 (4):377–382.
19. Laureys, S., Lemaire, C., Maquet, P., Phillips, C. and Franck, G. (1999) Cerebral metabolism during vegetative state and after recovery to consciousness. *J Neurol Neurosurg Psychiatr* 67:121.
20. Boly, M., Faymonville, M.E., Peigneux, P., *et al.* (2004) Auditory processing in severely brain injured patients: Differences between the minimally conscious state and the persistent vegetative state. *Arch Neurol* 61 (2):233–238.
21. Agardh, C.D., Rosen, I. and Ryding, E. (1983) Persistent vegetative state with high cerebral blood flow following profound hypoglycemia. *Ann Neurol* 14 (4):482–486.
22. Laureys, S., Faymonville, M.E., Goldman, S., *et al.* (2000) Impaired cerebral connectivity in vegetative state. In *Physiological Imaging of the Brain with PET* A. Gjedde, S.B. Hansen, G.M. Knudsen, and O.B. Paulson, (eds.) San Diego, CA: Academic Press. pp. 329–334.

23. Schiff, N., Ribary, U., Plum, F. and Llinás, R. (1999) Words without mind. *J Cogn Neursci* 11 (6):650–656.

24. Baars, B., Ramsoy, T. and Laureys, S. (2003) Brain, conscious experience the observing self. *Trends Neurosci* 26:671–675.

25. Rudolf, J., Sobesky, J., Grond, M. and Heiss, W.D. (2000) Identification by positron emission tomography of neuronal loss in acute vegetative state. *Lancet* 355:155.

26. Laureys, S., Faymonville, M.E., Luxen, A., Lamy, M., Franck, G. and Maquet, P. (2000) Restoration of thalamocortical connectivity after recovery from persistent vegetative state. *Lancet* 355 (9217):1790–1791.

27. Gould, E., Reeves, A.J., Graziano, M.S. and Gross, C.G. (1999) Neurogenesis in the neocortex of adult primates. *Science* 286 (5439):548–552.

28. de Jong, B., Willemsen, A.T. and Paans, A.M. (1997) Regional cerebral blood flow changes related to affective speech presentation in persistent vegetative state. *Clin Neurol Neurosurg* 99 (3):213–216.

29. Haxby, J.V., Grady, C.L., Horwitz, B., Ungerleider, L.G., Mishkin, M., Carson, R.E., Herscovitch, P., Schapiro, M.B. and Rapoport, S.I. (1991). Dissociation of object and spatial visual processing pathways in human extrastriate cortex. *Proc Natl Acad Sci USA* 88:1621–1625.

30. Haxby, J.V., Horwitz, B., Ungerlieder, L.G., Maisog, J.M., Pietrini, P. and Grady, C.L. (1994) The functional organization of human extrastriate cortex: A PET-rCBF study of selective attention to faces and locations. *J Neurosci* 14:6336–6353.

31. Owen, A.M., Menon, D.K., Johnsrude, I.S., *et al.* (2002) Detecting residual cognitive function in persistent vegetative state. *Neurocase* 8 (5):394–403.

32. Laureys, S., Faymonville, M.E., Peigneux, P., *et al.* (2002) Cortical processing of noxious somatosensory stimuli in the persistent vegetative state. *Neuroimage* 17 (2):732–741.

33. Laureys, S., Faymonville, M.E., Degueldre, C., *et al.* (2000) Auditory processing in the vegetative state. *Brain* 123 (Pt 8):1589–1601.

34. Owen, A.M., Coleman, M.R., Menon, D.K., Berry, E.L., Johnsrude, I.S., Rodd, J.M., Davis, M.H., and Pickard, J.D. (2005) Using a hierarchical approach to investigate residual auditory cognition in persistent vegetative state. In Laureys, S. (eds.). *The Boundaries of Consciousness: Neurobiology and Neuropathology. Progress in Brain Research*, Vol. 150, pp. 461–476. London: Elsevier.

37. Owen, A.M., Coleman, M.R., Menon, D.K., Johnsrude, I.S., Rodd, J.M., Davis, M.H., Taylor, K. and Pickard, J.D. (2005) Residual auditory function in persistent vegetative state: A combined PET and fMRI study. *Neuropsychol Rehabil* 15 (3–4):290–306.

38. Coleman, M.R., Rodd, J.M., Davis, M.H., Johnsrude, I.S., Menon, D.K., Pickard, J.D. and Owen, A.M. (2007) Do vegetative patients retain aspects of language? Evidence from fMRI. *Brain* 130:2494–2507.

39. Wu, H.M., Huang, S.C., Hattori, N., *et al.* (2004) Selective metabolic reduction in gray matter acutely following human traumatic brain injury. *J Neurotrauma* 21 (2):149–161.

40. Hamlin, G.P., Cernak, I., Wixey, J.A. and Vink, R. (2001) Increased expression of neuronal glucose transporter 3 but not glial glucose transporter 1 following severe diffuse traumatic brain injury in rats. *J Neurotrauma* 18 (10):1011–1018.

41. Bergsneider, M., Hovda, D.A., McArthur, D.L., *et al.* (2001) Metabolic recovery following human traumatic brain injury based on FDG-PET: Time course and relationship to neurological disability. *J Head Trauma Rehabil* 16 (2):135–148.

40. Goodman, J.C., Valadka, A.B., Gopinath, S.P., Uzura, M. and Robertson, C.S. (1999) Extracellular lactate and glucose alterations in the brain after head injury measured by microdialysis. *Crit Care Med* 27 (9):1965–1973.

41. Hovda, D.A., Becker, D.P. and Katayama, Y. (1992) Secondary injury and acidosis. *J Neurotrauma* 9 (Suppl 1):S47–S60.

42. Herscovitch, P., Auchus, A.P., Gado, M., Chi, D. and Raichle, M. E. (1986) Correction of positron emission tomography data for cerebral atrophy. *J Cereb Blood Flow Metab* 6 (1):120–124.

43. Videen, T.O., Perlmutter, J.S., Mintun, M.A. and Raichle, M. E. (1988) Regional correction of positron emission tomography data for the effects of cerebral atrophy. *J Cereb Blood Flow Metab* 8 (5):662–670.

44. Sakatani, K., Murata, Y., Fukaya, C., Yamamoto, T. and Katayama, Y. (2003) BOLD functional MRI may overlook activation areas in the damaged brain. *Acta Neurochir Suppl* 87:59–62.

45. Gsell, W., De Sadeleer, C., Marchalant, Y., MacKenzie, E.T., Schumann, P. and Dauphin, F. (2000) The use of cerebral blood flow as an index of neuronal activity in functional neuroimaging: Experimental and pathophysiological considerations. *J Chem Neuroanat* 20 (3–4):215–224.

46. Hamzei, F., Knab, R., Weiller, C. and Rother, J. (2003) The influence of extra- and intracranial artery disease on the BOLD signal in FMRI. *Neuroimage* 20 (2):1393–1399.

47. Rossini, P.M., Altamura, C., Ferretti, A., *et al.* (2004) Does cerebrovascular disease affect the coupling between neuronal activity and local haemodynamics? *Brain* 127 (Pt 1):99–110.

48. Owen, A.M., Coleman, M.R., Davis, M.H., Boly, M., Laureys, S. and Pickard, J.D. (2006) Detecting awareness in the vegetative state. *Science* 313:1402.

49. Owen, A.M., Coleman, M.R., Davis, M.H., Boly, M., Laureys, S. and Pickard, J.D. (2007) Response to Comments on 'Detecting awareness in the vegetative state'. *Science* 315:1221c.

50. Bates, D. (2005) Incidence and prevalence of the vegetative and minimally conscious states. *Neuropsychol Rehabil* 15:175.

51. Royal College of Physicians (2003) *The Vegetative State: Guidance on Diagnosis and Management [Report of a Working Party]*, London: Royal College of Physicians.

52. Boly, M., Coleman, M.R., Davis, M.H., *et al.* (2007) When thoughts become actions: An fMRI paradigm to study volitional brain activity in non-communicative brain injured patients. *Neuroimage* 36(3):979–992.

53. Fins, J.J. (2003) Constructing an ethical stereotaxy for severe brain injury: Balancing risks, benefits and access. *Nat Rev Neurosci* 4 (4):323–327.

54. Turkstra, L.S. (1995) Electrodermal response and outcome from severe brain injury. *Brain Injury* 9 (1):61–80.

The Minimally Conscious State: Clinical Features, Pathophysiology and Therapeutic Implications

Joseph T. Giacino and Nicholas D. Schiff

ABSTRACT

The minimally conscious state (MCS) is a condition of severely altered consciousness that is distinguished from the vegetative state (VS) by the presence of minimal but clearly discernible behavioural evidence of self or environmental awareness. There is increasing evidence from neurobehavioural and neuroimaging studies that important differences in clinical presentation, neuropathology and functional outcome exist between MCS and VS. This chapter describes the characteristic features of MCS, discusses specialized assessment techniques required for accurate diagnosis and outlines potential pathophysiological mechanisms underlying MCS which may provide important clues for the development of effective treatment interventions.

Clinicians specializing in the care of patients with severe brain injury are well acquainted with the clinical features of coma and the vegetative state (VS).

Both of these disorders are characterized by the complete absence of behavioural signs of self and environmental awareness. VS can be readily distinguished from coma by observing for spontaneous or elicited eye-opening which occurs in VS and not in coma [1]. The reemergence of eye-opening signals that the reticular system has regained control over wakefulness, although individuals in VS remain completely unaware of self or environment. In VS, the brainstem also resumes control over vital bodily functions including respiration, heart rate and thermal regulation. Although these functions may still be compromised during VS, life-sustaining interventions such as mechanical ventilation are usually not required.

Recovery from VS is variable in rate and degree [2, 3]. Some individuals rapidly recover behavioural signs of consciousness within the first few weeks of injury while others demonstrate slower, more gradual recovery of cognitive function over a period of months. In a minority of cases, cognitive functions fail to reemerge and VS evolves into a permanent condition [2]. In those who do recover, the transition from unconsciousness to consciousness is characteristically subtle, often marked by ambiguous signs of consciousness. During this transitional period, command-following is often difficult to differentiate from random movement on bedside assessment [4]. Further complicating matters, even when clear signs of conscious behaviour have been observed, they may be difficult to replicate within or across examinations [5].

Until recently, patients demonstrating minimal or intermittent signs of consciousness were not distinguished diagnostically from patients in VS and coma. In 1995, the American Congress of Rehabilitation introduced the term, *minimally responsive state (MRS)*, to describe patients manifesting inconsistent but clearly discernible signs of conscious behaviour [6]. A key element of this new diagnostic category was the requirement that behaviours thought to be indicative of consciousness be viewed as unequivocally 'meaningful' by the examiner. In view of concerns that patients in coma and VS also display some degree of behavioural (albeit reflexive) responsiveness, an expert panel known as the Aspen Workgroup recommended that the term, MRS, be replaced by *minimally conscious state (MCS)* to emphasize the partial preservation of consciousness that distinguishes this condition from coma and VS [7]. In 2002, following an extended period of literature review and discussion among professional organizations in rehabilitation, neurology and neurosurgery, a consensus-based case definition of MCS was published in association with recommendations for specific diagnostic criteria [8]. These recommendations were subsequently endorsed by the American Association of Neurological Surgeons, American Congress of Rehabilitation Medicine, American Academy of Physical Medicine and Rehabilitation, the Child Neurology Society and the Brain Injury Association of America, Inc.

Motivated in part by alarming published estimates of misdiagnosis of VS ranging from 15–43% [9–11], a primary aim of the Aspen Workgroup was to establish operationally defined criteria for MCS to facilitate differentiation of this condition from VS. A closely aligned aim was to provide a common frame of reference for researchers involved in the scientific study of this condition. Since publication of the MCS case definition, the number of reports addressing assessment, prognosis, pathophysiology, outcome and ethical issues has increased steadily [12]. The objective of this chapter is to provide a broad overview of the clinical and pathophysiological features of MCS, and to consider the therapeutic implications of these characteristics.

DEFINITION AND DIAGNOSTIC CRITERIA

MCS is a condition of severely altered consciousness in which minimal but definite behavioural evidence of self or environmental awareness is demonstrated on clinical examination [8]. To establish the diagnosis, there must be an evidence of least one clear-cut behavioural sign of cognitive processing *and* the behaviour must be reproduced at least once within the same examination. Because behavioural fluctuation is common during MCS, it is generally necessary to conduct serial examinations before an accurate diagnosis can be made. Complicating diagnosis further, patients may vacillate between VS and MCS before level of consciousness (LOC) stabilizes [13].

MCS is diagnosed when there is clear evidence of *one or more* of the following behaviours:

- simple command-following;
- gestural or verbal yes/no responses (regardless of accuracy);
- intelligible verbalization;
- movements or affective behaviours that occur in contingent relation to relevant environmental stimuli and are not attributable to reflexive activity.

Examples of contingent motor and affective responses include (1) episodes of crying, smiling or laughter produced by the linguistic or visual content of emotional but not neutral stimuli; (2) vocalizations or gestures that occur in direct response to verbal prompts; (3) reaching for objects with a clear relationship between object location and direction of reach; (4) touching or holding objects in a manner that accommodates the size and shape of the object; and (5) visual pursuit or sustained fixation in response to moving or salient stimuli.

Because the diagnostic criteria for MCS depend largely on the integrity of the language and motor systems, aphasia and apraxia may confound bedside assessment and should always be considered before the final diagnosis is established.

Behavioural parameters have also been defined to mark emergence from MCS [8]. Resolution of MCS is signalled by the return of one of two complex behaviours:

- *Reliable and consistent interactive communication*: Communicative responses may occur through speech, writing, yes/no signals or augmentative communication devices.

or

- *Functional object use*: This requires discrimination and appropriate use of two or more objects presented by the examiner. In MCS, there may be evidence of object manipulation but there is no apparent awareness of how the object is used.

The criteria for emergence from MCS were intended to reflect recovered capacity for meaningful environmental interaction. The clinical appropriateness of these behavioural benchmarks has been questioned by some authors. Taylor *et al.* [14] have suggested that the requirements for *reliable* communication and *functional* object use conflate features of post-traumatic amnesia (PTA) with MCS. They note that loss of executive control during PTA may cause disturbances in language and practic functions which are likely to interfere with satisfaction of the diagnostic criteria for emergence from MCS, consequently prolonging the duration of this condition. Moreover, they suggest that if a patient is able to follow simple instructions and attempts to answer yes/no questions, regardless of accuracy, these behaviours no longer represent 'minimal' evidence of consciousness but rather, an ability to actively engage in environmental interactions. They propose that it is more appropriate to describe the impact of PTA and confusion on behavioural performance at this point, rather than maintain the diagnosis of MCS. This issue

will need to be investigated empirically before the existing criteria are modified. Table 14.1 compares the clinical features of coma, VS, MCS and emergence from MCS.

TABLE 14.1 Comparison of Behavioural Features of MCS, VS and Coma

Behaviour	MCS	VS	Coma
Eye opening	Spontaneous	Spontaneous	None
Spontaneous movement	Automatic/object manipulation	Reflexive/patterned	None
Response to pain	Localization	Posturing/withdrawal	Posturing/none
Visual response	Object recognition/pursuit	Startle/pursuit (rare)	None
Affective response	Contingent	Random	None
Commands	Inconsistent	None	None
Verbalization	Intelligible words	Random vocalization	None

BEDSIDE ASSESSMENT METHODS

The approach to assessment of patients with disorders of consciousness (DOC) must consider two factors that may influence examination findings and lead to misdiagnosis. In light of the fluctuations in behaviour that commonly occur in this population, evaluations should be repeated over time and measures should be sensitive enough to detect subtle but prognostically important changes in neurobehavioural responsiveness. Conventional bedside assessment procedures and neurosurgical rating scales such as the Glasgow Coma Scale (GCS) [15] have limited utility when used to monitor progress in patients with prolonged disturbance in consciousness as they were built to detect fairly gross changes in behaviour and are not designed to distinguish random or reflexive behaviours from those that are purposeful. To address these shortcomings, both standardized and individualized assessment procedures have been devised. Standardized rating scales assess a broad range of neurobehavioural functions and rely on fixed administration and scoring procedures. Alternatively, individualized behavioural assessment protocols are intended to address case-specific questions using principles of single subject research design.

Standardized neurobehavioural assessment measures include the Coma Recovery Scale-R (CRS-R) [16, 17]), the Coma-Near Coma Scale (CNC) [18], the Western Neurosensory Stimulation Profile (WNNSP) [19], the Western Head Injury Matrix (WHIM) [20] and the Sensory Modality and Rehabilitation Technique (SMART) [21]. Although item content varies across measures, all evaluate behavioural responses to a variety of auditory, visual, motor and communication prompts. All of these instruments have been shown to have adequate reliability and validity; however, there is considerable variability in their psychometric properties and clinical utility. Of these measures, the CRS-R is the only one that directly incorporates the existing diagnostic criteria for coma, VS and MCS into the administration and scoring scheme. Giacino et al. [16] compared the CRS-R to the Disability Rating Scale (DRS) in 80 patients with DOC and found that although the two scales produced the same diagnosis in 87% of cases, the CRS-R identified 10 patients in MCS who were classified as VS on the DRS. There were no cases in which the DRS detected features of MCS missed by the CRS-R. A more recent study by Schnakers and co-workers administered the GCS, CRS-R and the Full Outline of Unresponsiveness [22] to 60 patients with acute (i.e., trauma centre) and subacute (i.e., rehabilitation centre) brain injury resulting in disturbance in consciousness. Among the 29 patients diagnosed with VS on the GCS, four were found to have at least one sign of consciousness on the FOUR. However, the CRS-R detected evidence of MCS in 7 additional patients diagnosed with VS on the FOUR. All seven of these patients showed visual fixation, a clinical sign heralding recovery from the VS.

Clinicians involved in the care of MCS patients often encounter situations in which the patients' behavioural responses are ambiguous or occur too infrequently to clearly discern their significance. These problems are often due to injury-related sensory, motor and drive deficits. For this reason, a technique referred to as Individualized Quantitative Behavioural Assessment (IQBA) was developed by Whyte and colleagues [23, 24]. IQBA is intended to address case-specific questions using individually tailored assessment procedures, operationally defined target responses and controls for examiner and response bias. Once the target behaviour (e.g., command-following, visual tracking) has been operationalized, the frequency of the behaviour is recorded following administration of an appropriate command, an incompatible command and during a rest interval.

Data are analysed statistically to determine whether the target behaviour occurs significantly more often in one condition relative to the others. When the frequency of the behaviour is greater during the 'rest' condition relative to the 'command' condition, for example, this suggests that the behaviour represents random movement rather than a direct response to the command.

IQBA can be applied across a broad array of behaviours and can address virtually any type of clinical question. McMillan [25] employed an IQBA protocol to determine whether a minimally responsive, traumatically brain-injured patient could reliably communicate a preference concerning withdrawal of life-sustaining treatment. Responses to questions were executed using a button press. Results indicated that the number of affirmative responses to 'wish to live' questions was significantly greater than chance suggesting that the patient could participate in end-of-life decision-making. McMillan's findings were subsequently replicated in a second IQBA assessment conducted by different group of examiners [26].

When behavioural responses are equivocal on bedside examination, the examiner should assure that the patient is adequately aroused prior to conducting the examination, potentially sedating medications should be discontinued and the patient should be screened for subclinical seizure activity. Arousal facilitation techniques that incorporate tactile stimulation, deep pressure or vestibular stimulation [27] should be administered to augment arousal and alertness. To increase the likelihood of detecting volitional responses, response modalities compromised by sensory or motor impairment should be avoided, unnecessary sources of distraction should be eliminated and a broad range of environmental stimuli should be presented. Observations of nursing staff, family members and paraprofessionals should be integrated into the examination. When evaluating young children, assessment procedures may require adaptation to account for immature language and motor development.

INCIDENCE AND PREVALENCE

The incidence and prevalence of MCS are difficult to estimate because of the lack of adequate surveillance outside of primary care settings. In the United States, most patients with DOC are transferred to long-term care facilities following relatively brief stays at a trauma (7–14 days) or inpatient rehabilitation (30 days) centre. Long-term care facilities are often ill-equipped to manage patients in MCS as clinical staff generally lack specialized training in assessment which may allow subtle but diagnostically important changes to go undetected. Further complicating surveillance efforts, there is no International Classification of Diseases (ICD) diagnostic code for MCS and the prevalence of MCS is influenced by survival, which is dependent upon access to care, quality of care and decisions to withdraw care.

The only published study concerning the prevalence of MCS was completed by Strauss and colleagues [28]. These researchers developed an operational definition for MCS based on a large state registry used by the California Department of Developmental Services to track medical care and services administered to residents between the ages of 3 and 15. Of the 5075 individuals in the registry who met criteria for VS or MCS, 11% were in VS and 89% in MCS. Extrapolating from US census data for the general adult population, the prevalence of MCS was estimated to be between 112 000 and 280 000. If these figures are correct, the prevalence of MCS may be sevenfold higher than VS.

PROGNOSIS AND OUTCOME

Few outcome predictors specific to MCS have been identified. It is likely that this is because outcome studies completed prior to establishing the diagnostic criteria for MCS in 2002 failed to distinguish patients in VS from those with minimal or inconsistent evidence of conscious behaviour. There is growing evidence that outcome from MCS may be associated with recovery of specific behaviours. A number of investigators have reported that reemergence of visual pursuit may presage recovery of other signs of consciousness. Among 104 patients admitted to an inpatient rehabilitation centre with a diagnosis of VS or MCS, Giacino and Kalmar [29] found intact visual pursuit in 82% of the MCS patients relative to 20% of the VS group. More importantly, 73% of the VS group with visual pursuit recovered other clear-cut signs of consciousness by 12 months, as compared to 45% of those without pursuit. Ansell and Keenan [19] reported that patients who demonstrated late improvement performed significantly better on tests of visual pursuit completed on admission to rehabilitation when compared to those who did not improve. Similarly, Shiel and colleagues

[20] found that acutely brain-injured patients who showed visual pursuit on hospital admission were more likely to demonstrate social interaction and communicative behaviour later in their course than those who did not.

Outcome following MCS also appears to be linked to rate of recovery. Whyte and colleagues [30] found that rate of improvement on the DRS [31] over the first 2 weeks of inpatient rehabilitation was highly predictive of subacute functional outcome. Patients with better DRS scores at enrolment and faster rates of initial improvement tended to have better DRS scores at 16 weeks. The combination of rate of DRS recovery, the time between injury and enrolment and the DRS score at enrolment accounted for nearly 50% of the variance in DRS score at 16 weeks and were highly significant predictors of time until commands were followed. An earlier study by Giacino and co-workers [17] found that change scores on three different assessment scales administered during the first month of rehabilitation were more predictive of functional outcome at discharge when compared to admission scores alone. While 19 of 20 patients with low change scores on the DRS were 'extremely severely disabled' to 'extremely vegetative' at discharge, only 1 of 8 patients with high change scores fell into one of these unfavourable outcome categories. Although neither of these studies stratified patients by diagnosis, both included cases diagnosed with MCS.

Studies consistently show that functional outcome is significantly more favourable for patients diagnosed with MCS during the acute recovery phase as compared to those diagnosed with VS. Giacino and Kalmar [29] found that 50% of patients in MCS, vs. 3% of those in VS, had 'no disability' to 'moderate disability' on the DRS at 1-year post-injury. Additionally, while 43% of patients in the traumatic VS subgroup fell between the 'VS' and 'extreme VS' categories, none of the patients in the traumatic MCS subgroup had scores in this range. Lammi et al. [32] followed 18 patients diagnosed with traumatic MCS and compared DRS outcome scores at 2–5 years post-injury (mean = 3.6 years) to those reported by Giacino and Kalmar at 1-year post-injury. Findings indicated that 15% of Lammi et al.'s sample had partial disability or less on the DRS, compared to 23% of the sample described by Giacino and Kalmar. The percentage of patients with scores in the extremely severe to vegetative range was also similar in both studies (Lammi et al. = 20%; Giacino and Kalmar = 17%). In both studies, the majority of patients were classified in the moderate to moderately severe ranges (55% and 50%, respectively). Interestingly, the duration of MCS

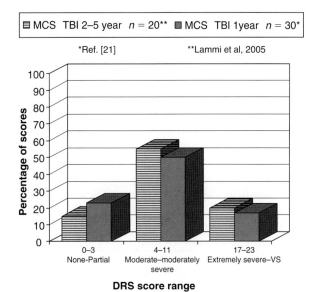

FIGURE 14.1   Comparison of mean DRS scores at 1 and 2–5 years post-injury as reported in the studies by Giacino and Kalmar [29, 32], respectively. The horizontal-patterned bars depict the percentage of late DRS outcome scores noted in the Lammi *et al.* study while the solid bars represent the percentage of early DRS scores reported by Giacino and Kalmar.

was not significantly correlated with overall level of recovery on the DRS or with a measure of psychosocial outcome. It is also important to note that one-third of Lammi's sample was deemed 'independent' in either cognitive or motor function at follow-up. Figure 14.1 compares mean DRS scores in the two samples.

Eilander and colleagues [33] investigated the relationship between LOC on admission to rehabilitation (i.e., conscious and able to communicate consistently, MCS or VS) and outcome at discharge in a cohort of 145 patients with traumatic and non-traumatic injuries. In the traumatic group, 86% of patients who were in MCS on admission were able to communicate consistently by discharged, as compared to 43% of patients in VS. The disparity was wider in the non-traumatic group (MCS: 65% and 11%, respectively). Using a set of predictor variables including LOC at admission, time between injury and admission, type of trauma, age at injury, team treatment and gender, the investigators correctly classified 88% of patients who regained consciousness and 62% of cases that failed to do so.

Although rare, significant late functional recovery from MCS has been reported. In one well-documented case, a 38-year-old man who sustained a severe traumatic brain injury (TBI) recovered from MCS after 19

years and regained fluent speech and lower extremity motor function. Diffusion tensor imaging showed evidence of axonal sprouting in the cerebellum over an 18-month period that correlated with the late improvement in motor function [34]. An additional area of increased anisotropy in the mesial parieto-occipital region normalized following recovery of speech suggesting ongoing plasticity despite injury onset 20 years earlier.

LIFE EXPECTANCY

Strauss and co-workers [28] estimated mortality risk and survival rates in patients diagnosed with VS and MCS. The investigators subdivided the MCS group into patients who were mobile and those without mobility, based on ability to lift the head while lying prone, roll forward or backward or maintain a sitting position for at least 5 minutes. The primary question addressed in this study was whether immobile MCS patients had a more favourable survival rate than patients in VS. The authors found little difference in survival time between the two groups suggesting that mobility is a better predictor of survival than the presence of consciousness. The percentage of patients in mobile MCS surviving for 8 years was 81% as compared to 65% and 63% for immobile MCS and VS, respectively. Duration of survival was also found to be longer for patients with acquired vs. congenital brain injury and shorter for those dependent upon gastrostomy feeding.

MODELLING THE MCS: NEUROIMAGING STUDIES AND THERAPEUTIC POSSIBILITIES

The diagnostic category of MCS canvasses a wider range of clinical phenotypes and structural pathologies than VS. In view of the recency of nosological criteria, conceptual models must accordingly be seen as tentative. It is anticipated that as additional investigational studies are done this category will become further refined, hopefully based on mechanistic distinctions. Nonetheless, existing data provide evidence that brain function in VS and MCS may be well separated at the extremes if not more generally.

In considering the available data from functional imaging, pathology and observational studies, a model is proposed that frames MCS primarily in terms of instability of the initiation, maintenance and completion of behavioural sets. These critical functions depend on the interaction of brainstem arousal systems and mesencephalic and diencephalic 'gating systems' (see below) with other cerebral structures. Pathological studies and observational data of fluctuations observed in severely brain-injured patients suggest that relatively subtle measurements of brain function may be necessary to identify the underlying mechanisms of failure to organize goal-directed behaviours and communication in MCS. Mechanisms identified in MCS patients with limited structural injuries will likely also apply to understanding problems of cognitive recovery of patients with less severe or moderate disabilities following brain injuries.

CORRELATIONS OF MCS WITH STRUCTURAL PATHOLOGY

Comprehensive studies of specific anatomic pathologies associated with MCS are unavailable. Autopsy studies of patients with severe disability following brain injuries show wide variations in underlying neuroanatomical substrates. Jennett and colleagues [35] reported 65 autopsies of patients with TBI leading either to a VS or severe disability. This study included 12 patients with histories consistent with MCS at the time of death. Over half of the severely disabled group demonstrated only focal brain injures, without diffuse axonal injury (DAI) or focal thalamic infarction (including 2 of the MCS patients). Structural brain imaging studies also demonstrate that the behavioural level ultimately achieved by a patient following severe brain injuries often cannot be simply graded by the degree of vascular, DAI, and direct ischaemic brain damage. Kampfl *et al.* [36] described indirect volumetric magnetic resonance imaging (MRI) indices that provide reasonable predictive accuracy (~84%), when combined with time in VS, for a permanently vegetative outcome of overwhelming traumatic brain injuries. Unfortunately, many patients fulfilling these criteria can recover after long intervals. In our own ongoing studies we have identified one MCS patient with a structural injury pattern on MRI fulfilling all of the Kampfl *et al.*

criteria who emerged at 8 months and is now near an independent functional level (unpublished observations). Danielsen *et al.* [37] report detailed MRI and magnetic resonance spectroscopy (^{1}H-MRS) findings from a patient with severe DAI measured over several timepoints while the patient remained in coma for 3 months and 21 months later when the patient had slowly recovered to a near independent level. In this patient ^{1}H-MRS revealed characteristic regional reductions of NAA (N-acetyl aspartate)/choline ratios associated with severe DAI that normalized by the study done at 21 months and correlated with cognitive recovery. McMillan and Herbert [38] recently reported a 10-year follow-up on an MCS patient who continued to recover 7–10 years following a TBI to a point of regaining the capacity to initiate conversation, express clear preferences and spontaneous humour. These observations suggest that some slow variables of recovery may exist and should be quantified through further structural imaging and longitudinal analysis of brain dynamics (see below).

Attempts to correlate outcome with structural injuries are further complicated by the potentially disproportionate impact of certain focal injury patterns. It is well known that enduring global DOC can result from relatively discrete injuries concentrated in the paramedian mesencephalon and thalamus [39]. The structures involved in these lesions include the thalamic intralaminar nuclei (ILN) and the mesencephalic reticular formation (MRF), which together with their connections to the thalamic reticular nucleus appear to play a key role linking arousal states to the control of moment-to-moment intention or attentional gating [40–52]. These structures can be considered 'gating' systems that control interactions of the cerebral cortex, basal ganglia and thalamus through their patterns of innervation within the cortex as well as rich innervation from the brainstem arousal systems [39, 53, 54]. Patients who recover from bilateral paramedian thalamic injuries typically demonstrate persistent instability of arousal level and within-state fluctuations of the selective gating of different cognitive functions [55–57]. Thus, even incomplete injuries to the gating systems may produce unique deficits in maintaining adequate cerebral activation and patterns of brain dynamics necessary to establish, maintain and complete behavioural set formation ([34]; see discussion below).

Enduring VS or MCS produced by such focal injuries will typically include bilateral damage to the MRF extending bilaterally into the intralaminar thalamic nuclei [58, 59]. However, en passant damage to the thalami and upper brainstem commonly follows both TBI and stroke as result of the selective vulnerability of this region to the effects of diffuse brain swelling that leads to herniation of these midline structures through the base of the skull (see [60]). It is likely that most patients who recover from severe brain injuries may represent mixed outcomes resulting from intermediate pathologies that combine moderately diffuse injuries with limited focal damage to paramedian structures [35, 61]. Pathophysiological mechanisms arising in the setting of such mixed pathologies have not been the subject of systematic study. It is known, however, that damage to the paramedian brainstem worsens prognosis following TBI and is associated with MCS and other poor outcomes [62].

In aggregate, clinical and pathological findings suggest significant variability in both the underlying mechanisms of cognitive disabilities and residual brain function accompanying severe brain injuries associated with MCS and other outcomes. It appears that severe disabilities may arise under at least two different conditions: (1) extensive, relatively uniform DAI or hypoxic–ischaemic damage and (2) focal cerebral injuries combined with minimal diffuse axonal or ischaemic damage with possible coexisting functional alteration of subcortical gating systems and their interaction with cortical association areas.

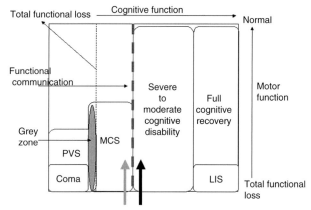

FIGURE 14.2   Conceptual scheme for global DOC. PVS: persistent vegetative state; MCS: minimally conscious state; LIS: locked-in state. Green and blue arrows indicate functional levels just below and above emergence from MCS. *Source*: Adapted from [75].

FUNCTIONAL BRAIN IMAGING IN MCS

Recent functional imaging studies have examined patients using the Aspen criteria for MCS [8]. Boly *et al.* [63] studied five MCS patients using the same functional positron emission tomography (fPET) auditory stimulation paradigm applied by [64] to study vegetative patients. In their studies, MCS patients and healthy controls both showed activation of auditory association regions in the superior temporal gyrus that did not activate in the persistent vegetative state (PVS) patients and strong correlation of the auditory cortical responses with frontal cortical regions providing evidence for preservation of cerebral processing associated with higher-order integrative function. The majority of the MCS patients were scanned approximately 1 month after initial injury and at time that electroencephalography (EEG) examinations revealed significant bilateral abnormalities

(mostly slowing in the theta and delta range). Boly *et al.* [63] have also identified a normal pain network response to somatosensory stimulation in their MCS patients.

Menon *et al.* [65] described selective cortical activation patterns using a ^{15}O-PET subtraction paradigm in a 26-year-old woman described as in a PVS 4 months following an attack of acute disseminated encephalomyelitis. The patient later improved to an MCS level by 6 months; emergence from MCS occurred sometime after 8 months and the patient eventually made a full cognitive recovery [66]. Imaging studies done during the PVS period demonstrated selective activations of right occipital–temporal regions. This pattern of activity was interpreted as indicating a recovery of minimal awareness without behavioural manifestation. Such an interpretation is limited by the lack of any evidence of behavioural response from the patient. It is generally agreed that the present state of imaging technologies cannot provide alternative markers of awareness [67–69]. The findings of Menon *et al.* [65] contrast with those of [64, 70] and suggest that ultimately neuroimaging studies may be able to elucidate underlying differences between PVS and MCS patients. Bekinschtein *et al.* [71] recently reported brain activations obtained using functional magnetic resonance imaging (fMRI) in an MCS patient recovering from TBI. A subtraction comparison of responses to presentations of the patient's mother's voice and a neutral control voice revealed selective activation of the amygdala and insular cortex suggesting emotional processing associated with the mother's voice. As in the interpretation of responses in VS, in patients without the ability to communicate we can only speculate about whether such activations indicate awareness.

We studied two MCS patients near the border of emergence more than 18 months after injury (green arrow in Figure 14.2) using fMRI, fluorodeoxyglucose-positron emission tomography (FDG-PET) and quantitative EEG [72, 73]. The patients and 7 control subjects were studied with fMRI language activation paradigms similar to paradigms used in normal subjects and neurosurgical candidates to map language networks [74]. Two 40 second narratives were prerecorded by a familiar relative and presented as normal speech and also played time reversed. Forward presentations generated robust activity in several language-related areas in both patients. Figure 14.3 shows cortical activity maps associated with the presentation of linguistic stimuli in a single patient. While wide network activation occurred with the forward presentations, time-reversed narratives only activated early sensory cortices in the left hemisphere. This pattern

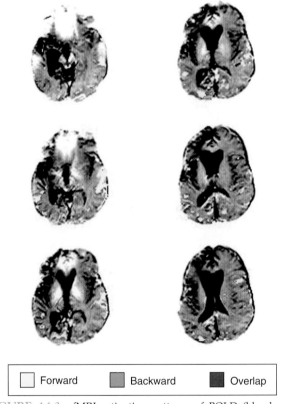

| ☐ Forward | ▨ Backward | ■ Overlap |

FIGURE 14.3 fMRI activation patterns of BOLD (blood oxygenation level dependent) signal in response to passive language presentations (see text for further details). *Source*: Reproduced with permission from MIT Press.

differs from that of normal subjects, where large activations for both stimulus types were observed, with time-reversed language presentation showing slightly more activation than forward presentations. These preliminary fMRI results have now been confirmed in further studies of MCS patients (unpublished data). The findings indicate that some MCS patients may retain large-scale cortical networks that underlie language comprehension and expression despite their inability to execute motor commands or communicate reliably.

In both patients studied we correlated fMRI findings with FDG-PET and quantitative EEG measurements. The patients demonstrated low global resting metabolic rates with significant differences in hemispheric resting metabolic rates and baseline thalamic activity. EEG studies in both patients reveal significant reductions in inter-regional coherence of the more damaged hemisphere in wakefulness [73]. In one patient this inter-regional coherence pattern showed a marked dependence on arousal state with coherence decreases observed across frequencies only in the state of wakefulness. The abnormalities of EEG coherence measures indicate a significant alteration of the functional integration of cortical regions in the more damaged hemisphere. This is all the more striking in that the EEG power spectrum showed no differences in the distribution of power across frequencies for both hemispheres in the two patients. Traditional EEG and MRI evaluations are known to be insensitive to detection of mild and moderate disabilities following brain injuries and to be poor predictors of gradation of severe TBI [76]. The observation of marked coherence abnormalities is consistent with experimental studies that indicate that coherence measures can provide a more direct reflection of behaviourally relevant dynamics than changes in the power spectrum (cf. [77]).

BRAIN DYNAMICS UNDERLYING BEHAVIOURAL FLUCTUATIONS IN MCS

It is notable that the low level of behavioural responses represented by MCS can be associated in some patients with intact large-scale network responses as observed in normal human subjects (shown in Figure 14.4). These observations lead naturally to the question of how to model the coexistence of recruitable large-scale networks and severely

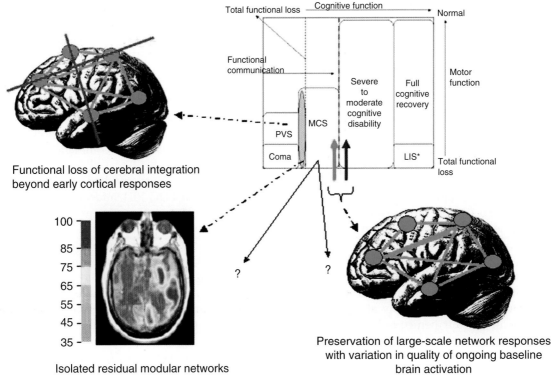

FIGURE 14.4   Mechanism underlying functional level across spectrum of VS and MCS patients. Co-registered FDG-PET and MRI image from patient in Figure 14.2 with colour scale indicating percentage of normal regional metabolic rates (from Schiff [59]; see text for further discussion).

limited behavioural repertoires? A systematic approach to this question is likely to require both consideration of normal mechanisms studied in cognitive neuroscience and a variety of clinical neurological disorders. As noted above, correlations of structural injuries and functional outcomes are not as strong as naïve assumptions would suggest, as widely differing structural pathologies may correlate with the same poor functional level. Moreover, functional measurements offer only snapshots of brain function in time. Baseline metabolic assessments or functional activation studies cannot adequately identify the frequency of the resting brain state sampled or likelihood of response at the time the measurements are taken. In patients with widely varying responsiveness these limitations present an important methodological concern and emphasize the need for more careful consideration of ongoing brain dynamics. What kinds of dynamical measures are needed? At least two different kinds of measurements suggest themselves. Dynamical structures arising in the EEG that correlate with elementary cognitive functions underlying behavioural set formation may quantify fluctuating responsiveness in MCS.

Alongside these measurements there is also a need to develop more sensitive diagnostics that can identify dynamical signatures of several abnormal processes that may arise in the setting of severe brain injuries and limit recovery.

Beginning with the observations above that, the shape of the spectrum of the EEG can be relatively normal in MCS patients, it is reasonable to next consider the fine correlation structure of the EEG as a potential indicator of mechanisms. In our preliminary studies discussed above, hemispheric coherence abnormalities have been identified [73] but such observations are only starting points for more detailed consideration of markers of cognition. The background activity of ongoing EEG during different arousal states can be precisely described as shifts in spectral content of the activity of distributed forebrain networks [78]. Combined studies of intralaminar thalamic neurons and EEG power spectra show that these neurons in concert with the brainstem arousal systems support the shift away from low frequencies characteristic of sleep to a mixed state including increased synchronized high frequency activity in natural awake attentive states [79, 80]. A recent theoretical model of the EEG demonstrates that most of the features of the shape of the EEG spectrum as it evolves across wakefulness and sleep stages can be captured in a partial differential equation system constructed from physiologically realistic parameters and the connectivity of only three major neuronal populations: thalamic relay and reticular neurons and cortical pyramidal neurons [81]. This architecture is consistent with experimentally based models of EEG generation. Simply recovering the shape of the EEG spectrum may therefore only indicate that an essential substrate of thalamocortical connectivity remains to produce this signal – not that the brain has re-established organized activity across widely distributed networks correlated with goal-directed behaviour and cognition.

Importantly, the long lasting changes of ongoing EEG background activity and thalamic firing patterns associated with the arousal state of wakefulness are episodically shaped at a finer temporal scale by brief phasic modulations of the rhythms that organize behavioural set formation. The aggregate abnormalities of resting coherence spectra observed in our two MCS patients likely reflect loss of this fine structure within their resting wakeful EEG. In wakeful states, quantitative EEG studies in normal subjects and experimental studies suggest several potential surrogate markers of elementary cognitive processes underlying the formation of behavioural sets. Among such measures that may prove relevant are regional excitation of high frequencies seen in primate cortical recordings in the 30–80 Hz range associated with working memory and attention [82, 83]. Similar patterns of frequency-specific, event-related synchronization and desynchronization events are identified in the human EEG [84] and in the dynamical structure associated with the contingent negative variation (CNV), a measure of expectancy generated by paramedian thalamic structures and medial frontal cortices in response to a warning cue CNV (cf. [85, 86]).

Although most studies of the correlation structure of the EEG examine dynamic patterns elicited by specific goal-directed tasks, such activations may only reflect half of the necessary fine structure typically present in a normal subject (and therefore possibly required for emergence from MCS). Raichle and colleagues have proposed that the very high resting metabolic rates in the normal human brain reflect 'default self-monitoring' activity that characterizes the conscious goal-directed brain [87, 88]. This

baseline activity is identified by specific patterns of reduction of brain oxygen extraction fraction (OEF) measured at rest across brain regions in a wide variety of goal-directed tasks. Maximum reductions in OEF arise in midline regions of the posterior medial parietal cortex (posterior cingulate cortex and precuneus) and mesial prefrontal cortex. The baseline mode is proposed to depend on tonically active processing in these areas and to correlate with the overall metabolic demands of resting wakeful states. The very low overall resting cerebral metabolic rates in MCS patients may reflect a severe deficit of such tonically active processes. The dissociation of low resting cerebral metabolism despite recruitable networks raises the possibility that patients who remain near the border of emergence from MCS are characterized by a loss of ongoing self-monitoring with fluctuation of recruitment of these large-scale networks under varying internal conditions of arousal and appearance of environmentally salient stimuli.

In a study including 10 MCS patients, Laureys and colleagues observed relatively increased metabolic activity in these medial posterior parietal regions compared to VS patients. As noted above, this may indicate a partial re-establishing of baseline metabolic activity. It is interesting that although these regions are the most metabolically active regions in the resting human brain, bilateral injuries in these locations are not known to produce global DOC. Focal injuries producing states of globally impaired consciousness and cognition, such as VS, MCS and other forms of severe disability, are typically associated with bilateral injuries of the paramedian mesencephalon and thalamus, medial frontal cortical systems or posterior-lateral temporal–parietal regions [39]. A possible interpretation of this difference, consistent with the proposed functions of these cortical regions, is that the self-monitoring activity thought to drive this high metabolic demand may not be necessary for goal-directed behaviour and awareness *per se*.

In addition to quantifying incompletely or insufficiently established dynamic phenomena associated with normal cognition, a systematic evaluation of abnormal dynamics arising in the severely injured brain will be required in evaluating MCS patients. A large variety of pathophysiological mechanisms producing abnormal dynamics have been catalogued in the context of severe brain injuries. At present few diagnostic efforts are applied to assess the contribution of such mechanisms in patients recovering

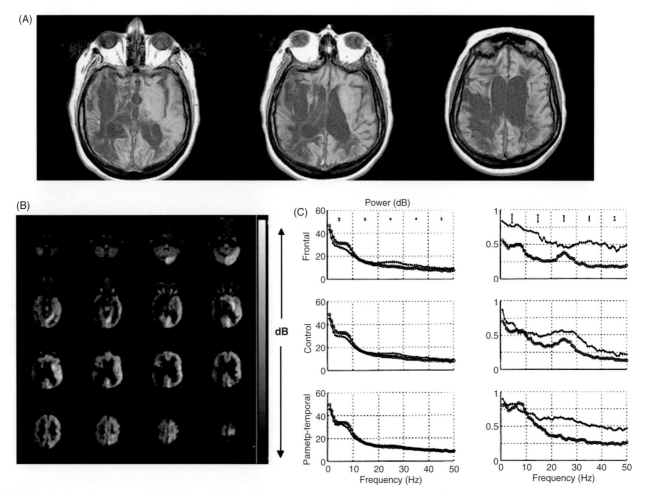

FIGURE 14.5   Figure shows MRI, PET and EEG studies for patient described in text. (A) MRI structural images show severe asymmetric brain damage with loss of right sided basal ganglia and thalamic structures [69]. (B) Positron emission tomography images of resting glucose metabolism across entire cerebrum. Marked asymmetry of right and left hemisphere metabolism is seen. (C) Dissociation of hemispheric variations of coherence measurements and regional power spectrum measurements (from [95]; see text). *Source*: Reproduced with permission from Elsevier Press.

from severe brain injury. A relatively common finding following focal brain injuries is a reduction in cerebral metabolism in brain regions remote from the site of injury [89]. Disproportionately large reductions of neuronal firing rates are associated with modest reduction of cerebral blood flow produced by these crossed-synaptic effects [90]. The cellular basis of this effect appears to be a loss of excitatory drive to neuronal populations that results in a form of inhibition known as disfacilitation in which hyperpolarization of neuronal membrane potentials arises from absence of excitatory synaptic inputs allowing remaining leak currents (principally potassium) to dominate [91]. Disfacilitation may play a large role in changing resting brain activity levels given

recent evidence [92] that cortical neurons may change fundamental firing properties based on levels of depolarization (considered here as a proxy for excitatory drive). Multifocal injuries may therefore result in wide passive inhibition of networks due to loss of background activity. Note that selective structural injuries to the paramedian thalamus are unique in producing hemisphere-wide metabolic reductions presumably through this mechanism [93, 94]. Similarly, herniation injuries may generally produce some level of hemisphere-wide disfacilitation. Thus, the broadband, hemispheric, reductions in EEG coherence observed in the MCS patients discussed above may reflect ongoing functional alteration of common thalamic driving inputs to the cerebral cortex, as opposed to complete structural thalamic injury as seen in Figure 14.5.

In addition to disfacilitation, which may arise on the basis of non-selective injuries across many different cerebral structures, other specific dynamical abnormalities may be associated with severe brain injuries. In some patients selective structural injuries may damage pathways of the brainstem arousal systems where the fibers emanate or run close together. Consequent withdrawal of broad cortical innervation by a neuromodulator could produce significant dynamical effects on the EEG and behaviour. In a small series of VS patients with isolated MRI findings of axonal injuries near the cerebral peduncle (including substantia nigra and ventral tegmental area) and Parkinsonism, the patients made late recoveries following administration of levodopa. The ascending cholinergic pathway also runs in tight bundles at points along its initial trajectory to the cerebral cortex and a role for focal injuries along this pathway has been proposed [96].

Epileptiform or similar hypersynchronous phenomena may arise in severe brain injuries without obvious traditional EEG markers. Williams and Parsons-Smith [97] described local epileptiform activity in the human thalamus that appeared only as surface slow waves in the EEG in a patient with a neurological exam alternating between a state consistent with MCS and interactive communication following an encephalitic injury. A similar mechanism might underlie a case of episodic recovery of communication in a severely disabled patient that intermittently resolved following occasional generalized seizures [98]. Experimental studies have shown increased excitability following even minor brain trauma that may promote epileptiform or other forms of hypersynchronous activity in both cortical and subcortical regions [99]. Other observed phenomena in severe brain injuries that may reflect hypersynchrony include several syndromes with features of dystonia such as oculogyric crises [100, 101], obsessive compulsive disorder [102] and paroxysmal autonomic phenomena (reviewed in [103]). These phenomena typically show selective responses to different pharmacotherapies.

Recently, a fascinating series of cases has been reported in which patients respond paradoxically to sedative medication with arousal responses. Although these cases could reflect epileptiform activity not seen on surface EEG, two studies suggest a different mechanism. Clauss et al. [104] described emergence from MCS in a 28-year-old man with DAI after a stable 3-year period following administration of the gamma-amino butyric acid (GABA) agonist zolpidem which correlated with 35–40% increases in blood flow measured by single photon emission computed tomography (SPECT) in the medial frontal cortex bilaterally and left middle frontal and supramarginal gyri. Brefel-Courbon et al. [105] reported that zolpidem given for nocturnal insomnia to a conscious patient who neither moved nor spoke after hypoxic injury but followed simple commands (possibly MCS) allowed the patient to stand and walk and eat (otherwise fed by gastrostomy), and to repeat single words and sentences, but not to exhibit spontaneous speech. FDG-PET studies showed a marked and reproducible increase in frontal and thalamic metabolism with application of zolpidem. Schiff and Posner [106] have proposed a circuit mechanism to account for these observations suggesting that the striatum may be failing to inhibit tonic pallidal inhibitory outflow to the thalamocortical system as a result of multiple areas of impaired neuronal function in the frontal cortex and basal ganglia. Zolpidem, by directly acting on the neurons in the globus pallidus, which have a high concentration of binding sites for the drug may inhibit the pallidal outflow, thus activating the thalamocortical system. This circuit model suggests mechanisms for dopaminergic agents and N-methyl-D-Aspartate (NMDA) antagonist to improve function in some patients as is occasionally reported.

It is not yet possible to accurately predict the presence and influence of reversible dynamical phenomena that may arise in the setting of novel connective topologies induced by structural brain injuries. However, it may be possible to begin to identify specific dynamical signatures of such state-dependent phenomena using quantitative EEG and MEG (magnetoencephalography) methods. Llinas et al. [107] demonstrated examples of spectral abnormalities in cross-frequency interactions in several different disorders including epilepsy, dystonia and tremor. At present, however, no systematic methods have been developed to screen for these mechanisms. The brief review above suggests that to accurately model recovery from severe brain injuries it will be necessary to attempt to isolate brain dynamics across different structural pathologies and possibly even patterns of resting metabolic activity. Available studies reviewed above indicate that structural pathology and resting metabolism may provide only limited guides to understanding cerebral integrative processes associated with consciousness and cognition in severe brain injury. Given these limitations complementary EEG measures need to be developed to track longitudinal changes in correlation with behavioural patterns and functional imaging.

DIRECTIONS FOR FUTURE RESEARCH

The last 10 years have been witness to important advances in our understanding of DOC. The development of a case definition for MCS, the availability of novel functional neuroimaging strategies, the refinement of neurobehavioural assessment tools and the identification of reliable prognostic indicators of functional recovery represent examples of such achievements. These accomplishments have given rise to many new questions and have helped forge a new research agenda. Some of the key questions that will need to be addressed are listed below:

- *Should we continue to rely on behaviour as the 'gold standard' for evidence of consciousness?* Functional neuroimaging studies suggest that cognitive processing capacity may be underestimated in patients in MCS [65, 108]. This may be related to sensory, motor and drive deficits which may mask signs of consciousness. fMRI and PET (positron emission tomography) studies are expected to clarify the relationship between behavioural signs of consciousness and the integrity of underlying neural networks.
- *What is the natural history of MCS?* Preliminary data suggest that MCS usually represents a transitional state between coma/VS and normal consciousness but may also be a permanent outcome. The natural history of MCS will need to be investigated further so that there is a reference against which the effectiveness of rehabilitative interventions can be measured.
- *What accounts for the fluctuation in cognitive responsiveness that defines MCS?* To solve the fluctuation problem, a multidimensional assessment approach that incorporates electrophysiological recordings (EEG, evoked potentials), structural and functional neuroimaging techniques (MRI, fMRI) and behavioural measures (standardized rating scales, video logs) will be required. The resources required to accomplish this will likely require multicentre collaboration.
- *Is it possible to improve functional outcome following MCS?* At present, there are no proven

treatments for promoting recovery from MCS. There are some promising drug studies although these are comprised by methodological weaknesses [109, 110]. Deep brain stimulation of carefully selected neuromodulatory targets has also been proposed to facilitate cognitive recovery [111]. Clinical trials will require multicentre protocols to assure adequate sample size and sufficient power.

CONCLUSIONS

Until it is possible to precisely map the neural substrate underlying consciousness, its borders will remain arbitrary. At present, diagnostic assessment of DOC must continue to be guided by behavioural criteria that can be assessed at the bedside. Prognostic accuracy and treatment effectiveness rest largely on diagnostic accuracy. The development of a case definition for MCS offers the clinician and researcher a means by which to distinguish those patients who demonstrate some evidence of consciousness from those who never show such signs.

Since the diagnostic criteria for MCS were published, an emerging body of research has begun to show clear differences in pathophysiology, residual cerebral activity and functional outcome between VS and MCS. There is also theoretical and empirical support for the premise that patients in MCS may respond more favourably to treatment interventions than those in VS. Neuroimaging studies have begun to map the pathophysiological substrate underlying MCS offering clues to the development of novel treatment interventions.

ACKNOWLEDGEMENTS

Portions of this article were originally presented at The Satellite Symposium on Coma and Impaired Consciousness, University of Antwerp, Antwerp, Belgium, 24 June 2004. The authors thank Dr Steven Laureys, the Association for the Scientific Study of Consciousness and the Mind Science Foundation for the invitation to speak at this symposium. We also wish to thank Dr Kathleen Kalmar for her boundless support of all aspects of our work concerning assessment and treatment of patients with DOC, Dr Joseph Fins and Andrew Hudson for comments on the manuscript. The support of the National Institute on Disability and Rehabilitation Research, Charles A. Dana Foundation and the NIH-NINDS (NS02172, NS43451) are gratefully acknowledged.

References

1. Jennett, B. and Plum, F. (1972) Persistent vegetative state after brain damage: A syndrome in search of a name. *Lancet* 1:734–737.
2. Multi-Society Task Force Report on PVS (1994) Medical aspects of the persistent vegetative state. *New Engl J Med* 330:1499–1508. 1572–1579.
3. Giacino, J.T. and Whyte, J. (2005) The vegetative state and minimally conscious state: Current knowledge and remaining questions. *J Head Trauma Rehabil* 20 (1):30–50.
4. Giacino, J.T. and Zasler, N.D. (1995) Outcome after severe traumatic brain injury: Coma, the vegetative state, and the minimally responsive state. *J Head Trauma Rehabil* 10 (1):40–56.
5. Giacino, J. and Smart, C. (2007). *Curr Opin Neurol* 20:614–619.
6. American Congress of Rehabilitation Medicine (1995) Recommendations for use of uniform nomenclature pertinent to persons with severe alterations in consciousness. *Arch Phys Med Rehabil* 76:205–209.
7. Giacino, J.T., Zasler, N.D., Katz, D.I., Kelly, J.P., Rosenberg, J.H. and Filley, C.M. (1997) Development of practice guidelines for assessment and management of the vegetative and minimally conscious states. *J Head Trauma Rehabil* 12 (4):79–89.
8. Giacino, J.T., Ashwal, S.A., Childs, N., Cranford, R., Jennett, B., Katz, D.I., Kelly, J., Rosenberg, J., Whyte, J., Zafonte, R.A. and Zasler, N.D. (2002) The minimally conscious state: Definition and diagnostic criteria. *Neurology* 58:349–353.
9. Andrews, K., Murphy, L., Munday, R. and Littlewood, C. (1996) Misdiagnosis of the vegetative state: Retrospective study in a rehabilitation unit. *BMJ* 313:13–16.
10. Childs, N.L., Mercer, W.N. and Childs, H.W. (1993) Accuracy of diagnosis of persistent vegetative state. *Neurol* 43:1465–1467.
11. Tresch, D.D., Sims, F.H., Duthie, E.H., Goldstein, M.D. and Lane, P.S. (1991) Clinical characteristics of patients in the persistent vegetative state. *Arch Internal Med* 151:930–932.
12. Laureys, S., Giacino, J., Schiff, N., Schabus, M. and Owen, A. (2006) How should functional imaging of patients with disorders of consciousness contribute to their clinical rehabilitation needs? *Curr Opin Neurol.* 19:520–557.
13. Giacino, J.T. and Trott, C. (2004) Rehabilitative management of patients with disorders of consciousness: Grand rounds. *J Head Trauma Rehabil* 19 (3):262–273.
14. Taylor, C., Aird, V., Tate, R. and Lammi, M. (2007) Sequence of recovery during the course of emergence from the minimally conscious state. *Arch Phys Med Rehabil* 88:521–525.
15. Teasdale, G. and Jennett, B. (1974) Assessment of coma and impaired consciousness. *Lancet* 2:81–84.
16. Giacino, J.T., Kalmar, K. and Whyte, J. (2004) The JFK Coma Recovery Scale – Revised: measurement characteristics and diagnostic utility. *Arch Phys Med Rehabil* 85:2020–2029.
17. Giacino, J.T., Kezmarsky, M.A., DeLuca, J. and Cicerone, K.D. (1991) Monitoring rate of recovery to predict outcome in minimally responsive patients. *Arch Phys Med Rehabil* 72:897–901.
18. Rappaport, M., Dougherty, A.M. and Kelting, D.L. (1992) Evaluation of coma and vegetative states. *Arch Phys Med Rehabil* 73:628–634.
19. Ansell, B.J. and Keenan, J.E. (1989) The Western Neuro Sensory Stimulation Profile: A tool for assessing slow-to-recover head-injured patients. *Arch Phys Med Rehabil* 70:104–108.
20. Shiel, A., Horn, S.A., Wilson, B.A., Watson, M.J., Campbell, M.J. and McLellan, D.L. (2000) The Wessex Head Injury Matrix (WHIM) main scale: A preliminary report on a scale to assess and monitor patient recovery after severe head injury. *Clin Rehabil* 14 (4):408–416.
21. Wilson, S.L. and Gill-Thwaites, H. (2000) Early indications of emergence from vegetative state derived from assessment with the SMART – a preliminary report. *Brain Injury* 14 (4): 319–331.
22. Wijdicks, E.F.M., Bamlet, W.R., Maramattom, B.V., Manno, E.M. and McLelland, R.L. (2005) Validation of a new coma scale: the FOUR score. *Ann Neurol* 58:585–593.
23. Whyte, J. and DiPasquale, M. (1995) Assessment of vision and visual attention in minimally responsive brain injured patients. *Arch Phys Med Rehabil* 76 (9):804–810.
24. Whyte, J., DiPasquale, M. and Vaccaro, M. (1999) Assessment of command-following in minimally conscious brain injured patients. *Arch Phys Med Rehabil* 80:1–8.
25. McMillan, T.M. (1996) Neuropsychological assessment after extremely severe head injury in a case of life or death. *Brain Injury* 11 (7):483–490. 313.
26. Shiel, A. and Wilson, B. (1998) Assessment after extremely severe head injury in a case of life or death: Further support for McMillan. *Brain Injury* 12 (10):809–816.
27. Giacino, J.T., Sharlow-Galella, M., Kezmarsky, M.A., McKenna, K., Nelson, P., King, M., Cowhey-Brown, A. and Cicerone, K. (1992) *The JFK Coma Recovery Scale and Coma Intervention Program Treatment Procedures Manual.* Edison, NJ: Center for Head Injuries, pp. 1–24.
28. Strauss, D.J., Ashwal, S., Day, S.M. and Shavelle, R.M. (2000) Life expectancy of children in vegetative and minimally conscious states. *Pediatr Neurol* 23 (4):1–8.
29. Giacino, J.T. and Kalmar, K. (1997) The vegetative and minimally conscious states: A comparison of clinical features and functional outcome. *J Head Trauma Rehabil* 12 (4):36–51.
30. Whyte, J., Katz, D., DiPasquale, M.C., Polansky, M., Kalmar, K., Childs, N., Mercer, W., Novak, P. and Eifert, B. (2005) Predictors of outcome and effect of psychoactive medications in prolonged posttraumatic disorders of consciousness: A multicenter center. *Arch Phys Med Rehabil* 86:453–462.
31. Rappaport, M., Hall, K.M., Hopkins, K., Belleza, T. and Cope, D.N. (1982) Disability Rating Scale for severe head trauma: Coma to community. *Arch Phys Med Rehabil* 63:118–123.
32. Lammi, M.H., Smith, V.H., Tate, R.L. and Taylor, C.M. (2005) The minimally conscious state and recovery potential: A follow-up study 2 to 5 years after traumatic brain injury. *Arch Phys Med Rehabil* 86:746–754.
33. Eilander, H.L., Wijnen, V.J.M., Scheirs, J.G.M., De Kort, P.L.M. and Prevo, A.J.H. (2005) Children and young adults in a prolonged unconscious state due to severe brain injury: Outcome after an early intensive neurorehabilitation program. *Brain Injury* 19 (6):425–436.
34. Voss, H.U., Aziz, M.U., Dyke, J.P., Watts, R., Kobylarz, E., McCandliss, B.D., Heier, L.A., Beattie, B.J., Hamacher, K.A., Vallabhajosula, S., Goldsmith, S.J., Ballon, D., Giacino, J.T. and Schiff, N.D. (2006) Possible axonal regrowth in late recovery from the minimally conscious state. *J Clin Invest* 116 (7):2005–2011.
35. Jennett, B., Adams, J.H., Murray, L.S. and Graham, D.I. (2001) Neuropathology in vegetative and severely disabled patients after head injury. *Neurology* 56:486–489.

36. Kampfl, A., Schmutzhard, E., Franz, G., Pfausler, B., Haring, H.P., Ullmer, H., Felber, F., Golaszewski, S. and Aichner, F. (1998) Prediction of recovery from post-traumatic vegetative state with cerebral magnetic-resonance imaging. *Lancet* 351:1763–1767.

37. Danielsen, E.R., Christensen, P.B., Arlien-Soborg, P. and Thomsen, C. (2003) Axonal recovery after severe traumatic brain injury demonstrated *in vivo* by 1H MR spectroscopy. *Neuroradiology* 45 (10):722–724.

38. McMillan, T.M. and Herbert, C.M. (2004) Further recovery in a potential treatment withdrawal case 10 years after brain injury. *Brain Injury* 18 (9):935–940.

39. Schiff, N.D. and Plum, F. (2000) The role of arousal and 'gating' systems in the neurology of impaired consciousness. *J Clin Neurophysiol* 17:438–452.

40. Jones, E.G. (2001) The thalamic matrix and thalamocortical synchrony. *Trends Neurosci* 24:595–601.

41. Kinomura, S., Larssen, J., Gulyas, B. and Roland, P.E. (1996) Activation by attention of the human reticular formation and thalamic intralaminar nuclei. *Science* 271:512–515.

42. Llinas, R., Ribary, U., Joliot, M. and Wang, X.J. (1994) Content and context in temporal thalamocortical binding. In Buzsaki, G. *et al.* (eds.) *Temporal Coding in the Brain*, Heidelberg: Springer-Verlag. pp. 252–272.

43. Llinas, R.R., Leznik, E. and Urbano, F.J. (2002) Temporal binding via cortical coincidence detection of specific and nonspecific thalamocortical inputs: A voltage-dependent dye-imaging study in mouse brain slices. *Proc Natl Acad Sci* 99:449–454.

44. Matsumoto, N., Minamimoto, T., Graybiel, A.M. and Kimura, M. (2001) Neurons in the thalamic CM-Pf complex supply striatal neurons with information about behaviorally significant sensory events. *J. Neurophysiol.* 85:960–976.

45. Minamimoto, T. and Kimura, M. (2002) Participation of the thalamic CM-Pf complex in attentional orienting. *J Neurophysiol* 87:3090–3101.

46. Paus, T., Zatorre, R., Hofle, N., Caramanos, Z., Gotman, J., Petrides, M. and Evans, A. (1997) Time-related changes in neural systems underlying attention and arousal during the performance of an auditory vigilance task. *J Cogn Neurosci* 9:392–408.

47. Purpura, K.P. and Schiff, N.D. (1997) The thalamic intralaminar nuclei: role in visual awareness. *Neuroscientist* 3:8–14.

48. Schiff, N.D. and Purpura, K.P. (2002) Towards a neurophysiological basis for cognitive neuromodulation through deep brain stimulation. *Thalamus Relat Syst* 2 (1):51–69.

49. Schlag-Rey, M. and Schlag, J. (1984) Visuomotor functions of central thalamus in monkey. I. Unit activity related to spontaneous eye movements. *J Neurophysiol* 40:1149–1174.

50. Steriade, M. (1997) Thalamic substrates of disturbances in states of vigilance and consciousness in humans. In Steriade, M., Jones, E. and McCormic, D. (eds.) *Thalames*, Oxford, UK: Elsevier Publishers.

51. Wyder, M.T., Massoglia, D.P. and Stanford, T.R. (2003) Quantitative assessment of the timing and tuning of visual-related, saccade-related, and delay period activity in primate central thalamus. *J Neurophysiol* 90 (3):2029–2052.

52. Wyder, M.T., Massoglia, D.P. and Stanford, T.R. (2004) Contextual modulation of central thalamic delay-period activity: Representation of visual and saccadic goals. *J Neurophysiol* 91 (6):2628–2648.

53. Groenewegen, H. and Berendse, H. (1994) The specificity of the 'nonspecific' midline and intralaminar thalamic nuclei. *Trends Neurosci* 17:52–66.

54. Van Der Werf, Y.D., Witter, M.P. and Groenewegen, H.J. (2002) The intralaminar and midline nuclei of the thalamus. Anatomical and functional evidence for participation in processes of arousal and awareness. *Brain Res Rev* 39 (2–3):107–140.

55. Meissner, I., Sapir, S., Kokmen, E. and Stein, S.D. (1987) The paramedian diencephalic syndrome: A dynamic phenomenon. *Stroke* 18 (2):380–385.

56. Van Der Werf, Y.D., Weerts, J.G., Jolles, J., Witter, M.P., Lindeboom, J. and Scheltens, P. (1999) Neuropsychological correlates of a right unilateral lacunar thalamic infarction. *J Neurol Neurosurg Psychiatr* 66 (1):36–42.

57. Mennemeier, M., Crosson, B., Williamson, D.J., Nadeau, S.E., Fennell, E., Valenstein, E. and Heilman, K.M. (1997) Tapping, talking and the thalamus: possible influence of the intralaminar nuclei on basal ganglia function. *Neuropsychologia* 35 (2):183–193.

58. Plum, F. (1991) Coma and related global disturbances of the human conscious state. In Jones, E. and Peters, P. (eds.) *Cerebral Cortex*, Vol. 9:. New York: Plenum Press.

59. Schiff, N., Ribary, U., Moreno, D., Beattie, B., Kronberg, E., Blasberg, R., Giacino, J., McCagg, C., Fins, J.J., Llinas, R. and Plum, F. (2002) Residual cerebral activity and behavioral fragments in the persistent vegetative state. *Brain* 125:1210–1234.

60. Plum, F. and Posner, J. (1982) The pathologic physiology of signs and symptoms of coma. *The Diagnosis of Stupor and Coma*, 3rd Edition. Philadelphia, PA: FA Davis.

61. Adams, J.H., Graham, D.I. and Jennett, B. (2001) The structural basis of moderate disability after traumatic brain damage. *J Neurol Neurosurg Psychiatr* 71:521–524.

62. Wedekind, C., Hesselmann, V., Lippert-Gruner, M. and Ebel, M. (2002) Trauma to the pontomesencephalic brainstem – a major clue to the prognosis of severe traumatic brain injury. *Br J Neurosurg* 16:256–260.

63. Boly, M., Faymonville, M.E., Peigneux, P., Lambermont, B., Damas, P., Del Fiore, G., Degueldre, C., Franck, G., Luxen, A., Lamy, M., Moonen, G., Maquet, P. and Laureys, S. (2004) Auditory processing in severely brain injured patients: Differences between the minimally conscious state and the persistent vegetative state. *Arch Neurol* 61:233–238.

64. Laureys, S., Faymonville, M.E., Degueldre, C., Del Fiore, G., Damas, P., Lambermont, B., Jannsens, N., Aerts, J., Franck, G., Luxen, A., Moonen, G., Lamy, M. and Maquet, P. (2000) Auditory processing in the vegetative state. *Brain* 123:1589–1681.

65. Menon, D.K., Owen, A.M., Williams, E.J., Minhas, P.S., Allen, C.M.C., Boniface, S.J. and Pickard, J.D. (1998) Wolfson Brain Imaging Centre Team. Cortical processing in persistent vegetative state. *Lancet* 352:1148–1149.

66. Macniven, J.A., Poz, R., Bainbridge, K., Gracey, F. and Wilson, B.A. (2003) Emotional adjustment following cognitive recovery from 'persistent vegetative state': Psychological and personal perspectives. *Brain Injury* 17 (6):525–533.

67. Menon, D.K., Owen, A.M. and Pickard, J.D. (1999) Response from Menon, Owen and Pickard. *Trends Cogn Sci* 3 (2):44–46.

68. Schiff, N.D. and Plum, F. (1999) Cortical processing in the vegetative state. *Trends Cogn Sci* 3 (2):43–44.

69. Schiff, N.D., Ribary, U., Plum, F. and Llinas, R. (1999) Words without mind. *J Cogn Neurosci* 11 (6):650–656.

70. Laureys, S., Faymonville, M.E., Peigneux, P., Damas, P., Lambermont, B., Del Fiore, G., Degueldre, C., Aerts, J., Luxen, A., Franck, G., Lamy, M., Moonen, G. and Maquet, P. (2002) Cortical processing of noxious somatosensory stimuli in the persistent vegetative state. *Neuroimage* 17 (2):732–741.

71. Bekinschtein, T., Leiguarda, R., Armony, J., Owen, A., Carpintiero, S., Niklison, J., Olmos, L., Sigman, L. and Manes, F.J.

(2004) Emotion processing in the minimally conscious state. *J Neurol Neurosurg Psychiatr* 75 (5):788.

72. Schiff, N., Rodriguez-Moreno, D., Kamal, A., Petrovich, N., Giacino, J., Plum, F. and Hirsch, J. (2005) fMRI reveals intact large-scale networks in two minimally conscious patients. *Neurology* 64:514–523.

73. Kobylarz, E., Kamal, A. and Schiff, N.D. (2003) Power spectrum and coherence analysis of the EEG from two minimally conscious patients with severe asymmetric brain damage. ASSC Meeting.

74. Hirsch, J., Ruge, M.I., Kim, K.H., Correa, D.D., Victor, J.D., Relkin, N.R., Labar, D.R., Krol, G., Bilsky, M.H., Souweidane, M.M., DeAngelis, L.M. and Gutin, P.H. (2000) An integrated functional magnetic resonance imaging procedure for preoperative mapping of cortical areas associated with tactile, motor, language, and visual functions. *Neurosurgery* 47 (3):711–721.

75. Schiff, N.D. (2004) The neurology of impaired consciousness: Challenges for cognitive neuroscience. In Gazzaniga, M.S. (eds.) *The Cognitive Neurosciences,* 3rd Edition, Cambridge, Mass: MIT Press.

76. Thatcher, R.W., North, D.M., Curtin, R.T., Walker, R.A., Biver, C.J., Gomez, J.F. and Salazar, A.M. (2001) An EEG severity index of traumatic brain injury. *Neuropsychiatr Clin Neurosci* 13 (1):77–87.

77. Vaadia, E., Haalman, I., Abeles, M., Bergman, H., Prut, Y., Slovin, H. and Aertsen, A. (1995) Dynamics of neuronal interactions in monkey cortex in relation to behavioural events. *Nature* 373 (6514):515–518.

78. Steriade, M. (2000) Corticothalamic resonance, states of vigilance and mentation. *Neuroscience* 101:243–276.

79. Steriade, M. and Glenn, L.L. (1982) Neocortical and caudate projections of intralaminar thalamic neurons and their synaptic excitation from midbrain reticular core. *J Neurophysiol* 48:352–371.

80. Steriade, M., Contreras, D., Amzica, F. and Timofeev, I. (1996) Synchronization of fast (30–40Hz) spontaneous oscillations in intrathalamic and thalamocortical networks. *J Neurosci* 16:2788–2808.

81. Robinson, P.A., Rennie, C.J. and Rowe, D.L. (2002) Dynamics of large-scale brain activity in normal arousal states and epileptic seizures. *Phys Rev E Stat Nonlinear Soft Matter Phys* 65 (4):041924.

82. Pesaran, B., Pezaris, J.S., Sahani, M., Mitra, P.P. and Andersen, R. A. (2002) Temporal structure in neuronal activity during working memory in macaque parietal cortex. *Nat Neurosci* 5:805–811.

83 Fries, P., Reynolds, J.H., Rorie, A.E. and Desimone, R. (2001 Feb 23) Modulation of oscillatory neuronal synchronization by selective visual attention. *Science* 291 (5508):1560–1563.

84 Pfurtscheller, G. and Lopes da Silva, F.H. (1999) Event-related EEG/MEG synchronization and desynchronization: basic principles. *Clin Neurophysiol* 110 (11):1842–1857.

85. Nagai, Y., Critchley, H.D., Featherstone, E., Fenwick, P.B.C., Trimble, M.R. and Dolan, R.J. (2004) Brain activity relating to the contingent negative variation: An fMRI investigation. *NeuroImage* 21 (4):1232–1241.

86. Slobounov, S.M., Fukada, K., Simon, R., Rearick, M. and Ray, W. (2000) Neurophysiological and behavioral indices of time pressure effects on visuomotor task performance. *Cogn Brain Res* 9:287–298.

87. Raichle, M.E., MacLeod, A.M., Snyder, A.Z., Powers, W.J., Gusnard, D.A. and Shulman, G.L. (2001) A default mode of brain function. *Proc Natl Acad Sci* 98 (2):676–682.

88. Gusnard, D.A., Raichle, M.E. and Raichle, M.E. (2001) Searching for a baseline: Functional imaging and the resting human brain. *Nat Rev Neurosci* 2 (10):685–694.

89. Nguyen, D.K. and Botez, M.I. (1998) Diaschisis and neurobehavior. *Can J Neurol Sci* 25:5–12.

90. Gold, L. and Lauritzen, M. (2002) Neuronal deactivation explains decreased cerebellar blood flow in response to focal cerebral ischemia or suppressed neocortical function. *Proc Natl Acad Sci* 99 (7):699–704.

91. Timofeev, I., Grenier, F. and Steriade, M. (2001) Disfacilitation and active inhibition in the neocortex during the natural sleep–wake cycle: An intracellular study. *Proc Natl Acad Sci* 98:1924–1929.

92. Steriade, M. (2004) Neocortical cell classes are flexible entities. *Nat Rev Neurosci* 5 (2):121–134.

93. Szelies, B., et al. (1991) Widespread functional effects of discrete thalamic infarction. Arch Neurol 48:178–182.

94. Caselli, R.J., Graff-Radford, N.R. and Rezai, K. (1991) Thalamocortical diaschisis: Single-photon emission tomographic study of cortical blood flow changes after focal thalamic infarction. *Neuropsychiatr Neuropsychol Behav Neurol* 4:193–214.

95. Davey, M.P., Victor, J.D. and Schiff, N.D. (2000) Power spectra and coherence in the EEG of a vegetative patient with severe asymmetric brain damage. *Clin Neurophysiol* 111 (11):1949–1954.

96. Selden, N.R., Gitelman, D.R., Salamon-Murayama, N., Parrish, T.B. and Mesulam, M.M. (1998) Trajectories of cholinergic pathways within the cerebral hemispheres of the human brain. *Brain* 121:2249–2257.

97. Williams, D. and Parsons-Smith, G. (1951) Thalamic activity in stupor. *Brain* 74:377–398.

98. Burrus, j., Chacko Burruss, J.W. and Chacko, R.C. (1999) Episodically remitting akinetic mutism following subarachnoid hemorrhage. *J Neuropsychiatry Clin. Neurosci.* 11:100–102.

99. Santhakumar, V., Ratzliff, A.D., Jeng, J., Toth, Z. and Soltesz, I. (2001) Long-term hyperexcitability in the hippocampus after experimental head trauma. *Ann Neurol* 50:708–717.

100. Leigh, R.J., Foley, J.M., Remler, B.F. and Civil, R.H. (1987) Oculogyric crisis: A syndrome of thought disorder and ocular deviation. *Ann Neurol* 22:13–17.

101. Kakigi, R., Shibasaki, H., Katafuchi, Y., Iyatomi, I. and Kuroda, Y. (1986) The syndrome of bilateral paramedian thalamic infarction associated with an oculogyric crisis. *Rinsho Shinkeigaku* 26:1100–1105.

102. Berthier, M.L., Kulisevsky, J.J., Gironell, A. and Lopez, O.L. (2001) Obsessive compulsive disorder and traumatic brain injury: Behavioral, cognitive, and neuroimaging findings. *Neuropsychiatr Neuropsychol Behav Neurol* 14:23–31.

103. Blackman, J.A., Patrick, P.D., Buck, M.L. and Rust, R.S. Jr. (2004) Paroxysmal autonomic instability with dystonia after brain injury. *Arch Neurol* 61 (3):321–328.

104. Clauss, R.P., van der Merwe, C.E. and Nel, H.W. (2001) Arousal from a semi-comatose state on zolpidem. *S Afr Med J* 91 (10):788–789.

105. Brefel-Courbon, C., et al. (2007) Clinical and imaging evidence of zolpidem effect in hypoxic encephalopathy. *Ann Neurol.* 62 (1):102–105.

106. Schiff, N.D. and Posner, J.P. (2007) Another "Awakenings". *Annals of Neurology* 62:5–7.

107. Llinas, R.R., Ribary, U., Jeanmonod, D., Kronberg, E. and Mitra, P.P. (1999) Thalamocortical dysrhythmia: A neuro-logical and neuropsychiatric syndrome characterized by magnetoencephalography. *Proc Natl Acad Sci* 96: 15222–15227.

108. Hirsch, J., Kamal, A., Rodriguez-Moreno, D., Petrovich, N., Giacino, J., Plum, F. and Schiff, N. (2001) fMRI reveals intact cognitive systems in two minimally conscious patients. *Abst Soc Neurosci* 271:1397.

109. Schneider, W.N., Drew-Cates, J., Wong, T.M. and Dombovy, M.L. (1999) Cognitive and behavioural efficacy of amantadine in acute traumatic brain injury: An initial double-blind placebo-controlled study. *Brain Injury* 13:863–872.

110. Meythaler, J.M., Brunner, R.C., Johnson, A. and Novack, T.A. (2002) Amantadine to improve neurorecovery in traumatic brain injury – associated diffuse axonal injury: A pilot double-blind randomized trial. *J Head Trauma Rehabil* 17 (4):300.

111. Schiff, N.D., Rezai, A.R. and Plum, F.P. (2000) A neuromodulation strategy for rational therapy of complex brain injury states. *Neurol Res* 22:267–272.

Consciousness in the Locked-in Syndrome

Olivia Gosseries, Marie-Aurélie Bruno, Audrey Vanhaudenhuyse,
Steven Laureys and Caroline Schnakers

ABSTRACT

Patients in a locked-in syndrome (LIS) are selectively deefferented, that is, have no means of producing speech, limb, or face movements. Usually the anatomy of the responsible lesion in the brainstem is such that locked-in patients are left with the capacity to use vertical eye movements and blinking to communicate their awareness. The syndrome is subdivided as: (a) *classical* LIS is characterized by total immobility except for vertical eye movements or blinking; (b) *incomplete* LIS permits remnants of voluntary motion; and (c) *total* LIS with complete immobility including all eye movements combined with preserved consciousness. Eye-controlled computer-based communication technology currently allows these patients to control their environment, use a word processor coupled to a speech synthesizer and access the worldwide net.

'Thirty years ago a stroke left me in a coma. When I awoke I found myself completely paralyzed and unable to speak… I didn't know what paralysis was until I could move nothing but my eyes. I didn't know what loneliness was until I had to wait all night in the dark, in pain from head to foot, vainly hoping for someone to come with a teardrop of comfort. I didn't know what silence was until the only sound I could make was that of my own breath issuing from a hole drilled into my throat' [1].

DEFINITION

Plum and Posner first introduced the term 'locked-in syndrome' (LIS) in 1966 referring to the constellation of quadriplegia and anarthria brought about by the disruption of the brainstem's corticospinal and corticobulbar pathways, respectively [2]. In the LIS, unlike coma, the vegetative state or akinetic mutism, consciousness remains intact. The patient is locked inside his body, able to perceive his environment but extremely limited to voluntarily interact with it.

The American Congress of Rehabilitation Medicine most recently defined LIS by (i) the presence of sustained eye opening (bilateral ptosis should be ruled out as a complicating factor); (ii) preserved basic cognitive abilities; (iii) aphonia or severe hypophonia; (iv) quadriplegia or quadriparesis; and (v) a primary mode of communication that uses vertical or lateral eye movement or blinking of the upper eyelid [3].

Bauer *et al.* [4] subdivided the syndrome on the basis of the extent of motor and verbal impairment: (a) *classical* LIS is characterized by total immobility except for vertical eye movements or blinking; (b) *incomplete* LIS permits remnants of voluntary motion; and (c) *total* LIS consists of complete immobility including all eye movements combined with preserved consciousness.

AETIOLOGY

LIS is most frequently caused by a bilateral ventral pontine lesion (e.g., [2, 5]) (Figure 15.1). In rarer instances, it can be the result of a mesencephalic lesion (e.g., [4, 6, 7]). The most common aetiology of LIS is vascular pathology, either a basilar artery occlusion or a pontine haemorrhage [8]. Another relatively frequent cause is traumatic brain injury [9–14]. Following trauma, LIS may be caused either directly by brainstem lesions, secondary to vertebral artery damage and vertebrobasilar arterial occlusion, or to compression of the cerebral peduncles from tentorial herniation [13]. It has also been reported secondary to subarachnoid haemorrhage and vascular spasm of the basilar artery, a brainstem tumour, central pontine myelinolysis, encephalitis, pontine abscess, brainstem drug toxicity, vaccine reaction, and prolonged hypoglycemia [8].

A comparable awake conscious state simulating unresponsiveness may also occur in severe cases of peripheral polyneuropathy as a result of total paralysis of limb, bulbar, and ocular musculature. Transient LIS cases have been reported after Guillain-Barré polyradiculoneuropathy [15–17] and severe post-infectious polyneuropathy [18, 19]. Unlike basilar artery stroke,

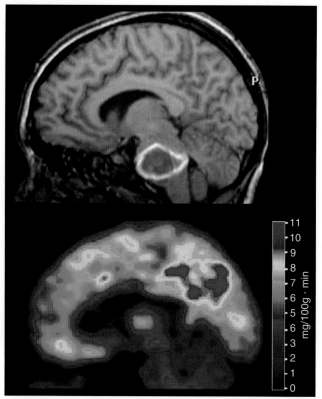

FIGURE 15.1 Upper panel: Magnetic resonance image (sagittal section) showing a massive hemorrhage in the brainstem (circular hyperintensity) causing LIS in a 13-year old girl. Lower panel: ^{18}F-fluorodeoxyglucose-Positron Emission Tomography illustrating intact cerebral metabolism in the acute phase of the LIS when eye-coded communication was difficult due to fluctuating vigilance. The colour scale shows the amount of glucose metabolized per 100 g of brain tissue per minute. Statistical analysis revealed that metabolism in the supra-tentorial gray matter was not significantly lower as compared to healthy controls (taken from Laureys *et al.*, [8]).

vertical eye movements are not selectively spared in these extensive peripheral disconnection syndromes. Another important cause of complete LIS can be observed in end-stage amyotrophic lateral sclerosis, that is, motor neuron disease [20–22]. Finally, temporary pharmacologically induced LIS can sporadically be observed in general anaesthesia when patients receive muscle relaxants together with inadequate amounts of anaesthetic drugs (e.g., [23]). Testimonies from victims relate that the worst aspect of the experience was the anxious desire to move or speak while being unable to do so [24–26]. Awake-paralyzed patients undergoing surgery may develop post-traumatic stress disorder (for recent review, see [27]).

MISDIAGNOSIS

Unless the physician is familiar with the signs and symptoms of the LIS, the diagnosis may be missed

BOX 15.1

FAMOUS LOCKED-IN PATIENTS

The LIS first described in Alexandre Dumas's novel the Count of Monte Cristo (1844–1845) [28]. Herein, Monsieur Noirtier de Villefort, was depicted as 'a corpse with living eyes'. Mr. Noirtier had been in this state for more than 6 years, and he could only communicate by blinking his eyes. His helper pointed at words in a dictionary and the monsignor indicated with his eyes the words he wanted. Some years later, Emile Zola wrote in his novel Thérèse Raquin [29] (1868) about a paralyzed woman who 'was buried alive in a dead body' and 'had language only in her eyes'. Dumas and Zola highlighted the locked-in condition before the medical community did.

For a long time, LIS has mainly been a retrospective diagnosis based on post-mortem findings [5, 30]. Medical technology now can achieve long survival in such cases – the longest history of this condition being 29 years (French ALIS). Computerized devices now allow the LIS patient and other patients with severe motor impairment to 'speak'. The preeminent physicist Stephen Hawking, author of the best-sellers *A Brief History of Time* and *The Universe in a Nutshell*, is able to communicate solely through the use of a computerized voice synthesizer. With one finger, he selects words presented serially on a computer screen; the words are then stored and later presented as a synthesized and coherent message (http://www.hawking.org.uk). The continuing brilliant productivity of Hawking despite his failure to move or speak illustrates that locked-in patients can be productive members of the society.

In December 1995, Jean-Dominique Bauby, aged 43 and editor-in-chief of the fashion magazine 'Elle', had a brainstem stroke. He emerged from a coma several weeks later to find himself in a LIS only able to move his left eyelid and with very little hope of recovery. Bauby wanted to show the world that this pathology, which impedes movement and speech, does not prevent patients from living. He has proven it in an extraordinary book in which he composed each passage mentally and then dictated it, letter by letter, to an amanuensis who painstakingly recited a frequency-ordered alphabet until Bauby chose a letter by blinking his left eyelid once to signify 'yes'. His book [31] *The diving bell and the butterfly* became a best-seller only weeks after his death due to septic shock on March 9, 1997. Bauby created an ALIS aimed to help patients with this condition and their families (http://www.alis-asso.fr).

Since its creation in 1997, ALIS has registered 438 locked-in patients in France (situation in May 2007).

and the patient may erroneously be considered as being in a coma, vegetative state, or akinetic mutism [32]. In a recent survey in 44 LIS patients belonging to the French Association for Locked-in Syndrome (ALIS, see Box 15.1) the first person to realize the patient was conscious and could communicate via eye movements most often was a family member (55% of cases) and not the treating physician (23% of cases) [33]. Most distressingly, the time elapsed between brain insult and LIS diagnosis was on an average of 2.5 months (78 days). Several patients were not diagnosed for more than 4 years. Leon-Carrion *et al.* [33] believed that this delay in the diagnosis of LIS mainly reflected initial misdiagnosis. Clinical experience indeed shows how difficult it is to recognize unambiguous signs of conscious perception of the environment and of the self in severely brain-injured patients. Voluntary eye movements and/or blinking can erroneously be interpreted as reflexive in anarthric and nearly completely paralyzed patients who classically show decerebration posturing (i.e., stereotyped extension reflexes).

However, part of the delay could be explained by an initial lower level neurological state (e.g., decreased or fluctuating arousal levels) or even psychiatric symptoms which would mask residual cognitive functions at the outset of LIS.

SURVIVAL AND MORTALITY

It has been stated that long-term survival in LIS is rare [34]. Mortality is indeed high in acute LIS (76% for vascular cases and 41% for non-vascular cases) with 87% of the deaths occurring in the first 4 months [5]. In 1987, Haig *et al.* first [35] reported on the life expectancy of persons with LIS, showing that individuals can actually survive for significant periods of time. Encompassing 29 patients from a major US rehabilitation hospital who had been in a LIS for more than 1 year they reported formal survival curves at 5-year [36] and 10-year follow-up [37]. These authors have shown that once a patient has medically stabilized in LIS for more than a year, 10-year survival is 83% and 20-year survival is 40% [37].

Data from the ALIS database (*n* = 320) show that survivors are younger at onset than those who die (Figure 15.2). The mean time spent in locked-in is 6 ± 4 years (range 14 days to 29 years, the latter patient still being alive). Reported causes of death for the 42 deceased subjects are predominantly infectious (40%, most frequently pneumonia), primary brainstem stroke (25%), recurrent brainstem stroke (10%), patient's refusal of artificial nutrition and hydration (10%), and other causes (i.e., cardiac arrest, gastrostomy surgery, heart failure, and hepatitis). It should be noted that the ALIS database does not contain the many LIS patients who die in the acute setting without being reported to the association. Recruitment of the ALIS database is based on case reporting by family and health care workers prompted by the exceptional media publicity of ALIS in France and tracked by continuing yearly surveys. This recruitment bias should, however, be taken into account when interpreting the presented data.

PROGNOSIS AND OUTCOME

Classically, the motor recovery of LIS of vascular origin is very limited [5, 37] even if rare cases of good recovery have been reported [38, 39]. Chang and Morariu [40] reported the first transient LIS caused by a traumatic damage of the brainstem. In their milestone paper, Patterson and Grabois [5], reviewed 139 patients – 6 cases from the author's rehabilitation centre in Texas, USA and 133 taken from 71 published studies from 1959 to 1983 and reported earlier and more complete recovery in non-vascular LIS compared to vascular LIS. Return of horizontal pursuit eye movements within 4 weeks post-onset are thought to be predictive of good recovery [6]. Richard *et al.* [41] followed 11 LIS patients for 7 months to 10 years and observed that despite the persisting serious motor deficit, all patients did recover some distal control of fingers and toe movements, often allowing a functional use of a digital switch. The motor improvement occurred with a distal to proximal progression and included a striking axial hypotonia.

LIS is uncommon enough that many clinicians do not know how to approach rehabilitation and there are no existing guidelines as how to organize the revalidation process. Casanova *et al.* [42] recently followed 14 LIS patients in three Italian rehabilitation centres for a period of 5 months to 6 years. They reported that intensive and early rehabilitative care improved functional outcome and reduced mortality rate when compared to the older studies by Patterson and Grabois [5] and Haig *et al.* [35].

Often unknown to physicians caring for LIS in the acute setting and despite the limited motor recovery of LIS patients, many patients can return living at home. The ALIS database shows that out of 245 patients, 108

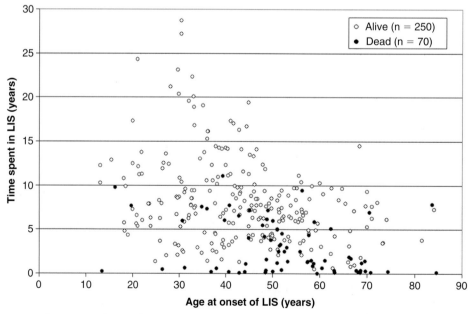

FIGURE 15.2   Age at insult vs. survival time of 320 locked-in patients registered in the ALIS database, 70 of whom died (filled circles).

(44%) are known to live at home (21% are staying in a hospital setting and 17% in a revalidation centre). Patients return home after a mean period of 2±16 years (range 2 months to 6 years, data obtained on $n = 55$). Results obtained in 95 patients show a moderate to significant recovery of head movement in 92% of patients, 65% showed small movement in one of the upper limbs (finger, hand, or arm) and 74% show a small movement in lower limbs (foot or leg). Half of the patients has recovered some speech production (limited to single comprehensible words) and 95% can vocalize unintelligible sounds (data obtained on $n = 50$). Some kind of electrical communication device is used by 81% of the LIS patients (data obtained on $n = 95$) [8].

COMMUNICATION

In order to functionally communicate, it is necessary for the LIS patient to be motivated and to be able to receive (verbally or visually; i.e., written commands) and emit information. The first contact to be made with these patients is through a code using eyelid blinks or vertical eye movements. In cases of bilateral ptosis the eyelids need to be manually opened in order to verify voluntary eye movements on command. To establish a yes/no eye code, the following instruction can suffice: 'yes' is indicated by one blink and 'no' by two or look indicates 'yes' and look down 'no'. In practice, the patient's best eye movement should be chosen and the same eye code should be used by all interlocutors. Such a code will only permit to communicate via closed questions (i.e., yes/no answers on presented questions). The principal aim of reeducation is to reestablish a genuine exchange with the LIS patient by putting into place various codes to permit them to reach a higher level of communication and thus to achieve an active participation. With sufficient practice, it is possible for LIS patients to communicate complex ideas in coded eye movements. Feldman [43] has first described a LIS patient who used jaw and eyelid movements to communicate in Morse Code.

Most frequently used are alphabetical communication systems. The simplest way is to list the alphabet and ask the LIS patient to make a pre-arranged eye movement to indicate a letter. Some patients prefer a listing of the letters sorted in function of appearance rate in usual language (i.e., in the English language: E-T-A-O-I-N-S-R-H-L-D-C-U-M-F-P-G-W-Y-B-V-K-X-J-Q-Z). The interlocutor pronounces the letters beginning with the most frequently used, E, and continues until the patient blinks after hearing the desired letter which the interlocutor then notes. It is necessary to begin over again for each letter to form words and phrases. The rapidity of this system depends upon practice and the ability of patient and interlocutor to work together. The interlocutor may be able to guess at a word or a phrase before all the letters have been pronounced. It is sufficient for him to pronounce the word or the rest of the sentence. The patient than confirms the word by making his eye code for 'yes' or disproves by making his eye code for 'no'. Other systems have been discussed elsewhere [8].

The above discussed communication systems all require assistance from others. Recent developments in informatics are drastically changing the lives of patients with LIS. Instead of passively responding to the requests of others, new communication facilitation devices couplet to computers now allow the patient to initiate conversations [8]. Experts in rehabilitation engineering and speech-language pathology are continuingly improving various brain–computer interfaces (BCI). BCIs (also named thought translation devices) are a mean of communication in which messages or commands that an individual sends to the external world do not pass through the brain's normal output pathways of peripheral nerves and muscles [44]. These patient–computer interfaces such as infrared eye movement sensors which can be coupled to on-screen virtual keyboards allowing the LIS survivor to control his environment, use a word processor (which can be coupled to a text-to-speech synthesizer), operate a telephone of fax, or access the Internet and use e-mail (Figure 15.3; Box 15.2).

Wilhelm et al. [45] have shown that mental manipulation of salivary pH may be an alternative way to document consciousness in acute LIS (see Figure 15.4). Birbaumer et al. [46] reported that chronic near-complete LIS and end-stage amyotrophic lateral sclerosis, patients were able to communicate without any verbal or motor report but solely by modulating their electroencephalographic (EEG). In the future, more widely available access to enhanced communication computer prosthetics should additionally enhance the quality of life of LIS survivors (also see Chapter 17).

RESIDUAL BRAIN FUNCTION

Neuropsychological Testing

Surprisingly, there are no systematic neuropsychological studies of the cognitive functions in patients living with a LIS. Most case reports, however, failed to show any significant cognitive impairment when LIS patients were tested 1 year or more after the brainstem

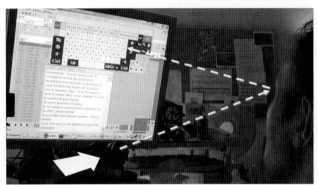

FIGURE 15.3   A locked-in person updates the database of ALIS, moving the cursor on screen by eye movements. An infrared camera (white arrow) mounted below the monitor observes one of the user's eyes, an image processing software continually analyzes the video image of the eye and determines where the user is looking on the screen. The user looks at a virtual keyboard that is displayed on the monitor and uses his eye as a computer-mouse. To 'click' he looks at the key for a specified period of time (typically a fraction of a second) or blinks. An array of menu keys allow the user to control his environment, use a speech synthesizer, browse the worldwide web or send e-mail independently (picture used with kind permission from DT).With a similar device Philippe Vigand, locked-in since 1990, has written a testimony of his LIS experience in an astonishing book 'Putain de silence' translated as 'Only the eyes say yes' [48].

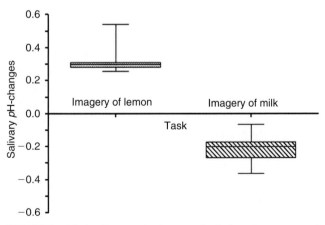

FIGURE 15.4   Communication method based on mental imagery and measurement of salivary pH changes. Imagery of lemon increases salivary pH and is used to communicate 'yes' while imagery of milk decreases pH and communicates 'no'. Result obtained in one healthy volunteer box and whiskers represent mean, SD and minimum/maximum measurements. *Source*: Adapted from Vanhaudenhuyse *et al.* [49].

insult. Allain *et al.* [50] performed extensive neuropsychological testing in two LIS patients studied 2 and 3 years after their basilar artery thrombosis. Patients communicated via a communication PrintWriter system and showed no impairment of language, memory, and intellectual functioning. Cappa *et al.* [51, 52] studied one patient who was LIS for over 12 years and observed intact performances on language, calculation, spatial orientation, right–left discrimination, and personality testing. Recently, New and Thomas [53] assessed cognitive functioning in a LIS patient 6 months after basilar artery occlusion and noted significant reduction in speed of processing, moderate impairment of perceptual organization and executive skills, mild difficulties with attention, concentration, and new learning of verbal information. Interestingly, they subsequently observed progressive improvement in most areas of cognitive functioning until over 2 years after his brainstem stroke.

In a survey conducted by ALIS and Léon-Carrion *et al.* [33] in 44 chronic LIS patients, 86% reported a good attentional level, all but two patients could watch and follow a film on TV and all but one were well-oriented in time (mean duration of LIS was 5 years). More recently, ALIS and Schnakers *et al.* [54] adapted a standard battery of neuropsychological testing

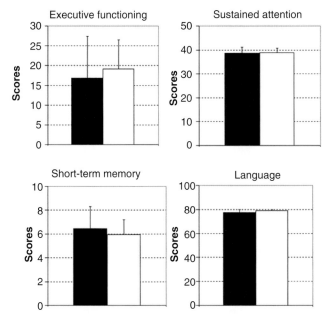

FIGURE 15.5 Neuropsychological testing data from six LIS patients (three males; mean age 42 ± 16 years) and 40 healthy adults (matched according to age and level of education). Note that LIS patients show cognitive functioning not significantly different from controls. *Source*: Data adapted from Schnakers *et al.* [54].

(i.e., sustained and selective attention, working and episodic memory, executive functioning, phonological and lexico-semantic processing and vocabulary knowledge) to an eye-response mode for specific use in LIS patients. Overall, performances in the LIS patients studied 3 to 6 years after their brainstem insult were not significantly different from matched healthy controls who, like the LIS patients, had to respond solely via eye movements (Figure 15.5). These data re-emphasize the fact that LIS due to purely pontine lesions is characterized by the restoration of a globally intact cognitive potential.

Electrophysiologic Measurements

Markland [55] reviewed EEG recordings in eight patients with LIS and reported it was normal or minimally slow in seven and showed reactivity to external stimuli in all patients. These results were confirmed by Bassetti *et al.* [56] who observed a predominance of reactive alpha activity in six LIS patients. In their seminal paper, Patterson and Grabois [5] reported normal EEG findings in 39 (45%) and abnormal (mostly slowing over the temporal or frontal leads or more diffuse slowing) in 48 (55%) patients out of 87 reviewed patients. Jacome and Morilla-Pastor [57], however, reported three patients with acute brainstem strokes and LIS whose repeated EEG recordings exhibited an 'alpha coma' pattern including an unreactive alpha rhythm to multimodal stimuli. Unreactive EEG in LIS was also reported by Gutling *et al.* [58] confirming that lack of alpha reactivity is not a reliable indicator of unconsciousness and cannot be used to distinguish the 'locked-in' patients from those comatose due to a brainstem lesion. Nevertheless, the presence of a relatively normal reactive EEG rhythm in a patient that appears to be unconscious should alert one to the possibility of a LIS.

Somatosensory evoked potentials are known to be unreliable predictors of prognosis [56, 59] but motor evoked potentials have been proposed to evaluate the potential motor recovery (e.g., [56]).

Cognitive event-related potentials (ERPs) in patients with LIS may have a role in differential diagnosis of brainstem lesions [60] and have also shown their utility to document consciousness in total LIS due to end-stage amyotrophic lateral sclerosis [22] and fulminant Guillain-Barré syndrome [16]. Figure 15.6 shows ERPs in locked-in patients showing a positive 'P3' component only evoked by the patient's own name (thick line) and not by other names (thin line). It should, however, be noted that such responses can also be evoked in minimally conscious patients [61]

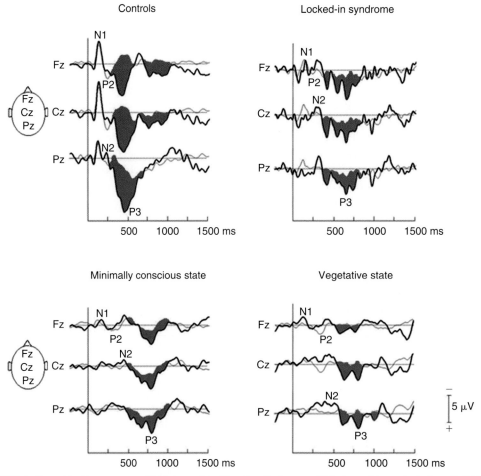

FIGURE 15.6 ERPs to the subject's own name (thick traces) and to other first names (thin traces) in controls ($n = 5$), LIS ($n = 4$), minimally conscious state ($n = 6$) and vegetative state ($n = 5$) patients. Note that a P3 response (pink) is no reliable marker of consciousness as it could be obtained in well-documented vegetative patients who never recovered. *Source*: Adapted from Perrin *et al.* [69].

and that they even persist in the vegetative state [62] and sleeping normal subjects [63].

Functional Neuroimaging

Classically, structural brain imaging (MRI) may show isolated lesions (bilateral infarction, haemorrhage, or tumour) of the ventral portion of the basis pontis or midbrain (e.g., [64]). PET scanning has shown significantly higher metabolic levels in the brains of patients in a LIS compared to patients in the vegetative state [65]. Preliminary results PET studies [66, 67] indicate that no supra-tentorial cortical area show significantly lower metabolism in acute and chronic LIS patients when compared to age-matched healthy controls (Figure 15.2). Conversely, a significantly hyperactivity was observed in bilateral amygdala of acute, but not chronic, LIS patients [8]. The absence of metabolic signs of reduced function in any area of the gray matter re-emphasizes

the fact that LIS patients suffer from a pure motor deefferentation and recover an entirely intact intellectual capacity. Previous PET studies in normal volunteers have demonstrated amygdala activation in relation to negative emotions such as fear and anxiety (e.g., [69]). It is difficult to make judgments about patient's thoughts and feelings when they awake from their coma in a motionless shell. However, in the absence of decreased neural activity in any cortical region, we assume that the increased activity in the amygdala in acute non-communicative LIS patients, relates to the terrifying situation of an intact awareness in a sensitive being, experiencing frustration, stress and anguish, locked in an immobile body. These preliminary findings emphasize the need to quickly make the diagnosis and also recognize the terrifying situation of a pseudocoma (i.e., LIS) at the intensive care or coma unit. Health care workers should adapt their bedside-behaviour and consider pharmacological anxiolytic therapy of locked-in patients, taking into account the intense emotional state they go through.

DAILY ACTIVITIES

For those not dealing with these patients on a daily basis it is surprising to see how chronic LIS patients, with the help of family and friends, still have essential social interaction and lead meaningful lives. Doble et al. [37] reported that most of their chronic LIS patients continued to remain active through eye and facial movements. Listed activities included: TV, radio, music, books on tape, visiting with family, visit vacation home, e-mail, telephone, teaching, movies, shows, the beach, bars, school, and vocational training. They also reported an attorney who uses Morse code eye blinks to provide legal opinions and keeps up with colleagues through fax and e-mail. Another patient taught math and spelling to third graders using a mouth stick to trigger an electronic voice device. The authors reported being impressed with the social interactions of chronic LIS patients and stated it was apparent that the patients were actively involved in family and personal decisions and that their presence was valued at home. Only four out of the 13 patients used computers consistently, two accessed the internet and one was able to complete the telephone interview by himself using a computer and voice synthesizer. A survey by ALIS showed that out of 17 questioned chronic LIS patients living at home, 11 (65%) used a personal computer [8].

QUALITY OF LIFE

A study conducted by the French ALIS assessed the quality of life in LIS. Chronic LIS survivors ($n = 17$, LIS duration 6±4 years) who did not show major motor recovery (i.e., used eye movements or blinking as the major mode of communication) and who lived at home were asked to fill in the Short Form-36 (SF-36) questionnaire [70] on quality of life. On the basis of this questionnaire LIS patients unsurprisingly showed maximal limitations in physical activities (all patients scoring zero). Interestingly, self-scored perception of mental health (evaluating mental well-being and psychological distress) and personal general health were not significantly lower than values from age-matched French control subjects [8, 71]. Note that the perception of mental health and the presence of physical pain was correlated to the frequency of suicidal thought [8]. This stresses the importance of managing

pain in chronic LIS patients. Our results confirm earlier reports on quality of life assessments in chronic LIS patients. Leon-Carrion et al. [33] and the French ALIS showed that about half of the assessed patients ($n = 44$) regarded their mood as good. Similarly, Doble et al. [37] studied 13 LIS patients and reported that more than half note were satisfied with life in general. In 2007, we have assessed the quality of life of 11 patients (LIS duration 7±3 years) (unpublished data) using the ACSA scale (Anamnestic Comparative Self Assessment) [72]. ACSA estimates overall well-being on a scale from −5 (worst period in the respondent's life) to +5 (best period). As show in Figure 15.7, LIS patients' overall quality of life was not significantly different from healthy matched controls.

THE RIGHT TO DIE OR THE RIGHT TO LIVE?

As stated by The American Academy of Neurology (AAN), patients with profound and permanent paralysis have the right to make health care decisions about themselves including to accept or refuse life-sustaining therapy [73]. Bruno et al. have questioned 97 clinicians: At the affirmation: 'Being LIS is worse than being in a vegetative state or in a minimally conscious state?', 66% said 'yes', 34% 'no' [74]. The unfortunate consequence of this might be that biased clinicians provide less aggressive medical treatment and influence families in ways not appropriate to the situation [37]. Some health care professionals who have no experience with chronic LIS survivors might believe that LIS patients want to die but many studies have shown that patients typically have a wish to live. In 1993, Anderson et al. [75] reported that all questioned LIS patients wanted life-sustaining treatment. A previous study by the French ALIS showed that 75% of chronic LIS patients without motor recovery rarely or never had suicidal thoughts. The question: 'would you like to receive antibiotics in

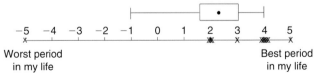

FIGURE 15.7 ACSA [72] showing self-rated quality of life in 11 LIS patients (crosses; mean age 37±6 year; eight males). Box and whiskers represent mean, SD, minimum and maximum of self-rated quality of life in 22 controls (mean age 43±10 year; eight males). Note that on average LIS patients self-rated quality of life is not significantly lower than in controls. Source: Adapted from Bruno, Pellas and Laureys [74].

case of pneumonia', 80% answered 'yes' and in reply to the question *'would you like reanimation to be tempted in case of cardiac arrest'*, 62% said 'yes'[8]. Similarly, in a recent survey conducted by Bruno *et al.* nearly two-thirds of studied LIS patients (*n* = 54) never had suicidal thoughts (see Figure 15.8) [74]. In line with these findings, Doble *et al.* [37] reported that none of the questioned chronic LIS patients had a 'do not resuscitate' order, more than a half had never considered or discussed euthanasia. These authors also noted that none of the 15 deaths of their study cohort of chronic LIS patients (*n* = 29) could be attributed to euthanasia. Since its creation, the French ALIS has registered over 400 patients with LIS in France. Only five reported deaths were related to the patient's wish to die.

In accordance with the principle of patient autonomy, physicians should respect the right of LIS patients to accept or refuse any treatment. At least two conditions are necessary for full autonomy, patients need to have intact cognitive abilities and they must be able to communicate their thoughts and wishes.

Likewise, in amyotrophic lateral sclerosis, ill-informed patients are regularly advised by physicians to refuse intubation and withhold life-saving interventions [76, 77]. However, ventilator users with neuromuscular disease report meaningful life satisfaction [78]. Bach [79] warns that 'virtually no patients are appropriately counselled about all therapeutic options' and states that advance directives, although

appropriate for patients with terminal cancer, are inappropriate for patients with severe motor disability.

Katz *et al.* [36] cite the Hastings Centre Report, 'Who speaks for the patient with LIS?'. With the initial handicap of communicating only through eyeblink who can decide whether the patient is competent to consent or to refuse treatment? [80]. With regard to end-of-life decisions taken in LIS patients, an illustrative case is reported by Fred [81]. His 80-year old mother became locked-in. In concert with the attending physician, without consent of the patient herself, the decision was made to 'have her senses dulled' and provide supportive care only. She died shortly thereafter with a temperature of 109°F (43°C). In the accompanying editorial, Stumpf [82] commented that 'human life is to be preserved as long as there is consciousness and cognitive function in contrast to a vegetative state or neocortical death'.

CONCLUSION

The discussed data stress the need for critical care physicians who are confronted to acute LIS to recognize this infrequent syndrome as early as possible. Health care workers who take care of acute LIS patients need a better understanding of the long-term outcome of LIS. Opposite to the beliefs of many physicians, LIS patients self-report a meaningful quality

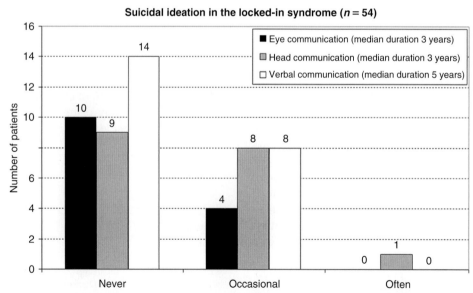

FIGURE 15.8 Frequency of suicide thoughts in 54 patients with chronic LIS (age 22–60 years), 14 communicate with their eyes, 18 have recovered some communication using their head, and 22 have recovered some verbal communication. Note that 33 patients never had suicidal thoughts, 20 had some occasionally and only one patient presented frequent suicide thoughts. *Source*: Adapted from Bruno, Pellas and Laureys [74].

of life and the demand of euthanasia existing but is uncommon. Studies emphasize LIS patients' right to autonomy and demonstrate their ability to exercise it, including taking end-of-life decisions. The strength of medical and communication-technological progress for patients with severe neurological conditions is that it makes them more and more like all the rest of us [83]. Clinicians should realize that quality of life often equates with social rather than physical interaction. It's important to emphasize that only the medically stabilized, informed LIS patient is able to accept or to refuse life-sustaining treatment. LIS patients should not be denied the right to die –and to die – but also, and more importantly, they should not be denied the right to live – and to live with dignity and the best possible care.

ACKNOWLEDGEMENTS

This research was supported by the European Commission, the Belgian Fonds National de la Recherche Scientifique (FNRS), the Centre Hospitalier Universitaire Sart Tilman, Liège, the University of Liège, the French Association Locked-in Syndrome (ALIS), and the Mind Science Foundation, San Antonio, Texas, USA. OG and MAB are Research Fellows and SL is Senior Research Associate at FNRS. AV is supported by the Concerted Research Action of the French Speaking Community of Belgium and CS is supported by EU Mindbridge funding.

The authors thank all participating LIS patients, their families and their physicians and acknowledge Fabien Perrin (Lyon), Jacques Berré and Serge Goldman (Brussels), Marie-Elisabeth Faymonville, Maurice Lamy, Gustave Moonen and Francois Damas (Liège), Frederic Pellas, Philippe Van Eeckhout, Sofiane Ghorbel and Véronique Blandin (ALIS France), and Karl-Heinz Pantke (LIS eV Germany).

References

1. Tavalaro, J. and Tayson, R. (1997) *Look Up for Yes*, New York, NY: Kodansha America, Inc.
2. Plum, F. and Posner, J.B. (1983) *The Diagnosis of Stupor and Coma*, Davis, F.A. (ed.) 3rd Edition. Philadelphia: Davis, F.A.
3. American Congress of Rehabilitation Medicine (1995) Recommendations for use of uniform nomenclature pertinent to patients with severe alterations of consciousness. *Arch Phys Med Rehabil* 76:205–209.
4. Bauer, G., Gerstenbrand, F. and Rumpl, E. (1979) Varieties of the locked-in syndrome. *J Neurol* 221:77–91.
5. Patterson, J.R. and Grabois, M. (1986) Locked-in syndrome: A review of 139 cases. *Stroke* 17:758–764.
6. Chia, L.G. (1991) Locked-in syndrome with bilateral ventral mid-brain infarcts. *Neurology* 41:445–446.
7. Meienberg, O., Mumenthaler, M. and Karbowski, K. (1979) Quadriparesis and nuclear oculomotor palsy with total bilateral ptosis mimicking coma: A mesencephalic 'locked-in syndrome'? *Arch Neurol* 36:708–710.
8. Laureys, S., *et al.* (2005) The locked-in syndrome: What is it like to be conscious but paralyzed and voiceless? *Prog Brain Res* 150:495–511.
9. Britt, R.H., Herrick, M.K. and Hamilton, R.D. (1977) Traumatic locked-in syndrome. *Ann Neurol* 1:590–592.
10. Golubovic, V., Muhvic, D. and Golubovic, S. (2004) Posttraumatic locked-in syndrome with an unusual three day delay in the appearance. *Coll Antropol* 28:923–926.
11. Fitzgerald, L.F., Simpson, R.K. and Trask, T. (1997) Locked-in syndrome resulting from cervical spine gunshot wound. *J Trauma* 42:147–149.
12. Rae-Grant, A.D., *et al.* (1989) Post traumatic extracranial vertebral artery dissection with locked-in syndrome: A case with MRI documentation and unusually favourable outcome. *J Neurol Neurosurg Psychiatr* 52:1191–1193.
13. Keane, J.R. (1986) Locked-in syndrome after head and neck trauma. *Neurology* 36:80–82.
14. Landrieu, P., *et al.* (1984) Locked in syndrome with a favourable outcome. *Eur J Pediatr* 142:144–145.
15. Bakshi, N., *et al.* (1997) Fulminant demyelinating neuropathy mimicking cerebral death. *Muscle Nerve* 20:1595–1597.
16. Ragazzoni, A., Grippo, A., Tozzi, F. and Zaccara, G. (2000) Event-related potentials in patients with total locked-in state due to fulminant Guillain-Barre syndrome. *Int J Psychophysiol* 37:99–109.
17. Loeb, C., Mancardi, G.L. and Tabaton, M. (1984) Locked-in syndrome in acute inflammatory polyradiculoneuropathy. *Eur Neurol* 23:137–140.
18. Carroll, W.M. and Mastaglia, F.L. (1979) 'Locked-in coma' in postinfective polyneuropathy. *Arch Neurol* 36:46–47.
19. O'Donnell, P.P. (1979) 'Locked-in syndrome' in postinfective polyneuropathy. *Arch Neurol* 36:860.
20. Hayashi, H. and Kato, S. (1989) Total manifestations of amyotrophic lateral sclerosis. ALS in the totally locked-in state. *J Neurol Sci* 93:19–35.
21. Kennedy, P.R. and Bakay, R.A. (1998) Restoration of neural output from a paralyzed patient by a direct brain connection. *Neuroreport* 9:1707–1711.
22. Kotchoubey, B., Lang, S., Winter, S. and Birbaumer, N. (2003) Cognitive processing in completely paralyzed patients with amyotrophic lateral sclerosis. *Eur J Neurol* 10:551–558.
23. Sandin, R.H., Enlund, G., Samuelsson, P. and Lennmarken, C. (2000) Awareness during anaesthesia: A prospective case study. *Lancet* 355:707–711.
24. Anonymous (1973). Awareness during anaesthesia. *Lancet* 2:1305.
25. Brighouse, D. and Norman, J. (1992) To wake in fright. *BMJ* 304:1327–1328.
26. Peduto, V.A., Silvetti, L. and Piga, M. (1994) An anesthetized anesthesiologist tells his experience of waking up accidentally during the operation. *Minerva Anestesiol* 60:1–5.
27. Sigalovsky, N. (2003) Awareness under general anesthesia. *AANA J* 71:373–379.
28. Dumas, A. (1997) *The Count of Monte Cristo*, London: Wordworth Editions Limited.
29. Zola, E. (1979) *Thérère Raquin*, Paris: Ed. Gallimard, 352.
30. Haig, A.J., Katz, R.T. and Sahgal, V. (1986) Locked-in syndrome: A review. *Curr Concepts Rehabil Med* 3:12–16.
31. Bauby, J.-D. (1997) In E.R. Laffont (ed.) *The Diving Bell and the Butterfly (Original Title: Le scaphandre et le papillon)*.

32. Gallo, U.E. and Fontanarosa, P.B. (1989) Locked-in syndrome: Report of a case. *Am J Emerg Med* 7:581–583.

33. Leon-Carrion, J., van Eeckhout, P., Dominguez-Morales Mdel, R. and Perez-Santamaria, F.J. (2002) The locked-in syndrome: A syndrome looking for a therapy. *Brain Injury* 16:571–582.

34. Ohry, A. (1990) The locked-in syndrome and related states. *Paraplegia* 28:73–75.

35. Haig, A.J., Katz, R.T. and Sahgal, V. (1987) Mortality and complications of the locked-in syndrome. *Arch Phys Med Rehabil* 68:24–27.

36. Katz, R.T., Haig, A.J., Clark, B.B. and DiPaola, R.J. (1992) Long-term survival, prognosis, and life-care planning for 29 patients with chronic locked-in syndrome. *Arch Phys Med Rehabil* 73:403–408.

37. Doble, J.E., Haig, A.J., Anderson, C. and Katz, R. (2003) Impairment, activity, participation, life satisfaction, and survival in persons with locked-in syndrome for over a decade: Follow-up on a previously reported cohort. *J Head Trauma Rehabil* 18:435–444.

38. McCusker, E.A., Rudick, R.A., Honch, G.W. and Griggs, R.C. (1982) Recovery from the 'locked-in' syndrome. *Arch Neurol* 39:145–147.

39. Ebinger, G., Huyghens, L., Corne, L. and Aelbrecht, W. (1985) Reversible 'locked-in' syndromes. *Intens Care Med* 11:218–219.

40. Chang, B. and Morariu, M.A. (1979) Transient traumatic 'locked-in' syndrome. *Eur Neurol* 18:391–394.

41. Richard, I., *et al.* (1995) Persistence of distal motor control in the locked in syndrome. Review of 11 patients. *Paraplegia* 33:640–646.

42. Casanova, E., Lazzari, R.E., Lotta, S. and Mazzucchi, A. (2003) Locked-in syndrome: Improvement in the prognosis after an early intensive multidisciplinary rehabilitation. *Arch Phys Med Rehabil* 84:862–867.

43. Feldman, M.H. (1971) Physiological observations in a chronic case of 'locked-in' syndrome. *Neurology* 21:459–478.

44. Kubler, A. and Neumann, N. (2005) Brain-computer interfaces – the key for the conscious brain locked into a paralyzed body. *Prog Brain Res* 150:513–525.

45. Wilhelm, B., Jordan, M. and Birbaumer, N. (2006) Communication in locked-in syndrome: Effects of imagery on salivary pH. *Neurology* 67:534–535.

46. Birbaumer, N., *et al.* (1999) A spelling device for the paralysed. *Nature* 398:297–298.

47. Vigand, P. (2002) *Promenades Immobiles*, Le Livre de Poche.

48. Vigand, P. and Vigand, S. (2000) *Only the Eyes Say Yes (Original Title: Putain de silence)*, Arcade Publishing.

49. Vanhaudenhuyse, A., *et al.* (2008) The challenge of disentangling reportability and phenomenal consciousness in post-comatose states. *Behav Brain Sci* (in press).

50. Allain, P., *et al.* (1998) Cognitive functions in chronic locked-in syndrome: A report of two cases. *Cortex* 34:629–634.

51. Cappa, S.F., Pirovano, C. and Vignolo, L.A. (1985) Chronic 'locked-in' syndrome: Psychological study of a case. *Eur Neurol* 24:107–111.

52. Cappa, S.F. and Vignolo, L.A. (1982) Locked-in syndrome for 12 years with preserved intelligence. *Ann Neurol* 11:545.

53. New, P.W. and Thomas, S.J. (2005) Cognitive impairments in the locked-in syndrome: A case report. *Arch Phys Med Rehabil* 86:338–343.

54. Schnakers, C., *et al.* (2005) Neuropsychological testing in chronic locked-in syndrome. *Psyche, abstracts from the Eighth Conference of the Association for the Scientific Study of Consciousness (ASSC8)*, University of Antwerp, Belgium, 26–28 June 2004, 11.

55. Markand, O.N. (1976) Electroencephalogram in 'locked-in' syndrome. *Electroencephalogr Clin Neurophysiol* 40:529–534.

56. Bassetti, C., Mathis, J. and Hess, C.W. (1994) Multimodal electrophysiological studies including motor evoked potentials in patients with locked-in syndrome: Report of six patients. *J Neurol Neurosurg Psychiatr* 57:1403–1406.

57. Jacome, D.E. and Morilla-Pastor, D. (1990) Unreactive EEG: Pattern in locked-in syndrome. *Clin Electroencephalogr* 21:31–36.

58. Gutling, E., Isenmann, S. and Wichmann, W. (1996) Electrophysiology in the locked-in-syndrome. *Neurology* 46:1092–1101.

59. Towle, V.L., Maselli, R., Bernstein, L.P. and Spire, J.P. (1989) Electrophysiologic studies on locked-in patients: Heterogeneity of findings. *Electroencephalogr Clin Neurophysiol* 73:419–426.

60. Onofrj, M., *et al.* (1997) Event related potentials recorded in patients with locked-in syndrome. *J Neurol Neurosurg Psychiatr* 63:759–764.

61. Laureys, S., *et al.* (2004) Cerebral processing in the minimally conscious state. *Neurology* 14:916–918.

62. Perrin, F., *et al.* (2006) Brain response to one's own name in vegetative state, minimally conscious state, and locked-in syndrome. *Arch Neurol* 63:562–569.

63. Perrin, F., Garcia-Larrea, L., Mauguiere, F. and Bastuji, H. (1999) A differential brain response to the subject's own name persists during sleep. *Clin Neurophysiol* 110:2153–2164.

64. Leon-Carrion, J., van Eeckhout, P. and Dominguez-Morales Mdel, R. (2002) The locked-in syndrome: A syndrome looking for a therapy. *Brain Injury* 16:555–569.

65. Levy, D.E., *et al.* (1987) Differences in cerebral blood flow and glucose utilization in vegetative versus locked-in patients. *Ann Neurol* 22:673–682.

66. Laureys, S., *et al.* (2003) Brain function in acute and chronic locked-in syndrome. *Presented at the 9th Annual Meeting of the Organisation for Human Brain Mapping (OHBM)*, NY, USA, June 18–22, 2003, NeuroImage CD ROM, 19 (2, Suppl 1).

67. Laureys, S., Owen, A.M. and Schiff, N.D. (2004) Brain function in coma vegative state, and related disorders. *Lancet Neurol* 3:537–546.

68. Calder, A.J., Lawrence, A.D. and Young, A.W. (2001) Neuropsychology of fear and loathing. *Nat Rev Neurosci* 2:352–363.

69. Perrin, F., *et al.* (2005). Evaluation of preserved linguistic processing in brain damaged patients, *submitted*.

70. Ware, J.E., Snow, K.K. and Kosinski, M. (1993) *SF-36 Health Survey Manual and Interpretation Guide*, Boston, MA: The Health Institute, New England Medical Center.

71. Ghorbel, S. (2002) Statut fonctionnel et qualité de vie chez le locked-in syndrome a domicile, In *DEA Motricité Humaine et Handicap*, Montpellier, France: Laboratory of Biostatistics, Epidemiology and Clinical Research, Université Jean Monnet Saint-Etienne.

72. Bernheim, J.L. (1999) How to get serious answers to the serious question: 'How have you been?': Subjective quality of life (QOL) as an individual experiential emergent construct. *Bioethics* 13:272–287.

73. Ethics and Humanities Subcommittee of the AAN (1993) Position statement: Certain aspects of the care and management of profoundly and irreversibly paralyzed patients with retained consciousness and cognition. Report of the Ethics and Humanities Subcommittee of the American Academy of Neurology. *Neurology* 43:222–223.

74. Bruno, M.A., Pellas, F. and Laureys, S. (2008) Quality of life in locked-in syndrome. In Vincent, J.L. (eds.) *Yearbook of Intensive Care and Emergency Medicine*, pp. 881–890. Berlin: Springer-Verlag.

75. Anderson, C., Dillon, C. and Burns, R. (1993) Life-sustaining treatment and locked-in syndrome. *Lancet* 342:867–868.

76. Christakis, N.A. and Asch, D.A. (1993) Biases in how physicians choose to withdraw life support. *Lancet* 342:642–646.

77. Trail, M., *et al.* (2003) A study comparing patients with amyotrophic lateral sclerosis and their caregivers on measures of quality of life, depression, and their attitudes toward treatment options. *J Neurol Sci* 209:79–85.

78. Kübler, A., Winter, S., Ludolph, A.C., Hautzinger, M. and Birbaumer, N. (2005) Severity of depressive symptoms and quality of life in patients with amyotrophic lateral sclerosis. *Neurorehabil Neural Repair* 19(3):182–193.

79. Bach, J.R. (2003) Threats to 'informed' advance directives for the severely physically challenged? *Arch Phys Med Rehabil* 84:S23–S28.

80. Steffen, G.E. and Franklin, C. (1985) Who speaks for the patient with the locked-in syndrome? *Hastings Cent Rep* 15:13–15.

81. Fred, H.L. (1986) Helen. *South Med J* 79:1135–1136.

82. Stumpf, S.E. (1986) A comment on 'Helen'. *South Med J* 79:1057–1058.

83. Bruno, M., Bernheim, J.L., Schnakers, C. and Laureys, S. (2008) Locked-in: Don't judge a book by its cover. *J Neurol Neurosurg Psychiatr* 79:2.

Consciousness and Dementia: How the Brain Loses Its Self

Pietro Pietrini, Eric Salmon and Paolo Nichelli

ABSTRACT

Consciousness is based on the ability to rapidly integrate information and requires the optimal functioning of neural networks widely distributed between the thalami and the whole cortical mantle. Neurodegenerative processes that occur in dementing disorders, including Alzheimer's disease, frontotemporal dementia and Lewy Body Disease, lead to a progressive disruption of the brain functional and anatomical connectivity that sustains complex mental activity in the human brain. Not only different dementia syndromes affect the brain in different ways but also patients with the same disease may show distinctive clinical features. By combining clinical, neuropsychological and functional brain imaging studies in selected patients, scientists are gaining new insights on the cerebral bases of conscious mental activity and of the neural events that make awareness of the surrounding world and of ourselves to dissolve.

According to the information integration theory of consciousness [1, 2], consciousness corresponds to the brain's ability to rapidly integrate information. This ability to integrate information requires a well-functioning thalamocortical system [2, 3]. Indeed, extensive lesions of the thalamocortical system are usually associated with a global loss of consciousness, such as that seen in comatose patients [4]. Also, in patients who have undergone the surgical section of the corpus callosum for therapeutic purposes, leading to a splitting of the thalamocortical system, consciousness is split as well [2]. Neural activity that correlates with conscious experience appears to be widely distributed over the cortex, indicating that consciousness is based on the optimal functioning of a distributed thalamocortical network rather than on the activity of a specific single cortical region [2]. This also is in line with the observation that lesions of selected cortical areas result in the impairment of specific submodalities of conscious experience, such as the perception of faces, but do not produce any alteration of global consciousness [5].

Alzheimer's disease is the most common form of dementing disorders in the elderly, affecting more than 5% of individuals aged 65 years and older and almost one out of two individuals over 85 years of age [6]. Patients with Alzheimer's disease show a progressive, multivariate and irreversible deterioration of cognitive abilities. Different aspects of consciousness also may be impaired, including conscious processing of information and awareness of disease condition [7, 8].

Cognitive impairment in Alzheimer's disease is the consequence of the functional and anatomical disruption of cortical integrity due to the progressive development of the neuropathological process. The availability of modern brain imaging methodologies, including positron emission tomography (PET) and magnetic resonance imaging, in combination with sophisticated experimental paradigms, has made it possible to examine in a non-invasive manner the neurometabolic bases of mental function in healthy human subjects and in patients with dementia [7–10]. Because the neuropathological process may progress to affect preferentially different cortical areas in individual patients, dementia represents a valuable "natural model" to investigate the effects of distinct patterns of disruption of cortical integrity on consciousness.

In this chapter we will review what we have learned in this respect from combined behavioural and *in vivo* brain imaging studies in patients with Alzheimer's disease and frontotemporal dementia.

COGNITIVE IMPAIRMENT AND DISRUPTION OF BRAIN FUNCTIONAL INTEGRITY IN ALZHEIMER'S DISEASE

Disturbances of attention and memory typically are the first clinical manifestations in patients with Alzheimer's disease and may remain the only symptoms for a long time. Impairments in attentional and executive functions, abstract reasoning, semantic memory, visuoperceptual skills along with alterations in personality and behaviour and loss of insight into the disease condition then occur in different combinations in individual patients [8, 9, 11–14].

Cognitive impairment is due to the insidious development of a neuropathological process characterized by the presence of senile plaques, neurofibrillary tangles and loss of neurons and their synaptic projections [15, 16]. These neuropathological lesions affect mostly the neocortical association areas of the parietal, temporal and frontal lobes and limbic regions and show a regional distribution that may vary among individual patients [15, 17–19]. Typically, the neuropathological process starts in the medial temporal lobe structures, including the entorhinal cortex and the hippocampal formation, and subsequently spreads to the neocortical association areas of the temporal, parietal and frontal lobes, leading to the disruption of various mental functions [17, 18, 20].

Over the past three decades, many studies have been conducted with PET to measure regional cerebral glucose metabolism and blood flow in patients with Alzheimer's disease examined at rest (eyes patched, ears plugged, no sensory stimulation) as well as during a variety of cognitive tasks (see [10] for a review). Measures of both cerebral glucose metabolism and blood flow are reliable indices of neuronal synaptic activity, as they reflect the brain metabolic need for glucose and oxygen in order to produce adenosine triphosphate (ATP). ATP in the central nervous system is mostly required for maintenance and restoration of ionic gradients and cell membrane potentials due to electrical activity associated with action potentials and transmission of impulses from neuron to neuron [21, 22]. Therefore, changes in synaptical activity lead to parallel changes in the demand for ATP and, in turn, for glucose utilization and capillary blood flow in the same brain regions. Indeed, the frequency of action potentials and the rate of glucose utilization show a direct linear correlation [22–26].

Overall, the PET studies conducted in several laboratories across the world have been consistent in providing the following pieces of evidence (Figure 16.1):

1. *Cerebral glucose metabolism is impaired in Alzheimer's disease*. Regional cerebral glucose metabolism measured at rest is significantly reduced in patients with Alzheimer's disease, compared to matched healthy individuals, mostly in the association neocortical areas, with a relative sparing of primary neocortical and subcortical regions and cerebellum, at least until the later stages of the disease [9, 10, 27–30].
2. *Metabolic abnormalities worsen with progression of dementia*. With progression of dementia severity, brain metabolic reductions in patients with

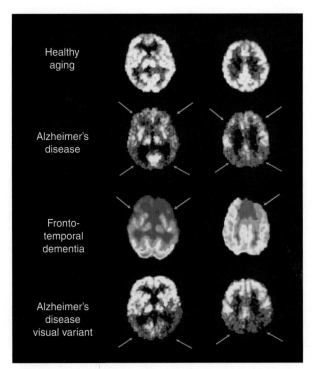

FIGURE 16.1   Regional cerebral glucose utilization as measured by PET in a healthy control subject, in a representative patient
with the classical form of Alzheimer's disease, in a frontotemporal
dementia patient, and in a patient suffering from the visual variant
of Alzheimer's disease. Brain metabolism was determined with subjects in the resting state (eyes patched and ears plugged, no sensory
stimulation). For each subject, two horizontal brain slices taken parallel and above the inferior orbito-meatal line are shown, approximately 45 mm left side of the figure, and 90 mm right, respectively.
For each individual slice, the right side corresponds to the right side
of the brain, and the left to the left side, respectively. Compared to
the healthy control subject, the patient with Alzheimer's disease
show reduction in cerebral glucose metabolism in the frontal, temporal and parietal neocortical association areas, the patient with
frontotemporal dementia in prefrontal and frontotemporal areas,
and the patient suffering from the visual variant of Alzheimer's disease in occipito-temporal areas with a sparing of the most anterior
portion of the brain. *Source*: Adapted from [10].

Alzheimer's disease become more and more
severe and extend to include the remainder
of the neocortical mantle, with only a relative
preservation of the sensorimotor and primary
visual cortices, subcortical structures and
cerebellum [10, 27–30]. Furthermore, progression
of dementia is associated with a progressive
decline in the ability to increase synaptic activity
in response to stimulation up to a point when, in
the advanced stages of disease, there is minimal
or null synaptic metabolic increment over rest,
indicating that synapses in those brain regions are
no longer functional [31].

3. *Cerebral metabolic alterations are heterogeneous.*
Metabolic abnormalities may show a different

topographic distribution across individual
patients, that is, some patients show a greater
involvement of the left hemisphere whereas
others may show more reductions in the right
hemisphere. For instance, in a large sample of
Alzheimer patients in the mild to moderate stages
of dementia severity, a principal component
analysis showed that the most common pattern
involved metabolic reductions in superior and
inferior parietal lobules and in the posterior medial
temporal regions. A second subgroup had reduced
glucose utilization in orbitofrontal and anterior
cingulate areas, with a relative sparing of parietal
regions. Metabolic reductions affected more
selectively the left hemisphere in a third group
of patients, and the fourth group had reduced
metabolism in frontal, temporal and parietal
cortical areas [32].

4. *Patterns of cerebral metabolic alteration are related
to patterns of cognitive impairment.* These patterns
of metabolic alterations are related to and may
even precede and predict the pattern of cognitive
impairment in individual patient subgroups [12,
33]. For example, the group of patients showing
reduced metabolism in orbitofrontal cortex,
a brain region known to be involved in the
modulation of aggressive behaviour [34], showed
agitation, anger outbursts, inappropriate social
behaviour, and personality and mood changes [32].
Similarly, patients with visuospatial dysfunction
showed greater right- than left-hemisphere
hypometabolism while patients with language
deficits had predominant left-hemisphere
hypometabolism [12, 30, 33]. In some cases, the
pattern of cerebral hypometabolism could be
detected several months before the appearance of
the related picture of cognitive impairment.

Furthermore, the relative pattern of regional
distribution of metabolic alterations is maintained
across progression of dementia severity, that is,
patients who reveal a greater left- than right-
hypometabolism in the early phases of the disease
will show a relatively more severe left-hemisphere
metabolic impairment also in the later/end stages,
indicating that the pathological process maintains
a relatively more selective effect on the same brain
regions across the different stages of dementia
progression [11, 12, 35].

5. *Distinct cognitive and cerebral metabolic features
characterize clinical subtypes of Alzheimer's disease.*
Clinical subtypes of Alzheimer's disease are
characterized by the predominant involvement
as well as the relative sparing of selected cortical
regions as compared to the classical form of

Alzheimer's disease. For instance, patients with the so-called *visual variant of Alzheimer's disease* [9, 36] show a remarkable metabolic impairment of posterior cortical regions, including primary visual cortex – which is typically spared in Alzheimer's disease – in contrast with a peculiar sparing of the more anterior parts of the brain, including the entorhinal cortex and the limbic cortex which, on the contrary, are considered the hallmark feature in patients with classical Alzheimer's disease [37]. Compared to the classical Alzheimer patients, the visual variant patients show early and prominent disturbances of visual consciousness, including visual agnosia and Balint's syndrome but retain awareness of their cognitive deficits until the end stages of the disease, as we will discuss later [9, 36].

6. *Regional functional connectivity is altered in Alzheimer's disease.* The correlation coefficient between the regional cerebral metabolic rates for glucose (as well as between regional cerebral blood flow values) provides a measure for the functional association between distinct brain regions [38]. The pattern of such interregional correlations reflects the integrated cerebral activity either at rest or during a specific cognitive task. Patients with Alzheimer's disease show abnormal patterns of interregional metabolic correlations both in the resting state and during the cognitive tasks [14, 38–45]. The alterations in functional connectivity may even precede the onset of significant reductions in regional glucose metabolism and indicate the progressive disruption of cerebral integrity in patients with Alzheimer's disease.

In summary, the dementing process in patients with Alzheimer's disease – as well as in patients with other forms of dementia, such as frontotemporal dementia or Lewy Body Disease, as we will discuss later – is associated with a heterogeneous and progressive disruption of the brain functional integrity. These alterations that can be measured in individual patients as dementia worsens and the patterns of abnormal neural functioning can be related to distinct changes in cognition and consciousness. These observations can shed new light on the understanding of the brain functional architecture that makes us aware of the surroundings and of ourselves.

HOW THE BRAIN GETS LOST IN DEGENERATIVE DEMENTIA

"This disease is worse than cancer", is among the most frequent comments that a clinician may hear from

family members of a patient with dementia. *"Because it destroys the self"*, is usually the explanation that follows. And indeed, this is what happens in patients with Alzheimer's disease or with another similar dementia syndrome. Patients become more and more unaware of the world and of themselves, until they eventually slide in a meaningless present with a fading past and no future. If this is the inevitable final destination for all patients who reach a severe stage, they may take different routes to arrive there. While these routes certainly share some way and intersecte, they also present some distinctive features, so that by following step by step the descending march of patients along these pathways, scientists may begin to understand how the brain gets lost.

In degenerative diseases, the patients progressively lose not only their cognitive or behavioural abilities, but also the awareness of the functioning of these abilities, and frequently the awareness of their own incapacities. For example, patients with frontotemporal dementia may know that eating too much is bad for health (preserved common knowledge), but they cannot avoid eating quickly (impaired awareness of the application of common knowledge in society), and they do not see themselves as behaving abnormally (impaired awareness of self behaviour).

LOSS OF INSIGHT VS. LOSS OF SIGHT

Lack of awareness for the disease, anosognosia, or loss of insight are used interchangeably to indicate the patient inability to properly recognize their clinical condition, as it is frequently observed in patients with Alzheimer's disease or frontotemporal dementia [7, 8, 46–48]. Anosognosia may be limited to some aspects of the disease and may be more pronounced for cognitive deficits than for behavioural dysfunction [48, 49]. Also, patients may be aware of their symptoms but not of their severity. In some patients with Alzheimer's disease insight into the disease condition may be retained until the most advanced stages of dementia whereas in others may be lost since the early phases [7–9], that may explain why correlations between loss of insight and dementia severity or illness duration in patients with Alzheimer's disease remain controversial [50–52]. In patients with frontal lobe dementia, the inability to accurately perceive changes in behaviour and personality is indeed one of the core clinical features that lead to the diagnosis [53].

Recently, Salmon and colleagues [8] investigated the neural basis of anosognosia for cognitive impairment in a large sample of patients with Alzheimer's disease

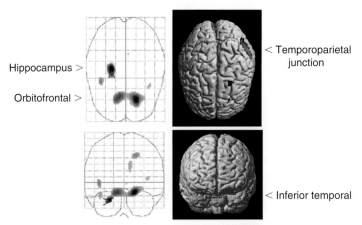

FIGURE 16.2　PET data showing brain region with a significant correlation between glucose metabolism and anosognosia for cognitive impairment in patients with Alzheimer's disease. Anosognosia was measured in 209 Alzheimer's disease patients either using patient's (erroneous) assessment of cognitive performances (on the left side) or by a discrepancy score between patient's and relative's assessment (on the right side). Correlations were obtained in cerebral glucose metabolic data measured in the resting state. *Source*: Adapted from [8].

in the mild to moderate range of dementia severity by examining the relation between regional cerebral glucose utilization at rest and two measures of anosognosia. They used a research questionnaire that covered 13 cognitive domains, including memory, attention, temporal and spatial orientation, abstract thinking, word finding, calculation and others [46] and obtained three dependent variables: the caregiver evaluation of the patient's cognitive dysfunction, the self-evaluation by the patient and the discrepancy score between the caregiver and the patient's evaluation. In this manner, the authors had two measures of anosognosia: the self-assessment of cognitive impairment by the patient and the discrepancy score between caregiver's and patent's evaluation [54]. The patient's self-assessment alone has the major limitation that a score indicating mild cognitive difficulties would be reported both by Alzheimer patients with truly mild cognitive deficit and by more severely demented patients with anosognosia. The discrepancy score, on the contrary, makes it possible to distinguish these two cases, as patients with anosognosia will receive a greater impairment score by their caregivers. It is interesting to note that a high discrepancy score, indicating greater informant than self-reported cognitive difficulties, in individuals with mild cognitive impairment (MCI) but no dementia may predict the risk of conversion to Alzheimer's disease [55].

Correlation analyses showed that impaired self-evaluation was related to reduced cerebral glucose metabolism in the right parahippocampal cortex and in the orbitofrontal cortex. The discrepancy score was negatively correlated with glucose metabolism in the temporoparietal junction, inferior temporal cortex and left superior frontal sulcus, that is, patients with

greater lack of insight in their cognitive deficits had lower glucose utilization in these associative cortical regions [8] (Figure 16.2). These findings are particularly robust, as the authors examined over 200 patients with Alzheimer's disease recruited at many European centres and the analyses took into consideration several potential confounding variables.

In another study, patients with Alzheimer's disease failed to activate the ventromedial prefrontal cortex as elderly controls did for assessing self-relevance of personality traits adjectives [56]. As a whole, these results indicate that anosognosia in Alzheimer's disease is associated with dysfunction in frontal and temporoparietal associative structures that subserve perspective taking on self and others [57]. This observation is consistent also with data from patients with frontotemporal dementia who show an early loss of insight and have a selective functional damage of frontal and temporal cortical regions, with a relative sparing of the posterior parts of the brain, including the parietal lobes that are instead severely damaged in Alzheimer's disease [53, 58]. In a recent study in a group of patients with frontotemporal dementia, the degree of metabolic activity in the left temporal pole was related to the severity of anosognosia for behavioural changes in social situations, in the sense that the greater was the lack of insight, the lower was glucose utilization in the temporal pole [47] (Figure 16.3). Dysfunction of the left temporal pole would prevent patients with frontotemporal dementia to get access to a script of their social behaviour to correctly assess their personality.

On the other hand, demented patients with Alzheimer's disease who show a metabolic preservation of the frontal and temporal cortex maintain

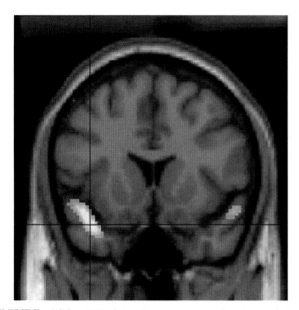

FIGURE 16.3 PET data showing a significant correlation between glucose metabolism in the superior temporal pole and anosognosia for behavioural changes in patients with frontotemporal dementia. Anosognosia was measured by a discrepancy score between 16 frontotemporal dementia patients' and their relative's assessment of social behaviour. Correlations were obtained in cerebral glucose metabolic data measured in the resting state. *Source*: Adapted from [47].

insight into their condition until the very late stages of dementia. This preservation can be appreciated particularly in a relatively rare subgroup of patients with the so-called visual variant of Alzheimer's disease [9, 59, 60]. The peculiarities of the clinical, neuropsychological and neurometabolic pictures make it possible to separate these patients from the classical Alzheimer patients. Unlike the classical Alzheimer patients, patients with the visual variant of Alzheimer's disease show early and prominent disturbances of visual abilities in the absence of any memory difficulties. They often have difficulties driving, including being unable to drive in a straight line, to maintain the proper distance from other cars, or to make turns without hitting the curb [59, 60]. The clinical picture may progress to include difficulties in keeping track of a written line while reading, in reading an analogic watch, decreased hand–eye coordination, alexia, agraphia, visual agnosia and Balint's syndrome (oculomotor apraxia, optic ataxia, visual inattention and simultagnosia). These visual difficulties are usually the first and only complaint for a long time and remain prominent also after the appearance of other cognitive deficits and until the end stages of the disease [9, 36, 61]. From a brain metabolic point of view, patients with the visual variant of Alzheimer's disease show reduced cerebral glucose

utilization bilaterally in primary and association visual cortices, posterior cingulate, parietal, superior and middle temporal areas and sensorimotor cortex relative to matched healthy control subjects. In contrast, they have no reduction in frontal, inferior temporal, anterior and posterior medial temporal regions, or subcortical structures. In comparison to matched patients with the classical form of Alzheimer's disease, the visual variant patients show significantly reduced glucose utilization in bilateral occipital association cortex, and significantly higher metabolism bilaterally in frontal, anterior medial temporal and anterior cingulate regions, inferior temporal and basal ganglia [9]. Thus, in this pathology where the dementing process spares frontal and temporal cortex, patients do not lose awareness of their condition and of the severity of their cognitive deficits.

On the other hand, patients like those with the visual variant of Alzheimer's disease clearly show impairment in distinct aspects of consciousness and often since the initial phases of the disease. While these patients retain insight, moral judgement, abstract thinking and even a sense of humour, they progressively lose the ability to perceive visually the surrounding world. They may describe one by one each detail of what they see in front of them, recognize the colours and even faces of people but be unable to grab the whole scene, so that a picture of a living room only becomes a boring list of pieces of furniture.

Neuropathological examinations in patients with the visual variant of Alzheimer's disease indicated a specific loss of functional connections between the primary visual cortex and regions in the posterior parietal cortex, whereas the connections between the primary visual cortex and the inferior temporal cortex does not appear more damaged than in typical Alzheimer patients [37, 62]. Thus, the pattern of cerebral metabolism found in our sample of patients with the visual variant of Alzheimer's disease mirrors at a functional level, and extends to earlier stages of disease, the cerebral distribution of neurofibrillary tangles seen at autopsy [37] and indicates a more selective involvement of the dorsal visual pathway and a relative sparing of the ventral pathway. Considered the distinctive functional organization of the dorsal and ventral visual pathways in the human brain [63, 64], this preferential involvement of the dorsal visual pathway and the relative sparing of the ventral one may account for the visuospatial dysfunction shown by these patients and the preservation of their ability to perceive a face or a colour [9].

While neuropathological examinations have confirmed the diagnosis of Alzheimer's disease in most patients with these prominent visual disturbances

[37, 59, 65], other neurodegenerative disorders, such as Creutzfeldt–Jakob disease and subcortical gliosis, may give rise to similar patterns of visual impairment early in the course of the disease [65]. These different dementia syndromes which preferentially affect the more posterior parts of the brain have in common also a much greater incidence of visual hallucinations than that usually observed in patients with typical Alzheimer's disease, suggesting that visual hallucinations may be related to the prominent loss of integrity in the occipital-parietal visual cortical structures that occurs in these patients [66, 67].

HALLUCINATIONS IN DEMENTIA: WHERE DO THEY COME FROM?

Visual hallucinations are the most common type of hallucinations in patients with Alzheimer's disease and are significantly associated with disorders of the visual system, including decreased visual acuity and visual agnosia, and appear to be related to the neuropathological damage in the occipital cortex [66, 67]. A structural magnetic resonance imaging study showed a significantly reduced ratio of occipital volume to whole brain volume in Alzheimer patients with visual hallucinations as compared to age- and severity-matched Alzheimer patients without visual hallucinations [67]. Alteration in visual association cortical areas (Brodmann area 18 and 19) rather than in primary calcarine cortex (BA 17) seems to be more relevant in the genesis of visual hallucinations. Indeed, complex visual hallucinations have been induced by the electrical stimulation of BA 19 but not BA 17 [68] and, in patients with Alzheimer's disease, neurofibrillary tangles and neuritic plaques are 20–40 times more concentrated in visual association cortical areas than in calcarine cortex [18].

Visual hallucinations, however, are also relatively frequent in Lewy Body Disease, the second most common form of dementia in the elderly, in which Lewy bodies, which are the hallmark neuropathological feature of Parkinson's disease, are found in the cortex and subcortical structures of the affected patients [69]. Patients with Lewy Body Disease present a fluctuating cognitive impairment that affects memory and higher cognitive functions, recurrent visual hallucinations and Parkinsonian-like motor disturbances [70]. Disturbances of consciousness include mainly visual hallucinations associated in some instances to paranoid delusions. Auditory hallucinations are rare [69, 71].These disturbances of consciousness

have been found in up to 70% of patients with Lewy Body Disease, and thus are much more frequent than in patients with Alzheimer's disease who present these features only in 5–30% of the cases [69, 71, 72]. Typically, visual hallucinations are complex images with people and animals and may be very vivid and rich of details. Neuropathological studies have found no correlation between visual hallucinations or the other mental disturbances and the distribution of Lewy bodies or senile plaques in the cortex of the affected patients [71]. This lack of correlation is not surprising, as the fluctuating nature of the cognitive impairment and alteration of consciousness in these patients suggest that the true cause of visual hallucinations may be not at an anatomical level, but rather be linked to some other mechanisms than simply the prominent functional and anatomical disgregation of visual cortical areas found in patients with the visual variant of Alzheimer's disease or similar dementing disorders.

Lewy Body Disease is associated with a remarkable impairment of the cholinergic neurotransmission due to the loss of acetyltransferase, the enzyme that synthetizes acetylcholine [71, 73]. The cholinergic impairment in the neocortex of patients with Lewy body dementia is greater than that found in patients with Alzheimer's disease, in which archicortical deficits (e.g., in the hippocampal regions) are more severe. A neurochemical study in patients with Lewy body dementia showed that acetyltransferase activity in the parietal and temporal cortex of patient with visual hallucinations was less than 20% of healthy control values whereas patients who did not experience visual hallucinations had values around 50% of the normal range [73].

Cholinergic activity in the cortex modulates signal-to-noise in neuronal firing, by increasing the firing of postsynaptic potentials and increasing their probability of being distinguished from background cortical activity [74]. In an fMRI study in young healthy subjects we showed that pharmacological potentiation of cholinergic neurotransmission by physostigmine, which inhibits the enzyme acetylcholinesterase, lead to an improved processing of information in visual cortical areas as compared to the placebo condition during a visual working memory task [75]. Specifically, neuronal activity, as measured by the fMRI-BOLD signal, during cholinergic enhancement was significantly greater in response to the target visual stimuli (faces to be remembered) than to the distractor (a non-sense scrambled picture). In contrast, during placebo, neural responses to the target and the distractor were identical [75] (Figure 16.4). Thus, cholinergic modulation appears to

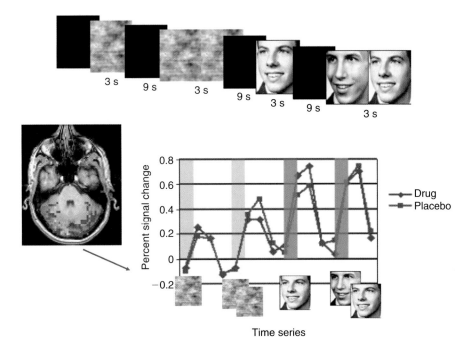

FIGURE 16.4   Effects of cholinergic potentiation on neural response in ventral extrastriate visual cortical areas that are activated in a visual working memory for faces task. (Top) For each scan series, subjects performed a task that alternated between a sensorimotor control item and a working memory item. For each working memory item, a picture of a face was presented for 3 seconds, followed by a 9-second delay, and by a 3-second presentation of two faces. Subjects indicated which of the two faces they had seen previously. For each sensorimotor control item, identical scrambled faces were presented to control for spatial frequency, brightness, and contrast, and subjects were instructed to press both buttons simultaneously when shown two scrambled faces. (Bottom) An axial slice of ventral occipital cortex from a single representative subject is reported with the voxels that showed a significant response to the task. The panel shows time series averaged across subjects, hemispheres, and all trials for the voxels that showed significant face-selectivity or encoding-selectivity. The figures show percent change in signal from baseline. The light gray bars indicate when the control stimuli (scrambled faces) were presented and the dark gray bars illustrate when the memory stimuli (faces) were presented. Data acquired during placebo (red) and during physostigmine (blue) are shown in each panel. Note the enhancement in signal-to-noise neuronal response during cholinergic potentiation as compared to the placebo condition. *Source*: Adapted from [75].

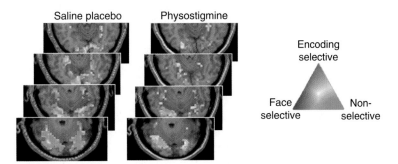

FIGURE 16.5   Improved signal-to-noise neuronal response during cholinergic enhancement. Axial slices of the ventral temporo-occipital cortex from representative subjects during a working memory for faces task during the administration either of placebo saline or physostigmine. Face-selective voxels are shown in blue, encoding-selective voxels in red, while non-selective voxels in green. Note the generalized increased selectivity of response across the ventral temporo-occipital cortex during cholinergic enhancement as compared to administration of placebo saline.

be important in allowing the brain to select relevant information from the background [76] (Figure 16.5).

It has been proposed that visual hallucinations that occur in patients with impaired cholinergic neurotransmission may be due to an inability to suppress intrinsic cortical activity during perception [71]. According to this hypothesis, when the cortical cholinergic modulation is diminished, there would be a failure to focus on the most relevant information and to maintain an appropriate conscious stream of awareness, with the intrusion of irrelevant information from the subconscious into consciousness [71]. The role of the cholinergic deficit in the genesis of visual hallucinations is also supported by the evidence that the pharmacological blockade of muscarinic receptors results in complex and vivid visual hallucinations which resemble those experienced by patients with Lewy body dementia [71]. On the other hand, visual hallucinations respond, at least to some extent, to treatments with cholinergic potentating drugs [77, 78].

Considering that cholinergic terminals are spread across the whole cortex, one could speculate that the diffuse deficit in cholinergic activity may precipitate a functional impairment in those cortical regions that are more selectively targeted by the neuropathological process. Thus, in patients with a predominant compromission of the occipital and parietal association cortical areas, the lack of an efficient cholinergic modulation might lead to visual hallucinations [78] whereas in others it might determine the appearance of different alterations of consciousness.

DELUSIONAL MISIDENTIFICATION SYNDROMES

The term delusional misidentification syndromes refers to a false belief in doubles and duplicates, and includes the syndromes of Capgras [79] and Fregoli, their variants, reduplicative paramnesia and other reduplicative phenomena.

Reduplication of person is the belief that a person has more than one identity, or that someone has been replaced by a close double. Patients with temporal reduplication are convinced that a current event or period of time has already taken place in the past, a sort of prolonged déjà fait experience. The first case of reduplicative paramnesia, reported by Arnold Pick in 1903 [80], was a woman with senile dementia who was convinced that there were two clinics in Prague, an "old" clinic and a "new" one, each directed by a Professor Pick. In the Capgras syndrome, the patient is convinced that a family member or a close friend is an impostor.

Delusional misidentification syndromes are frequently observed in patients with severe close head traumas and have been described also in association with vascular and neoplastic lesions and epilepsy, especially when affecting the frontal and temporal poles especially of the right hemisphere [81].

Delusional misidentification syndromes are selective, that is, only a few people, places or objects are misidentified, and also specific, that is, the misidentification always regards the same person and only that person. For instance, if a patient is convinced that her husband is an impostor, she will recognize him and only him as an impostor and will not misdesignate any other person.

From a brain functional point of view, demented patients with Alzheimer's disease and delusional misidentification syndrome showed a significant metabolic impairment in bilateral orbitofrontal and cingulate cortex and sensory association areas, including the superior temporal and inferior parietal cortex, as compared to severity-matched patients with Alzheimer's disease but no delusional syndrome [81]. The pattern of metabolic alterations is consistent with the hypothesis that delusional misidentification syndromes may be rooted in a disruption of the connections between multimodal cortical association areas and paralimbic and limbic structures [82] that are thought to relate intermodal sensory information with emotional tone to validate experience [83]. This could result in a sensory – affective dissonance so that the patient perceives the stimulus but not its emotional significance and relevance to the self [81]. In the example cited above, the patient with Capgras delusion may recognize her husband but she does not feel that he is really her spouse.

Delusional misidentification syndromes are often associated with other delusions, anosognosia, environmental disorientation, depersonalization and derealization, in which similar mechanisms of disrupted sensory – emotional connection may occur. As we discussed earlier, patients with anosognosia reveal a cerebral metabolic impairment that greatly overlaps with that found in patients with delusional misidentification syndrome.

IN DEMENTIA LOSING THE MIND MAY BE LOOSENING THE BRAIN

Impairments in cognitive and behavioral functions and disturbances of consciousness in patients with Alzheimer's disease or other neurodegenerative dementias are not only the consequence of the well-documented functional and morphological compromission of specific cortical regions but also of a breakdown in the brain functional connectivity. While most studies have used univariate analyses that considered each region separately and therefore could only determine specific metabolic alterations as compared to healthy control subjects, a few studies have employed a more sophisticated approach to examine the patterns of interregional metabolic correlations in the human brain and the alterations associated with the dementing process [39–42, 45, 84].

Overall, these studies have demonstrated that in the brain of patients with Alzheimer's disease there is a decrease in functional interactions among several brain regions, indicating a disconnection likely due to lesions in the associative pathways. Alterations in the pattern of functional interactions have been showed between anterior and posterior cortical regions, between the right and the left hemisphere [38, 85] and between medial temporal structures, including the hippocampus and the entorhinal cortex, and the posterior cingulate cortex [84] as well as between the hippocampus and a number of regions in frontal, temporal and parietal cortex [42, 44]. Because the medial temporal cortex typically is affected early and heavily in the course of dementia in patients with Alzheimer's disease, the disruption of functional connectivity between its neural structures and other cortical systems not only may account for the early and prominent memory deficits but might also contribute to some of the non-memory cognitive disturbances. From a neurometabolic viewpoint, reductions in glucose metabolism in several cortical association areas, including the posterior cingulate cortex, which is commonly affected since the initial stages in patients with Alzheimer's disease [86], could be the consequence, at least in part, of the alterated connectivity with medial temporal structures [42, 84]. This is supported by the observation that neurotoxic lesions in the entorhinal and perirhinal cortex in baboons determine a reduction in cerebral glucose metabolism in regions of the temporal, parietal and occipital association cortex and in the posterior cingulate cortex [87]. More recently, however, the posterior cingulate cortex was shown to be part of three principal components in patterns of cerebral metabolism obtained from 225 patients with Alzheimer's disease [14]. Posterior cingulate activity covaried not only with metabolism in the Papez's circuit, comprising the medial temporal lobe (PC2, 12% of the total variance), but it was also independently correlated with activity in the posterior cerebral cortices (PC1, 17% of the variance) and in frontal associative cortices (PC3, 9% of the variance), confirming a central role of the posterior cingulate region in Alzheimer's disease. Moreover, all principal components were correlated with controlled cognitive performances, suggesting that impaired interregional functional connectivity is related to decreased controlled (conscious) processes in Alzheimer's disease.

Disruption of the physiological functional connectivity in patients with Alzheimer's disease has been found not only in the default-mode network, that is, in the resting brain, but also while the brain is engaged in tasks that involve attention, perception and memory [42, 85, 88]. Horwitz and colleagues [85] found that during a face perception task healthy older control subjects showed a strong correlation between neural activity in the occipitotemporal region and in the right prefrontal cortex, whereas in the patients with Alzheimer's disease the activity in the right prefrontal area was correlated only with activity in other regions of the prefrontal cortex, indicating that the interaction between the face processing area in extrastriate visual cortex and the frontal cortex was disrupted. A similar loss of functional connectivity was found in patients with Alzheimer's disease when they were asked to perform a visual working memory for faces task in which memory delay was varied systematically [42]. While healthy controls engaged a correlated functional network that included prefrontal, visual extrastriate and parietal areas and the hippocampus across the different memory delays, the Alzheimer patients failed to show any correlated activity between the prefrontal cortex and the hippocampus at any memory delay and had reduced correlations between the prefrontal cortex and visual cortical areas [42].

The results of these studies are consistent with and extend the observation of a disconnection between anterior and posterior cortical regions in the brain of patients with Alzheimer's disease found in the resting state [38, 39, 84].

Moreover, in patients in the initial or even in the preclinical phases of Alzheimer's disease abnormal patterns in the brain interregional metabolic correlations may be detectable even before significant changes in the neural activity of any specific cortical or subcortical structure become evident [39–41]. This suggests that the earliest effects of the developing neuropathological process are those of loosening the brain functional integrity and therefore affect the ability to rapidly integrate information that corresponds to the definition of consciousness itself [1, 2]. In this respect, a recent fMRI study showed that the functional connectivity between the hippocampus of both the hemispheres and posterior cingulate cortex present in healthy elderly controls was absent in individuals with amnestic mild cognitive impairment, who have a high risk of developing Alzheimer's disease but do not have dementia [89].

To conclude with a more positive note, we should say that the brain is not merely a passive bystander towards the neuropathological process. So, if many cortical regions loosen their functional connections, other areas may tighten theirs in an attempt to compensate for the losses attributable to the degenerative process, at least temporarily. In a study of semantic and episodic memory, patients with Alzheimer's disease in the mild stage of dementia recruited a unique and more extensive network of regions that included bilateral prefrontal and temporal cortex as compared to matched healthy subjects who showed a functional network between frontal and occipital areas in the left hemisphere [90]. Of note, neural activity in this network of regions was correlated with the ability of patients to perform the memory tasks, indicating that this extended functional network may compensate the disruption of the physiological network by facilitating the interactions among posterior storage regions and prefrontal areas that mediate executive and monitoring functions [90].

CONCLUSIONS

Awareness of what happens around us and of ourselves is rooted in the complexity of the functional and anatomical networks of the thalamocortical system that enables the brain to rapidly integrate information [1, 2]. If the integrity of the thalamocortical connectivity is altered, cognition and consciousness are impaired as well. Patients with dementing disorders represent a precious model to investigate the effects of the disruption of different brain structures and networks on the distinct components of consciousness. In this chapter, we have reviewed work by our own labs and other groups that have combined clinical, neuropsychological, neurochemical and post-mortem examinations with *in vivo* brain functional and structural measures in patients with Alzheimer's disease and other dementia syndromes in the effort to gain novel insights in the neural mechanisms that sustain consciousness and its dysfunction.

We have shown that distinct components of consciousness may be affected or spared selectively in individual patients according to the differential development of the neuropathological process within the brain. Sophisticated functional brain imaging studies have proved that the earliest effects of the neuropathological process are the loosening of the connections that enable different parts of the cortex to communicate among themselves. This impairment of functional connectivity is detectable even before any specific cortical region may reveal any metabolic or functional sign of dysfunction. Impairments in cholinergic neurotransmission, as seen in patients with Alzheimer's disease or Lewy Body Disease, may compromise neuronal information processing by decreasing signal-to-noise.

Obviously, here we have considered only some aspects of the topic and several important issues have only been mentioned or even ignored, including evidence from other forms of dementia or other neurological disorders, the role of other neurotransmitter systems and so on. While many questions remain widely open, the journey that scientist have begun in the dementing brain is providing new stimulating insights on how the mind arises and falls [91].

ACKNOWLEDGEMENTS

Research work by our groups reported in this chapter has been supported by the intramural National Institute on Aging/NIH program, a Young Investigator Award from the National Alliance for Research on Schizophrenia and Depression, the Italian Minister of Health (RF-TOS-2005-146663 to P.P.), the Italian Ministry of Education, University and Research (9706104230_003, 9806103083_002, 9906104777_008, MM06244347_003 to P.P.), and by Fondazione IRIS, Castagneto Carducci (Livorno, Italy to P.P.). Research work in the Cyclotron Research Centre, University of Liège, was supported by the National Fund for Scientific Research (FNRS), by the University of Liège, by the InterUniversity Attraction Pole P 6/29 (Belgian State-Belgian Science Policy) and by the EC-FP6-project DiMI, LSHB-CT-2005-512146. We thank Emiliano Ricciardi for comments on an earlier version of the chapter and Roberta Lariucci and Caterina Iofrida for assistance in the preparation of the manuscript.

References

1. Tononi, G. (2001) Information measures for conscious experience. *Arch Ital Biol* 139:367–371.
2. Tononi, G. (2005) Consciousness, information integration, and the brain. In *The Boundaries of Consciousness: Neurobiology and Neuropathology* S. Laureys (eds.) Elsevier Science. pp. 109–126.
3. Plum, F. (1991) Coma and related global disturbances of the human conscious state. In Peters, A. (eds.) *Normal and Altered States of Function Vol. 9*, pp. 359–425. New York: Plenum.
4. Laureys, S., *et al.* (2004) Brain function in coma, vegetative state, and related disorders. *Lancet Neurol* 3:537–546.
5. Kolb, B. and Whishaw, I.Q. (1996) *Fundamentals of Human Neuropsychology*, New York: Wh Freeman.
6. Bachman, D.L., *et al.* (1992) Prevalence of dementia and probable senile dementia of the Alzheimer type in the Framingham Study. *Neurology* 42:115–119.
7. Salmon, E., *et al.* (2005) Two aspects of impaired consciousness in Alzheimer's disease. *Prog Brain Res* 150:287–298.
8. Salmon, E., *et al.* (2006) Neural correlates of anosognosia for cognitive impairment in Alzheimer's disease. *Hum Brain Map* 2:588–597.
9. Pietrini, P., *et al.* (1996) Preferential metabolic involvement of visual cortical areas in a subtype of Alzhimer's disease: Clinical implications. *Am J Psychiatr* 153:1261–1268.
10. Pietrini, P., *et al.* (2000) The neurometabolic landscape of cognitive decline: *In vivo* studies with positron emission tomography in Alzheimer's disease. *Int J Psychophysiol* 37:87–98.

11. Grady, C.L., *et al.* (1988) Longitudinal study of the early neuropsychological and cerebral metabolic changes in dementia of the Alzheimer type. *J Clin Exp Neuropsychol* 10:576–596.

12. Haxby, J.V., *et al.* (1990) Longitudinal study of cerebral metabolic asymmetries and associated neuropsychological patterns in early dementia of the Alzheimer type. *Arch Neurol* 47:753–760.

13. Mendez, M.F., *et al.* (1990) Complex visual disturbances in Alzheimer's disease. *Neurology* 40:439–443.

14. Salmon, E., *et al.* (2007) On the multivariate nature of brain metabolic impairment in Alzheimer's disease. *Neurobiol Aging.* . doi:10.1016/j.neurobiolaging.2007.06.010

15. Terry, R.D. and Katzman, R. (1983) Senile dementia of the Alzheimer type. *Ann Neurol* 14 (5):497–506.

16. Whitehouse, P.J., *et al.* (1981) Alzheimer disease: Evidence for selective loss of cholinergic neurons in the nucleus basalis. *Ann Neurol* 10:122 126.

17. Braak, H. and Braak, E. (1991) Neuropathological stageing of Alzheimer-related changes. *Acta Neuropathol* 82:239–259.

18. Lewis, D.A., *et al.* (1987) Laminar and regional distributions of neurofibrillary tangles and neuritic plaques in Alzheimer's disease: A quantitative study of visual and auditory cortices. *J Neurosci* 7:1799–1808.

19. Hof, P.R., *et al.* (1995) The morphologic and neurochemical basis of dementia: Aging, hierarchical patterns of lesion distribution and vulnerable neuronal phenotype. *Rev Neurosci* 6 (2):97–124.

20. Van Hoesen, G.W., *et al.* (1991) Entorhinal cortex pathology in Alzheimer's disease. *Hippocampus* 1:1–8.

21. Whittam, R. (1962) The dependence of the respiration of brain cortex on active cation transport. *Biochem J* 82:205–212.

22. Jueptner, M. and Weiller, C. (1995) Review: Does measurement of regional cerebral blood flow reflect synaptic activity? Implications for PET and fMRI. *Neuroimage* 2:148–156.

23. Sokoloff, L. (1981) Relationships among local functional activity, energy metabolism and blood flow in the central nervous system. *Fed Proc* 40:2311–2316.

24. Schwartz, W.J., *et al.* (1979) Metabolic mapping of functional activity in the hypothalamo-neurohypophysial system of the rat. *Science* 205:723–725.

25. Kadekaro, M., *et al.* (1985) Differential effects of electrical stimulation of sciatic nerve on metabolic activity in spinal cord and dorsal root ganglion in the rat. *Proc Natl Acad Sci USA* 82:6010–6013.

26. Kadekaro, M., *et al.* (1987) Effects of antidromic stimulation of the ventral root on glucose utilization in the ventral horn of the spinal cord in the rat. *Proc Natl Acad Sci USA* 84:5492–5495.

27. Pietrini, P., *et al.* (2000) Brain metabolism in Alzheimer's disease and other dementing illnesses. In *Functional Neurobiology of Aging* P. Hof, and C. Mobbs, (eds.) San Diego, CA: Academic Press. pp. 227–242.

28. Duara, R., *et al.* (1986) Positron emission tomography in Alzheimer's disease. *Neurology* 36:879–887.

29. Grady, C.L. and Rapoport S.I. (1992) Cerebral metabolism in aging and dementia. *Handbook of Mental Health and Aging*, 201–208. Academic press.

30. Kumar, A., *et al.* (1991) High-resolution PET studies in Alzheimer's disease. *Neuropsychopharmacology* 4:35–46.

31. Pietrini, P., *et al.* (2000) Cerebral metabolic response to passive audiovisual stimulation in patients with Alzheimer's disease and healthy volunteers assessed by PET. *J Nucl Med* 41:575–583.

32. Grady, C.L., *et al.* (1990) Subgroups in dementia of the Alzheimer type identified using positron emission tomography. *J Neuropsychiatr Clin Neurosci* 2:373–384.

33. Haxby, J.V., *et al.* (1985) Relations between neuropsychological and cerebral metabolic asymmetries in early Alzheimer's disease. *J Cereb Blood Flow Metab* 5:193–200.

34. Pietrini, P., *et al.* (2000) The neurometabolic bases of aggressive behavior assessed by positron emission tomography in humans. *Am J Psychiatr* 157:1772–1781.

35. Haxby, J.V., *et al.* (1988) Heterogenous anterior-posterior metabolic patterns in dementia of the Alzheimer type. *Neurology* 38:1853–1863.

36. Furey-Kurkjian, M.L., *et al.* (1996) Visual variant of Alzheimer disease: Distinctive neuropsychological features. *Neuropsychology* 10:294–300.

37. Hof, P.R., *et al.* (1993) Posterior cortical atrophy in Alzheimer's disease: Analysis of a new case and revaluation of a historical report. *Acta Neuropatol* 86:215–223.

38. Horwitz, B., *et al.* (1987) Intercorrelations of regional cerebral glucose metabolic rates in Alzheimer's disease. *Brain Res* 407:294–306.

39. Azari, N.P., *et al.* (1992) Patterns of interregional correlations of cerebral glucose metabolic rates in patients with dementia of Alzheimer type. *Neurodegeneration* 1:101–111.

40. Azari, N.P., *et al.* (1993) Early detection of Alzheimer's disease: A statistical approach using positron emission tomographic data. *J Cereb Blood Flow Metab* 13:438–447.

41. Pietrini, P., *et al.* (1993) Pattern of cerebral metabolic interactions in a subject with isolated amnesia at risk for Alzheimer's disease: A longitudinal evaluation. *Dementia* 4:94–101.

42. Grady, C.L., *et al.* (2001) Altered brain functional connectivity and impaired short-term memory in Alzheimer's disease. *Brain* 124 (4):739–756.

43. Rombouts, S.A., *et al.* (2005) Altered resting state networks in mild cognitive impairment and mild Alzheimer's disease: An fMRI study. *Hum Brain Map* 26 (4):231–239.

44. Wang, L., *et al.* (2006) Changes in hippocampal connectivity in the early stages of Alzheimer's disease: Evidence from resting state fMRI. *Neuroimage* 31 (2):496–504.

45. Allen, G., *et al.* (2007) Reduced hippocampal functional connectivity in Alzheimer's disease. *Arch Neurol* 64:1482–1487.

46. Kalbe, E., *et al.* (2005) Anosognosia in very mild Alzheimer's disease but not in mild cognitive impairment. *Dement Geriatr Cogn Disord* 19:349–356.

47. Ruby, P., *et al.* (2007) Social mind representation: Where does it fail in frontotemporal dementia? *J Cogn Neurosci* 19 (4):671–683.

48. Salmon, E., *et al.* (2008) A comparison of unawareness in frontotemporal dementia and Alzheimer's disease. *J Neurol Neurosurg Psychiatr* 79:176–179.

49. Kotler-Cope, S. and Camp, C.J. (1995) Anosognosia in Alzheimer disease. *Alzheimer Dis Assoc Disord* 9:52–56.

50. Sevush, S. (1999) Relationship between denial of memory deficit and dementia severity in Alzheimer disease. *Neuropsychiatr Neuropsychol Behav Neurol* 12:88–94.

51. Gil, R., *et al.* (2001) Self-consciousness and Alzheimer's disease. *Acta Neurol Scand* 104 (5):296–300.

52. Zanetti, O., *et al.* (1999) Insight in dementia: When does it occur? Evidence for a nonlinear relationship between insight and cognitive status. *J Gerontol B Psychol Sci Soc Sci* 54:100–106.

53. O'Keeffe, F.M., *et al.* (2007) Loss of insight in frontotemporal dementia, corticobasal degeneration and progressive supranuclear palsy. *Brain* 130:753–764.

54. Cummings, J.L., *et al.* (1995) Depressive symptoms in Alzheimer disease: Assessment and determinants. *Alzheimer Dis Assoc Disord* 9:87–93.

55. Tabert, M.H., *et al.* (2002) Functional deficits in patients with mild cognitive impairment: Prediction of AD. *Neurology* 58:758–764.

56. Ruby, P., *et al.* (2008) Perspective taking to assess self-personality: What's modified in Alzheimer's disease? *Neurobiol Aging.* doi:10.1016/j.neurobiolaging.2007.12.014.

57. Frith, U. and Frith, C.D. (2003) Development and neurophysiology of mentalizing. *Philos Trans R Soc Lond B Biol Sci* 358 (1431):459–473.

58. Salmon, E., *et al.* (2003) Predominant ventromedial frontopolar metabolic impairment in frontotemporal dementia. *Neuroimage* 20:435–440.

59. Levine, D.N., *et al.* (1993) The visual variant of Alzheimer's disease: A clinicopathologic case study. *Neurology* 43:305–313.

60. Graff-Radford, N.R., *et al.* (1993) Simultagnosia as the initial sign of degenerative dementia. *Mayo Clin Proc* 68:955–964.

61. Pietrini, P., *et al.* (1993) A longitudinal PET study of cerebral glucose metabolism in patients with Alzheimer's disease and prominent visuospatial impairment. *Adv Biosci* 87:69–70.

62. Hof, P.R., *et al.* (1990) Selective disconnection of specific visual association pathways in cases of Alzheimer's disease presenting with Balint's syndrome. *J Neuropathol Exp Neurol* 2:168–184.

63. Haxby, J.V., *et al.* (1994) The functional organization of human extrastriate cortex: A PET-rCBF study of selective attention to faces and locations. *J Neurosci* 14:6336–6353.

64. Haxby, J.V., *et al.* (2001) Distributed and overlapping representations of faces and objects in ventral temporal cortex. *Science* 293:2425–2430.

65. Victoroff, J., *et al.* (1994) Posterior cortical atrophy. Neuropathologic correlations. *Arch Neurol* 51:269–274.

66. Holroyd, S. and Sheldon-Keller, A. (1995) A study of visual hallucinations in Alzheimer's disease. *Am J Geriatr Psychiatr* 3:198–205.

67. Holroyd, S., *et al.* (2000) Occipital atrophy is associated with visual hallucinations in Alzheimer's disease. *J Neuropsychiatr Clin Neurosci* 12:25–28.

68. Foerster, O. (1931) The cerebral cortex in man. *Lancet* 2:309–319.

69. Perry, R.H., *et al.* (1990) Senile dementia of Lewy body type: A clinically and neuropathologically distinct form of Lewy body dementia in the elderly. *J Neurol Sci* 95:119–139.

70. McKeith, I.G., *et al.* (1992) Operational criteria for senile dementia of Lewy body type (SDLT). *Psychol Med* 22:911–922.

71. Perry, E.K. and Perry, R.H. (1995) Acetylcholine and hallucinations: Disease-related compared to drug-induced alterations in human consciousness. *Brain Cogn* 28:240–258.

72. Ropacki, S.A. and Jeste, D.V. (2005) Epidemiology of and risk factors for psychosis of Alzheimer's disease: A review of 55 studies published from 1990 to 2003. *Am J Psychiatr* 162 (11):2022–2030.

73. Perry, R.H., *et al.* (1993) Cholinergic transmitter and neurotrophic activities in Lewy body dementia: Similarity to Parkinson's and distinction from Alzheimer disease. *Alzheimer Dis Assoc Disord* 7:69–79.

74. Drachman, D.A., Sahakian, B.J. (1979) Effects of cholinergic agents on human learning and memory, Nutrition and the Brain, 351–366.

75. Furey, M.L., *et al.* (2000) Cholinergic enhancement and increased selectivity of perceptual processing during working memory. *Science* 290:2315–2319.

76. Furey, M.L., *et al.* (2008) Selective effects of cholinergic modulation on task performance during selective attention. *Neuropsychopharmacology* 33:913–923.

77. Onofri, M., *et al.* (2007) New approaches to understanding hallucinations in Parkinson's disease: Phenomenology and possible origins. *Expert Rev Neurother* 7:1731–1750.

78. Nestor, P.J. (2007) The Lewy body, the hallucination, the atrophy and the physiology. *Brain* 130 (Pt 10):e81, .

79. Capgras, J. and Reboul-Lachaux, J. (1923) Illusion des sosies dans un délire systémisé chronique. *Bulletin de la Société Clinique de Médicine Mentale* 2:6–16.

80. Pick, A. (1903) Clinical studies: III. On reduplicative paramnesia. *Brain* 26:260–267.

81. Mentis, M.J., *et al.* (1995) Abnormal brain glucose metabolism in the delusional misidentification syndromes: A Positron Emission Tomography study in Alzheimer disease. *Biol Psychiatr* 38:438–449.

82. Price, B.H. and Mesulam, M. (1985) Psychiatric manifestations of right hemisphere infarctions. *J Nerv Ment Dis* 173:610–614.

83. Pandya, D.P. and Seltzer, B. (1982) Association areas of the cerebral cortex. *Trends Neurosci* 53:386–439.

84. Greicius, M.D., *et al.* (2004) Default-mode network activity distinguishes Alzheimer's disease from healthy aging: Evidence from functional MRI. *Proc Natl Acad Sc USA* 101:4637–4642.

85. Horwitz, B., *et al.* (1995) Network analysis of PET-mapped visual pathways in Alzheimer type dementia. *Neuroreport* 6 (17):2287–2292.

86. Minoshima, S., *et al.* (1994) Posterior cingulate cortex in Alzheimer's disease. *Lancet* 344:895, .

87. Meguro, K., *et al.* (1999) Neocortical and hippocampal glucose hypometabolism following neurotoxic lesions of the entorhinal and perirhinal cortices in the non-human primate as shown by PET. Implications for Alzheimer's disease. *Brain* 122 (8):1519–1531.

88. Bokde, A.L., *et al.* (2006) Functional connectivity of the fusiform gyrus during a face-matching task in subjects with mild cognitive impairment. *Brain* 129:1113–1124.

89. Sorg, C., *et al.* (2007) Selective changes of resting-state networks in individuals at risk for Alzheimer's disease. *Proc Natl Acad Sci USA* 104:18760–18765.

90. Grady, C.L., *et al.* (2003) Evidence from functional neuroimaging of a compensatory prefrontal network in Alzheimer's disease. *J Neurosci* 23:986–993.

91. Pietrini, P. (2003) Toward a biochemistry of mind? *Am J Psychiatr* 160:1907–1908.

Brain–Computer Interfaces for Communication in Paralysed Patients and Implications for Disorders of Consciousness

Andrea Kübler

ABSTRACT

Brain–computer interfaces (BCI) are direct connections between the brain and a computer. Regulation of neuroelectrical activity or brain activity as a response to sensory stimulation are used to select items, words, or letters in a communication programme or for neuroprosthesis control. Ten years work with severely paralysed and locked-in patients demonstrated that BCI can be utilized for communication and interaction with the environment if control of the motor periphery is lost. Recent non-visual BCI render this technology feasible for patients who even lost control of eye movement due to injury or disease. In addition to passive stimulation and volitional paradigms to assess cognitive processing in patients with disorders of consciousness (DOC), who may appear quite similar to patients with motor paralysis, the use of BCI is suggested in this article. This review of BCI and future prospects is a proposal to merge the so far independent streams of research – BCI in patients with paralysis and cognitive processing in patients with DOC – for the benefit of the patients and to further elucidate how much brain needs the mind.

BRAIN–COMPUTER INTERFACES: WHAT, WHY, AND WHERETO

Brain–computer interfaces (BCI) allow us to interact between the brain and artificial devices (for reviews see for example [1, 24–26]). They rely on continuous, real-time interaction between living neuronal tissue and artificial effectors (Box 17.1). Neuronal activity of few neurons or large cell assemblies is sampled and processed in real time and converted into commands

---

BOX 17.1

BCI FOR COMMUNICATION AND PROSTHESIS CONTROL

A BCI system can be depicted as a series of functional components [1, 2]. The starting point is the user, whose intent is coded in the neural activity of his or her brain (input). The end point is the device which is controlled by the brain activity of the user (output) and provides him or her with feedback of the current brain activity (closed-loop systems).

Invasive recording methods allow us recording of: (1) action potentials of single neurons with electrodes containing neurotrophic factors inducing nerve growth into the glass tip [3]; (2) patterns of neural activity with few or multiple electrode arrays [4–6]; (3) local field potentials [4, 7]; (4) electrocorticogram (ECoG) with electrode grids or stripes sub- or epidurally [8–10]); all invasive methods require surgery.

The *non-invasive recording* of the EEG is the most frequently used method in BCI research. Components most often used are (a) sensorimotor rhythms (SMR) [11–15], (b) slow cortical potentials [16, 17], and (c) event-related potentials (ERPs) as a response to sensory, auditory, or tactile stimulation, namely the P300, a positive deflection in the EEG about 300 ms after presentation of rare target stimuli within a stream of frequent standard stimuli [18, 19], and steady-state visually or somatosensorily evoked potentials [20, 21] as response to visual or tactile stimulation between 6–24 Hz [22].

The acquired signals are digitized and subjected to a variety of feature extraction procedures, such as spatial filtering, amplitude measurement, spectral analysis, or single-neuron separation [23]. In the following step a specific algorithm translates the extracted features into commands that represent the users' intent. These commands can either control effectors directly such as robotic arms or indirectly via cursor movement on a computer screen to activate switches for interaction with the environment or to select items, words, or letters from a menu for communication or to surf the Internet.

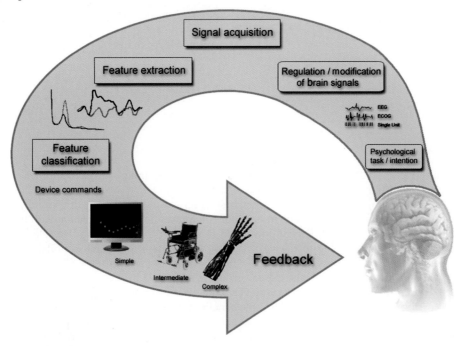

to control an application, such as a robot arm or a communication programme (e.g., [4, 16, 27]).

Brain activity is either recorded intracortically with multielectrode arrays or single electrodes, epi- or subdurally from the cortex or from the scalp. A variety of non-invasive technologies for monitoring brain activity may serve as a BCI (Boxes 17.1 and 17.2). In addition to electroencephalography (EEG) and invasive electrophysiological methods (Box 17.1), these include magnetoencephalography (MEG), positron emission tomography (PET), functional magnetic resonance imaging (fMRI, Box 17.2), and optical imaging (functional near infrared spectroscopy, fNIRS). As MEG, PET, and fMRI are demanding, tied to the laboratory, and expensive, these technologies are more suitable to address basic research questions and short-term intervention to localize sources of brain activity and to modify brain activity in diseases with known neurobiological dysfunction. In contrast, EEG, NIRS, and invasive systems are portable, and thus may offer practical BCI for communication and control in daily life.

In many studies it has been shown that patients with severe motor impairment and patients in the locked-in state (LIS), in which only residual muscular movement such as eye blinking is possible, were able to achieve control over a BCI and to use this ability for communication [16, 17, 28, 29]. In exemplary patients, control of a neuroprosthetic arm [4, 30] and the patient's own paralysed limb by means of an orthosis [31] or functional electric stimulation [27] has been demonstrated. In all these patients communication and control was restricted due to motor impairment, and a BCI can provide a key for the conscious brain locked into a paralysed body.

Patients with disorders of consciousness (DOC) may phenomenologically be similar to LIS patients or patients in the complete locked-in state (CLIS) in which no voluntary muscular movement is possible due to complete motor paralysis. The reason for the non-responsiveness, however, is quite different. The connections between the brain and its motor effectors may be intact, yet the commanding centres and their interaction are disturbed or destroyed due to traumatic or non-traumatic brain injury [32].

To date the vast majority of studies with DOC patients use passive stimulation paradigms to infer cortical processing [33–35]. Patients are confronted with auditory or tactile stimulation and the related brain activity is recorded with EEG, PET, or fMRI. From a comparison with the brain activity seen in healthy volunteers with the same stimulation it is deduced how much cerebral processing is maintained. Impressive abilities – in relation to the brain

injury – were found in those studies including semantic differentiation of auditorily presented sentences [34]. The question whether conscious and intentional processing is still possible and may not be expressed due to motor impairment, aphasia, akinesia, or disturbed arousal cannot be answered with such paradigms. The decipherment of consciousness is still one of the major challenges of neuroscience [36]. The high diagnostic insecurity with regards to DOC patients [37, 38] adds to the urgency of the matter. BCI may offer a new tool for intervention and interaction with DOC patients as they proved their feasibility in many severely disabled patients.

In this chapter I will give an overview of the traditional patient groups targeted by BCI research. Subsequently I will present a review of the state-of-the-art in BCI research with patients. A section follows on non-visual BCI which I consider indispensable if BCI are to be used with DOC patients. The issue of learning in the complete locked-in (=non-responsive) state will be discussed, I will suggest a hierarchical approach to cognitive processing in DOC patients including volitional tasks and BCI, and I will end with a critical discussion of prospects for BCI in DOC patients.

BCI FOR COMMUNICATION AND CONTROL: TARGETED PATIENTS

A variety of neurological diseases with different neuropathology may lead to the so-called LIS in which only residual voluntary muscular control is possible. In the 'classic' locked-in syndrome (see Chapter 15), vertical eye movement and eye blinks remain intact [39], whereas in the CLIS, patients lose all ability to move and communicate [40, 41]. Haemorrhage or an ischaemic stroke in the ventral pons can cause a locked-in syndrome, which includes tetraplegia and paralysis of cranial nerves [42]. The syndrome can also occur due to traumatic brainstem injury [39], encephalitis [43], or tumour [44]. Other causes of the LIS are degenerative neurological diseases [45], the most frequent being amyotrophic lateral sclerosis, which involves a steadily progressive degeneration of central and peripheral motoneurons [46].

Despite the variable disease aetiology the affected patients are very similar such that they can hardly communicate, have no control over limb movement, depend on intensive care, are artificially fed and often also ventilated, and lack immediate reinforcement of thoughts and intentions [40, 41]. In most cases residual muscular control like blinking and eye movement

BOX 17.2

REAL-TIME FMRI: THE BOLD RESPONSE AS INPUT SIGNAL FOR BCI

Since approximately 7 years it has been possible to use the blood oxygen level-dependent (BOLD) response as input signal for a BCI (top figure). State-of-the-art real-time fMRI may employ tailored magnetic resonance imaging (MRI) acquisition techniques for optimal speed and data quality, such as multiecho echo-planar imaging (mEPI) or adaptive multiresolution EPI [47]. Online pre-processing techniques include distortion correction, prospective or retrospective 3D motion correction, temporal filtering, spatial smoothing and spatial normalization to stereotactic space. The real-time implemented data analysis and statistical methods includes *t*-tests, correlation analysis, general linear model (GLM) and multiple regression, and independent component analysis [47]. The result of pre-processing, data analysis, and statistical analysis is then fed back to the participant. Feedback can be provided via a 'thermometer' (top Figure). The blue bar moves up and gets red for activation and moves down for deactivation of the region-of-interest. The background colour indicates the task: red for activation, blue for deactivation [48, 49].

Compared to EEG, fMRI allows us spatial resolution in the range of millimetres and a more precise allocation of neuronal activity. Additionally activation in subcortical areas can be recorded. Target areas for feedback were sensory (S1, e.g., [50]) and motor areas (M1, e.g., [51], or supplementary motor area, SMA [52]), the parahippocampal place area [52], and rostral anterior cingulate cortex (ACC) [53]. Learning of regulation of the BOLD response proved possible and behavioural effects were reported in relation to activation or deactivation of targeted areas: for example, decreased reaction time in a motor task after up-regulation of the SMA was demonstrated [52]. Regulation of the insula, an area involved in emotional processing, proved also possible and was shown to increase the negative valence of participants when confronted with negative stimuli such as pictures of violence or mutilated bodies [48]. Specific effects on pain perception as a function of self-regulation of the rostral part of the ACC was reported in the first clinical study including patients with chronic pain, and reduced pain ratings after deactivation of ACC was found [53].

In a pilot study regulation of ACC which is also involved in inhibitory control and error monitoring [54], and its effect on behaviour was demonstrated in six healthy subjects (bottom Figure). When confronted with a Go-NoGo task after up-regulation, the number of commission errors (failed inhibitions) was reduced (the figure is with kind permission of Ralf Veit, Ute Strehl, and Tilman Gaber from the Institute of Medical Psychology and Behavioural Neurobiology, University of Tübingen, who conducted the experiment and data analysis). The region-of-interest is encircled; the lighter the colour the higher the activation compared to baseline. The *T*-value of activity is given in the adjacent colour scale. Other areas were co-activated depending on the strategy used for regulation.

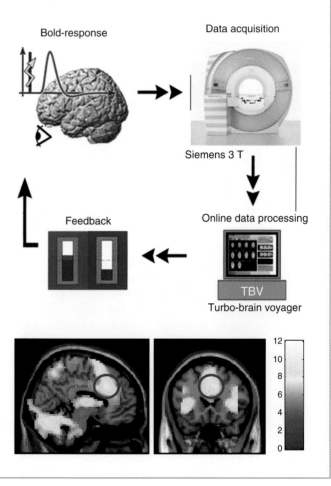

remains available. However, patients may also be or enter – with disease progression – in the CLIS in which no muscular control and thus, no communication is possible [41]. I further refer to non-responsive patients, regardless of aetiology, as CLIS patients.

BRAIN–COMPUTER INTERFACING IN PATIENTS WITH MOTOR DISABILITY

Table 17.1 lists the number and type of patients who have been involved in BCI research for the past 10 years. Patients with epilepsy and facial pain are clearly not in need of a BCI, but are targeted, because they are implanted with an electrode grid for ECoG before surgery.

Two approaches to BCI control exist, although almost all BCI realize a mixture of both approaches: (1) learning to voluntarily regulate brain activity by means of neurofeedback and operant learning principles [16]. Following training different brain states can be produced on command and thus, become suitable to control devices. (2) Machine learning procedures which enable us to infer the statistical signature of specific brain states or intentions within a calibration session; decoding algorithms are individually adapted to the users that perform the task [11, 25].

In the following I will give a summary of BCI research with patients; that is, work with healthy subjects, with BCI for other purposes than communication and control, and animals will not be included; the reader is referred to existing reviews [24, 26, 55, 56].

Non-invasive BCI with the EEG as Input Signal (EEG-BCI)

Non-invasive BCI use the electrical activity of the brain (EEG) recorded with single or multiple electrodes from the scalp surface as input signal for BCI control. Participants are presented with stimuli or are required to perform specific mental tasks while the electrical activity of their brains is being recorded. Extracted and relevant EEG features can then be fed back to the user by so-called closed-loop BCI. Specific features of the EEG are either regulated by the BCI user (SCP, SMR) or are elicited by sensory stimulation (ERPs).

SCP as Input Signal for BCI (SCP-BCI)

The vertical arrangement of pyramidal cells in the cortex is essential for the generation of SCP. Most apical dendrites of pyramidal cells are located in cortical layers I and II. Depolarization of the apical dendrites giving rise to SCP is dependent on sustained afferent intracortical or thalamocortical input to layers I and II,

TABLE 17.1   Disease and Number of Patients Who Have Participated in BCI Training for Communication and Control since 1997

Disease	Number of patients	BCI input signal	Published in
Amyotrophic lateral sclerosis	37	EEG (SCP, SMR, ERP) ECoG, intracortical (action potentials)	[3, 10, 12, 16–19, 29, 57–65]
Spinal cord injury	15	EEG (SMR, ERP) intracortical (neural ensemble activity)	[4, 13, 19, 27, 30, 66–69]
Guillan-Barré syndrome	2	EEG (SMR, ERP)	[10, 68]
Muscular dystrophy	1	EEG (SCP)	[70]
Cerebral paresis	1	EEG (SCP, SMR)	[28]
Classic locked-in syndrome (after stroke in the pons)	3	EEG (SCP, ERP)	[64, 68, 71]
Stroke (other)	1	EEG (SMR)	[10]
Cerebral palsy	2	EEG (SMR, ERP)	[19, 72]
Multiple sclerosis	2	EEG (ERP)	[19, 68]
Post-anoxic encephalopathy	2	EEG (SMR, ERP)	[10, 19]
Epilepsy	14	ECoG	[8, 9, 73, 74]
Intractable facial pain	1	ECoG	[8]
Factor-Q deficiency	1	Intracortical (action potentials)	[75]

Note: If the same patients were published in several articles, the patient – if identifiable – was counted only once and only one article is cited in the table.

and on simultaneous depolarization of large pools of pyramidal neurons [76]. The SCP amplitude recorded from the scalp depends upon the synchronicity and intensity of the afferent input to layers I and II. The depolarization of cortical cell assemblies reduces their excitation threshold. Firing of neurons in regions responsible for specified motor or cognitive tasks is facilitated. Negative amplitude shifts grow with increasing attentional or cognitive resource allocation. Cortical positivity may result from active inhibition of apical dendritic neural activity or simply from a reduction of afferent inflow and subsequent reduced post-synaptic activity. A strong relationship between self-induced cortical negativity and reaction time, signal detection, and short-term memory performance has been reported in several studies in humans and monkeys [76].

Over the past 10 years 28 paralysed patients were trained with the SCP-BCI [41] (Figure 17.1). Twenty-three were diagnosed with amyotrophic lateral sclerosis (ALS), one with chronic Guillan-Barré syndrome, one with muscular dystrophy, one with cerebral paresis, and one had post-anoxic encephalopathy. Twenty of the patients were either tetraplegic with severely impaired speech, in the LIS or CLIS (6) [41]. Eighteen of the patients achieved significant cursor control within a few training sessions [41] and learned to use this ability for communication, which required to regulate the SCP amplitude with at least 70% accuracy [16, 17, 77]; performance above 70% correct is referred to as criterion level control [41, 55]. Although the SCP-BCI takes quite a while until patients are able to communicate, messages of considerable length were communicated [16, 70, 77]. The number of training sessions needed to achieve significant cursor control was moderately predictive for the time needed to achieve criterion level control [57]; other reliable predictors could not be found [78]. Learning occurred in the early stages of training and patients remained stable around the performance level, which they achieved in the first 10 to 20 training sessions [57, 78]. Having predictors of BCI training outcome is desirable, because BCI training with patients is a substantial effort for both patients and trainers.

In summary, regulation of the SCP amplitude can be achieved by patients with severe paralysis. SCP-BCI training may require a substantial amount of time, but has the advantage that it can be initiated without the presence of a classifiable brain response. Following a shaping schedule [17] every response in accordance with the task requirement has to be positively reinforced (operant conditioning). SCP-BCI were used for verbal communication and Internet surfing: all the links of one website are assigned to either the top or

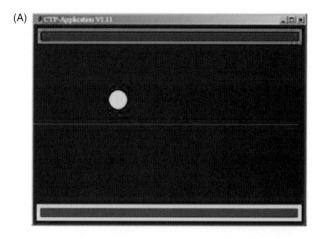

(A)

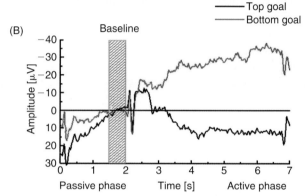

(B)

FIGURE 17.1   *The SCP-BCI*: The EEG was recorded with single electrodes. (A) To learn regulation of the SCP amplitude, patients were presented with two targets one at the top and one at the bottom of the screen. Continuous feedback was provided from the Cz electrode in discrete trials via cursor movement on a computer screen. Patients' task was to move the cursor (yellow dot) towards the target with the highlighted frame. The cursor moved steadily from left to right and its vertical deflection corresponded to the SCP amplitude. (B) Time course of the SCP amplitude averaged across 200 trials separated by task requirement. A negative SCP amplitude (red line) moved the cursor towards the top, positive SCP amplitude (black line) towards the bottom target. At time point −2 seconds the task was presented, at 500 ms the baseline was recorded, and at 0 cursor movement started. Positive and negative SCP amplitude shifts were clearly distinguishable indicating that the participant learned to manipulate the SCP amplitude.

bottom half of the screen. The number of links per target is divided after selection until a single link is presented for selection [79].

SMR as Input Signal for BCI (SMR-BCI)

SMR include arch-shaped mu-rhythm usually with a frequency of 10 Hz (range 8–11 Hz) often mixed with a beta (around 20 Hz) and a gamma component (around 40 Hz) recorded over somatosensory cortices, most preferably over C3 and C4 [80]. Spreading to parietal leads is frequent and is also seen in patients with ALS [12]. The SMR is related to the motor cortex with contributions of somatosensory areas such that the beta component arises from the motor, the alphoid mu-component from sensory cortex. SMR desynchronizes with movement, movement imagery, and movement preparation (event-related desynchronization, ERD), and increases or synchronizes (event-related synchronization, ERS) in the post-movement period or during relaxation [81]. Thus, it is regarded as 'idling' rhythm of the cortical sensory region.

Operant learning of SMR regulation is achieved through activation and deactivation of the central motor loops. To learn to modulate the power of SMR, patients are also presented with feedback, for example, cursor movement on a computer screen in one or two dimensions [82, 83] and instructed to imagine a movement of, for example, fingers or legs (Figure 17.2). Using the SMR-BCI it was shown that ALS patients were able to achieve SMR regulation of more than 75% accuracy within less than 20 training sessions [12]. To date, Wolpaw and his colleagues trained patients with spinal cord injury, cerebral palsy, and ALS to control cursor movement in one or two dimensions towards 2 to 8 targets via regulation of the SMR amplitude [13, 58, 66, 72, 83]. In one study participants (including one minor impaired ALS patient) used SMR regulation to answer yes/no questions, such that the two targets were replaced by the words YES and NO [59].

Neuper and colleagues reported results of a patient with infantile cerebral paresis, who was trained over a period of several months with the SMR-BCI [28]. The patient was trained with a two-target task. Eventually, the targets were replaced by letters and the patient could spell with the system, using a so-called virtual keyboard. The spelling rate varied between 0.2 and 2.5 letters per minute. Although this rate may seem slow, Neuper and colleagues showed for the first time that SMR-BCI could provide communication for patients in the LIS. During training of this patient a telemonitoring system was implemented allowing the experimenter to control and supervise BCI training from the laboratory [60, 84]. This is particularly important if patients wish to use a BCI for daily communication and are located far away from the BCI laboratory.

Besides communication, SMR-BCI mediated neuroprosthesis control was implemented in two exemplary patients. First, a tetraplegic patient after spinal cord injury whose residual muscle activity of the upper limbs was restricted to the left biceps learned to open and close his hand with the aids of an orthosis which reacted upon changes in SMR [31]. The authors report an accuracy of almost 100%. In a second study with the same patient grasping movement was realized via SMR-BCI controlled functional electric stimulation [27].

(A)
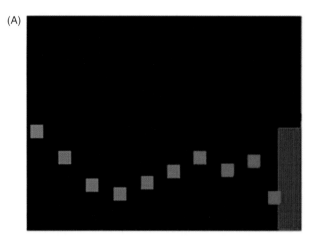

(B)
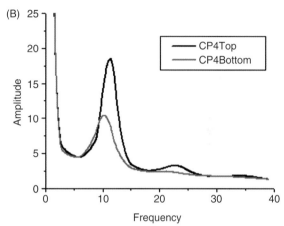

FIGURE 17.2 *SMR-BCI*: (A) During each trial of one-dimensional control, users were presented with a target consisting of a red vertical bar that occupied the top or bottom half of the right edge of the screen and a cursor on the left edge. The cursor moved steadily across the screen, with its vertical movement controlled by the SMR amplitude. Patients' task was to move the cursor into the target. Cursor movement is indicated by the squares; during feedback of SMR amplitude, only one square was visible. Low SMR amplitude following movement imagery moved the cursor to the bottom bar, high SMR amplitude following thinking of nothing in particular (relaxation) moved the cursor towards the top bar. Cursor movement into different targets could also be achieved by different movement imagery (e.g., left vs. right hand or feet vs. hand movement). (B) Amplitude of the EEG as a function of frequency power spectrum averaged across 230 trials separated by task requirement (top vs. bottom target). Black line indicates frequency power spectrum when the cursor had to be moved towards the top target; red line when the cursor had to be moved towards the bottom target. A difference in amplitude can be clearly seen around the 10 Hz SMR peak.

Another patient with spinal cord injury (below C5) used the SMR-BCI system for neuroprosthesis control [30]. The patient was trained with the so-called Basket paradigm. A trial consisted of a ball descending from the top to the bottom of a black screen. Baskets (serving as cues) positioned either on the left or the right half of the screen indicated by their colour (red: target; green: non-target) which type of imagery the patient should perform to move the ball into the basket. Then the BCI was coupled with the neuroprosthesis. Each detection of left hand motor imagery switched the neuroprosthesis subsequently to grasping movement. Krausz and colleagues trained four wheelchair-bound paraplegic patients with the 'Basket paradigm'. After a few sessions, within weeks, all patients learned to control the BCI with the best session between 77–95% accuracy [67].

In summary, SMR-BCI have been successfully tested in ALS, cerebral paresis, and spinal cord injury patients and may provide communication or rudimentary restoration of lost motor function. With the SMR-BCI patients learnt cursor control faster than with the SCP-BCI. Supposedly, suitable strategies are provided via the specific instruction to imagine a movement; therefore, these strategies are more readily available.

ERPs as Input Signals for BCI (ODDBALL-BCI)

ERPs are electrocortical potentials that can be measured in the EEG before, during, or after a sensory, motor, or psychological event. They have a fixed time delay to the stimulus and their amplitude is usually much smaller than the ongoing spontaneous, EEG activity. To detect ERP averaging techniques are used. An averaged ERP is composed of a series of large, biphasic waves, lasting a total of 500–1000 ms [85]. The P300 component of the ERP and steady-state visually or somatosensorily (see section on 'Non-visual BCI') evoked potentials have been used as input signal for BCI.

The P300 is a positive deflection in the EEG time-locked to stimuli presentation. It is typically seen when participants are required to attend to a stream of rare target stimuli and frequent standard stimuli, an experimental design referred to as an oddball paradigm [86]. It is mostly observed in central and parietal regions (Box 17.3). It is seen as a correlate of an extinction process in short-term memory when new stimuli require an update of representations [85].

Although the prototype of a P300-BCI (Figure 17.3) was published in 1988 [87], it was not until recently, that ERPs were tested and used in BCI for paralysed patients. Presented with a 6 × 6 matrix (Figure 17.3) ALS patients achieved accuracies up to 100% [88]. Nijober and colleagues showed that patients with ALS can use the P300-BCI for free and independent communication [29]. The P300 response was also demonstrated to remain stable over a period from 12 to more than 50 daily sessions in healthy volunteers as well as in ALS patients [18, 29]. Sellers and Donchin introduced a visual and auditory 4-choice spelling system which allowed patients yes/no communication [18] (see also section on 'Non-visual BCI'). Piccione and

colleagues required their participants (five patients with paralysis of different aetiology among healthy participants) to choose one of four arrows pointing to top, down, left, and right on a monitor to move a virtual object from a starting to an end point along a specific path pre-set by the trainer. Patients' mean accuracy was about 69% [68]. In a 6-choice paradigm Hoffmann and colleagues achieved 100% accuracy for both healthy participants and severely disabled patients with paralysis and speech impairment of different origin [19], as did Neshige and colleagues with ALS patients in a 4-choice paradigm, a 5 × 5 matrix with symbols and even a 5 × 10 sounds matrix (Japanese) [61] (see Table 17.1 for patients' diagnosis).

In most patients classification of ERP to target and non-target stimuli was possible [18, 29, 68]. However, shape and latency of the ERP may differ from that of potentials in healthy controls [18]. In two of the patients of Sellers and Donchin large and late positive and negative potentials were found as response to the targets [18]. Similarly, one of the patients of Nijboer and colleagues controlled the 'P300-BCI' with a negative potential of 200 ms latency [29]. Altered waveforms, latencies, and topographies are typically seen in LIS and CLIS patients [89]. Thus, it might be more appropriate to refer to the P300-BCI or P300-speller as ODDBALL-BCI or Oddball-speller.

Taken together, to achieve control of the SCP- and SMR-BCI is more time consuming than that of the ODDBALL-BCI, because the latter requires no learning to regulate the EEG. With the ODDBALL-BCI 100% accuracy and selection rates of up to 10 items per minute were achieved. If classifiable ERP can be detected, the ODDBALL-BCI is the method of choice for communication. The SCP- and SMR-BCI are advantageous if a specific brain response is not readily available, because they allow the user learning on the basis of operant conditioning.

INVASIVE BCI

Invasive recording methods (Box 17.1) have strong advantages in terms of signal quality and dimensionality [73], but issues of long-term stability of implants and protection from infection arise [4]; all require surgery. Intracortical recording methods require electrodes that penetrate the brain whereas electrode grids for ECoG remain on the cortical surface.

Intracortical Signals as Input for BCI

Studies with invasive recordings for the purpose of communication and control with a BCI are sparse.

BOX 17.3

AN AUDITORY BCI IN A LIS/CLIS PATIENT

In the auditory 5 × 5 letter matrix (top left) the rows and columns are auditorily coded by numbers from 1 to 10. Selection occurs by attending to those stimuli which are corresponding to the coordinate of the target letter in the matrix. Presentation of the stimuli coding the rows (1–5) is followed by a classification and continues with the presentation of the stimuli coding the columns of the matrix (6–10) followed by a second classification [90]. In future, after selection of a row, the letters will be presented directly. In addition to presenting the numbers which code the letters auditorily, the matrix is also displayed on a monitor placed in front of the BCI user. If all vision is lost, users have to learn the structure of the matrix by heart. For initial training users have to spell a pre-set word given by the trainer (top line above the matrix). In each of the trials the letter in parenthesis has to be selected and selected letters appear in the line below and are also presented auditorily.

GR, a 39 years old man, was diagnosed with first symptoms of ALS in 1996. When we met him first January 2006, he was able to communicate yes/no with a twitch of the right corner of the mouth. He controlled a mouse with thumb movement, which enabled him to use digital programs for communication, emailing, and Internet surfing. Control of eye movement was unreliable.

To date (July 2007), GR lost thumb control and communication by means of twitching with the lip is unreliable. On first encounter we used a simple oddball paradigm to test GR for P300. Having already the 4-choice speller [18] in mind, we confronted him with a sequence of 4 tones of different pitch in random order; each tone had a probability of 25%. GR's task was to count the lowest tones and he had 'textbook' P300 to the target tones (solid line in top right graph – thanks to Eric Sellers, Wadsworth Center, New York State Department of Health, Albany, New York, for this figure). Within the following 1½ years we presented him with a German version of the 4-choice speller (middle right) and the 5 × 5 auditory letter matrix (bottom right) (solid line shows averaged EEG to target words or letters, dashed line to non-targets). The P300 was typically most prominent at parietal sites (bottom left). His performance varied strongly across days and even within a day but approached 100% accuracy in some sessions. These encouraging results indicate that patients who are partially in the CLIS can communicate with an auditory BCI (thanks to PhD students Adrian Furdea, Sebastian Halder, Eva-Maria Hammer, and Femke Nijboer, at the Institute of Medical Psychology and Behavioural Neurobiology, University of Tübingen, for data acquisition, analysis, and graphs).

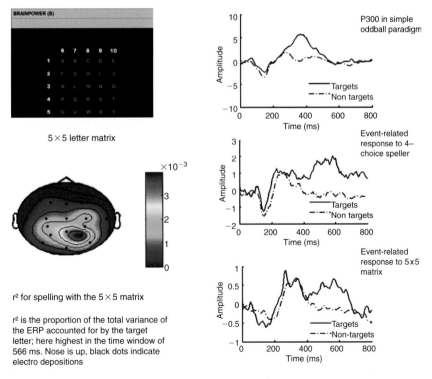

5 × 5 letter matrix

r^2 for spelling with the 5 × 5 matrix

r^2 is the proportion of the total variance of the ERP accounted for by the target letter; here highest in the time window of 566 ms. Nose is up, black dots indicate electro depositions

(A)

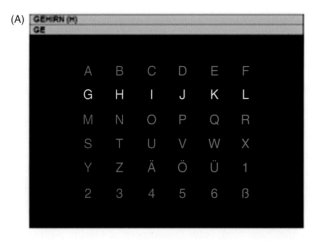

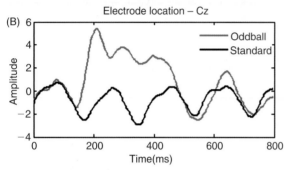

FIGURE 17.3 *P300-BCI/ODDBALL-BCI*: For communication with a P300-BCI users were typically presented with matrices where each of the matrix cell contained a character or a symbol. (A) This figure depicts a 6 × 6 letter matrix. This design becomes an oddball paradigm by first, intensifying each row and column for 100 ms in random order and second, by instructing participants to attend to only one of the cells. In one sequences of flashes (one flash for each row and each column), the target cell will flash only twice constituting a rare event compared to the flashes of all other rows and columns and will therefore elicit a P300 [87]. Selection occurs by detecting the row and column which elicit the largest P300 [91]. The P300-BCI did not require self-regulation of the EEG. All that was required from the users was that they were able to focus attention and gaze on the target letter albeit for a considerable amount of time. In the copy spelling mode [17], the patients' task was to copy the word presented in the top line (GEHIRN = German for 'brain'). In each trial, patients had to count how often the target letter flashed. The target letter was presented in parenthesis at the end of the word. Selected letters were presented in the second line below the word to copy. (B) This panel depicts EEG to target letters (red line) averaged across 43 trials comprising 430 flashes of the target letter and 2150 flashes of all rows and columns not containing the target letter. Black line indicates the course of the EEG to all the non-target rows and columns (for an exact description of letter selection see for example [88]). EEG to target letters was clearly distinguishable from non-target letters.

Kennedy and Bakay showed in few ALS patients that humans were able to modulate the action potential firing rate when provided with feedback [3, 71]. The authors implanted into the motor cortex a single electrode with a glass tip containing neurotrophic

factors. Adjacent neurons grew into the tip and after few weeks action potentials were recorded. One patient was able to move a cursor on a computer screen to select presented items. However, a quadriplegic patient with factor-Q deficiency who had significant atrophy in sensorimotor cortices failed to achieve control of the action potential firing rate [75].

Hochberg and colleagues implanted a multielectrode array in the hand motor area of two patients with tetraplegia following spinal cord injury [4]. Neural activity from field potentials was translated into movement of a robotic arm and continuous mouse movement on a computer monitor. However, none of the invasive procedures allowed restoration of skilful movement in daily life situations.

The ECoG as Input Signal for BCI (ECoG-BCI)

The ECoG is measured with strips or arrays epidurally or subdurally from the cortical surface. ECoG-BCI have been tested with epilepsy patients in whom electrode grids were implanted for the purpose of later brain surgery to treat epilepsy. Modulation of the ECoG as a function of actual or imagined movement or both was recorded [8, 9]. Presented with a one-dimensional binary task, patients achieved 74–100% accuracy by imagery of speech, hand, and tongue movement [73, 74]. Encouraged by these results it was tried to reinstall communication in an ALS patient in the CLIS [56]. The patient responded to sensory stimulation (finger and mouth) and the corresponding areas in S1 were perfectly localizable, but when regulation of this activity was required by imagery of finger and tongue movement no classification of the signal was possible. This underlines convincingly and dramatically that results of healthy BCI users or patients diagnosed with other diseases which do not lead to paralysis of the motor system or otherwise to non-responsiveness, are not sufficient to claim that a BCI is suitable to maintain communication and control in LIS and non-responsive CLIS patients.

NON-VISUAL BCI

Almost all approaches to BCI rely on intact vision. Intact gaze and reliable control of eye movement are the pre-requisite for all these BCI which render them unsuitable for CLIS patients. BCI based on auditory and tactile information presentation may provide a solution to this problem. Visual BCI allow us the presentation of the task requirement, the items to select and the feedback of brain activity simultaneously on a monitor; likewise selected items or hit targets and positive reinforcement (in BCI that use operant conditioning to learn regulation of a brain response) can also be presented simultaneously. The difficulty for auditory BCI is that all information about the task, the items to select, the feedback of brain activity, the results of selection and positive reinforcement has to be presented consecutively. To date, SCP, SMR, and ERPs where used as input signals for non-visual BCI.

Hinterberger and colleagues compared learning to regulate the SCP amplitude of the EEG by means of visual or auditory feedback or a combination of the two modalities [92]. Visual feedback was superior to the auditory and combined feedback, but BCI control could be also achieved with auditory feedback. Presentation of combined feedback prevented learning. The superiority of visual over auditory feedback was also found in the first study that used auditory feedback of SMR [93]. SMR desynchronization was represented by bongo sounds and synchronization by harp sounds. With visual feedback participants achieved high performance already in the first training session. In contrast, with auditory feedback, participants started at chance level indicating that they had no control over their SMR amplitude. After three training sessions, however, performance was the same in both groups. Thus, auditory feedback required more training, but lead to approximately the same level of performance at the end of training. The authors concluded that a 2-choice BCI based on auditory feedback is feasible for communication provided sufficient time for learning [93].

Hill and co-workers attempted to classify P300 evoked responses to two simultaneously presented auditory stimulus streams [94]. Both streams constituted an auditory oddball paradigm. To choose one of two possible targets, the participant had to focus on either one of the streams. When attention was focused on the target stimuli (e.g., by counting them), EEG responses to target stimuli and standard stimuli could be classified. Although variation between participants existed, classification results suggested that it was possible for a user to direct conscious attention, and thereby to modulate the ERPs to auditory stimuli reliably enough, in single trials, to provide a useful basis for an auditory BCI.

Sellers and Donchin tested healthy volunteers and patients with ALS with a 4-choice ODDBALL-BCI (4-choice speller). Patients were presented either visually or auditorily or both with the words 'yes', 'no', 'pass', and 'end' [18]. The patients' task was to focus their attention on either 'yes' or 'no'. The authors were able to show that a target probability of 25%

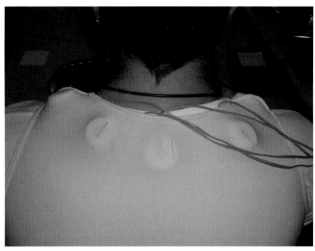

FIGURE 17.4 *The vibrotactile BCI*: Feedback was provided via vibrotactile transducers mounted around the neck between two T-Shirts. A contactor in the centre of a magnetic coil through which current was flowing moved against the skin and back at a frequency of 200 Hz. Imagery of right hand movement activated the contactors on the right hand side of the neck and imagery of left hand movement those of the left hand side. *Source*: The photograph is with kind permission from Dr. Febo Cincotti, Laboratory of Neuroelectrical Imaging and Brain Computer Interface, Fondazione Santa Lucia IRCCS, Rome, Italy.

was low enough to reliably elicit a P300. In contrast to combined feedback in the SCP-BCI [92], simultaneous presentation of auditory and visual stimuli with the 4-choice speller did not lead to a decrement in classification.

An auditory ERP based spelling system was also proposed [90]. This system is simulating a 5×5 matrix containing letters (Box 17.3). Healthy subjects achieved an accuracy above 70% which is the criterion level for spelling [17, 41]. The auditory 4-choice speller and the 5×5 letter matrix were tested in an LIS patient on the border of becoming completely locked-in (Box 17.3).

A BCI based on steady-state evoked potentials independent of vision was introduced by Müller-Putz and colleagues [20]. The authors used vibratory stimulation of left and right hand finger tips to elicit somatosensory steady-state evoked potentials (SSSEP). The EEG was recorded from central electrodes (C3, Cz, and C4). In each trial both index fingers were stimulated simultaneously at different frequencies and participants were instructed via arrows on a computer screen to which finger they should pay attention. Online accuracies of four participants varied between 53% (chance level) and 83%.

Most recently, vibrotactile feedback of SMR was realized by Cincotti and colleagues [95] (Figure 17.4). Accuracy for six subjects was with 56–77% comparable to visual feedback (58–80%).

Taken together, studies with non-visual BCI imply that learning to regulate brain activity such as SCP and SMR when provided with auditory or tactile feedback is possible albeit slower than with visual feedback. ERPs in response to auditory or tactile stimulus presentation were also classifiable with a BCI. Non-visual BCI allowed the users to achieve accuracies high enough to use the BCI for communication and control. These BCI await testing with LIS and CLIS patients, but first results with a patient on the border of becoming completely paralysed (Box 17.3) are encouraging.

BCI IN DOC

To date, BCI have not been tested or used in patients diagnosed with DOC. From the review provided above, it is clear that to operate a BCI, understanding of instruction, volition, and sustained attention and decision making are necessary at least for a period of time. In the case of the SCP- and SMR-BCI susceptibility to operant conditioning including reinforcement is necessary.

Learning in LIS and Non-responsive CLIS Patients

Little is known about learning in locked-in or completely locked-in patients. In an N100 (mismatch negativity, MMN) paradigm applied to 33 patients in the vegetative state Kotchoubey and colleagues showed habituation to the deviant tone indicating the presence of an elementary learning process [96]. With neuropsychological tests Schnakers and colleagues found slightly impaired learning and long-term memory in 2 of 10 LIS patients after brainstem stroke [97]. In a group of 11 severely impaired patients with ALS (including 6 LIS patients) Lakerveld and colleagues demonstrated learning and memory in a verbal and non-verbal learning test being as good as in matched healthy controls and as compared to normative data [98].

Piccione and colleagues found that with the visual ODDBALL-BCI paralysed patients' performance (68.6%) was worse than that of healthy participants (76.2%) [68]. In particular, those patients who were more impaired performed worse, whereas there was no difference between less impaired patients and healthy participants [68]. However, Nijboer and colleagues could not confirm such a relation between ODDBALL-BCI performance and physical impairment [29]. An important difference between the two

studies was that Nijboer and colleagues required the patients to select letters from a 6 × 6 matrix, whereas Piccione and colleagues used a spatial orientation task which required an additional cognitive effort.

Kübler and Birbaumer performed a meta-analysis of BCI performance across 51 patients in all stages of paralysis and found no relation between performance level and physical impairment provided that CLIS patients were excluded from analysis [41]. From seven patients in the CLIS only two acquired regulation of the SCP amplitude above chance level, but communication could not be re-established. Taking an operant conditioning view, the authors speculated that after a longer period of time in the CLIS, the loss of contingency between intention and consequences may lead to an extinction of goal-directed thinking and learning. Except 2, all 11 patients in the LIS learned BCI control. All CLIS patients who were trained with a BCI were already in this state when training started. Whether patients who learn BCI control in the LIS can retain this ability when they enter the CLIS is still an open empirical question. The data presented from one LIS patient (Box 17.3) indicate that this might be possible.

A Hierarchical Approach to Cognitive Processing in Non-responsive Patients Including BCI

Hierarchical approaches to cognitive processing in DOC patients were suggested with regards to passive stimulation paradigms [34, 89]. According to the underlying idea of all such approaches, processing of physically simple stimuli is necessary for the processing of more complex material including semantic stimulation which requires processing of verbal material. Typically, paradigms on the basis of auditory stimulation are used to elicit the MMN as indicator of pre-attentive cortical orientation, the P300 for deeper cortical analysis of the physical properties of stimuli, and responses to semantic stimulation leading to a P300, N400, or P600 [89]. A pre-requisite for all these paradigms is the presence of the N1–P2 complex to ensure processing of auditory stimuli in primary auditory cortices. In a large group of vegetative state and minimally conscious patients, which could be categorized along the continuum of consciousness [99] from completely non-responsive with a pathological rest EEG below 4 Hz to severely brain damaged, but responsive with fast theta or slow alpha oscillations which were suppressed by light, a hierarchy of information processing could not be confirmed [89]. This result is in line with the idea that islands of cortical processing may remain intact in patients with DOC, but that the connectivity between cortical and subcortical areas is lost [100].

Passive stimulation paradigms allow us to infer which cortical areas are still involved in cognitive processing, but bottom line they will not tell us anything about possible conscious awareness in nonresponsive patients. It was suggested to address this issue with volitional paradigms which require understanding of instruction, volition to perform as required (by the experimenter), and the capability to perform as required [38, 101]. Owen and colleagues distinguished successfully activation patterns related to motor imagery (playing tennis) and spatial navigation (through one's own house starting at the front door) in a patient diagnosed with persistent vegetative state, and could thus show that she was conscious [38]. The ODDBALL-BCI, namely the auditory 4-choice speller constitutes another volitional paradigm, which does not require the ability to imagine movements, but the focus of attention to one of two possible responses YES and NO as pre-set by the experimenter. The pre-requisite for this paradigm is the classification of ERP to the target stimuli. The lateralized Bereitschaftspotenzial could also be used for such volitional tasks: in a classic S1–S2 paradigm [76] participants are at S1 (warning stimulus) instructed to *prepare* for left or right hand movement imagery and at S2 (imperative stimulus) to *imagine* the movement. Typically, a negative SCP shift (contingent negative variation) is seen over central leads (hand motor areas) of the contralateral hemisphere as a correlate of depolarized cell assemblies preparing for movement imagery [76, 102].

Between passive stimulation and volitional paradigms is a tremendous gap with regards to cognitive requirement: the first requires only listening whereas the latter necessitates understanding, compliance, and ability (see above). To bridge this gap, it is suggested to add the instruction to pay attention to target stimuli presented in the passive stimulation paradigms. It was demonstrated that if participants followed this instruction, implying understanding and compliance, but not the ability of mental imagery or verbal processing during stimulation, the amplitude of the P300 was considerably increased [103, 104].

If patients in a non-responsive state performed above chance level in any of the volitional paradigms, then it may be inferred that higher cognitive processing is still possible and volition can be exerted, meaning that such patients are not unconscious. It may then be investigated whether those patients can use one or any of these brain responses to control a BCI (Figure 17.5). Above the requirements of volitional paradigms, a BCI necessitates decision making. In the

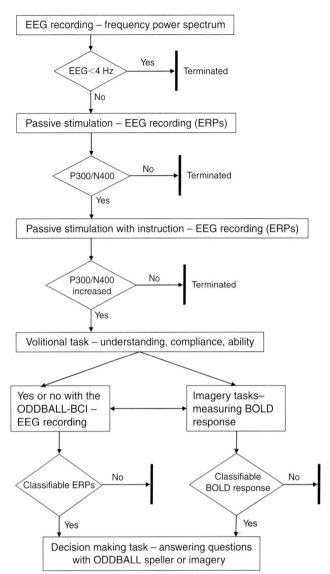

FIGURE 17.5   Flow chart of the hierarchical approach to the use of BCI in DOC. Each level involves higher demands on cognitive processing: first, *simple EEG recording* is necessary and patients with a rest EEG below 4 Hz are excluded [89]. If *passive stimulation* leads to classifiable ERPs, instruction to *focus attention* on target stimuli is added to the passive stimulation task. If amplitudes of ERP are increased, *volitional tasks* are presented: the EEG is recorded during presentation of the 4-choice oddball-speller or the BOLD response during mental imagery or both. If above chance level performance is obtained, the highest level of cognitive performance requiring *decision making* by means of a BCI can be tested.

volitional paradigm YES or NO responses are preset by the experimenter. Decision making with a BCI would include intentionally choosing either the one or the other response. ODDBALL-BCI allow users to directly answer questions, whereas BCI on the basis of imagery require the patient to relate a specific imagery, for example, 'playing tennis' to a specific answer, for example, YES. This is an additional step requiring cognitive resources, and it is an empirical question how well this can be accomplished. In any case, state-of-the-art real-time fMRI (Box 17.2) allows us to online decipher distinct brain states.

Problems and Prospects

From a technical point of view several issues have to be resolved before BCI can be utilized across a wide range of clinical or daily life settings. Sensors are the bottleneck of today's invasive and non-invasive BCI. Invasive sensors last only a limited time before they loose signal [4], and non-invasive sensors need long preparation time due the still necessary conductive gel. First results of classification of SMR modulation with dry electrodes are promising [105]. Machine learning and advanced signal processing methods play a key role in BCI research as they allow us decoding of different brain states within the noise of the spontaneous neuronal activity in real time [106]. Particularly, higher robustness of recording, online adaptation to compensate for non-stationarities, sensor fusion strategies, and techniques for transferring classifier or filter parameters from session to session are among the burning topics [25].

BCI research also has to face open neurobiological questions. Only little is known about how the brain instantiates regulation of EEG components as required in the SCP- and SMR-BCI. It was demonstrated that during voluntary produced negative SCP a widespread fronto-parietal network was activated including bilateral precentral gyrus, SMA, and middle frontal gyrus (areas under the feedback electrode) as well as dorsolateral prefrontal cortex, insula, supramarginal gyrus, and inferior parietal lobule. In contrast, positive SCP were accompanied by deactivations in central, temporal–hippocampal, and prefrontal areas. The putamen as a part of the striatum and the input nuclei of the basal ganglia were only activated in preparation for positive SCP amplitudes. The inability to voluntarily produce positive SCP was attributed to failed deactivation of frontal areas [107]. In about 20% of participants (healthy and patients) trained with a BCI, regulation of the targeted brain response was not achieved or ERP patterns could not be classified, and the reason for this failure is not known [25, 41]. Thus, to infer cognitive processing or even conscious cognition from the hierarchical procedure suggested (Figure 17.5), the predictive value of ERPs recorded during passive stimulation paradigms for successful (above chance level) performance in volitional ERP paradigms such as the 4-choice speller has to be defined in normative studies with healthy participants. Likewise,

the ability to generate classifiable mental imagery has to be assessed. Next, it has to be investigated how predictive successful imagery or successful ERP classification is for the use of BCI which requires decision making for meaningful communication.

From a psychological point of view, three models were proposed on how humans learn to regulate an autonomous response such as the electrical activity of the brain. The *operant conditioning* approach is based on the increasing probability of a behaviour if it is followed by reinforcement which can be positive or negative [108]. According to this model, learning occurs such that a spontaneous behaviour that is already in the individual's behavioural repertoire is selectively reinforced and thus, its occurrence increases. The *two-process theory* of biofeedback learning is based on the assumption, that regulation of the EEG is learned such that the user searches for a successful strategy [109]. Which strategy is chosen depends strongly on the instruction. As soon as there is only a minimal success with the chosen strategy, the user will stick to and optimize it. Only if users find no appropriate strategy in their behavioural repertoire, they create – in a second process – a new motor activation pattern. To achieve control over the to-be-learned behaviour, the users have to pay attention which internal stimuli such as heart rate or blood pressure accompany the motor activation pattern. This is enacted by means of the feedback signal which is controlled by the motor activation pattern and which occurs always together with the same internal stimuli. Those internal stimuli which occur always together with the activation pattern are referred to as *response image*. If a response image has been learned, it can be activated and the related brain response will be produced automatically. According to Lang, learning to regulate a physiological parameter is comparable to *motor learning* [110]. This approach assumes that regulation of the EEG requires an organized sequence of activities and symbolic information, which are also necessary to learn how to hit a tennis ball. Consequently, regulation of the EEG is influenced by the users' sensorimotor abilities and capacities. These three models overlap tremendously. The first learning process of the two-process theory – the search for a successful strategy – is comparable with operant conditioning. The second learning process can also be regarded as motor learning.

To date, it is not known whether non-responsive patients are susceptible to operant conditioning including reinforcement. Susceptibility to reinforcers is the pre-requisite to achieve regulation of SCP or SMR if motor imagery does not provide classifiable results in the first session. Processing of aversive stimuli has been investigated in patients in the vegetative state [111].

Primary sensory areas and the thalamus were activated in response to painful stimulation whereas secondary sensory cortices were not. The authors concluded that patients in the vegetative state perceived but did not 'feel' pain. By contrast, processing of pleasant stimulation in DOC patients has never been investigated. One reason for this shortfall may be the difficulty to find out what may be experienced as pleasant by the individual patient. With regards to aversive stimulation consent exists that painful stimulation is generally perceived aversive; however, with pleasant stimulation the situation is less clear cut. Although it appears evident that sexual stimulation is generally perceived as pleasant, the ethical and practical difficulties of such stimulation in DOC patients are obvious.

CONCLUSION

BCI proved successful for communication and control in patients with severe paralyses or in the LIS. BCI allow users to directly communicate their intention without any involvement of the motor periphery. The development of non-visual BCI renders this technology feasible for patients who lost control of eye movement due to disease progression or injury. Before the suggested hierarchical approach to cognitive processing can be applied to DOC patients, normative studies have to clarify the predictive value of ERP or mental imagery classification for BCI use. Studies with DOC patients will then demonstrate whether BCI can be purposefully utilized to investigate cognitive processing, to improve diagnosis, or even for social interaction in patients with DOC. It is unknown how much structural and functional integrity and connectivity of the brain is necessary to use a BCI for at least minimal (yes/no) communication. But the time is ripe to gather empirical data and to merge the so far independent research streams of BCI and cortical processing in DOC patients.

ACKNOWLEDGEMENTS

I gratefully acknowledge the patient help of Adrian Furdea with designing and making the figures. I thank Boris Kotchoubey, Steven Laureys, Adrian Owen, and Niels Birbaumer for fruitful discussions on the use of BCI in patients with DOC. Thanks to Femke Nijboer, Tamara Matuz, Sebastian Halder, Adrian Furdea, Eva-Maria Hammer, Sonja Häcker, Ursula Mochty, Slavica von Hartlieb, Seung-Soo Lee, Miguel Jordan, Emily Mugler, and Jacqueline Bocanfuso from the Tübingen BCI group for their commitment to BCI research with patients. I am strongly indebted to the patients who made this research possible. Supported by the Deutsche Forschungsgemeinschaft, Germany, and the National Institutes of Health, USA.

References

1. Kübler, A. and Neumann, N. (2005) Brain–computer interfaces – the key for the conscious brain locked into a paralysed body. *Prog Brain Res* 150:513–525.
2. Mason, S.G. and Birch, G.E. (2003) A general framework for brain–computer interface design. *IEEE Trans Neural Syst Rehabil Eng* 11:70–85.
3. Kennedy, P.R. and Bakay, R.A. (1998) Restoration of neural output from a paralyzed patient by a direct brain connection. *Neuroreport* 9:1707–1711.
4. Hochberg, L.R., *et al.* (2006) Neuronal ensemble control of prosthetic devices by a human with tetraplegia. *Nature* 442:164–171.
5. Nicolelis, M.A., *et al.* (2003) Chronic, multisite, multielectrode recordings in macaque monkeys. *Proc Natl Acad Sci USA* 100:11041–11046.
6. Taylor, D.M., *et al.* (2002) Direct cortical control of 3D neuroprosthetic devices. *Science* 296:1829–1832.
7. Schalk, G., *et al.* (2007) Decoding two-dimensional movement trajectories using electrocorticographic signals in humans. *J Neural Eng* 4:264–275.
8. Felton, E.A., *et al.* (2007) Electrocorticographically controlled brain–computer interfaces using motor and sensory imagery in patients with temporary subdural electrode implants. Report of four cases. *J Neurosurg* 106:495–500.
9. Leuthardt, E.C., *et al.* (2006) Electrocorticography-based brain computer interface – the Seattle experience. *IEEE Trans Neural Syst Rehabil Eng* 14:194–198.
10. Hill, N.J., *et al.* (2006) Classifying EEG and ECoG signals without subject training for fast BCI implementation: Comparison of nonparalyzed and completely paralyzed subjects. *IEEE Trans Neural Syst Rehabil Eng* 14:183–186.
11. Blankertz, B., *et al.* (2007) The non-invasive Berlin Brain–computer interface: Fast acquisition of effective performance in untrained subjects. *Neuroimage* 37:539–550.
12. Kübler, A., *et al.* (2005) Patients with ALS can use sensorimotor rhythms to operate a brain–computer interface. *Neurology* 64:1775–1777.
13. Wolpaw, J.R. and McFarland, D.J. (2004) Control of a two-dimensional movement signal by a noninvasive brain–computer interface in humans. *Proc Natl Acad Sci USA* 101:17849–17854.
14. Neuper, C., *et al.* (2005) Imagery of motor actions: Differential effects of kinesthetic and visual-motor mode of imagery in single-trial EEG. *Cogn Brain Res* 25:668–677.
15. Cincotti, F., *et al.* (2003) The use of EEG modifications due to motor imagery for brain–computer interfaces. *IEEE Trans Neural Syst Rehabil Eng* 11:131–133.
16. Birbaumer, N., *et al.* (1999) A spelling device for the paralysed. *Nature* 398:297–298.
17. Kübler, A., *et al.* (2001) Brain–computer communication: Self-regulation of slow cortical potentials for verbal communication. *Arch Phys Med Rehabil* 82:1533–1539.
18. Sellers, E.W. and Donchin, E. (2006) A P300-based brain–computer interface: Initial tests by ALS patients. *Clin Neurophysiol* 117:538–548.
19. Hoffmann, U., *et al.* (2008) An efficient P300-based brain–computer interface for disabled subjects. *J Neurosci Meth.* 167:115–125.

20. Müller-Putz, G.R., *et al.* (2006) Steady-state somatosensory evoked potentials: Suitable brain signals for brain–computer interfaces? *IEEE Trans Neural Syst Rehabil Eng* 14:30–37.

21. Müller-Putz, G.R., *et al.* (2005) Steady-state visual evoked potential (SSVEP)-based communication: Impact of harmonic frequency components. *J Neural Eng* 2:123–130.

22. Gao, X., *et al.* (2003) A BCI-based environmental controller for the motion-disabled. *IEEE Trans Neural Syst Rehabil Eng* 11:137–140.

23. Wolpaw, J.R., *et al.* (2002) Brain–computer interfaces for communication and control. *Clin Neurophysiol* 113:767–791.

24. Birbaumer, N. and Cohen, L.G. (2007) Brain–computer interfaces: Communication and restoration of movement in paralysis. *J Physiol* 579:621–636.

25. Kübler, A., and Müller, K.-R. (2007) An introduction to brain–computer interfacing. In Dornhege, G., Millan, J.D.R., Hinterberger, T., McFarland, D. and Müller, K.-R. (eds.) *Towards Brain-Computer Interfacing*. Cambridge, MA: MIT press, pp. 1–25.

26. Lebedev, M.A. and Nicolelis, M.A. (2006) Brain–machine interfaces: Past, present and future. *Trends Neurosci.* 29:536–46.

27. Pfurtscheller, G., *et al.* (2003) 'Thought' – control of functional electrical stimulation to restore hand grasp in a patient with tetraplegia. *Neurosci Lett* 351:33–36.

28. Neuper, C., *et al.* (2003) Clinical application of an EEG-based brain–computer interface: A case study in a patient with severe motor impairment. *Clin Neurophysiol* 114:399–409.

29. Nijboer, F., *et al.* (in press) A brain–computer interface (BCI) for people with amyotrophic lateral sclerosis (ALS). *Clin Neurophysiol*.

30. Müller-Putz, G.R., *et al.* (2005) EEG-based neuroprosthesis control: A step towards clinical practice. *Neurosci Lett* 382:169–174.

31. Pfurtscheller, G., *et al.* (2000) Brain oscillations control hand orthosis in a tetraplegic. *Neurosci Lett* 292:211–214.

32. Laureys, S., *et al.* (2004) Brain function in coma, vegetative state, and related disorders. *Lancet Neurol* 3:537–546.

33. Boly, M., *et al.* (2004) Auditory processing in severely brain injured patients: Differences between the minimally conscious state and the persistent vegetative state. *Arch Neurol* 61:233–238.

34. Owen, A.M., *et al.* (2005) Using a hierarchical approach to investigate residual auditory cognition in persistent vegetative state. *Prog Brain Res* 150:457–471.

35. Schiff, N.D., *et al.* (2005) fMRI reveals large-scale network activation in minimally conscious patients. *Neurology* 64:514–523.

36. Buzsaki, G. (2007) The structure of consciousness. *Nature* 446:267.

37. Andrews, K., *et al.* (1996) Misdiagnosis of the vegetative state: Retrospective study in a rehabilitation unit. *BMJ* 313:13–16.

38. Owen, A.M., *et al.* (2006) Detecting awareness in the vegetative state. *Science* 313:1402.

39. Smith, E. and Delargy, M. (2005) Locked-in syndrome. *BMJ* 330:406–409.

40. Birbaumer, N. (2006) Breaking the silence: Brain–computer interfaces (BCI) for communication and motor control. *Psychophysiology* 43:517–532.

41. Kübler, A., and Birbaumer, B. (in press) Brain-computer interfaces for communication in paralysis. *Clin Neurophysiol*.

42. Chia, L.G. (1991) Locked-in syndrome with bilateral ventral midbrain infarcts. *Neurology* 41:445–446.

43. Acharya, V.Z., *et al.* (2001) Enteroviral encephalitis leading to a locked-in state. *J Child Neurol* 16:864–866.

44. Breen, P. and Hannon, V. (2004) Locked-in syndrome: A catastrophic complication after surgery. *Br J Anaesth* 92:286–288.

45. Karitzky, J. and Ludolph, A.C. (2001) Imaging and neurochemical markers for diagnosis and disease progression in ALS. *J Neurol Sci* 191:35–41.

46. Leigh, P.N., *et al.* (2004) Amyotrophic lateral sclerosis: A consensus viewpoint on designing and implementing a clinical trial. *Amyotroph Lateral Scler Other Motor Neuron Disord* 5:84–98.

47. Weiskopf, N., *et al.* (2007) Real-time functional magnetic resonance imaging: Methods and applications. *Magn Reson Imaging* 25:989–1003.

48. Caria, A., *et al.* (2007) Regulation of anterior insular cortex activity using real-time fMRI. *Neuroimage* 35:1238–1246.

49. Sitaram, R., *et al.* (2005) Real-time fMRI based brain–computer interface enhanced by interactive virtual worlds. *Psychophysiology* 42 (Suppl 1):115.

50. Yoo, S.S., *et al.* (2004) Brain–computer interface using fMRI: Spatial navigation by thoughts. *Neuroreport* 15:1591–1595.

51. deCharms, R.C., *et al.* (2004) Learned regulation of spatially localized brain activation using real-time fMRI. *Neuroimage* 21:436–443.

52. Weiskopf, N., *et al.* (2004) Principles of a brain-computer interface (BCI) based on real-time functional magnetic resonance imaging (fMRI). *IEEE Trans Biomed Eng* 51:966–970.

53. deCharms, R.C., *et al.* (2005) Control over brain activation and pain learned by using real-time functional MRI. *Proc Natl Acad Sci USA* 102:18626–18631.

54. Fassbender, C., *et al.* (2004) A topography of executive functions and their interactions revealed by functional magnetic resonance imaging. *Cogn Brain Res* 20:132–143.

55. Schwartz, A.B. (2004) Cortical neural prosthetics. *Annu Rev Neurosci* 27:487–507.

56. Kübler, A., *et al.* (2007) Brain–computer interfaces for communication and motor control – perspectives on clinical application. In Dornhege, G., Millan, J.D.R.,Hinterberger, T., McFarland, D. and Müller, K.-R. (eds.) *Towards Brain–Computer Interfacing*. Cambridge, MA: MIT press. pp. 373–391.

57. Kübler, A., *et al.* (2004) Predictability of brain–computer communication. *J Psychophysiol* 18:121–129.

58. Wolpaw, J.R., *et al.* (1997) Timing of EEG-based cursor control. *J Clin Neurophysiol* 14:529–538.

59. Miner, L.A., *et al.* (1998) Answering questions with an electroencephalogram-based brain–computer interface. *Arch Phys Med Rehabil* 79:1029–1033.

60. Müller-Putz, G., *et al.* (2004) EEG-basierende Kommunikation: Erfahrungen mit einem Telemonitoring system zum Patiententraining. *Biomedizinische Technik. Beiträge zur 38. Jahrestagung der Deutschen Gesellschaft für Biomedizinische Technik im VDE - BMT*, Berlin, pp. 230–231.

61. Neshige, R., *et al.* (2006) Optimal methods of stimulus presentation and frequency analysis in P300-based brain–computer interfaces for patients with severe motor impairment. *Suppl Clin Neurophysiol* 59:35–42.

62. Hinterberger, T., *et al.* (2005) Assessment of cognitive function and communication ability in a completely locked-in patient. *Neurology* 64:1307–1308.

63. Kübler, A., *et al.* (1999) The thought translation device: A neurophysiological approach to communication in total motor paralysis. *Exp Brain Res* 124:223–232.

64. Kuebler, A., *et al.* (1998) Self-regulation of slow cortical potentials in completely paralyzed human patients. *Neurosci Lett* 252:171–174.

65. Neumann, N., *et al.* (2001) Self-regulation of slow cortical potentials: Prediction of performance. *Psychophysiology* 38:S71–S71.

66. McFarland, D.J., *et al.* (2005) Brain–computer interface (BCI) operation: Signal and noise during early training sessions. *Clin Neurophysiol* 116:56–62.

67. Krausz, G., *et al.* (2003) Critical decision-speed and information transfer in the 'Graz Brain-Computer Interface'. *Appl Psychophysiol Biofeedback* 28:233–240.

68. Piccione, F., et al. (2006) P300-based brain computer interface: Reliability and performance in healthy and paralysed participants. Clin Neurophysiol 117:531–537.

69. Kauhanen, L., et al. (2006) EEG and MEG brain–computer interface for tetraplegic patients. IEEE Trans Neural Syst Rehabil Eng 14:190–193.

70. Kübler, A. (2000) Brain–Computer Communication – Development of a Brain–Computer Interface for Locked-in Patients on the Basis of the Psychophysiological Self-regulation Training of Slow Cortical Potentials (SCP), Tübingen: Schwäbische Verlagsgesellschaft.

71. Kennedy, P.R., et al. (2000) Direct control of a computer from the human central nervous system. IEEE Trans Neural Syst Rehabil Eng 8:198–202.

72. McFarland, D.J., et al. (2003) Brain–computer interface (BCI) operation: Optimizing information transfer rates. Biol Psychol 63:237–251.

73. Leuthardt, E., et al. (2004) Brain–computer interface using electrocorticographic signals in humans. J Neural Eng 1:63–71.

74. Lal, T.N., et al. (2005) Methods towards invasive human brain computer interfaces. In Soul, L.K. Weiss, Y. and Bottou, L. (eds.) Advances in Neural Information Processing Systems, pp. 737–744. Cambridge, MA.: MIT Press.

75. Bakay, R.A. (2006) Limits of brain–computer interface. Case report. Neurosurg Focus 20:E6.

76. Birbaumer, N., et al. (1990) Slow potentials of the cerebral cortex and behavior. Physiol Rev 70:1–41.

77. Neumann, N., et al. (2003) Conscious perception of brain states: Mental strategies for brain–computer communication. Neuropsychologia 41:1028–1036.

78. Neumann, N. and Birbaumer, N. (2003) Predictors of successful selfcontrol during brain–computer communication. J Neurol Neurosurg Psychiatr 74:1117–1121.

79. Karim, A.A., et al. (2006) Neural Internet: Web surfing with brain potentials for the completely paralyzed. Neurorehabil Neural Repair 20:508–515.

80. Niedermeyer, E. (2005) The normal EEG of the waking adult. In Niedermeyer, E. and Lopes da Silva, F.H. (eds.) Electroencephalography – Basic Principles, Clinical Applications, and Related Fields, pp. 167–192. Philadelphia, PA: Lippincott Williams & Wilkins.

81. Pfurtscheller, G. (2005) EEG event-related desynchronization (ERD) and event-related synchronization (ERS). In Niedermeyer, E. and Lopes da Silva, F.H. (eds.) Electroencephalography – Basic Principles, Clinical Applications, and Related Fields, pp. 958–967. Philadelphia, PA: Lippincott Williams & Wilkins.

82. Wolpaw, J.R., et al. (1991) An EEG-based brain–computer interface for cursor control. Electroencephalogr Clin Neurophysiol 78:252–259.

83. Wolpaw, J.R. and McFarland, D.J. (1994) Multichannel EEG-based brain–computer communication. Electroencephalogr Clin Neurophysiol 90:444–449.

84. Müller, G.R., et al. (2003) Implementation of a telemonitoring system for the control of an EEG-based brain–computer interface. IEEE Trans Neural Syst Rehabil Eng 11:54–59.

85. Birbaumer, N. and Schmid, R.F. (2006) Methoden der Biologischen Psychologie. In Birbaumer, N. and Schmid, R.F. (eds.) Biologische Psychologie, pp. 483–511. Berlin: Springer Verlag.

86. Fabiani, M., et al. (1987) Definition, identification, and reliability of measurement of the P300 component of the event-related brain potential. Adv Psychophysiol 2:1–78.

87. Farwell, L.A. and Donchin, E. (1988) Talking off the top of your head: Toward a mental prosthesis utilizing event-related brain potentials. Electroencephalogr Clin Neurophysiol 70:512–523.

88. Sellers, E.W., et al. (2006) Brain–computer interface research at the University of South Florida cognitive psychophysiology laboratory: The P300 Speller. IEEE Trans Neural Syst Rehabil Eng 14:221–224.

89. Kotchoubey, B., et al. (2005) Information processing in severe disorders of consciousness: Vegetative state and minimally conscious state. Clin Neurophysiol 116:2441–2453.

90. Furdea, A., et al. (submitted) An auditory oddball (P300) spelling system for brain-computer interfaces (BCI), submitted after revision, Psychophysiology.

91. Krusienski, D.J., et al. (2006) A comparison of classification techniques for the P300 Speller. J Neural Eng 3:299–305.

92. Hinterberger, T., et al. (2004) A multimodal brain-based feedback and communication system. Exp Brain Res 154: 521–526.

93. Nijboer, F., et al. (2008) An auditory brain–computer interface (BCI). J Neurosci Meth. 167:43–50.

94. Hill, N.J., et al. (2005). An auditory paradigm for brain–computer interfaces, pp. 569–76. Advances in Neural Information Processing Systems. Cambridge, MA: MIT Press.

95. Cincotti, F., et al. (2007) Vibrotactile feedback for brain–computer interface operation. Comput Intell Neurosci. 48937.

96. Kotchoubey, B., et al. (2006) Evidence of cortical learning in vegetative state. J Neurol 253:1374–1376.

97. Schnakers, C., et al. (2008) Cognitive function in the locked-in syndrome. J Neurol. 255:323–330.

98. Lakerveld, J., et al. (2008) Cognitive function in late stage ALS patients. J Neurol Neurosurg Psychiatr. 79:25–29.

99. Kübler, A., and Kotchoubey, B. (2007) Brain–computer interfaces in the continuum of consciousness. Curr Opin Neurol. 20:643–649.

100. Giacino, J.T., et al. (2006) Functional neuroimaging applications for assessment and rehabilitation planning in patients with disorders of consciousness. Arch Phys Med Rehabil 87:S67–S76.

101. Boly, M., et al. (2007) When thoughts become action: An fMRI paradigm to study volitional brain activity in non-communicative brain injured patients. Neuroimage 36:979–992.

102. Hinterberger, T., et al. (2005) A device for the detection of cognitive brain functions in completely paralyzed or unresponsive patients. IEEE Trans Biomed Eng 52:211–220.

103. Lang, S., et al. (1997) What are you doing when you are doing nothing? ERP components without a cognitive task. Z Exp Psychol 44:138–162.

104. Lang, S. and Kotchoubey, B. (2002) Brain responses to number sequences with and without active task requirement. Clin Neurophysiol 113:1734–1741.

105. Popescu, F., et al. (in press) Single trial classification of motor imagination using 6 dry EEG electrodes. PLoS ONE 2(7), e637.

106. Haynes, J.D. and Rees, G. (2006) Decoding mental states from brain activity in humans. Nat Rev Neurosci 7:523–534.

107. Hinterberger, T., et al. (2004) An EEG-driven brain–computer interface combined with functional magnetic resonance imaging (fMRI). IEEE Trans Biomed Eng 51:971–974.

108. Skinner, B.F. (1945) The operational analysis of psychological terms. Psychol Rev 52:270–277.

109. Lacroix, J.M. (1981) The acquisition of autonomic control through biofeedback: The case against an afferent process and a two-process alternative. Psychophysiology 18:573–587.

110. Lang, P.J. (1975) Acquisition of heart-rate control: Method, theory, and clinical implications. In Fowles, D.C. (eds.) Clinical Applications of Psychophysiology, pp. 167–191. New York: Columbia University Press.

111. Laureys, S., et al. (2002) Cortical processing of noxious somatosensory stimuli in the persistent vegetative state. Neuroimage 17:732–741.

Neuroethics and Disorders of Consciousness: A Pragmatic Approach to Neuropalliative Care

Joseph J. Fins

ABSTRACT

Unravelling the mysteries of consciousness, lost and regained, and perhaps even intervening so as to prompt recovery are advances for which neither the clinical nor the lay community are prepared. These advances will shake existing expectations about severe brain damage and will find an unprepared clinical context, perhaps even one inhospitable to what should clearly be viewed as important advances. This could be the outcome of this line of enquiry, if this exceptionally imaginative research can continue at all. This work faces a restrictive research environment that has the potential to imperil it. Added to the complexity of the scientific challenges that must be overcome is the societal context in which these investigations must occur. Research on human consciousness goes to the heart of our humanity and asks us to grapple with fundamental questions about the self. Added to this is the regulatory complexity of research on subjects who may be unable to provide their own consent because of impaired decisionmaking capacity, itself a function of altered or impaired consciousness. These factors can lead to a restrictive view of research that can favor risk aversion over discovery. In this paper, I will attempt to explain systematically some of these challenges. I will suggest that some of the resistance might be tempered if we view the needs of patients with severe brain injury through the prism of palliative care and adopted that field's ethos and methods when caring for and conducting research with individuals with severe brain damage and disorders of consciousness. To make this argument I will draw upon the American pragmatic tradition and utilize *clinical pragmatism*, a method of moral problem solving that my colleagues and I have developed to address ethical challenges in clinical care and research.

INTRODUCTION

The world is not ready for the potential discoveries and innovations described in this collection. Unravelling the mysteries of consciousness, lost and regained, and novel interventions, such as the recent report of deep brain stimulation in the minimally conscious state (MCS) [1] so as to prompt recovery are possibilities for which neither the clinical nor the lay community are prepared. These developments will shake existing expectations about severe brain damage and will find an ambivalent clinical context.

This could be the outcome of this line of enquiry, if this exceptionally imaginative research can continue at all. This work faces a restrictive research environment that has the potential to imperil it [2, 3]. Added to the complexity of the scientific challenges that must be overcome is the societal context in which these investigations must occur. Research on human consciousness goes to the heart of our humanity and asks us to grapple with fundamental questions about the self [4]. Added to this is the regulatory complexity of research on subjects who may be unable to provide their own consent because of impaired decisionmaking capacity, itself a function of altered or impaired consciousness. These factors can lead to a restrictive view of research that can favor risk aversion over discovery.

In this paper, I will attempt to explain systematically some of these challenges. I will suggest that some of the resistance might be tempered if we view the needs of patients with severe brain injury through the prism of palliative care. To make this argument I will draw upon the American pragmatic tradition and utilize *clinical pragmatism*, a method of moral problem solving that I have developed with colleagues for clinical care and research [5–8, 9].

CLINICAL PRAGMATISM

Clinical pragmatism has its philosophical roots in the American pragmatic and the work of John Dewey (1859–1952) in particular [10–13]. Dewey was a leading American philosopher of the first half of the 20th century as well as a psychologist, democratic theorist and education reformer [14–17]. Deweyan pragmatism is an appealing philosophical method to assess the novel ethical challenges posed by neuroscience because Dewey sought to use the scientific method as a means to inductively address normative questions [18–20].

As a method of moral problem solving, clinical pragmatism begins with the recognition of the

TABLE 18.1   Clinical Pragmatism and Inquiry

I. Recognition of the problematic situation and the need for inquiry
II. Data collection: medical, narrative, contextual
   1. Medical facts
   2. Patient/surrogate preferences
   3. Family dynamics
   4. Institutional arrangements
   5. Broader societal issues and norms
III. Interpretation (ethics differential diagnosis)
IV. Negotiation
V. Intervention
VI. Periodic review/experiential learning

(Modified from): Fins, J.J. and Miller F.G. [21].

problematic situation. This prompts a process of enquiry which includes the collection of medical, narrative and contextual data. This information leads to the articulation of an ethics differential diagnosis. These speculations in turn inform a negotiation with stakeholders about a plan of action with this consensus leading to an intervention (Table 18.1). This process is completed with a periodic review that will foster experiential learning [22].

CLINICAL PRAGMATISM AND DISORDERS OF CONSCIOUSNESS

The Problematic Situation

The very clinical context of care encountered by patients with disorders of consciousness is a problematic situation, which generally goes unrecognized. I have previously characterized this as a *neglect syndrome*, borrowing the diagnostic category from clinical neurology [2]. Although notable exceptions exist amongst highly dedicated neurologists, neurosurgeons and rehabilitation specialists, the vast majority of patients with disorders of consciousness are a population who remain out of our gaze.

Without careful consideration or an evidence base, it is taken for granted that patients who have sustained severe brain damage are beyond hope of any remediation. This leads to a clinical context marked by errors of omission and a sense that ethically, nothing can or should be done for patients with catastrophic brain dysfunction. These prevailing sentiments have undermined the usual intellectual curiosity that marks other areas of practice. Surveys of neurologists' knowledge of diagnostic categories related to disorders of consciousness are rife with errors that would be intolerable elsewhere in practice [23], though they are tolerated here because of the sense that diagnostic clarity in the face of one form of futility or another just does not matter.

This is indeed paradoxical because while most in the clinical context are dismissive of these patients, questions related to consciousness are among the most fascinating topics in science and society [24–28]). Despite this interest outside of medicine, within the clinic disinterest and lack of intellectual curiosity have marked the clinical context. Even diagnostic rigour is lacking [29]. It is not uncommon for the same patient with impaired consciousness to be described as nearly brain-dead, vegetative or comatose.

These practices can create a problematic situation that can go unrecognized because such attitudes become so pervasive so as to become the norm. The potential recovery of a brain damaged patient goes unexamined because it is assumed that the intellectual consequences will be dire. Even survivors with intact cognitive abilities, like Jean Dominique Bauby – the author of *The Diving Bell and the Butterfly* a memoir of the Locked-in-State (LIS) – comments, 'But improved resuscitation techniques have prolonged the agony.' [30, p. 4]. These perceptions prevail despite the fact that evidence-based outcomes demonstrate a wide variety of outcomes depending upon a range of patient variables.

Although one would think that absence of careful diagnosis and informed prognostication would be an obvious deficit calling out for more precise assessment, confident pronouncements that there is 'no hope for meaningful recovery' are taken for granted, unexamined and without the requisite scepticism that marks prudential medicine. Meaningful to whom? The neurologist? The patient? Their family? [31] It is also critical to appreciate that notions of the life that might be worth living can evolve as disability is confronted. Quality of life considerations can also be informed by perspective [32, 33].

Another unarticulated problem which informs the care provided to these patients are the norms that inform decisions about life-sustaining therapy. Our views on do-not-resuscitate (DNR) orders and decisions to withdraw life-sustaining therapies have grown out of our experience in intensive care units and the provision of acute care [34]. In that setting the loss of consciousness may be taken as the ethical predicate to withdraw life-sustaining therapy because it signals the end-stage of a disease process. This is in contradistinction to the loss of consciousness that occurs at the outset of severe brain [35].

This is the context of care for critically ill patients who have sustained brain damage, where clinical routines can become an excuse for unreflective practice. It is a setting with decisional constructs that operate in days and weeks, not months. And these contextual factors lead to a paradox that also informs the problematic situation: decisions about withholding and forgoing life-sustaining therapy are made prematurely for patients with disorders of consciousness because options for withdrawals are increasingly abridged as the patient moves from the acute to chronic stage of illness, even though these decisions may become more justifiable once the prognosis becomes clearer.

As has been noted elsewhere in this collection of essays, the course of recovery from the vegetative states can take from 3 to 12 months, depending upon whether the etiology of the insult was anoxic or traumatic [36, 37]. Thus, to fully know whether recovery from the vegetative state is possible, a patient with traumatic brain injury might have to be observed for 12 months. By then he will have become *medically* stable and been extubated [38]. His only life-sustaining therapy might be his percutaneous gastrostomy tube and hence the paradox. While the legal and ethical norms clearly view a ventilator as an extraordinary measure that can be withdrawn within weeks of an injury, the ethical (and theological consensus) on decisions to withdraw artificial nutrition and hydration is less clear even after a patient is irreversibly in a permanent vegetative state.

These difficulties, coupled with the culture of the intensive care, lead to decisions to remove life-sustaining therapy while it remains feasible even though the dimensions of the patient's recovery remain unknown. This can lead to pronouncements about expected outcomes that may reflect personal biases and fall short on the evidence [31]. A better approach would be to be transparent with families and explain to them that the patient's prognosis and hope for recovery of consciousness will become clearer within weeks and months. Although we should not compel families to continue to treat patients who are persistently but not permanently vegetative in order to develop greater prognostic clarity, it seems prudent and ethically within the norm of informed consent *and* refusal, to be intellectually honest about what can be predicted so early in the course of care. At the very least clinicians need to be careful about making expedient claims that there is 'no hope for meaningful recovery' when the evidence is lacking in order to 'scientifically' justify decisions to forgo life-sustaining therapy.

Data Collection

Clarifying the Medical Facts: Brain Damage and the Challenge of Diagnosis and Prognosis

The first issue that will be seen as immediately different in the care of patients with disorders of consciousness is the fact that it may be difficult to clarify the medical facts. The diagnostic categories that inform practice in this area – the vegetative and MCS [39] – remain *descriptive*. Diagnoses are just on the cusp of becoming more physiologic and precise utilizing advanced imaging techniques and sophisticated electroencephalography, but our state of knowledge remains rudimentary compared with other domains in medicine.

A colleague suggested that our state of knowledge is just a bit more evolved from the time when infectious diseases were termed 'the fevers' [40]. A review of the history of medicine from Hippocrates and Galen to Osler and beyond indicates how etiology and prognostication evolved from rudimentary observations and theoretical speculations concerning fever [41]. Asserting that patients had a pattern of fevers carried less diagnostic and prognostic precision than linking these empirical manifestations of illness to an actual pathogen.

The state of affairs in neurological diagnosis, because of the complexity of the object of study, *is less evolved than other areas of medicine*. Families depend upon diagnostic clarity to make life-altering and family defining choices, but even this basic element of decisionmaking may be lacking clarity in disorders of consciousness. We take some semblance of diagnostic clarity elsewhere in medicine for granted. Clinicians counselling families about disorders of consciousness need to be careful to be as precise as possible and to acknowledge the limitations of what is currently known and predictable.

Although progress has been made since Jennett and Plum described the vegetative state as 'a syndrome in search of a name' [42], descriptive brain states are only now being refined in sub-categories such as the persistent and permanent vegetative states and the more recent MCS based on correlations between clinical observation neuropathological studies and neuroimaging studies [37, 43–54].

But as noteworthy as this work is, these efforts are rudimentary and fundamentally still descriptive with patients with variable injuries and outcomes clumped together into broad inclusive categories. This imprecision can lead to disorders of consciousness of different aetiologies being clinically indistinguishable, although their causes and potential course are dramatically different, making prediction and prognostication so difficult. Such diagnostic questions are further confounded by diagnostic error.

These issues create a challenging problem for clinical care which may be unique to this area in medicine, namely the difficulty of providing patients and families with a clear and meaningful diagnosis, which is an essential element of any ethical analysis about care. Families accustomed to diagnostic precision in other disciplines have similar expectations when a loved one has a disorder of consciousness. They expect precision and could easily mistake a magnetic resonance imaging (MRI) scan as meeting their expectations or misconstrue meanings of investigational work, such as the report by Owen *et al*. of a neuroimaging response in a patient who was behaviourally in the vegetative state [52].

This potential for misconstrual is heightened by popular articles on neuroethics, increasingly a mode of technological critique vs. a scholarly discipline, that warn of imaging studies that might be able to read your mind and monitor your thoughts [55–59]. If that is the case, they might logically ask, why can't my child's neurologist tell me if he is going to come out of his coma [57]?

And when we do return from the realm of science fiction to the less promising confines of the clinic, we appreciate how crude our categories are. Here families also encounter a profession and society that has yet to reach a clear consensus on emerging diagnostic domains, as demonstrated by the controversy over the status of the MCS. Minimally *contentious* to some, there is the scientific critique about the use of a consensus panel to create such categories [60, 61], as well as the political concerns of advocates asserting disability rights and the right to die. Some disability advocates have been wary of MCS because they fear that a new diagnostic category could equate patients with higher functioning to those in the vegetative state and lead to the devaluation of their lives [62]. Conversely, right to die advocates fear that the new category may open Pandora's box by suggesting that patients with impaired consciousness might be candidates for treatment and more aggressive care [60]. If they are, these advocates worry, will this erode society's willingness to accept withdrawal of care?

Despite the forces that might conspire to rob patients of the most accurate diagnosis currently available, establishing the medical facts and the diagnosis is a critical and necessary step in making ethical choices about patient care. This becomes clear if we consider the exceptional case of Terry Wallis who was misdiagnosed, or perhaps simply ignored, while in the (MCS) [63]. In 1984, Wallis was an unrestrained passenger in a motor vehicle accident and suffered severe head trauma. He received acute medical care, survived and was discharged to a nursing home only months after his injury [64]. He carried the diagnosis of the persistent vegetative state. But on July 11, 2003, he had what has been described as a miracle awakening while in 'custodial care' in a nursing home. He spoke tentatively, single words at a time like 'Mom' and 'Pepsi.' As the weeks passed, he spoke still haltingly but with greater fluency. In his mind he had never aged, and Reagan was still President.

Although Wallis had been labelled as being in the persistent vegetative state, the behaviours noted by family members – evidence of episodic but unreliable demonstrations of awareness and consciousness – went unheeded by the nursing home staff. Their views about him were codified by his diagnosis on transfer. He had been and would always remain vegetative. The family had requested that a neurologist reassess him during this period and were refused, so certain or indifferent were the staff to the question of his diagnosis. This neglect of Wallis was all the more poignant because subsequent diffusion tensor imaging (DTI) revealed what was described as the 'sprouting' of new axonal connections. It was hypothesized that these new connections between surviving neurons might have plated a role in the evolution of his brain state and his recovery [51]. Although these findings generated worldwide media attention, before his emergence from MCS, Mr Wallis went nearly two decades without a neurological assessment because he failed to demonstrate overt clinical improvement, a health policy question of great import [65].

This is a generic problem because patients who fail to meet medical necessity or demonstrate improvement with rehabilitative interventions are transferred to what is ungraciously described as 'custodial care,' where assessment is rare and incomplete. Given the exigencies of discharge planning, it is quite possible for a patient to be discharged while still in the persistent vegetative state and move to MCS once transferred to a nursing home within the first year of traumatic injury. If this occurs in an inattentive or disinterested setting, crossing this diagnostic demarcation may go unnoticed to the detriment of the patient and family.

Another pressure that makes the usually routine task of diagnosis so difficult is that these diagnoses have become so value laden. If we recall the Terri Schiavo case in Florida, we are reminded of how the objective process of diagnosis can be eroded by ideology [66]. That these diagnoses are prone to becoming so value laden has the potential to further complicate family counselling. Though each of us can place a different moral valuation on life in a vegetative state, we should not let these values turn the objective clinical evidence into something that it is not. Moral valuation should follow *upon* the clinical facts and *not transmute them* to meet political or ideological needs. Diagnostic clarity, or its distortion, has consequences beyond the patient. It also has implications for other patients and society in general [29]. Asserting by executive or legislative fiat, that Terri Schiavo was conscious when she was not obscures material differences between patients like Schiavo and Wallis. Such conflations have the potential to further the neglect of patients who retain residual elements of consciousness and who should be the object of intense study and clinical concern.

Patient and Surrogate Preferences

Once the medical facts have been clarified it is time to turn to the narrative dimensions of the case. Most patients do not engage in advance planning, that is talking with family and friends about their wishes in the event of decisional incapacity [67]. Of those who do, even fewer envision a cognitively altered state while still a young person, the demographic most affected by traumatic brain injury. Nonetheless strong views persist about cognitive impairment from Alzheimer's disease or following stroke later in life. In a study we recently concluded using structured vignettes to assess patient and proxy views on end-of-life decisionmaking, respondents were averse to continued life support following a stroke which left the patient with 'no hope for meaningful recovery' [31], a phrase as we have noted that is in the common prognostic discourse in the clinical setting. It is important to be cautious about these *background* views about impaired consciousness when they are analogized from the geriatric context and the setting of degenerative diseases to disorders of consciousness which are traumatic, occurring in an otherwise healthy younger patient cohort. Although analogic reasoning is how we often analyse difficult choices, it is important to appreciate the salient differences between various types of cognitive impairment throughout the life cycle and make these potential biases explicit.

Parents of young adults considering their own views about cognitive impairment later in life or in their parents may erroneously generalize these preferences to a context, which is biologically and developmentally quite different, at the risk of being too pessimistic about hopes for some modicum of recovery. It is worth remembering and counselling surrogates that recovery from brain damage is more variable than the inexorable decline that follows a diagnosis of Alzheimer's disease. And as the compelling account of the Central Park jogger's account of her experience shows, though statistically unusual, even patients who have a grim Glasgow Coma Scale of 4–5 have the potential to recover cognitive function, as Meli's account indicates [68].

In addition to pre-existing views of cognitive impairment analogized from other contexts, families will also bring their religious and cultural traditions to bear upon these deliberations. Life in the persistent vegetative state may look different to a family from a more fundamentalist religious tradition that holds that life itself is precious and which does not sanction quality of life distinctions. Such a vitalist approach, that any life is worth preserving, is often accompanied by an obligation to provide what, in the Catholic tradition, is called ordinary care such as artificial nutrition, hydration [69]. As has been noted, this becomes a critical point because late withdrawals will not likely involve ventilator support but simple feeding tubes, the subject of a 2004 Papal discourse [31, 70].

If surrogates are looking to forgo life-prolonging therapies, the process should be analogous to the process of an informed consent discussion, although in this context it would be an informed refusal of care. The practitioner should avoid value-laden statements that can engineer outcomes and preclude choice and provide surrogate decisionmakers with the best available evidence of the patient's outcome as well as its time course and any burdens associated with continued treatment. The patient's ability to perceive pain and experience suffering should be discussed and efforts to provide symptomatic relief should be reviewed [70].

Given the potential for confusion about the sequence of recovery, clinicians should carefully explain how a patient who is comatose, who neither dies nor regains consciousness, moves into the 'wakeful unresponsiveness' of the vegetative state after a couple of weeks. Clinicians should appreciate that families may perceive that eye opening is an improvement over the eyes-closed state of coma. This misconstrual needs to be clarified and families made aware that the failure to recover consciousness and awareness coming out of coma is a negative prognostic sign. The move into the vegetative state, though, needs to be tempered with information that a persistent vegetative state is not yet permanent and that prospects for the MCS and subsequent emergence can remain for months depending upon the etiology of injury. These discussions become even more complex if the patient recovers and is able to communicate preferences.

When the patient is able to participate in these decisions they are confronted with the challenge of being an altered self. Paradoxically an improvement in awareness and self-awareness may also bring a greater appreciation of how devastating an injury has been and how much farther one has to travel to regain skills and the ability for independent living [71].

Is the goal to recapture former self or approximate a reasonable facsimile? The literature is rife with narratives of brain injury survivors who provide first-hand accounts of this very private journey. Theirs are an admixture of physiology and psychology in which the nature of their injury determines *what* their deficits will be while their personal narratives will determine *who* they will now become. Claudia Osborn, a physician who sustained head trauma and lost much of her executive function characterized the psychological evolution necessitated by her injury [30, 68, 73].

The challenge of crafting a new future becomes even more formidable when the body has been paralyzed but the mind remains intact as in the LIS. In these cases it becomes especially important *to speak with the patient* using assistive devices or rudimentary efforts at blinking [74]. Indeed, if we take self-determination seriously, we need to ensure that those trapped in a lifeless body are not robbed of the opportunity to direct their care by turning to surrogates for guidance. Contrary to the expectations held by the able-bodied and anecdotal reports [75], a systematic assessment of the quality of life of patients in the LIS indicate that they can maintain a quality of life, enjoy social intercourse and that depression is not the norm [76].

Finally, it is important to appreciate that views about an acceptable existence are plastic. They evolve over time, often accommodating an increasing burden of disability. Studies have shown that patients are willing to continue treatments that physicians think are burdensome. Physician and patient views about quality of life can be discordant. These valuations can inform the clinicians' view of 'appropriate' end-of-life decisions even though patients may see things differently [32, 33]. Physicians must recognize these potential biases so as to enable neutral counselling about what might constitute proportionate care [76].

Family Dynamics

Thrown into this mix is the impact of care on the family. Having a family member with severe brain damage can lead to social isolation, or as one commentator put it, 'of the loneliness of the long-term care giver' [77]. Relationships change with the patient when the person has changed but one's marital status has not. For better or worse takes on a new connotation when one spouse no longer recognizes the other or when a frontal head injury has led to disinhibition and dramatic change in personality and temperament. When this occurs love can turn to compassion and compassion might turn to resentment. Spouses can feel as trapped as the patient, burdened by loving vows that may seem impossible to fill and tethering. It is important to appreciate the stress that families operate under when challenged by brain damage in a loved one. The patient's dependency, indeed fragility, becomes the epicentre of family life, altering roles and obligations.

Institutional Arrangements

Whatever the family dynamic, it will be played out within an institutional setting. For the most part, these institutions will not be geared to the chronic care needs of patients with severe head injury but rather to the provision of acute or what has been euphemistically called 'custodial care' [38]. These contextual factors can distort decisionmaking and engineer outcomes that may not be in the patient or family's best interest.

We have already described how the time frame of end-of-life decisions are discordant with the pace of recovery from head injury. Similar economic pressures exist, at least in the North American context, to discharge patients from acute care if they do not demonstrate what has been termed 'medical necessity' or more colloquially, show improvement. Although it is appreciated that recovery from brain damage can take months and that the trajectory of improvement may not be linear, the prevailing bureaucracy regulates length of stay in ways that may truncate admissions and deprive patients of adequate diagnostic assessment and proper placement in appropriate rehabilitation settings.

The pace of discharge from hospital, and the sequestration of the acute and rehabilitative medical communities, can lead to distortions among the former about what may be achievable with continued treatment over time. Because acute-academic and rehabilitative care centres are generally geographically separate, acute care practitioners can have a distorted view about patient outcomes. They suffer from what has been described as a 'bureaucratization of prognosis' [79, 80].

At its worst, institutional perceptions about what might constitute futile care can become objectionable. Consider the conflicting goals of caring for patients with severe brain damage and the need to obtain organs for transplantation. The contemporary example of organ procurement practices has historical roots that also inform our utilitarian views about severely brain injured and our societal obligations. In 1968, the diagnosis of brain death was justified by the greater good that might come from organ harvesting [81, 82]. These powerful perspectives have expanded to those who are still not brain dead and today it is not uncommon for organ procurement personnel to urge referrals of patients with Glasgow Coma Scales of three to five for assessment as potential donors, even though these patients may yet harbour the potential for recovery [68]. My goal is not to undermine laudable transplantation efforts but rather to illustrate how views about the viability and potential of patients with severe brain injury can be shaped by institutional practices that may go unexamined.

Societal Issues and Norms

All of the above factors are occurring against a broader societal backdrop as illustrated by the impact of cases like Schiavo and Wallis. I have addressed this broader context elsewhere at great length [2, 22, 29, 66], suffice it to say here that our collective views about disorders of consciousness are informed by the tangled history of brain damage and the evolution of the right to die in modern medical ethics. American bioethics since the 1960s has been predicated upon the evolution of self-determination and autonomy. This right evolved as the right to be left alone and to have life-sustaining therapy withdrawn. The important right to die, to direct one's care at the end of life autonomously, was founded upon a number of landmark cases involving patients in the vegetative state, most notably Quinlan and Cruzan [83, 84]. This is critical because the test cases to establish this *negative* right were in vegetative patients whose society concluded were beyond hope and beyond care. Further treatment in their case was, in a sense, the paradigmatic case of medical futility [85] simply geared at the preservation of vegetative functions and not as the Quinlan court put it a, 'cognitive sapient state' [86].

By considering the potential for recovery we are now asking society to intervene in a population which resembles those in whom the negative right to be left alone was first established. This has created a bit of cognitive dissonance – an oxymoron if you will – seen so dramatically in the cases of Schiavo and Wallis, in which the laudable goals of *preserving the right to die* and *affirming the right to care* have come into conflict [22].

Interpretation (Ethics Differential Diagnosis): Towards a Palliative Neuroethics

In considering how to reconcile these two conflicting obligations – preserving the hard-won right to direct care at the end of life and to care for those who may be helped – I would like to suggest that there may be a value in viewing these cases through the ethos of palliative care. The World Health Organization (WHO) defines palliative care as '… the active total care of patients whose disease is not responsive to curative treatment. Control of pain, of other symptoms, and of psychological, social and spiritual support is paramount. The goal of palliative care is the achievement of the best quality of life for patients and their families.' [87, pp. 11–12]. Conceptually palliative care can accommodate the oxymoron of affirming the right to die and preserving the right to care in patients with disorders of consciousness. Clinically, it does not preclude active care but at the same time it attends to symptom management and quality-of-life issues when the patient has eluded cure.

Palliation is an especially good metaphor to describe interventional strategies being developed for patients with disorders of consciousness. If we consider the philological origins of palliation we are reminded that to palliate means to cloak or disguise [88]. This is precisely what will occur if deep brain stimulation can restore impaired consciousness or [89] if brain–computer interfaces can help locked-in patients communicate [90]. Neither of these interventions are curative but rather assistive devices that palliate by *cloaking* or placing a *veneer* over underlying disability which remains. (Such is the case of deep brain stimulation in the MCS, making it a mosaic blend of the curative and palliative.) [1]

But more fundamentally palliative medicine is concerned with questions of meaning and suffering. At the most fundamental level disorders of consciousness are about the endangered and altered self, raising the possibility the potential for suffering as the patient contemplates what has been lost, what remains and what still might be. What aspect of the self-matters? Is the goal of care restoration or personal identity or a tolerable facsimile? Or is it the restoration of affect, memory and executive function? These are both empirical questions that will be relevant to emerging therapies such as DBS [1, 72].

It is vitally critical that practitioners attend to this alteration of the self and appreciate that there are indeed psychological connections between the patient before and after injury. Although some philosophers, like Derek Parfit, maintain that there is a discontinuity between the former and current self [91], this is more a theoretical argument than a pragmatic one as there is indeed continuity of memory and affect. Though these linkages may be tenuous at the margins, they do remain and inform relationships with intimates.

These sentiments remind us of the importance of appreciating that even as we distinguish differing brain states from another, there is a unique psychological element at each bedside, even when there are disorders of consciousness. Consciousness is about questions of meaning and though physiologically based, is psychological in its expression.

Negotiation and Intervention

In the absence of a particular patient narrative, it is difficult to script how to negotiate a plan of care with patients or their surrogates, but as a rule it is helpful to suggest plausible and achievable goals of care.

Surrogates confronted with the spectre of a loved one with brain damage may want to precipitously withdraw care or cling to hope when there is none. These emotional responses may reflect more about their preconceptions about brain injury than the clinical reality that they face. To temper these responses and help ensure that surrogates are adequately informed, it is essential that surrogates understand the patient's diagnosis, prognosis and prospects for recovery. It is important to avoid misconstruals that might distort the surrogate's thinking and help ensure that they appreciate the likelihood and time course of recovery, its scope and the foreseeable burdens that might be imposed by on-going care. This information needs to be conveyed empathically and with compassion, appreciating that most of us never consider the prospect of brain injury touching our families or close friends.

A palliative approach may help frame the goals of care by acknowledging both the right to die and the right to care while seeking an optimal quality of life through the mitigation of the patient's symptom burden. Palliative care, however, should be carefully introduced into the discourse, because it is generally associated with end-of-life care. To avoid this potential confusion, it may be best not to explicitly label care as 'palliative.' It would be more effective to be descriptive about the *elements* of palliative care including the right to withhold or withdraw life-sustaining therapies.

When offering palliation, or any other care strategy, it is important that the appropriate surrogate decisionmaker retains the ability to direct care. Ultimately, any decisionmaking authority resides in the patient's surrogate. This moral authority is based on what they know about the patient's preferences or values and their pre-existing relationship [92]. The practitioner's task is to help weave a consensus with the surrogate that takes account of the medical facts and the patient and surrogate's values and balances burdens and benefits.

Once a care plan has been agreed upon, it is helpful to suggest a *time trial* to see how and if the patient improves, leaving open the possibility that the goals of care can evolve as the situation changes. Time trials are also an important way to achieve a consensus and balance the power dynamic between clinician and family. They are essential to the *process of negotiation* and provide time for the surrogates to accommodate themselves to the sudden and often tragic reality of severe brain damage. Most importantly, they help safeguard the surrogate's authority and help them make decisions without being dictated to by the clinical team.

Periodic Review

The final step in the process of clinical pragmatism is periodic review. This is a critical step because it allows for the reassessment of decisions made in particular cases and modification of a course of action. As critically, this process allows us to organize empirical observations to reform practice and public policy. Public policy that governs research with individuals with disorders of consciousness is one critical issue that calls for reassessment in the wake of this consideration of the clinical care of such patients.

It is beyond the scope of this paper to address fully the challenge of engaging in clinical research with subjects who have decisional incapacity [93, 94]. These subjects are rightly considered a vulnerable population and subject to special protections because they are unable to provide their autonomous consent for enrolment in clinical trials. Although their next-of-kin or surrogates may authorize therapeutic procedures with demonstrated benefit, surrogates' ability to authorize enrolment in research is constrained when it has yet to demonstrate medical benefit, unless it was authorized prospectively by the patient before decisional incapacity. This severely limits the potential for phase I research in individuals who cannot provide consent [3, 20, 72, 95–98].

But unlike other vulnerable populations, the disorder that precludes autonomous consent is the object of the intervention when trying to restore consciousness. A compelling argument emerges that clinical trials to restore consciousness would be ethically proportionate, even with the challenges posed by surrogate consent, when we appreciate this critical distinction and the burdens imposed on these patients and families [1, 72].

While those with disorders of consciousness should be protected from harm, balancing and specifying the ethical principles of respect for persons, beneficence, and justice compel us to craft a responsible and responsive research ethic geared, for now, towards the pursuit of palliation [2, 93]. This becomes a fiduciary obligation grounded in a justice claim to meet the needs of patients society has so misunderstood and historically neglected [2].

CONCLUSION

The *terra nova* of neuroscience exploring disorders of consciousness is, to invoke an over-used phrase, paradigm breaking [99]. This line of enquiry will challenge assumptions, stir up misconceptions and engender both unrestrained hopes and unsubstantiated fears. If we are to grapple with the promise and peril of this work, it is critical to engage in a deliberative process of enquiry that allows us to see all sides of the argument, identify the range of stakeholders who may be affected by clinical and scientific developments, and to reach a societal consensus on how these efforts will proceed. An inductive approach which is reminiscent of diagnostics, clinical pragmatism can help constructively apply ethical principles to the context of care [96] and bring principled reasoning to complex ethical questions posed by cognitive neuroscience.

ACKNOWLEDGEMENTS

This essay is an abridged and updated version of 'Clinical pragmatism and the care of brain injured patients: towards a palliative neuroethics for disorders of consciousness' which appeared in *Prog Brain Res*, (2005)150, 565–582.

The author thanks Dr. Steven Laureys, the Mind Brain Foundation and the organizers of the Satellite Symposium on Coma and Impaired Consciousness at The Eighth Annual Conference of the Association for the Scientific Study of Consciousness for the invitation to present an earlier version of this paper at the University of Antwerp, Belgium on June 24, 2004.

Funded in part by a Robert Wood Johnson Foundation Investigator Award in Health Policy Research to Dr. Fins who also gratefully acknowledges support from The Charles A. Dana and Buster Foundations.

References

1. Schiff, N.D., Giacino, J.T., Kalmar, K., Victor, J.D., Baker, K., Gerber, M., Fritz, B., Eisenberg, B., O'Connor, J., Kobylarz, E.J., Farris, S., Machado, A., McCagg, C., Plum, F., Fins, J.J. and Rezai, A.R. (2007) Behavioral improvements with thalamic stimulation after severe traumatic brain injury. *Nature* 448 (7153):600–603.
2. Fins, J.J. (2003) Constructing an ethical stereotaxy for severe brain injury: Balancing risks, benefits and access. *Nat Rev Neurosci* 4:323–327.
3. Fins, J.J. (2003) From psychosurgery to neuromodulation and palliation: History's lessons for the ethical conduct and regulation of neuropsychiatric research. *Neurosurg Clin N Am* 14 (2):303–319.
4. Fins, J.J. (2004) Neuromodulation, free will and determinism: Lessons from the psychosurgery debate. *Clin Neurosci Res* 4 (1–2):113–118.
5. Fins, J.J. and Bacchetta, M.D. (1995) Framing the physician-assisted suicide and voluntary active euthanasia debate: The role of deontology, consequentialism and clinical pragmatism. *J Am Geriatr Soc* 43 (5):563–568.
6. Fins, J.J. (1996) From indifference to goodness. *J Relig Health* 35 (3):245–254.

7. Fins, J.J., Bacchetta, M.D. and Miller, F.G. (1997) Clinical pragmatism: A method of moral problem solving. *Kennedy Inst Ethic J* 7 (2):129–145.

8. Miller, F.G., Fletcher, J.C. and Fins, J.J. (1997) Clinical pragmatism: A case method of moral problem solving. In Fletcher, J.D., Lambardo, P.A., Marshall, M.F. and Miller, F.G., (eds.) *Introduction to Clinical Ethics*, 2nd edition. Frederick, Maryland: University Publishing Group.

9. Fins, J.J. (1998) Approximation and negotiation: Clinical pragmatism and difference. *Camb Quarterly Healthc Ethic* 7 (1):68–76.

10. Menand, L. (2001) *The Metaphysical Club*, New York: Farrar, Straus and Giroux.

11. Dewey, J. (1988) The Quest for Certainty. In *The Later Works, Vol. 4:1929*, Carbondale: Southern Illinois University Press.

12. Dewey, J. (1991) Theory of Valuation. In *The Later Works, Vol. 13: 1938–1939*, Carbondale: Southern Illinois University Press.

13. Dewey, J. (1991) Logic: The Theory of Inquiry. In *The Later Works, Vol. 12:1938*, Carbondale: Southern Illinois University Press.

14. Ryan, A. (1995) *John Dewey and the High Tide of American Liberalism*, New York: W.W. Norton.

15. Hook, S. (1995) *John Dewey: An Intellectual Portrait*, Amherst, New York: Prometheus Book.

16. Miller, F.G., Fins, J.J. and Bacchetta, M.D. (1996) Clinical pragmatism: John Dewey and clinical ethics. *J Contemp Health Law Policy* 13 (27):27–51.

17. Fins, J. J. (1999). Klinischer Pragmatismus und Ethik-Konsultation (Clinical pragmatism and ethics case consultation). Das Parlament 49.Jahrgang/Nr. 23.4 Juni: 18.

18. Dewey, J. (1997) *Experience and Nature*, Chicago and LaSalle Illinois: Open Court Publishing Company. pp. 134–137.

19. Dewey, J. (1998) The logic of judgments of practice. In Hickman, L.A. and Alexander, T.M. (eds.) *The Essential Dewey: Ethics, Logic, Psychology*, Vol. 2, pp. 236–271. Bloomington: Indiana University Press.

20. Miller, F.G. and Fins, J.J. (2006) Protecting human subjects in brain research: A pragmatic approach perspective. In *Neuroethics: Defining the Issues in Theory, Practice and Policy* J. Illes (eds.) New York: Oxford University Press. pp. 123–140.

21. Fins, J.J. and Miller, F.G. (2000) Clinical Pragmatism, Ethics Consultation and the Elderly. *Clinics in Geriatric Medicine* 16:71–81.

22. Fins, J.J. (2006) *A Palliative Ethic of Care: Clinical Wisdom at Life's End*. Sudbury, MA: Jones and Bartlett.

23. Childs, N.L., Mercer, W.N. and Childs, H.W. (1993) Accuracy of Diagnosis of Persistent Vegetative State. *Neurology* 43: 1465–1467.

24. Sacks, O. (1994) In the river of consciousness. *The New York Review of Books* 15:41–44.

25. Edelman, G.M. (2004) *Wider than the Sky: The Phenomenal Gift of Consciousness*, New Haven: Yale University Press.

26. Crick, F. (1994) *The Astonishing Hypothesis: The Scientific Search for the Soul*, New York: Scribner.

27. Searle, J.R. (2002) *Consciousness and Language*, New York: Cambridge University Press.

28. Koch, C. (2004) *The Quest for Consciousness: A Neurobiological Approach*, Englewood, Colorado: Roberts & Co.

29. Fins, J.J. and Plum, F. (2004) Neurological diagnosis is more than a state of mind: Diagnostic clarity and impaired consciousness. *Arch Neurol* 61 (9):1354–1355.

30. Bauby, J.-D. (1997) *The Diving Bell and the Butterfly*, New York: Vintage International.

31. Fins, J.J. (2005) Rethinking disorders of consciousness: New research and its implications. *Hast Cent Rep* 35 (2):22–24.

32. Uhlmann, R.F., Pearlman, R.A. and Cain, K.C. (1988) Physicians' and spouses' predictions of elderly patients' resuscitation preferences. *J Gerontol* 43:M115–121.

33. Uhlmann, R.F. and Pearlman, R.A. (1991) Perceived quality of life and preferences for life-sustaining treatment in older adults. *Arch Intern Med* 151:495–497.

34. Zussman, R. (1992) *Intensive Care: Medical Ethics and the Medical Profession*, Chicago: University of Chicago.

35. Fins, J.J. (2007) Ethics of clinical decision making and communication with surrogates. In Posner, J., Saper, C., Schiff, N.D. and plum, F. *Plum and Posner's Diagnosis of Stupor and Coma*, 4th edition, pp. 376–380. New York: Oxford University Press.

36. Kobylarz, E.J. and Schiff, N.D. (2004) Functional imaging of severely brain injured patients: Progress, challenges, and limitations. *Arch Neurol* 61 (9):1357–1360.

37. Jennett, B. (2002) *The Vegetative State*, Cambridge: Cambridge University Press.

38. Winslade, W. (1998) *Confronting Traumatic Brain Injury: Devastation, Hope and Healing*, New Haven: Yale University Press.

39. Giacino, J.T., Ashwal, S., Childs, N., Cranford, R., Jennett, B., Katz, D.I., Kelly, J.P., Rosenberg, J.H., Whyte, J., Zafonte, R.D. and Zasler, N.D. (2002) The minimally conscious state: Definition and diagnostic criteria. *Neurology* 58 (3):349–353.

40. Barondess, J.A. (2003) Personal communication to Joseph J. Fins.

41. Wilson, L.G. (1997) Fevers. In Bynum, W.F. and Porter, R. (eds.) *Companion Encyclopedia of the History of Medicine*, Vol. 1, pp. 382–411. London and New York: Routledge.

42. Jennett, B. and Plum, F. (1972) Persistent vegetative state after brain damage. A syndrome in search of a name. *Lancet* 1 (7753):734–737.

43. Jennett, B., Adams, J.H., Murray, L.S. and Graham, D.I. (2001) Neuropathology in vegetative and severely disabled patients after head injury. *Neurology* 56 (4):486–490.

44. Schiff, N.D., Ribary, U., Moreno, D.R., Beattie, B., Kronberg, E., Blasberg, R., Giacino, J., McCagg, C., Fins, J.J., Llinas, R. and Plum, F. (2002) Residual cerebral activity and behavioural fragments can remain in the persistently vegetative brain. *Brain* 125:1210–1234.

45. Menon, D.K., Owen, A.M., Williams, E.J., Minhas, P.S., Allen, C.M., Boniface, S.I. and Pickard, J.D. (1998) Cortical processing in persistent vegetative state Wolfson Brain Imaging Centre Team. *Lancet* 18:352 (9123):200.

46. Schiff, N.D. and Plum, F. (1999) Cortical function in the persistent vegetative state. *Trends in Cognitive Sciences* 3 (2):43–44.

47. Laureys, S., Faymonville, M.E., Moonen, G., Luxen, A. and Maquet, P. (2000) PET scanning and neuronal loss in acute vegetative state. *Lancet* 355 (9217):1825–1826.

48. Laureys, S., Antoine, S., Boly, M., Elincx, S., Faymonville, M. E., Berre, J., Sadzot, B., Ferring, M., De Tiege, X., van Bogaert, P., Hansen, I., Damas, P., Mavroudakis, N., Lambermont, B., Del Fiore, G., Aerts, J., Degueldre, C., Phillips, C., Franck, G., Vincent, J.L., Lamy, M., Luxen, A., Moonen, G., Goldman, S. and Maquet, P. (2002) Brain function in the vegetative state. *Acta Neurol Belg* 102 (4):177–185.

49. Schiff, N.D., Ribary, U., Moreno, D.R., Beattie, B., Kronberg, E., Blasberg, R., Giacino, J., McCagg, C., Fins, J.J., Llinas, R. and Plum, F. (2003) Residual cerebral activity and behavioural fragments can remain in the persistently vegetative brain. *Brain* 125 (pt 6):1210–1234.

50. Laureys, S., Owen, A.M. and Schiff, N.D. (2004) Brain function in coma, vegetative state and related disorders. *Lanc Neurol* 3 (9):537–546.

51. Voss, H.U., Uluc, A.M., Dyke, J.P., Watts, R., Kobylarz, E.J., McCandliss, B.D., Heier, L.A., Beattie, B.J., Hamacher, K.A., Vallabhajosula, S., Goldsmith, S.J., Ballon, D., Giacino, J.T. and Schiff, N.D. (2006) Possible axonal regrowth in late recovery from the minimally conscious state. *J Clin Invest* 116:2005–2011.

52. Owen, A.M., Coleman, M.R., Boly, M., Davis, M.H., Laureys, S. and Pickard, J.D. (2006) Detecting awareness in the vegetative state. *Science* 313 (5792):1402.

53. Wilson, B.A., Gracey, F. and Bainbridge, K. (2001) Cognitive recovery from 'persistent vegetative state': Psychological and personal perspectives. *Brain Inj* 15 (12):1083–1092.

54. Schiff, N.D., Rodriguez-Moreno, D., Kamal, A., *et al.* (2005) fMRI reveals large-scale network activation in minimally conscious patients. *Neurology* 64:514–523.

55. The Economist. (2004) Inside the mind of the consumer. June 10, 2004.

56. Farah, M.J. and Wolpe, P.R. (2004) Monitoring and manipulating brain function, new neuroscience technologies and their ethical implications. *Hast Cent Rep* 34 (3):35–45.

57. Fins, J.J. (2005) The Orwellian threat to emerging neurodiagnostic technologies. *Am J Bioteh* 5 (2):56–58.

58. Fins, J.J. (2007) Review, Mind Wars: Brain Research and National Defense. Moreno, J.D. Dana Press, New York. *JAMA* 297 (12):1382–1383.

59. Moreno, J.M., Mind Wars (2006) *Mind Wars: Brain Research and National Defense*, New York: Dana Press.

60. Cranford, R.E. (1998) The vegetative and minimally conscious states: Ethical implications. *Geriatrics* 53:S70–S73.

61. Shewmon, D.A. (2002) The minimally conscious state: Definition and diagnostic criteria. *Neurology* 58:506–507.

62. Coleman, D. (2002) The minimally conscious state: Definition and diagnostic criteria. *Neurology* 58:506–507.

63. Schiff, N.D. and Fins, J.J. (2003) Hope for 'comatose' patients. *Cerebrum* 5 (4):7–24.

64. Giacino, J.T. (2004) Personal communication with Joseph J. Fins.

65. Fins, J.J., Schiff, N.D. and Foley, K.M. (2007) Late Recovery from the Minimally Conscious State: Ethical and Policy Implications. *Neurology* 68:304–307.

66. Fins, J.J. (2006) Affirming the Right to Care, Preserving the Right to Die: Disorders of Consciousness and Neuroethics after Schiavo. *Supportive & Palliative Care* 4(2): 169–178.

67. The SUPPORT Investigators (1995) A controlled trial to improve care for seriously ill hospitalized patients: the Study to Understand Prognoses and Preferences for Outcomes and Risks of Treatment (SUPPORT). *JAMA* 274:1591–1598.

68. Meli, T. (2003) *I am the Central Park Jogger*, New York: Scribner, pp. 57–58.

69. Beauchamp, T.L. and Childress, J.F. (1994) *Principles of Biomedical Ethics*, 4th Edition. New York: Oxford University Press.

70. John Paul II (2004) Speech to the Participants at the International Congress, 'Life Sustaining Treatments and Vegetative State: Scientific Advances and Ethical Dilemmas'. March 20, 2004.

71. Schiff, N.D. (1999) Neurobiology, suffering, and unconscious brain states. *J Pain Symp Manag* 17 (4):303–304.

72. Fins, J.J. (2000) A proposed ethical framework for interventional cognitive neuroscience: A consideration of deep brain stimulation in impaired consciousness. *Neurologic Res* 22:273–278.

73. Osborn, C.L. (1998) *Over My Head*, Kansas City: Andrews McNeal Publishing.

74. Morris, K. (2004) Mind moves onscreen: Brain-computer interface comes to trial. *Lanc Neurol* 3:329.

75. Powell, T. and Lowenstein, B. (1996) Refusing life-sustaining treatment after catastrophic injury: Ethical implications. *J Law, Med Ethic* 24:54–61.

76. Leon-Carrion, J., van Eeckhourt, P., Dominguez-Morales, M.D.R. and Santamaria, F.J.P. (2002) Survey: The Locked-in-Syndrome: A syndrome looking for a therapy. *Brain Inj* 16 (7):571–582.

77. Fins, J.J. (1992) The Patient Self-Determination Act and patient–physician collaboration in New York State. *NY State J Med* 92 (11):489–493.

78. Levine, C. (1999) The loneliness of the long-term care giver. *N Eng J Med* 340 (20):1587–1590.

79. Christakis, N.A. (1999) *Death Foretold: Prophecy and Prognosis in Medical Care*, Chicago: The University of Chicago Press. pp. 41.

80. Fins, J.J. (2002) When the prognosis leads to indifference. *J Palliat Med* 5 (4):571–573.

81. Stevens, M.L. (1995) Redefining death in America, 1968. *Caduceus, 1995 Winter* 11 (3):207–219.

82. Beecher, H.K. (1968) Ethical problems created by the hopelessly unconscious patient. *N Eng J Med* 278 (26):1425–1430.

83. Cantor, N.L. (2001) Twenty-five years after Quinlan: A review of the jurisprudence of death and dying. *J Law Med Ethic 2001 Summer* 29 (2):182–196.

84. *Cruzan v Director* Missouri Department of Health, 110 S. Ct. 2841 (1990).

85. Cranford, R.E. (1994) Medical futility: Transforming a clinical concept into legal and social policies. *J Am Geriatr Soc* 42:894–898.

86. Annas, G.J. (1996) The 'right to die' in America: Sloganeering from Quinlan and Cruzan to Quill and Kevorkian. *Duquesne Law Rev* 34 (4):875–897.

87. World Health Organization (1990) *Cancer Pain Relief and Palliative Care*, Geneva, Switzerland: World Health Organization. pp. 11–12.

88. Fins, J.J. (1992) Palliation in the age of chronic disease. *Hast Cent Rep* 22 (1):41–42.

89. Fins, J.J. (2004) Deep Brain Stimulation. In Post, S.G. (ed.) *Encyclopedia of Bioethics (3rd Edition)*, Vol. 2, pp. 629–634. New York: MacMillan Reference.

90. Leon-Carrion, J., van Eeckhourt, P., Dominguez-Morales, M.D.R. and Santamaria, F.J.P. (2002) Review of subject: The Locked-in-Syndrome: A syndrome looking for a therapy. *Brain Inj* 16 (7):555–569.

91. Parfit, D. (1987) *Reasons and Persons*, New York: Clarendon Press-Oxford University Press.

92. Fins, J.J. (1999) From contract to covenant in advance care planning. *J Law, Med Ethic* 27:46–51.

93. National Bioethics Advisory Commission (1998) Research Involving Persons with Mental Disorders that May Affect Decision-making Capacity. Rockville, MD.

94. Fins, J.J. and Miller, F.G. (2000) Enrolling decisionally incapacitated subjects in neuropsychiatric research. *CNS Spect* 5 (10):32–42.

95. Michels, R. (1999) Are research ethics bad for our mental health? *N Eng J Med* 340 (18):1427–1430.

96. Miller, F.G. and Fins, J.J. (1999) Protecting vulnerable research subjects without unduly constraining neuropsychiatric research. *Archives of General Psychiatry* 56:701–702.

97. Miller, F.G. and Fins, J.J. (2005) Protecting human subjects in brain research: A pragmatic perspective. In Illes, J. (ed.) *Neuroethics: Defining the Issues in Theory, Practice and Policy*, pp. 123–140. New York: Oxford University Press.

98. Fins, J.J., Rezai, A.R. and Greenberg, B.D. (2006) Psychosurgery: Avoiding an ethical redux while advancing a therapeutic future. *Neurosurgery* 59 (4):713–716.

99. Kuhn, T.S. (1996) *The Structure of Scientific Revolutions*, 3rd Edition. Chicago: University of Chicago Press,

100. Schmidt-Felzmann, H. (2003) Pragmatic principles-methodological pragmatism in the principle-based approach to bioethics. *Journal of Medicine and Philosophy* 28 (5–6):581–596.

101. Fins, J.J., Maltby, B.S., Friedmann, E., Green, M., Norris, K., Adelman, R. and Byock, I. (2005) Contracts, covenants and advance care planning: An empirical study of the moral obligations of patient and proxy. *J Pain Symp Manag* 29 (1):55–68.

SEIZURES, SPLITS, NEGLECTS AND ASSORTED DISORDERS

Epilepsy and Consciousness

Hal Blumenfeld

ABSTRACT

Conscious information processing depends on synchronous network activity in the brain. The same network which evolved for the generation of normal consciousness can be exploited by abnormally intense and synchronous discharges, leading to epileptic seizures. By involving these networks, seizures often cause impaired consciousness. In analogy to sensory, motor, and other systems in the brain, we refer to brain networks involved in consciousness as the 'consciousness system.' We propose here that diverse seizure types share in common the involvement of specific anatomical structures in the consciousness system, leading to impaired consciousness. Thus, absence seizures, generalized tonic–clonic seizures, and temporal lobe complex partial seizures differ dramatically in their cause, behaviour, and electrophysiology. However, all the three seizure types cause impaired consciousness. Recent advances in neuroimaging and electrophysiology demonstrate that these seizures share a common pattern of disrupted activity in the consciousness system, involving the: (i) upper brainstem and medial thalamus, (ii) anterior and posterior interhemispheric regions (cingulate, medial frontal cortex, and precuneus), and (iii) lateral frontal and parietal association cortex. The physiology may differ between seizure types, causing either abnormal increases or decreases in neuronal activity and neuroimaging, but the anatomical regions involved when consciousness is impaired remain the same. Understanding the mechanisms for impaired consciousness in epilepsy has important practical applications for preventing patient injuries and social stigma, and may also shed light on mechanisms important for normal consciousness.

INTRODUCTION

Consciousness is something that every child understands, but that scientist and philosophers still struggle to explain. We are all intimately acquainted with what it means to be conscious or unconscious as we wake up in the morning, doze off briefly during a lecture, drive somewhere without thinking about the

TABLE 19.1   Seizures Associated with Impaired Consciousness

	Absence seizure (petit mal)	Generalized tonic-clonic seizure (grand mal)	Complex partial seizure
Classification	Generalized	Generalized	Partial
Typical behavior	Motionless stare, unresponsive, often with eyelid flutter, and minor hand movements	Bilateral tonic limb rigidity and extension lasting 10–20 second, then rhythmic bilateral clonic limb jerks for ~1 minute	Aura (vague premonition, fear, rising epigastric feeling, etc.), then stare, unresponsive, chewing or lip smacking, contralateral limb dystonia, ipsilateral repetitive automatisms (rubbing, picking, etc.)
Duration	Less than 10 seconds	1–2 minutes	1–2 minutes
Postical deficits	None	Sleepy or sleeping, weakness, confused	Confused
Scalp EEG	Generalized 3–4 Hz spike-wave discharge	**Tonic phase:** Generalized high-frequency polyspike discharge **Clonic phase:** Generalized polyspike-and-wave discharge **Postictal:** Generalized suppression or generalized slowing	**Ictal:** 5–7 Hz rhythmic temporal discharge, with some bilateral slowing **Postical:** Generalized slowing

route, or engage in a stimulating discussion requiring full awareness. Consciousness provides an important, human quality to our life experience, and we depend on consciousness as an efficient way to organize and prioritize our memories and actions [1]. In epilepsy, consciousness is suddenly and involuntarily taken away. During seizures, patients experience lapses in consciousness, which can have major negative impact including injuries, social stigma, and lost time.

Up until recently, the mechanisms for impaired consciousness in epilepsy were not known. Much work has been done, and is ongoing to elucidate the mechanisms of normal consciousness, and impaired consciousness in disease states (see other chapters in this volume). With advances in functional neuroimaging and neurophysiology it is now possible, for the first time, to identify specific networks that are affected in the brain during epileptic unconsciousness. Recent investigations suggest that epilepsy, like other disorders of consciousness, disrupts a core network of anatomical structures critical for the maintenance of normal consciousness. Because epileptic seizures cause transient, dynamic, deficits in consciousness which can range from mild impairment of attention to complete behavioural unresponsiveness, the study of seizures provides an opportunity to functionally localize specific aspects of consciousness in the brain. Impaired consciousness in epilepsy also has major practical significance, since most negative consequences of seizures (driving accidents, falls, burns,

social stigma, and work-related disability) are directly related to loss of consciousness.

Epileptic seizures are usually classified as either partial, meaning that they involve focal regions of the brain, or generalized, meaning that they involve widespread regions of the brain bilaterally [2]. Interestingly, impaired consciousness can be seen in both partial and generalized seizures. Thus, impaired consciousness is seen in generalized seizure types, such as absence (petit mal), and tonic–clonic (grand mal) seizures, as well as in partial seizure types, namely complex partial temporal lobe seizures (Table 19.1). These three types of seizures differ dramatically in terms of their usual causes, behavioural manifestations, and brain electrical activity (Table 19.1).

However, despite the differences between absence, tonic–clonic, and complex partial seizures, they all share a common thread of impaired consciousness, and affect the same specific brain networks (Figure 19.1). As we will discuss in this chapter, these seizure types cause changes in: (i) the upper brainstem and medial thalamus; (ii) the anterior and posterior cingulate, medial frontal cortex, and precuneus; (iii) lateral and orbital frontal cortex, and lateral parietal cortex. Epilepsy can disrupt brain function through either abnormal increases or abnormal decreases in neuronal activity [3]. Although the direction of regional activity increases or decreases differs between absence, tonic–clonic, and complex partial seizures, the specific anatomical networks affected are the same.

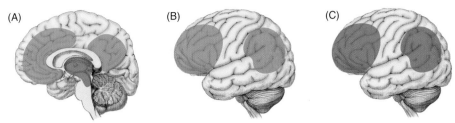

FIGURE 19.1   The 'consciousness system': a common network for consciousness. The depicted regions are important for normal consciousness. During seizures, bilateral abnormal activity in these regions is associated with impaired consciousness. (A) Bilateral abnormal increases in activity (red) are seen in the upper brainstem and medial thalamus (midline, mediodorsal, and intralaminar nuclei) during absence, generalized tonic–clonic, and temporal lobe complex partial seizures. Bilateral abnormal decreases in activity (blue) are seen in certain midline interhemispheric regions (anterior and posterior cingulate, medial frontal cortex, and precuneus) during these same three seizure types. Decreases in the interhemispheric regions persist in the postictal period, a time when patients often remain unconscious. (B) Bilateral abnormal decreases in activity occur in the lateral frontal and parietal cortex during absence and temporal lobe complex partial seizures. Decreases in these same regions are seen in the postictal period after temporal lobe complex partial seizures and after generalized tonic–clonic seizures. (C) Bilateral abnormal increased activity is seen in the lateral frontal and parietal cortex during generalized tonic–clonic seizures. Note that these same regions show decreased activity postictally following generalized tonic–clonic seizures. During absence seizures, these lateral frontal and parietal regions show some increases, as well as decreases (B). Brain illustrations modified with permission from [5].

Improved understanding of the specific brain regions involved during epileptic unconsciousness may allow therapeutic interventions, such as deep brain stimulation, or targeted medical therapies to be developed which will prevent this serious consequence of epilepsy. In addition, since the impaired consciousness in epilepsy is variable, careful study of specific deficits and involved brain areas during seizures may allow a greater understanding of the anatomy of consciousness. In this chapter we will first introduce the common anatomical networks of cortical and subcortical structures known to be important for consciousness in general and recently found to also be involved when seizures cause loss of consciousness. Next we will review the three main types of seizures causing impaired consciousness, and discuss each in turn, emphasizing recent neuroimaging and other results that suggest the mechanisms for impaired consciousness. Finally, we will discuss practical applications and future directions for work on impaired consciousness in epilepsy.

THE 'CONSCIOUSNESS SYSTEM': A COMMON NETWORK FOR CONSCIOUSNESS

As discussed elsewhere in this volume (Chapters 1, 2), consciousness depends on a network of cortical and subcortical structures. Many studies have been done in both normal states of alertness and attention, and in states of impaired consciousness such as sleep, anaesthesia, and brain lesions to reveal a common network of structures critically involved in the generation of consciousness. We refer to these structures, collectively, as the 'consciousness system' in analogy to other major systems (sensory, motor, limbic, etc.) in the brain. Consciousness has long been separated into structures necessary for controlling the *level* of consciousness, and those involved in generating the *content* of consciousness [4]. The content of consciousness can be considered the substrate (hierarchical sensorimotor, memory, and emotional systems) upon which level-of-consciousness systems act (Chapter 2, this volume [3, 5]). Here we define the 'consciousness system' as those structures directly involved in controlling the level of consciousness, which in turn, depends on multiple systems acting together. These include systems necessary for maintaining: (i) the alert, awake state, (ii) attention, and (iii) awareness of self and the environment. Therefore, the consciousness system at minimum includes regions of the frontal and parietal association cortex, cingulate gyrus, precuneus, thalamus (especially the medial, midline, and intralaminar nuclei), and multiple activating systems located in the basal forebrain, hypothalamus, midbrain, and upper pons. Some would also include the basal ganglia and cerebellum due to their possible roles in controlling attention [6–8].

Much previous work has demonstrated the importance of the midline subcortical structures, and association cortex in normal consciousness [1, 9–20]. Prior studies in states of impaired consciousness such as coma and vegetative state [21, 22], sleep [23–26], and anaesthesia [27, 28] have, likewise, shown involvement of similar regions of the upper brainstem and medial thalamus, interhemispheric regions (cingulate, medial frontal cortex, precuneus), and lateral frontal and parietal association cortex.

In this chapter we will review recent findings which suggest that absence, generalized tonic–clonic, and complex partial seizures all involve the same anatomical regions of the consciousness system (Figure 19.1). Recent neuroimaging studies have shown that all three types of seizures cause abnormal increases in activity in the upper brainstem and medial thalamus. Changes in the interhemispheric regions are also remarkably similar in these three seizure types, with *decreases* in activity seen in the anterior and posterior cingulate, medial frontal cortex, and precuneus, both during and following seizures. Changes in the lateral and orbital frontal cortex, and lateral parietal cortex are also anatomically similar in these three seizure types. However, the direction of changes in the lateral association cortex is more complicated. Absence seizures show both increases and decreases in frontal functional magnetic resonance imaging (fMRI) signals, and show mainly decreases in the parietal cortex. Generalized tonic–clonic seizures show cerebral blood flow (CBF) increases in the lateral frontal and parietal association cortex during seizures, and decreases in these same regions in the postictal period, when consciousness usually remains severely impaired. Complex partial seizures show decreases in the frontal and parietal association cortex, which persist along with impaired consciousness in the postictal period.

We will now discuss absence seizures, generalized tonic–clonic seizures, and complex partial seizures in greater detail, emphasizing recent studies which relate impaired consciousness to altered function in specific brain regions.

ABSENCE SEIZURES

In absence seizures, as the name implies, awareness briefly vanishes. Typical absence seizures consist of staring and unresponsiveness, often accompanied by subtle eyelid fluttering or mild myoclonic jerks. Duration is usually less than 10 seconds (Table 19.1). Absence seizures occur most commonly in childhood, and are accompanied by bilateral, frontal predominant 3–4 Hz spike–wave discharges on electroencephalography (EEG) [29, 30]. Both human and animal studies support the role of corticothalamic network oscillations in generating absence seizures [31–39].

Because motor manifestations are relatively mild, absence can be considered the 'purest' form of impaired consciousness in epilepsy. Patients appear as if someone has pushed the 'pause button' on their stream of consciousness, briefly interrupting their ongoing behaviour, and then resuming approximately

where they left off without significant postictal deficits. More behavioural studies of impaired consciousness have been performed with absence seizures than any other seizure type. This is, most likely, because absence seizures can occur in susceptible individuals up to several hundred times per day. These behavioural studies were performed mostly in the 1930s through 1970s, before functional neuroimaging was available, and were reviewed in [40]. Based on these behavioural studies, it can be concluded that: (i) Impaired consciousness during spike–wave seizures varies from one patient to the next, and even within individual patients. (ii) The severity of impairment also varies with the specific task used for testing. For example, patients often perform better during absence seizures with simple repetitive motor tasks, and have the most difficulty with tasks that require complex decision making or a verbal response [41–44]. (iii). Atypical, irregular, or slow (~2 Hz or less) spike–wave discharges, and prolonged absence status epilepticus in some cases, cause little or no impairment of consciousness [45, 46].

Although considered a form of generalized epilepsy, there is ample evidence based on both human and animal studies that so-called 'generalized' spike–wave discharges in fact arise from specific corticothalamic networks which are most intensely involved, while other regions are relatively spared [39]. The specific brain regions involved during absence seizures may have important implications for explaining why these seizures cause relatively selective impairment of consciousness.

Human EEG recordings during absence seizures have long shown that the spike–wave discharges are of largest amplitude in the frontal midline regions [29, 30, 47]. Animal models have also supported focal involvement of bilateral anterior cortical and subcortical brain regions during spike–wave discharges, based on electrophysiology [48–52], molecular changes [53], and more recently, neuroimaging with fMRI [54]. These investigations suggest that spike–wave seizures, which appear fairly generalized on scalp EEG recordings, in fact may intensely involve some corticothalamic networks, while other brain regions are relatively spared.

Early human imaging studies during absence seizures produced highly variable results, with some studies showing global increases in cerebral metabolism or blood flow [55–59], and others showing no change, biphasic changes, or generalized decreases [55, 60, 61]. Some of this variability may reflect technical limitations of the methods used. For example, Doppler flow studies have limited spatial resolution, and imaging methods such as positron emission tomography

(PET) or single photon emission computed tomography (SPECT) have limited temporal resolution relative to absence seizure duration. However, the variable results could at least in part also reflect the variable nature of absence seizures themselves. For example, even typical absence seizures have varying EEG amplitude, duration, and rhythmicity; and larger amplitude often fluctuates between the right and left side [62, 63].

The availability of simultaneous EEG-fMRI has greatly improved the spatial and temporal resolution of neuroimaging during spike–wave seizures. Several recent studies have investigated the fMRI changes during spike–wave seizures [64–72], some of which were performed in children with absence epilepsy [65, 66, 69]. These studies have shown bilateral fMRI changes in the consciousness system described above (Figure 19.1). Thus, during spike–wave seizures, fMRI increases have been reported in the thalamus (Figure 19.2A), with decreases seen in the anterior and posterior interhemispheric regions (Figure 19.2C), and decreases in the lateral frontal and parietal association cortex (Figure 19.2B). Most of these studies have also reported variable fMRI increases in the lateral frontal and parietal cortical regions in addition to the decreases.

Based on these results, we and others have hypothesized that loss of consciousness in absence seizures is not an 'all-or-none' phenomenon resulting from involvement of the entire brain in the seizure discharge [3, 37, 40]. Rather, focal involvement of the bilateral association cortex and related subcortical structures, disrupts normal information processing in specific brain regions leading to impaired consciousness. Variable involvement of different regions in different seizures may account for the variable severity of deficits seen during absence seizures. The detailed anatomical relationship of these changes to behaviour will need additional investigation.

GENERALIZED TONIC–CLONIC SEIZURES

Like absence seizures, grand mal (tonic–clonic) seizures are classified as 'generalized (Table 19.1).' Although it may appear obvious that generalized tonic–clonic seizures cause impaired consciousness through involvement of widespread brain regions, surprisingly little research has been done to investigate this claim. It is natural to ask whether, like in absence seizures, impaired consciousness in so-called 'generalized' tonic–clonic seizures may depend on abnormal activity in focal brain regions. Generalized tonic–clonic seizures are subdivided into primarily generalized, in which there is no obvious focal onset, and secondarily generalized, in which seizures begin in a focal brain region and then spread. In the tonic phase, there are sustained muscle contractions accompanied by high frequency activity on EEG recordings lasting 10–20 seconds (Table 19.1). This is followed by rhythmic clonic contractions of the limbs accompanied by polyspike-and-wave EEG discharges. After 1–2 minutes, clinical and EEG seizure activity usually abruptly stops, and the patient remains deeply lethargic, unresponsive, and with markedly suppressed EEG amplitude for a variable time in the postictal period.

Some previous studies, including those using electrophysiological, blood flow, and metabolic mapping, suggest that the entire brain may be homogeneously involved in generalized tonic–clonic seizures [58, 73–77]. However, other animal studies show more regional changes [78, 79]. Furthermore, secondarily generalized tonic–clonic seizures in humans often cause focal postictal deficits, reflecting impaired function in the regions of seizure onset [80, 81]. SPECT imaging studies of CBF in secondarily generalized tonic–clonic seizures have shown focal involvement as well, often in regions of seizure onset [82–87]. These findings suggest that secondarily generalized, and possibly also primary generalized tonic–clonic seizures do not involve

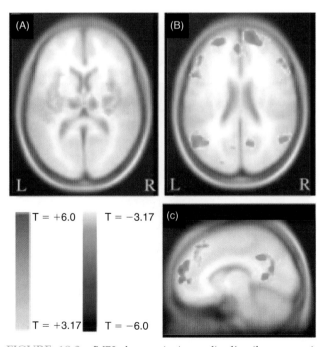

FIGURE 19.2 fMRI changes in 'generalized' spike–wave seizures. Group analysis of 15 patients with idiopathic generalized epilepsy. (A) Increases are seen in bilateral thalami, as well as several cortical areas. (B) Decreases are seen in bilateral interhemispheric regions, as well as in the lateral frontal and parietal association cortex. Modified with permission from [68].

the entire brain homogenously, but may instead affect certain regions most intensely. Like in absence seizures, identifying the specific regions involved may be important for understanding how generalized tonic–clonic seizures cause impaired consciousness.

SPECT ictal–interictal difference imaging is a useful method for investigating brain regions involved in human generalized tonic–clonic seizures, because this method can be used even when patients move during seizures [81, 86, 87]. This is because the SPECT radiopharmaceutical is injected during the seizure, but the actual imaging can be done later, when the patient is stable. The imaging done later reflects blood flow at the time of the injection, not at the time of imaging. Using this approach, we have imaged spontaneous secondarily generalized tonic–clonic seizures in patients with epilepsy [81, 86, 87], and generalized tonic–clonic seizures induced by electroconvulsive therapy (ECT) for treatment of refractory depression (in patients without epilepsy) [81, 88–90]. In all spontaneous and induced generalized tonic–clonic seizures we saw focal CBF increases in specific brain regions, not global increases. The regions involved were again in the consciousness system described above (Figure 19.1). During seizures, there were CBF increases in the thalamus and upper brainstem, and decreases in the cingulate gyrus. In the lateral frontal and parietal cortex there were large CBF increases during seizures. In the postictal period, when patients remain unconscious, there were large CBF decreases in the lateral frontal and parietal cortex, along with continued decreases in the anterior and posterior cingulate.

More recent work has shown that these brain regions undergo a complex sequence of changes at different times during and after generalized tonic–clonic seizures. For example, early on in bilateral ECT-induced seizures, focal increases are seen in the fronto-temporal association cortex, near the region of the stimulating electrodes, along with increases in the thalamus (Figure 19.3A). Thirty seconds later, large increases are seen in the bilateral parietal cortex, along with decreases in the cingulate gyrus (Figure 19.3B) [89]. In the postictal period, study of spontaneous secondarily generalized tonic–clonic seizures has shown an interesting progression of CBF increases in the cerebellum [86, 87]. Cerebellar CBF increases in the postictal period are correlated with increases in the thalamus, and with profound CBF *decreases* in frontal and parietal cortex. These findings suggest a possible role for inhibitory cerebellar outputs in seizure termination, and in postictal depression of consciousness [91, 92].

It is interesting that the regions most intensely involved in CBF increases during generalized tonic–clonic seizures were the bilateral frontal and parietal

association cortex, while intervening regions were relatively spared (Figure 19.3). Seizure propagation between frontal and parietal association cortex could occur through long association fiber pathways such as the superior longitudinal fasciculus [93, 94], or through cortical–thalamic–cortical interactions [95, 96]. Sparing of motor cortex supports the notion that the motor manifestations of generalized tonic–clonic seizures may be mediated primarily by brainstem circuitry [97–100]. Interestingly, the converse situation has also been reported in the literature. In other words, in the rare situation where seizures are confined to the sensorimotor areas bilaterally, patients exhibit generalized tonic–clonic seizures with complete sparing of consciousness [101].

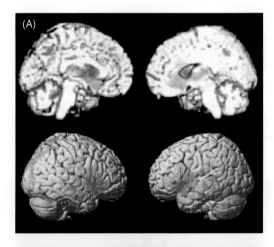

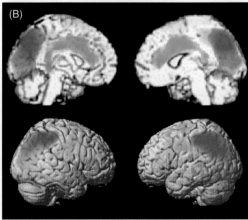

FIGURE 19.3 CBF changes in 'generalized' tonic–clonic seizures. SPECT ictal–interictal difference imaging from patients undergoing bilateral ECT. (A) CBF changes at seizure onset (0 second after ECT stimulus). Increases (red) occur in the bilateral inferior frontal gyrus, anterior insula, basal ganglia, and thalamus. No significant decreases were found (n = 4). (B) CBF changes 30 second after the ECT stimulus. Increases occur in bilateral parietal cortex, while decreases (green) occur in the bilateral interhemispheric regions (n = 7). Modified with permission from [89].

Additional work is needed to better understand the electrophysiological correlates of imaging changes seen during generalized tonic–clonic seizures. It has been shown, for example, that paradoxical imaging changes can occur during tonic clonic seizures, which do not always accurately reflect the underlying electrical activity [102]. It will, therefore, be crucial to verify neuroimaging findings during tonic–clonic seizures with direct electrical recordings from patients or animals models.

COMPLEX PARTIAL SEIZURES

While it is logical that absence and tonic–clonic seizures impair consciousness by involving the brain bilaterally, it has been more difficult to explain how a partial seizure, which involves a focal unilateral region such as the temporal lobe, can cause impaired consciousness. Partial seizures which spare consciousness are called simple partial seizures, while partial seizures accompanied by impaired consciousness are called complex partial seizures [2] (alternative classifications have been proposed [103, 104], but the terms 'simple partial' and 'complex partial' remain in wide use). Complex partial seizures most often arise from the temporal lobe, and are frequently accompanied by pathological changes referred to as mesial temporal sclerosis [105, 106]. Temporal lobe seizures typically begin with focal phenomena such as fear,

rising epigastric sensation, an indescribable premonition, or lip smacking automatisms [107, 108] (Table 19.1). Although consciousness may be spared initially, progression to impaired consciousness is common during temporal lobe seizures. In addition to impaired responsiveness and amnesia, temporal lobe complex partial seizures are often accompanied by automaton-like movements referred to by Penfield as 'automatisms,' dystonic posturing of the limbs [109], and neuroendocrine changes [110, 111]. Complex partial seizures usually last 1–2 minutes, and electrographically show 5–7 Hz rhythmic temporal lobe activity on scalp EEG recordings, with some bilateral slowing (Table 19.1). Impaired consciousness in complex partial seizures is usually most profound late in the seizure and can persist for up to several minutes after the seizure has ended (postictal period).

The diverse behavioural repertoire of temporal lobe seizures, and prior human and animal investigations, suggest that more widespread neural networks beyond the temporal lobe are recruited during these events [92, 112–116]. Based on EEG studies, it has been suggested that bilateral temporal lobe involvement is important for loss of consciousness in complex partial seizures [117–121]. However, while bilateral temporal lobe dysfunction may cause amnesia [122], it is unclear why this would cause impaired consciousness, manifested as loss of responsiveness and awareness during seizures.

To explain how impaired consciousness could occur with focal temporal lobe seizures, we proposed a 'network inhibition hypothesis' (Figure 19.4) [3, 92].

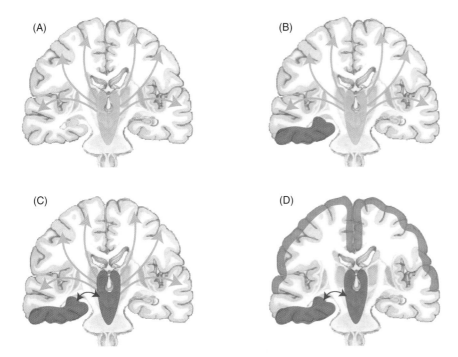

(A)

(B)

(C)

(D)

FIGURE 19.4   Network inhibition hypothesis for loss of consciousness in complex partial seizures. (A) Under normal conditions, the upper brainstem-diencephalic activating systems interact with the cerebral cortex to maintain normal consciousness (yellow represents normal activity). (B) A focal seizure (red) involving the mesial temporal lobe unilaterally. (C) Propagation of seizure activity from the mesial temporal lobe to midline subcortical structures. (D) Disruption of the normal activating functions of the midline subcortical structures leads to depressed activity (blue) in bilateral regions of the fronto-parietal association cortex, leading to loss of consciousness. Modified with permission from [3].

According to this model, impaired consciousness occurs in temporal lobe seizures due to spread of seizures to midline subcortical structures (Figure 19.4B, C). This in turn, blocks the normal activating function of these midline structures, and causes bilateral cortical suppression (Figure 19.4D). Note that the structures involved in this model, including the midline subcortical structures, anterior and posterior interhemispheric regions, and lateral fronto-parietal association cortex, again lie within the consciousness system discussed earlier (Figure 19.1).

Direct support for the network inhibition hypothesis would require complete investigation of the underlying physiological mechanisms. However, several studies provide indirect support for the network inhibition hypothesis. Work in animal models suggests an important role for the medial thalamus in limbic seizures [78, 116, 123–129]. In humans, the thalamus on the side of temporal lobe seizure onset has been shown to have functional decreases on interictal PET, SPECT, and magnetic resonance spectroscopy (MRS) imaging [130–133]; and reduced volume on MRI and postmortem studies [134–137].

Functional imaging with ictal SPECT further supports the importance of medial temporal and midline subcortical connections in limbic seizures. Mayanagi *et al.* initially reported involvement of the medial thalamus and upper brainstem on ictal SPECT in temporal lobe epilepsy [138]. Lee *et al.* subsequently found an association between medial thalamic and upper brainstem involvement on SPECT imaging during seizures, and loss of consciousness [115]. In addition to midline subcortical involvement, SPECT imaging has also identified frontal or parietal hypoperfusion during temporal lobe seizures [139–142].

In studying patients with temporal lobe epilepsy who had impaired consciousness during seizures, we found widespread changes outside the temporal lobe on ictal SPECT imaging [143, 144]. Increased CBF was present in the upper brainstem and medial thalamus. Interestingly, the increases in the medial thalamus were correlated with decreases in the anterior and posterior interhemispheric regions, and in the fronto-parietal association cortex (Figure 19.5A, B) [144]. In contrast, we found that simple partial seizures (consciousness spared), were associated with more focal changes confined to the temporal lobes, and did not show fronto-parietal or midline subcortical changes [144]. Several additional studies have shown similar involvement of midline subcortical structures on SPECT imaging during temporal lobe seizures [145–147].

These neuroimaging findings suggest that loss of consciousness during temporal lobe seizures may be caused by abnormal activity in the midline subcortical structures and depressed function of the fronto-parietal association cortex. What are the physiological

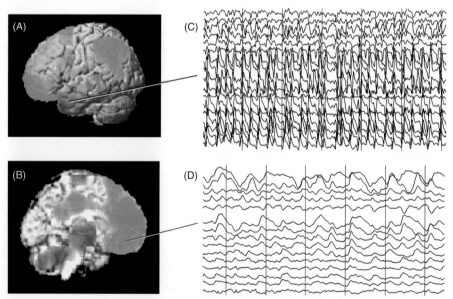

FIGURE 19.5   CBF and EEG changes in temporal lobe complex partial seizures. (A, B) Group analysis of SPECT ictal–interictal difference imaging during temporal lobe seizures. CBF increases are present in the temporal lobe (A) and in the medial thalamus (B). Decreases are seen in the lateral front-parietal association cortex (A) and in the interhemispheric regions (B). (C, D.) Intracranial EEG recordings from a patient during a temporal lobe seizure. High frequency polyspike-and-wave seizure activity is seen in the temporal lobe (C). The orbital and medial frontal cortex (and other regions, EEG not shown) do not show polyspike activity, but instead large amplitude, irregular slow rhythms resembling coma or sleep (D). Vertical lines in C, D denote one second intervals. Note that the EEG and SPECT data were from similar patients, but were not simultaneous, and are shown together here for illustrative purposes only. A, B modified with permission from [144]. C, D modified with permission from [149].

changes underlying the decreased CBF in the fronto-parietal cortex? Interestingly, human intracranial EEG studies have shown slow waves in the association cortex during temporal lobe seizures [138, 148, 149]. Some have interpreted this as 'propagation' of seizure activity outside the temporal lobe; however, unlike the high frequency seizure discharges seen in the temporal lobe (Figure 19.5C), the activity in the fronto-parietal association cortex consists of slow waves, without spike or sharp components (Figure 19.5D) [149]. We have argued that this slow rhythm on intracranial recordings does not represent seizure activity, but instead more closely resembles the EEG patterns seen in sleep, coma, or encephalopathy [149]. Further support for this has come from quantitative studies of intracranial EEG in temporal lobe epilepsy, confirming distinct activity patterns in the temporal lobe and the association cortex [150]. In addition, recent work in an animal model has shown that during limbic seizures there is slow activity in the frontal cortex, accompanied by decreased frontal neuronal firing, and decreased CBF which closely resembles deep anaesthesia and sleep in the same model [151]. Together, these findings suggest that focal seizure activity in the temporal lobe may, through spread to midline subcortical structures, put the rest of brain into a sleep-like state, resulting in loss of consciousness.

To recapitulate the network inhibition hypothesis discussed above (Figure 19.4), under normal conditions the upper brainstem-diencephalic activating systems interact with the cortex to maintain the normal conscious state (Figure 19.4A). A focal seizure in the temporal lobe (Figure 19.4B) may propagate through known pathways [116, 123, 124] to midline subcortical structures (Figure 19.4C). This disrupts the normal activating function of these circuits, leading to widespread inhibition of the fronto-parietal association cortex (Figure 19.4D). It remains unknown whether decreased activity in the fronto-parietal cortex is caused by increased inhibitory inputs, decreased excitatory inputs, or both. Further investigations in both humans and animal models [151] will be necessary to fully understand the behavioural details and physiological mechanisms of impaired consciousness in temporal lobe epilepsy.

SUMMARY AND CONCLUSIONS

We have seen that diverse seizure types cause impaired consciousness through involvement of common structures in the 'consciousness system,' including the medial thalamus and upper brainstem, interhemispheric regions (medial frontal cortex,

cingulate, and precuneus), and lateral frontal and parietal association cortex (Figure 19.1). Absence, generalized tonic–clonic, and temporal lobe complex partial seizures all cause abnormal increases in activity of the medial thalamus and upper brainstem. All the three seizure types also cause *decreased* activity in the interhemispheric regions. The lateral frontal and parietal cortex shows a mixture of abnormal increases and decreases in activity during absence seizures; increases during generalized tonic–clonic seizures; and decreases during temporal lobe complex partial seizures. In the postictal period which usually follows generalized tonic–clonic and temporal lobe complex partial seizures (but not absence), there is often lingering impairment of consciousness, accompanied by markedly decreased activity in wide regions of the frontal and parietal association cortex.

There is much remaining work to be done to more fully understand the mechanisms of impaired consciousness in epilepsy. Absence seizures, with their variable impact on the performance of different tasks [40], may provide a unique opportunity to investigate the anatomical basis of specific deficits in the consciousness system. For example, more regions may be involved on fMRI when seizures disrupt performance on easy repetitive motor tasks, than when seizures only disrupt harder discrimination tasks. In so-called 'generalized' tonic–clonic seizures, it will be crucial to determine if electrical recordings will confirm the focal bilateral network changes seen on neuroimaging. In temporal lobe complex partial seizures, the mechanisms of decreased frontal and parietal function will need more fundamental studies, likely in an animal model, to determine if the decreases arise from reduced excitation, increased inhibition, or some other mechanism. In all three seizure types, direct electrophysiological recordings are needed to better interpret the meaning of neuroimaging signals. For example, it is not known whether regions showing fMRI decreases during absence seizures will exhibit spike–wave discharges, relative silence, or some other pattern on electrophysiological measurements.

Impaired consciousness in epilepsy has a major negative effect on patient quality of life. For example, the amount of time that patient spend before returning to normal after seizures has been shown to have a strong correlation with reduced quality of life [152]. Impaired quality of life in patients with epilepsy includes a shorter life expectancy, and greater risk of injuries than the general population [152–154]. Epilepsy-related injuries such as burns, falls, and motor vehicle accidents are often caused by impaired consciousness during seizures. Patients with seizures causing impaired consciousness are not permitted to drive, which often has a large effect on self-esteem, and employability, contributing to the economic impact of epilepsy [155, 156]. Risk of motor vehicle accidents, including those causing death, is increased in patients with epilepsy [157–160]. Motor vehicle accident risk is highest in complex partial seizures and generalized tonic–clonic seizures, less in simple partial seizures [161, 162]. The stigma of suddenly losing conscious control of one's actions in public also has a large adverse effect [163].

With a greater understanding of the mechanisms of impaired consciousness in epilepsy it may be possible to devise new treatments to prevent these adverse consequences. Although the first goal is to stop all seizures, including both those do and don't cause impaired consciousness, in many cases this is not possible. Often a large improvement would be made if the seizures causing impaired consciousness could be stopped, even if some simple partial seizures remained. Implantation of deep brain stimulators is a growing field both for the treatment of epilepsy [164–166], and disorders of consciousness [167, 168]. It may be possible to devise stimulation protocols or electrode locations that if, unable to fully block seizures, will at least prevent impaired consciousness. Knowledge of the specific brain networks, and underlying biological changes in the regions causing impaired consciousness in epilepsy may also allow the targeting of improved medications to these regions. New drugs which help patients retain consciousness during seizures would be a very welcome addition for patients with medically refractory epilepsy.

In conclusion, investigation of impaired consciousness in epilepsy may have a large impact on improving quality of life in this disorder. In addition, by understanding the specific anatomical brain regions that are crucial for changes in consciousness, and how patterns of neuronal activity during seizures alter information flow, we may also gain important insights into normal mechanisms for human consciousness.

ACKNOWLEDGEMENTS

We thank Michael Purcaro for help in preparing the figures. This work was supported by NIH R01 NS049307, R01 NS055829, the Donaghue Foundation, and the Betsy and Jonathan Blattmachr family.

References

1. Koch, C. (2004) *The Quest for Consciousness: A Neurobiological Approach*, Denver, Colo.: Roberts and Co., xviii, 429 p.
2. ILAE (1981) Proposal for revised clinical and electroencephalographic classification of epileptic seizures. From the Commission on Classification and Terminology of the International League Against Epilepsy. *Epilepsia* 22 (4):489–501.
3. Blumenfeld, H. and Taylor, J. (2003) Why do seizures cause loss of consciousness? *Neuroscientist* 9 (5):301–310.
4. Plum, F. and Posner, J.B. (1980). The diagnosis of stupor and coma. Ed. 3. ed. *Contemporary Neurology Series*; 19, Philadelphia: Davis. xiii, 373.
5. Blumenfeld, H. (2002) *Neuroanatomy through Clinical Cases*, Sunderland, MA: Sinauer Assoc. Publ. Inc.
6. Ring, H.A. and Serra-Mestres, J. (2002) Neuropsychiatry of the basal ganglia. *J Neurol, Neurosurg Psychiatr* 72 (1):12–21.
7. Bischoff-Grethe, A., Ivry, R.B. and Grafton, S.T. (2002) Cerebellar involvement in response reassignment rather than attention. *J Neurosci* 22 (2):546–553.
8. Dreher, J.C. and Grafman, J. (2002) The roles of the cerebellum and basal ganglia in timing and error prediction. *Eur J Neurosci* 16 (8):1609–1619.
9. Leonards, U., *et al.* (2000) Attention mechanisms in visual search – an fMRI study. *J Cognitive Neurosci* 12 (Suppl 2): 61–75.
10. Penfield, W. and Erickson, T.C. (1941) *Epilepsy and Cerebral Localization*, Springfield: Charles Thomas.
11. Lumer, E.D., Friston, K.J. and Rees, G. (1998) Neural correlates of perceptual rivalry in the human brain. *Science* 280 (5371):1930–1934.
12. Moruzzi, G. and Magoun, H.W. (1949) Brain stem reticular formation and activation of the EEG. *Electroencephalogr Clin Neurophysiol* 1:455–473.
13. Kinomura, S., *et al.* (1996) Activation by Attention of the Human Reticular Formation and Thalamic INtralaminar Nuclei. *Science* 271:512–515.
14. Vogt, B.A. and Laureys, S. (2005) Posterior cingulate, precuneal and retrosplenial cortices: Cytology and components of the neural network correlates of consciousness. *Prog Brain Res* 150:205–217.
15. Singer, W. (1998) Consciousness from a neurobiological perspective. In *Brain and Mind: Evolutionary Perspectives* M. Gazzaniga, and J. Altman, (eds.) Strasbourg: HFSP. pp. 72–88.
16. Tononi, G. (2005) Consciousness, information integration, and the brain. *Prog Brain Res* 150:109–126.
17. Baars, B.J., Ramsoy, T.Z. and Laureys, S. (2003) Brain, conscious experience and the observing self. *Trends Neurosci* 26 (12):671–675.
18. Steriade, M., Jones, E.G., and McCormick, D.A. (1997) *Thalamus*, Amsterdam: Elsevier Science.
19. Steriade, M. and McCarley, R.W. (1990) *Brainstem Control of Wakefulness and Sleep*, New York: Plenum Press, xv, 499.
20. Llinás, R. and Paré, D. (1997) Coherent oscillations in specific and nonspecific thalamocortical networks and their role in cognition. In *Thalamus* M. Steriade, , E.G. Jones, and D.A. McCormick, (eds.) Oxford: Elsevier Science. pp. 501–516.
21. Laureys, S. (2005) Science and society: death, unconsciousness and the brain. *Nat Rev Neurosci* 6 (11):899–909.
22. Laureys, S. (2004) Functional neuroimaging in the vegetative state. *Neurorehabilitation* 19 (4):335–341.
23. Dang-Vu, T.T., *et al.* (2005) Cerebral correlates of delta waves during non-REM sleep revisited. *Neuroimage* 28 (1):14–21.
24. Maquet, P., *et al.* (2005) Human cognition during REM sleep and the activity profile within frontal and parietal cortices: A reappraisal of functional neuroimaging data. *Prog Brain Res* 150:219–227.
25. Kaufmann, C., *et al.* (2006) Brain activation and hypothalamic functional connectivity during human non-rapid eye movement sleep: an EEG/fMRI study. *Brain* 129 (Pt 3):655–667.

26. Czisch, M., *et al.* (2004) Functional MRI during sleep: BOLD signal decreases and their electrophysiological correlates. *Eur J Neurosc* 20 (2):566–574.

27. Alkire, M.T. and Miller, J. (2005) General anesthesia and the neural correlates of consciousness. *Prog Brain Res* 150:229–244.

28. White, N.S. and Alkire, M.T. (2003) Impaired thalamocortical connectivity in humans during general-anesthetic-induced unconsciousness. *Neuroimage* 19 (2 Pt 1):402–411.

29. Rodin, E. and Ancheta, O. (1987) Cerebral electrical fields during petit mal absences. *Electroencephalogr Clin Neurophysiol* 66 (6):457–466.

30. Weir, B. (1965) The morphology of the spike-wave complex. *Electroencephalogr Clin Neurophysiol* 19 (3):284–290.

31. Avoli, M. , *et al.* (1990) *Generalized Epilepsy*, Birkhauser: Boston.

32. Blumenfeld, H. (2002) The thalamus and seizures. *Arch Neurol* 59 (1):135–137.

33. Williams, D. (1953) A study of thalamic and cortical rhythms in petit mal. *Brain* 76:50–69.

34. Blumenfeld, H. (2003) From molecules to networks: Cortical/subcortical interactions in the pathophysiology of idiopathic generalized epilepsy. *Epilepsia* 44 (Suppl 2):7–15.

35. Blumenfeld, H. and McCormick, D.A. (2000) Corticothalamic inputs control the pattern of activity generated in thalamocortical networks. *J Neurosci* 20 (13):5153–5162.

36. Crunelli, V. and Leresche, N. (2002) Childhood absence epilepsy: Genes, channels, neurons and networks. *Nat Rev Neurosci* 3 (5):371–382.

37. Kostopoulos, G.K. (2001) Involvement of the thalamocortical system in epileptic loss of consciousness. *Epilepsia* 42 (Suppl 3):13–19.

38. McCormick, D.A. and Contreras, D. (2001) On the cellular and network bases of epileptic seizures. *Ann Rev Physiol* 63:815–846.

39. Blumenfeld, H. (2005) Cellular and network mechanisms of spike-wave seizures. *Epilepsia* 46 (Suppl 9):21–33.

40. Blumenfeld, H. (2005) Consciousness and epilepsy: why are patients with absence seizures absent? *Prog Brain Res* 150:271–286.

41. Goode, D.J., Penry, J.K. and Dreifuss, F.E. (1970) Effects of Paroxysmal Spike-Wave on Continuous Visual-Motor Performance. *Epilepsia* 11:241–254.

42. Goldie, L. and Green, J.M. (1961) Spike and wave discharges and alterations of conscious awareness. *Nature* 191:200–201.

43. Browne, T.R., *et al.* (1974) Responsiveness before, during and after spike-wave paroxysms. *Neurology* 24 (7):659–665.

44. Mirsky, A.F. and Buren, J.M.V. (1965) On the nature of the 'absence' in centrencephalic epilepsy: A study of some behavioral, electroencephalogrpahic, and autonomic factors. *Electroencephalogr Clin Neurophysiol* 18:334–348.

45. Vuilleumier, P., *et al.* (2000) Distinct behavioral and EEG topographic correlates of loss of consciousness in absences. *Epilepsia* 41 (6):687–693.

46. Gokygit, A. and Caliskan, A. (1995) Diffuse spike-wave status of 9-year duration without behavioral change or intellectual decline. *Epilepsia* 36 (2):210–213.

47. Holmes, M.D., Brown, M. and Tucker, D.M. (2004) Are 'generalized' seizures truly generalized? Evidence of localized mesial frontal and frontopolar discharges in absence. *Epilepsia* 45 (12):1568–1579.

48. Manning, J.P., *et al.* (2004) Cortical-area specific block of genetically determined absence seizures by ethosuximide. *Neuroscience* 123 (1):5–9.

49. Vergnes, M., Marescaux, C. and Depaulis, A. (1990) Mapping of spontaneous spike and wave discharges in Wistar rats with genetic generalized non-convulsive epilepsy. *Brain Res* 523 (1):87–91.

50. Nersesyan, H., *et al.* (2004) Relative changes in cerebral blood flow and neuronal activity in local microdomains during generalized seizures. *J Cereb Blood Flow Metab* 24 (9):1057–1068.

51. Meeren, H.K., *et al.* (2002) Cortical focus drives widespread corticothalamic networks during spontaneous absence seizures in rats. *J Neurosci* 22 (4):1480–1495.

52. van Luijtelaar, G. and Sitnikova, E. (2006) Global and focal aspects of absence epilepsy: The contribution of genetic models. *Neurosci Biobehav Rev* 30 (7):983–1003.

53. Klein, J.P., *et al.* (2004) Dysregulation of sodium channel expression in cortical neurons in a rodent model of absence epilepsy. *Brain Res* 1000:102–109.

54. Nersesyan, H., *et al.* (2004) Dynamic fMRI and EEG recordings during spike-wave seizures and generalized tonic-clonic seizures in WAG/Rij rats. *J Cereb Blood Flow Metab* 24 (6):589–599.

55. Theodore, W.H., *et al.* (1985) Positron emission tomography in generalized seizures. *Neurology* 35 (5):684–690.

56. Prevett, M.C., *et al.* (1995) Demonstration of thalamic activation during typical absence seizures using H2(15)O and PET. *Neurology* 45 (7):1396–1402.

57. Engel, J.Jr., *et al.* (1985) Local cerebral metabolic rate for glucose during petit mal absences. *Ann Neurol* 17 (2):121–128.

58. Engel, J.Jr., Kuhl, D.E. and Phelps, M.E. (1982) Patterns of human local cerebral glucose metabolism during epileptic seizures. *Science* 218:64–66.

59. Yeni, S.N., *et al.* (2000) Ictal and interictal SPECT findings in childhood absence epilepsy. *Seizure* 9 (4):265–269.

60. Ochs, R.F., *et al.* (1987) Effect of generalized spike-and-wave discharge on glucose metabolism measured by positron emission tomography. *Ann Neurol* 21 (5):458–464.

61. Diehl, B., *et al.* (1998) Cerebral hemodynamic response to generalized spike-wave discharges. *Epilepsia* 39 (12):1284–1289.

62. Ebersole, J.S. and Pedley, T.A. (2003) *Current Practice of Clinical Electroencephalography*, 3rd Edition Philadelphia, PA: Lippincott Williams & Wilkins.

63. Mirsky, A.F. and Van Buren, J.M. (1965) On the Nature of the 'Absence' in Centrencephalic Epilepsy: A Study of some Behavioral, Electroencephalographic, and Autonomic Factors. *Electroencephalogr Clin Neurophysiol* 18:334–348.

64. Laufs, H., *et al.* (2006) Linking generalized spike-and-wave discharges and resting state brain activity by using EEG/fMRI in a patient with absence seizures. *Epilepsia* 47 (2):444–448.

65. Berman, R., *et al.* (2005) Combined EEG and fMRI during typical childhood absence seizures at 3T. *Epilepsia* . AES abstracts.

66. Berman, R., *et al.* (2005) Simultaneous EEG and fMRI recordings of childhood absence seizures. *Soc Neurosci Abs* . Online at http://web.sfn.org/.

67. Hamandi, K., *et al.* (2006) EEG-fMRI of idiopathic and secondarily generalized epilepsies. *Neuroimage* 31 (4):1700–1710.

68. Gotman, J., *et al.* (2005) Generalized epileptic discharges show thalamocortical activation and suspension of the default state of the brain. *Proc Nat Acad Sci USA* 102 (42):15236–15240.

69. Labate, A., *et al.* (2005) Typical childhood absence seizures are associated with thalamic activation. *Epileptic Disord* 7 (4):373–377.

70. Aghakhani, Y., *et al.* (2004) fMRI activation during spike and wave discharges in idiopathic generalized epilepsy. *Brain* 127 (Pt 5):1127–1144.

71. Salek-Haddadi, A., *et al.* (2003) Functional magnetic resonance imaging of human absence seizures. *Ann Neurol* 53 (5):663–667.

72. Archer, J.S., *et al.* (2003) fMRI 'deactivation' of the posterior cingulate during generalized spike and wave. *Neuroimage* 20 (4):1915–1922.

73. Handforth, A. and Treiman, D.M. (1995) Functional mapping of the early stages of status epilepticus: A 14C-2-deoxyglucose

study in the lithium-pilocarpine model in rat. *Neuroscience* 64 (4):1057–1073.

74. Matsumoto, H. and Marsan, C.A. (1964) Cortical cellular phenomena in experimental epilepsy: Ictal manifestations. *Exp Neurol* 9:305–326.

75. Engel, J.Jr., Wolfson, L. and Brown, L. (1978) Anatomical correlates of electrical and behavioral events related to amygdaloid kindling. *Ann Neurol* 3 (6):538–544.

76. Andre, V., Henry, D. and Nehlig, A. (2002) Dynamic variations of local cerebral blood flow in maximal electroshock seizures in the rat. *Epilepsia* 43 (10):1120–1128.

77. McCown, T.J., *et al.* (1995) Metabolic and functional mapping of the neural network subserving inferior collicular seizure generalization. *Brain Res* 701 (12):117–128.

78. McIntyre, D.C., Don, J.C. and Edson, N. (1991) Distribution of [^{14}C]2-deoxyglucose after various forms and durations of status epilepticus induced by stimulation of a kindled amygdala focus in rats. *Epilepsy Res* 10 (2–3):119–133.

79. Ackermann, R.F., Engel, J.Jr. and Baxter, L. (1986) Positron emission tomography and autoradiographic studies of glucose utilization following electroconvulsive seizures in humans and rats. *Ann NY Acad Sci* 462:263–269.

80. Rolak, L.A., *et al.* (1992) Clinical features of Todd's post-epileptic paralysis. *J Neurol, Neurosurg Psychiatr* 55 (1):63–64.

81. Blumenfeld, H., *et al.* (2003) Selective frontal, parietal and temporal networks in generalized seizures. *Neuroimage* 19:1556–1566.

82. Green, C. and Buchhalter, J.R. (1993) Ictal SPECT in a 16-day-old infant. *Clin Nucl Med* 18 (9):768–770.

83. Shin, W.C., *et al.* (2002) Ictal hyperperfusion patterns according to the progression of temporal lobe seizures. *Neurology* 58 (3):373–380.

84. Koc, E., *et al.* (1997) Ictal and interictal SPECT in a newborn infant with intractable seizure. *Acta Paediatr* 86 (12):1379–1381.

85. Lee, B.I., *et al.* (1987) HIPDM single photon emission computed tomography brain imaging in partial onset secondarily generalized tonic-clonic seizures. *Epilepsia* 28 (3):305–311.

86. Varghese, G.I., *et al.* (2005) Localizing value of ictal SPECT in secondarily generalized tonic-clonic seizures. *Soc Neurosci Abs*. Online at http://web.sfn.org/.

87. Varghese, G.I., *et al.* (2005) Comparisons between ictal and postictal changes in cerebral blood flow in secondarily generalized tonic-clonic seizures. *Epilepsia*. AES abstracts

88. Blumenfeld, H., *et al.* (2003) Targeted prefrontal cortical activation with bifrontal ECT. *Psychiat Res Neuroimag* 123 (3):165–170.

89. Enev, M., *et al.* (2007) Imaging Onset and Propagation of ECT-induced Seizures. *Epilepsia* 48 (2):238–244.

90. McNally, K.A. and Blumenfeld, H. (2004) Focal network involvement in generalized seizures: new insights from electroconvulsive therapy. *Epilepsy Behav* 5 (1):3–12.

91. Salgado-Benitez, A., Briones, R. and Fernandez-Guardiola, A. (1982) Purkinje cell responses to a cerebral penicillin-induced epileptogenic focus in the cat. *Epilepsia* 23 (6):597–606.

92. Norden, A.D. and Blumenfeld, H. (2002) The role of subcortical structures in human epilepsy. *Epilepsy Behav* 3 (3):219–231.

93. Makris, N., *et al.* (2005) Segmentation of subcomponents within the superior longitudinal fascicle in humans: A quantitative, in vivo, DT-MRI study. *Cereb Cortex* 15 (6):854–869.

94. Schwartz, M.L., Dekker, J.J. and Goldman-Rakic, P.S. (1991) Dual mode of corticothalamic synaptic termination in the mediodorsal nucleus of the rhesus monkey. *J Comp Neurol* 309 (3):289–304.

95. Guillery, R.W. and Sherman, S.M. (2002) Thalamic relay functions and their role in corticocortical communication: generalizations from the visual system. *Neuron* 33 (2):163–175.

96. Weisman, D., *et al.* (2003) Going deep to cut the link: Cortical disconnection syndrome caused by a thalamic lesion. *Neurology* 60 (11):1865–1866.

97. Velasco, F., *et al.* (1985) Comparative effects of topical perfusions of pentylenetetrazol in the mesencephalon and cerebral cortex of cats. *Exp Neurol* 87 (3):533–543.

98. Browning, R.A. (1985) Role of the brain-stem reticular formation in tonic-clonic seizures: Lesion and pharmacological studies. *FASEB* 44 (8):2425–2431.

99. Faingold, C.L. (1999) Neuronal networks in the genetically epilepsy-prone rat. *Adv Neurol* 79:311–321.

100. Gale, K. (1992) Subcortical structures and pathways involved in convulsive seizure generation. *J Clin Neurophysiol* 9 (2):264–277.

101. Bell, W.L., *et al.* (1997) Painful generalised clonic and tonic-clonic seizures with retained consciousness. *J Neurol, Neurosurg Psychiatr* 63 (6):792–795.

102. Schridde, U., Khubchandani, M., Motelow, J.E., Sanganahalli, B.G., Hyder, F. and Blumenfeld, H. (2008) Negative BOLD with large increases in neuronal activity. *Cerebral Cortex*. 2007 Dec 5; [Epub ahead of print]

103. Engel, J. and International League Against Epilepsy (ILAE). (2001) A proposed diagnostic scheme for people with epileptic seizures and with epilepsy: Report of the ILAE Task Force on Classification and Terminology, *Epilepsia* 42(6) pp. 796–803.

104. Luders, H., *et al.* (1998) Semiological seizure classification.[comment]. *Epilepsia* 39 (9):1006–1013.

105. Williamson, P.D., *et al.* (1993) Characteristics of medial temporal lobe epilepsy: II. Interictal and ictal scalp electroencephalography, neuropsychological testing, neuroimaging, surgical results, and pathology. *Ann Neurol* 34 (6):781–787.

106. Engel, J. Jr. (1987) Outcome with respect to epileptic seizures. In *Surgical Treatment of the Epilepsies* J. Engel, Jr. (eds.) New York: Raven. pp. 553–571.

107. Janszky, J., *et al.* (2003) Automatisms with preserved responsiveness and ictal aphasia: Contradictory lateralising signs during a dominant temporal lobe seizure. *Seizure* 12 (3): 182–185.

108. Park, S.A., *et al.* (2001) Ictal automatisms with preserved responsiveness in a patient with left mesial temporal lobe epilepsy. *Epilepsia* 42 (8):1078–1081.

109. Marks, W.J.Jr. and Laxer, K.D. (1998) Semiology of temporal lobe seizures: value in lateralizing the seizure focus. *Epilepsia* 39 (7):721–726.

110. Quigg, M., *et al.* (2002) Interictal and postictal alterations of pulsatile secretions of luteinizing hormone in temporal lobe epilepsy in men.[comment]. *Ann Neurol* 51 (5):559–566.

111. Bauer, J. (2001) Interactions between hormones and epilepsy in female patients. *Epilepsia* 42 (Suppl 3):20–22.

112. Zhang, D.X. and Bertram, E.H. (2002) Midline thalamic region: widespread excitatory input to the entorhinal cortex and amygdale. *J Neurosci* 22 (8):3277–3284.

113. Newton, M.R., *et al.* (1992) Dystonia, clinical lateralization, and regional blood flow changes in temporal lobe seizures. *Neurology* 42 (2):371–377.

114. Shin, W.C., *et al.* (2001) Ictal hyperperfusion of cerebellum and basal ganglia in temporal lobe epilepsy: SPECT subtraction with MRI coregistration. *J Nucl Med* 42 (6):853–858.

115. Lee, K.H., *et al.* (2002) Pathophysiology of altered consciousness during seizures: Subtraction SPECT study. *Neurology* 59:841–846.

116. Cassidy, R.M. and Gale, K. (1998) Mediodorsal thalamus plays a critical role in the development of limbic motor seizures. *J Neurosci* 18 (21):9002–9009.

117. Inoue, Y. and Mihara, T. (1998) Awareness and responsiveness during partial seizures. *Epilepsia* 39 (Suppl 5):7–10.

118. Lux, S., *et al.* (2002) The localizing value of ictal consciousness and its constituent functions: A video-EEG study in patients with focal epilepsy. *Brain* 125 (Pt 12):2691–2698.

119. Gloor, P., Olivier, A. and Ives, J. (1980) Loss of consciousness in temporal lobe epilepsy: Observations obtained with stereotaxic depth electrode recordings and stimulations. In *Advances in Epileptology: The XIth Epilepsy International Symposium* R. Canger, F. Angeleri, and J.K. Penry, (eds.) New York: Raven Press. pp. 349–353.

120. Munari, C., *et al.* (1980) Impairment of consciousness in temporal lobe seizures: Astereoelectroencephalographic study. In *Advances in Epileptology: The XIth Epilepsy International Symposium* R. Canger, , F. Angeleri, and J.K. Penry, (eds.) New York: Raven Press. pp. 111–114.

121. Bancaud, J., *et al.* (1994) Anatomical origin of deja vu and vivid 'memories' in human temporal lobe epilepsy. *Brain* 117 (Pt 1):71–90.

122. Milner, B. (1972) Disorders of learning and memory after temporal lobe lesions in man. *Clin Neurosurg* 19:421–446.

123. Zhang, D.X. and Bertram, E.H. (2002) Midline thalamic region: Widespread excitatory input to the entorhinal cortex and amygdale. *J Neurosci* 22 (8):3277–3284.

124. Bertram, E.H. and Scott, C. (2000) The pathological substrate of limbic epilepsy: Neuronal loss in the medial dorsal thalamic nucleus as the consistent change. *Epilepsia* 41 (Supp 6):S3–S8.

125. Bruehl, C., Hagemann, G. and Witte, O.W. (1998) Uncoupling of blood flow and metabolism in focal epilepsy. *Epilepsia* 39 (12):1235–1242.

126. Redecker, C., *et al.* (1997) Coupling of cortical and thalamic metabolism in experimentally induced visual and somatosensory focal seizures. *Epilepsy Res* 27 (2):127–137.

127. Clifford, D.B., *et al.* (1987) The functional anatomy and pathology of lithium-pilocarpine and high-dose pilocarpine seizures. *Neuroscience* 23 (3):953–968.

128. Handforth, A. and Ackermann, R.F. (1988) Functional [^{14}C]2-deoxyglucose mapping of progressive states of status epilepticus induced by amygdala stimulation in rat. *Brain Res* 460 (1):96–102.

129. VanLandingham, K.E. and Lothman, E.W. (1991) Self-sustaining limbic status epilepticus. I. Acute and chronic cerebral metabolic studies: Limbic hypermetabolism and neocortical hypometabolism. *Neurology* 41 (12):1942–1949.

130. Henry, T.R., Mazziotta, J.C. and Engel, J.J. (1993) Interictal metabolic anatomy of mesial temporal lobe epilepsy. *Arch Neurol* 50 (6):582–589.

131. Yune, M.J., *et al.* (1998) Ipsilateral thalamic hypoperfusion on interictal SPECT in temporal lobe epilepsy. *J Nucl Med* 39 (2):281–285.

132. Newberg, A.B., *et al.* (2000) Ipsilateral and contralateral thalamic hypometabolism as a predictor of outcome after temporal lobectomy for seizures. *J Nucl Med* 41 (12):1964–1968.

133. Pan, J.W., *et al.* (2005) Regional energetic dysfunction in hippocampal epilepsy. *Acta Neurol Scand* 111 (4):218–224.

134. DeCarli, C., *et al.* (1998) Extratemporal atrophy in patients with complex partial seizures of left temporal origin. *Ann Neurol* 43 (1):41–45.

135. Chan, S., Erickson, J.K. and Yoon, S.S. (1997) Limbic system abnormalities associated with mesial temporal sclerosis: A model of chronic cerebral changes due to seizures. *Radiographics* 17 (5):1095–1110.

136. Deasy, N.P., *et al.* (2000) Thalamic changes with mesial temporal sclerosis: MRI. *Neuroradiology* 42 (5):346–351.

137. Margerison, J.H. and Corsellis, J.A.N. (1966) Epilepsy and the temporal lobes: A clinical, electroencephalographic and neuropathological study of the brain in epilepsy, with particular reference to the temporal lobes. *Brain* 89 (3):499–530.

138. Mayanagi, Y., Watanabe, E. and Kaneko, Y. (1996) Mesial temporal lobe epilepsy: Clinical features and seizure mechanism. *Epilepsia* 37 (Suppl 3):57–60.

139. Menzel, C., *et al.* (1998) Inhibitory effects of mesial temporal partial seizures onto frontal neocortical structures. *Acta Neurologica Belgica* 98 (4):327–331.

140. Chang, D.J., *et al.* (2002) Comparison of statistical parametric mapping and SPECT difference imaging in patients with temporal lobe epilepsy. *Epilepsia* 43 (1):68–74.

141. Rabinowicz, A.L., *et al.* (1997) Changes in regional cerebral blood flow beyond the temporal lobe in unilateral temporal lobe epilepsy. *Epilepsia* 38 (9):1011–1014.

142. Van Paesschen, W., *et al.* (2003) SPECT perfusion changes during complex partial seizures in patients with hippocampal sclerosis. *Brain* 126 (5):1103–1111.

143. McNally, K.A., Paige, A.L., Varghese, G., Zhang, H., Novotny, E.J., Spencer, S.S., Zubal, I.G. and Blumenfeld, H. (2005) Localizing Value of Ictal-Interictal SPECT Analyzed by SPM (ISAS). *Epilepsia* 46 (9):1450–1464.

144. Blumenfeld, H., *et al.* (2004) Positive and negative network correlations in temporal lobe epilepsy. *Cereb Cortex* 14 (8): 892–902.

145. Tae, W.S., Joo, E.Y., Kim, J.H., Han, S.J., Suh, Y.-L., Kim, B.T., Hong, S.C. and Hong, S.B. (2005) Cerebral perfusion changes in mesial temporal lobe epilepsy: SPM analysis of ictal and interictal SPECT. *Neuroimage* 24:101–110.

146. Kaiboriboon, K., *et al.* (2005) Quantitative analysis of cerebral blood flow patterns in mesial temporal lobe epilepsy using composite SISCOM. *J Nucl Med* 46 (1):38–43.

147. Kim, J.H., *et al.* (2007) Ictal hyperperfusion patterns in relation to ictal scalp EEG patterns in patients with unilateral hippocampal sclerosis: A SPECT study. *Epilepsia* 48 (2): 270–277.

148. Lieb, J.P., Dasheiff, R.B. and Engel, J.Jr. (1991) Role of the frontal lobes in the propagation of mesial temporal lobe seizures. *Epilepsia* 32 (6):822–837.

149. Blumenfeld, H., *et al.* (2004) Ictal neocortical slowing in temporal lobe epilepsy. *Neurology* 63:1015–1021.

150. Golomb, J.D., *et al.* (2005) Quantitative analysis of intracranial EEG patterns: Evidence for neocortical slowing in temporal lobe seizures. *Soc Neurosci Abs* . Online at http://web.sfn.org/.

151 Englot DJ, Mishra AM, Mansuripur PK, Herman P, Hyder F, Blumenfeld H. (2008). Remote effects of focal hippocampal seizures on the rat neocortex (in press).

152. Vickrey, B.G., *et al.* (2000) Relationships between seizure severity and health-related quality of life in refractory localization-related epilepsy. *Epilepsia* 41 (6):760–764.

153. Sperling, M.R. (2004) The consequences of uncontrolled epilepsy. *CNS Spect* 9 (2):98–101.

154. Theodore, W.H., *et al.* (2006) Epilepsy in North America: A report prepared under the auspices of the global campaign against epilepsy, the International Bureau for Epilepsy, the International League Against Epilepsy, and the World Health Organization. *Epilepsia* 47 (10):1700–1722.

155. Begley, C.E. and Beghi, E. (2002) The economic cost of epilepsy: A review of the literature. *Epilepsia* 43 (Suppl 4):3–9.

156. Begley, C.E., *et al.* (2002) ILAE Commission on the Burden of Epilepsy, Subcommission on the Economic Burden of Epilepsy: Final report 1998–2001. *Epilepsia* 43 (6):668–673.

157. Sheth, S.G., *et al.* (2004) Mortality in epilepsy: Sriving fatalities vs other causes of death in patients with epilepsy. *Neurology* 63

(6):1002–1007. [summary for patients in Neurology. 2004 Sep 28;63(6):E12–3; PMID: 15452331]

158. Krauss, G.L., *et al.* (1999) Risk factors for seizure-related motor vehicle crashes in patients with epilepsy. *Neurology* 52 (7):1324–1329. [see comment]

159. Hansotia, P. and Broste, S.K. (1991) The effect of epilepsy or diabetes mellitus on the risk of automobile accidents. *N Eng J Med* 324 (1):22–26. [see comment]

160. Taylor, J., Chadwick, D. and Johnson, T. (1996) Risk of accidents in drivers with epilepsy. *J Neurol, Neurosurg Psychiatr* 60 (6):621–627.

161. Gastaut, H. and Zifkin, B.G. (1987) The risk of automobile accidents with seizures occurring while driving: relation to seizure type. *Neurology* 37 (10):1613–1616.

162. Berkovic, S.F. (2000) Epilepsy syndromes: Effects on cognition, performance and driving ability. *Med Law* 19 (4):757–761.

163. Jacoby, A., Snape, D. and Baker, G.A. (2005) Epilepsy and social identity: the stigma of a chronic neurological disorder. *Lancet Neurology* 4 (3):171–178.

164. Theodore, W.H. and Fisher, R.S. (2004) Brain stimulation for epilepsy. *Lancet Neurol* 3 (2):111–118. [erratum appears in *Lancet Neurol* 2004 June 3(6): 332]

165. Murphy, J.V. and Patil, A. (2003) Stimulation of the nervous system for the management of seizures: Current and future developments. *CNS Drugs* 17 (2):101–115.

166. Morrell, M. (2006) Brain stimulation for epilepsy: can scheduled or responsive neurostimulation stop seizures? *Curr Opin Neurol* 19 (2):164–168.

167 Schiff, N.D., Giacino, J.T., Kalmar, K., Victor, J.D., Baker, K., Gerber, M., Fritz, B., Eisenberg, B., Biondi, T., O'Connor, J., Kobylarz, E.J., Farris, S., Machado, A., McCagg, C., Plum, F., Fins, J.J. and Rezai, A.R. (2007 Aug 2) Behavioural improvements with thalamic stimulation after severe traumatic brain injury. *Nature* 448 (7153):600–603.

168. Schiff, N.D., Giacino, J.T., Kalmar, K., Victor, J.D., Baker, K., Gerber, M., Fritz, B., Eisenberg, B., Biondi, T., O'Connor, J., Kobylarz, E.J., Farris, S., Machado, A., McCagg, C., Plum, F., Fins, J.J. and Rezai, A.R. (2007) Behavioural improvements with thalamic stimulation after severe traumatic brain injury. *Nature* 448 (7153):600–603.

The Left Hemisphere Does Not Miss the Right Hemisphere

Michael S. Gazzaniga and Michael B. Miller

ABSTRACT

Research over the past 45 years on split-brain patients have revealed unique specialized processes in each hemisphere, including some recently discovered specialized processes in the right hemisphere. Yet, the patients' speaking left hemisphere consistently denies any change in their conscious experience as a result of severing the corpus callosum. We argue that this phenomenon is consistent with similar observations in other neurological patients, and that it is indicative of a conscious system that is comprised of thousands of specialized local circuits. Our entire conscious experience from moment to moment is bound by the inputs of one or more of these specialized circuits, and it is seemingly coordinated by a specialized system we refer to as the interpreter.

INTRODUCTION

One of several qualities that make split-brain patients so astonishing is that they seem utterly unaware of their special status. The loss of the ability to transfer information from the left hemisphere to the right hemisphere and vice-versa seems to have no impact on their overall psychological state. For example,

the sudden loss of the ability to verbally describe the flash of an object to the left visual field seems to be of little concern to them. The truth is that the left brain in these patients does not seem to miss the right brain, despite recent discoveries of several specialized properties in the right hemisphere. That is one of the enduring truths that come out of split-brain research and we believe it has major implications for understanding the physical basis of conscious experience.

In what follows, we argue that consciousness does not constitute a single, generalized process, but that it is an emergent property that arises out of hundreds if not thousands of specialized systems (modules). These systems consist of a neural circuitry specialized to process-specific domains of information [1–3]. These specialized neural circuitries enable the processing and mental representations of a specific aspect of conscious experience, and these circuits are widely distributed throughout the brain. Many of these specialized circuits may be directly connected to some of the other specialized circuits, but not to most of them. Each component competes for attention. From moment to moment, different modules or systems will win and serve as the neural system underlying that moment of conscious experience. Again it is this dynamic, moment-to-moment cacophony of systems that comprises our consciousness. And, yet, we do not experience this as a thousand chattering voices, but as a unified experience. It appears to us as if our consciousness flows easily and naturally from one moment to the next with a single, unified, and coherent narrative. Our sense of a unified experience emerges out of a particular specialized system called the interpreter, which coordinates and continually interprets and makes sense of our behaviours, emotions, and thoughts after they occur. This interpreter appears to be uniquely human and specialized to the left hemisphere.

An important aspect of this view of consciousness is that it is completely dependent on local, specialized components, or modules. If a particular module is impaired or loses its inputs, it alerts the whole system that something is wrong. For example, if the optic nerve is severed, the patient will notice immediately that they are blinded. But if the module itself is removed, as in the case of cortical blindness, then no warning signal is sent and the specific information processed by that specialized system is no longer acknowledged (out of sight, out of mind – so to speak). This creates the peculiar phenomenon that has been observed in a variety of neurological patients that deny that anything is wrong with them despite the clearly observable effects of the brain injury. This aspect of their condition, the unawareness of or denying the existence of their deficit is referred to as anosognosia.

In the next few sections, we will (1) discuss how anosognosia observed in many neurological disorders is indicative of a conscious system that is bound by the inputs of thousands of specialized local modules; (2) review split-brain research, including some recent developments of specialized processes that may contribute to the conscious experience of each hemisphere uniquely; (3) update our understanding of a left hemisphere specialization that we refer to as the

'interpreter' that unifies and interprets our conscious experience; and (4) take a speculative look at the world from the point of view of the right hemisphere.

ANOSOGNOSIA: THE DENIAL OF A DEFICIT AND ITS RELATIONSHIP TO CONSCIOUSNESS

A well-known example of anosognosia is often found in hemispatial neglect patients. This condition is usually caused by a stroke to the right parietal lobe that causes disruption of attention and spatial awareness of the left side of space [4]. They often behave as if the left side of the world does not exist. For example, they will only dress the right side of their body or eat all the food on the right side of a plate but not the left. Yet, despite the obviousness of the deficit to people observing the patients, the patients themselves are not aware of their deficit. They do not sense that anything is wrong with them!

In the model of consciousness that we are proposing, the denial of a deficit is the logical result of damage to a specific set of circuits [5, 6]. Damage to most areas of the nervous system that result in the impairment or loss of function will be noticed immediately by patients. For example, the patient will notice paralysis that is due to the severing of a nerve that connects the parietal lobe to the limbs immediately. They still have the mental representation of the existence of their left hand and, therefore, the failure to move it will be registered immediately and the patient will experience that failure as a very disturbing event. The module that represents the left side of the body can notify the interpreter that something is wrong.

At the same time, neglect patients, with damage to the right parietal lobe that also result in hemiplegia (paralysis to the left side of their body), deny their paralysis because these patients no longer have the mental representations of the existence of the left side of their body. There is no system to sense that something is wrong, so the patient assumes that everything is normal. For example, when these patients are confronted with a bimanual task in which they cannot complete because they are unable to move their left hand, they may reply with a statement such as 'I didn't want to do that task' [7]. When the paralyzed hand is presented to them, they often respond with the rationalization 'that's not my hand'. The conscious awareness that emerges from this specialized module does not exist for these patients. Therefore, no signals from this module are sent to the interpreter and this localized conscious element does not compete for or command our awareness.

The inability to process information about specific aspects of conscious awareness could be overcome conceivably by other cognitive means. For example, a neglect patient with hemiplegia anosognosia may learn about their own condition by observing other patients with similar conditions. However, these patients not only have an inability to acknowledge their own deficit, but they often deny the deficit in others as well [8]. Their brains can no longer process information regarding the left side of their body or the bodies of others, so this information is excluded from their available range of conscious experience and they redefine their world accordingly. For example, one patient explained that, 'I knew the word "neglect" was a sort of medical term for whatever was wrong but the word bothered me because you can only neglect something that is actually there, don't you? If it's not there, how can you neglect it?' [9].

Another conceivable way to overcome the lack of conscious awareness about a particular realm of information after a lesion has occurred is to reconcile the current awareness with a memory of the pre-lesion awareness. For example, a neglect patient may draw a picture of their home, but the picture they draw will only include the right side of their house. How can their denial of the left side be reconciled with their memory of the left side of their house? It turns out that the neglect syndrome not only affects their current perceptual awareness but also their memory representations as well. Previous studies have demonstrated that the retrieval of a memory entails activation of the same perceptual circuits that were directly activated during the encoding of the original event [10, 11]. Although the information regarding the left visual field remains encoded in visual hemineglect patients, they neglect that information in the realm of memory just as they do in their current perceptual awareness [12]. In a classic experiment to demonstrate this phenomenon, Bisiach asked patients with visual hemineglect that were familiar with a particular piazza to describe the scene from a particular vantage point. The patient, as usual, neglected all the details from the contralesional side of space. Then, he had the patients imagined themselves from the opposite end of the piazza and describe the scene again. Again, the patients neglected all the details from the contralesional side of space, but this time it was the previously neglected side of the piazza. Clearly, the visual information that was originally encoded in the brain is still available, but that information is neglected when memory systems attempt to retrieve it.

We know from our studies of patients with damage to the right parieto-occipital cortex that while enough information had been processed about stimuli presented to the left visual field to make an accurate same/different judgement, the patients still did not have a conscious representation of that stimuli that would enable them to identify it or even acknowledge its existence [13]. In that experiment, four patients were shown pictures of objects in the right or left visual field. When shown a single object in the left visual field, the patients could identify it. However, when shown two objects simultaneously in both visual fields, the patients could only identify the objects presented to the right visual field (this is known as extinction). Yet, when asked to make a same/different judgement about the two objects, the patients were able to make the judgement accurately despite their inability to identify the object in the left visual field. Further, two of the patients insisted that the task was 'silly', since there was no stimulus (according to them) in the left visual field.

Of course, there are possibly hundreds of specialized systems in the human brain, from basic systems of perceptual processing (like discriminating tones [14] and perceiving faces [15]) to more higher-order systems (like recognizing emotions [16], sympathizing with others [17] and detecting cheaters [18]). As we have seen with neglect patients, the corruption of one of these systems can have a profound effect on our conscious experience. But the effect need not be simply the denial of information; it can also include many other forms of corruption. Just as the voices in the head of a schizophrenic patient can seem to them as real as the perception of actual voices, many distortions caused by brain injury can become incorporated into our conscious experience and not seem out of place.

One such example is patients with reduplicative paramnesia. These patients often have extensive damage throughout the right hemisphere and both frontal lobes. The damage appears to specifically affect a specialized memory system that codes for the familiarity of places and locations [19], but in a way that increases familiarity for otherwise novel or relatively new locations. These patients form delusional beliefs that a place or location has been duplicated. In one case that we observed, a woman that was being examined at a New York hospital insisted that she was in her own home. The woman was intelligent and aware that her doctors did not agree with her assessment, but she was quite persistent. When confronted with the fact that if she was in her own home then how could she explain the bank of elevators just outside her door that could be seen clearly from her bed, she calmly exclaimed, 'Doctor, do you know how much it cost me to have those put in?' [20].

A conscious system that is bounded by the interpreted confluence of specialized and localized neural circuits explains the classic finding that a callosotomy patient's left hemisphere does not miss the right hemisphere. But in order to fully understand the consequences of this disconnection on the conscious experience of a split-brain patient, it is important to first appreciate some of the basic differences between the left and right hemispheres that have been illuminated by split-brain research.

THE SPLIT-BRAIN: SPECIALIZATIONS UNIQUE TO EACH HEMISPHERE

The first callosotomy surgeries were conducted in the 1940s by a Rochester, New York neurosurgeon named William Van Wagenen. Van Wagenen [21] was inspired to perform the surgery on patients with severe intractable epilepsy after observing that one of his epileptic patients experienced considerable relief after developing a tumour in his corpus callosum. The corpus callosum is the largest fibre tract in the brain, and it contains over 200 million axons that originate from layers 2 and 3 of both hemispheres [22]. Epileptic seizures are caused by abnormal electrical discharges that reverberate across the brain from one hemisphere to the other. For reasons that are still unclear, severing all or part of the callosum can reduce seizure activity by 60–70% in 80% of the patients. Although the surgery is not as dangerous as it was in the 1940s, given the advent of microsurgery techniques, it is still a treatment of last resort. And, the procedure is even more rare now since pharmacological treatments have greatly improved, as well as presurgical techniques to localize the origin of seizures.

But the callosotomy surgery offers a lot of hope to patients with no other treatment options, and in the 1940s those other options were much fewer. At the time, the physical danger of the surgery was certainly a concern (the corpus callosum is separated from the ventricles by a very thin wall of cells). There was also a concern about a psychological danger. Van Wagenen and his colleagues feared that one of the side effects of the surgery would be that it might produce a split personality, or a dual consciousness. However, after 20 of the surgeries were conducted in the 1940s, researchers like A.J. Akelaitis never found this psychological side effect [23, 24]. The surgery did not appear to create two minds, each with its own personality and consciousness, fighting over control of the body.

This fact, the absence of a dual consciousness, continued to be observed when the surgery was revived by Joseph Bogen in the early 1960s in collaboration with Roger Sperry and his young graduate student (MG). The general view held at the time by brain researchers was that severing the callosum in humans had little functional effect, in marked contrast to the animal findings [23–25]. Indeed, I (MG) found in patient W.J. that, despite some initial akinesis and mutism that quickly cleared up, that the operation appeared to have little effect on his temperament or intellect [26]. Patient W.J. repeatedly reported that he felt better than he had in years.

It was the introduction of lateralized procedures in this early study that realized the unique research opportunity presented by split-brain patients. For example, tactual testing of the right hand showed no significant impairments of the dominant but disconnected left hemisphere. However, similar testing of the left hand (for instance, by placing a pencil in the hand) indicated severe agnosia, anomia, and agraphia. Prior to surgery, patient W.J. could write legibly with his left hand, but after surgery the writing became a meaningless scribble. We also presented visual stimuli using a tachistoscopic presentation. Again, the results showed no abnormality in response to stimuli presented to the right visual field, but the patient was severely impaired with stimuli presented to the left visual field.

Since the 1960s, research on split-brain patients has produced a wealth of information about the functional organization of the brain and hemispheric specialization. Severing the entire callosum blocks the interhemispheric transfer of sensory, motor, perceptual, gnostic and other forms of information in such a way that it allows us to study hemispheric differences and the unique ways in which the hemispheres must interact with each other [20, 27, 28]. The most obvious hemispheric difference is the capacity to learn language. It had been known prior to split-brain research that the left hemisphere is dominant for language and, particularly, speech production [29], and we have observed this phenomenon in split-brain patients as well. The left hemisphere is also specialized for written language (with the exception noted below). And, while the right hemisphere does have a limited capacity for reading and is able to read whole words (ideographic lexical/semantic access), it is unable to convert graphemes to phonemes as can the language-dominant left hemisphere [30, 31]. Although most of the findings from split-brain studies regarding language have been consistent with previous studies of patients with unilateral lesions, there have been some surprising discoveries as well. One of the more remarkable recent cases is patient V.J., who generates spoken language exclusively from the left hemisphere, but generates written language exclusively from the right hemisphere. Previously, it had been assumed that spoken and written language shared the same neural mechanisms, but this patient demonstrates that the output of these two functions can be operated by independent modules [32].

Are knowledge structures in each hemisphere different? Although each hemisphere appears to have redundant knowledge structures that support basic functioning (e.g., the right hemisphere knows just as well as the left hemisphere what a 'chair' is and what its functions are), the extent of the semantic systems in the right hemisphere is clearly impoverished compared to the left [33–36], including a limited lexical organization in the right [37]. What about knowledge about the 'self'? John Kihlstrom and Stan Klein have emphasized that the *self* is a knowledge structure, not some mystical entity [38]. Severing the corpus callosum raises an interesting issue about whether a disconnected half brain will still have the same sense of self. Does the left hemisphere see itself differently than the right hemisphere?

Our colleague Dave Turk recently studied this in patient J.W. by having him judge whether a picture of a face was himself or somebody other than himself that he was quite familiar with (author MG). The key manipulation was that the picture of J.W. and the picture of MG were morphed into each other by varying degrees. Some morphed faces were more like J.W., while others were more like MG. We found that the right hemisphere was biased to respond that the face was MG, while the left hemisphere was biased to respond that the face was himself [39]. Although it is very difficult to accurately assess the extent of the right hemisphere's knowledge (self and otherwise) given its limited language ability, there does appear to be hemispheric differences in knowledge systems that bias each hemispheres' responses.

Although the left hemisphere is clearly dominant for language, many problem-solving skills, and semantic knowledge [20], the right hemisphere does have some specializations as well. Studies with split-brain patients have revealed right hemisphere superiority for various tasks involving such components as part–whole relations [40], spatial relationships [41], apparent motion detection [42], mental rotation [43], spatial matching [44], and mirror image discrimination [45]. The right hemisphere also appears to be more veridical in its memory recollections [46, 47] and to be better at illusory contour perception and amodal boundary completion [48]. One of the more compelling recent findings regarding the right hemisphere is its superiority in causal perception, although the left hemisphere was found to be superior at causal inferences [49]. Understanding cause and effect is fundamental to making sense of the dynamic physical

world, and the perception of spatial and temporal contiguity of the movements of colliding objects is a critical component of this basic understanding. In a recent study, Matt Roser had split-brain patients observe three panels that depicted the motion of a ball (A) towards another ball (B), and the subsequent motion of B. The movements of the two balls were either contiguous in space or time, or it included a small spatial or temporal gap. The right hemisphere was better at perceiving these gaps than the left hemisphere.

A well-known specialization of the right hemisphere is the detection of upright faces [1]. In our studies of split-brain patients, it is clear that the left hemisphere can perceive and recognize faces and it can perform just as well as the right with familiar faces, but the right hemisphere is superior in its ability to perceive and recognize unfamiliar faces [50–52]. Interestingly, though, while both hemispheres can generate spontaneous facial expressions, only the dominant left hemisphere can generate voluntary facial expressions [53].

While the right hemisphere certainly has some specializations of its own, the asymmetries that favour the right hemisphere are subtler than those that favor the left hemisphere [54]. It should also be noted that many popular views of hemispheric asymmetry oversimplify the observed differences between the hemispheres and suggest that they serve very different functions. In fact, the cognitive functioning of each hemisphere is quite redundant. For example, both hemispheres are quite capable of encoding and retrieving memories of past events, despite a significant theory in the 1990s on the brain regions underlying episodic memory function based on neuroimaging work. The theory, called HERA (hemispheric encoding/retrieval asymmetry), stipulated that episodic encoding was predominantly a left hemisphere process while episodic retrieval was predominantly a right hemisphere process [55]. However, the asymmetries observed in the neuroimaging studies were based on the fact that most studies at the time used verbal material. We found in split-brain patients that manipulating the encoding of words led to greater effects in the left hemisphere than the right, and that manipulating the encoding of faces led to greater effects in the right hemisphere than the left [52]. Since that split-brain study, recent neuroimaging studies have confirmed that encoding and retrieval asymmetries are primarily due to the type of stimuli used and not general hemispheric differences in processing [56].

Despite some unique specializations in the right hemisphere, breaking up with the right hemisphere is not hard to do for the left hemisphere. Although some effects due to the callosotomy surgery have been observed (e.g., we found impairments in free recall but not in recognition performance on some memory tasks that may be due to limitations in strategic and search processes imposed by the severing of the corpus callosum [57]), most functions remain intact after the right hemisphere is disconnected from the left, including verbal IQ [27, 58] and many problem-solving skills [59]. The disconnection also does not seem to affect another critical component of our conscious system, the 'interpreter'.

THE LEFT HEMISPHERE INTERPRETER: UNIFYING THE CONSCIOUS EXPERIENCE

According to our model of consciousness, there may be hundreds, if not thousands, of modules contributing to our conscious experience, each contributing specialized bits of information. Yet, our phenomenological experience will naturally flow from moment to moment depending on the demands of the environment as one unified and coherent experience. We believe this is due to a specialized process in the left hemisphere that we refer to as the interpreter. As one of us has written elsewhere; 'The "interpreter" is a specialized system that makes sense of all the information bombarding the brain, interpreting our responses – cognitive or emotional – to what we encounter in our environment, asking how one thing relates to another, making hypothesis, bringing order out of chaos, creating a running narrative of our actions, emotions, thoughts, and dreams. The interpreter is the glue that keeps our story unified and creates our sense of being into a coherent, rational agent. It is the insertion of the interpreter into an otherwise functioning brain that enables such a rich experience.' [60]

We first demonstrated the left hemisphere's unique drive to interpret the world around it using the simultaneous concept test on a split-brain patient [61]. Patient P.S. was shown simultaneously a chicken claw to the speaking left hemisphere and a snow scene to the silent right hemisphere. Patient P.S. was then instructed to pick out the picture most related to the scene he just saw from a set of eight choices, using both hands. His left hand (controlled by his right hemisphere) chose a snow shovel, while his right hand chose a chicken. When asked why he chose those particular pictures, P.S. replied, 'Oh, that's simple. The chicken claw goes with the chicken, and you need a shovel to clean out the chicken shed'. While the speaking left hemisphere can easily explain that he chose the chicken with his right hand because it was

picture most related to the chicken claw that he saw, the speaking left hemisphere did not see the snow scene so it must concoct a rational and reasonable explanation for why his left hand chose the snow shovel as well.

As demonstrated in the simultaneous concept test above, the left hemisphere quickly interprets the actions of its left hand controlled by the disconnected right hemisphere in a way that makes sense for the patient. It has no internal representation available to explain why he is moving his left hand in that way. Yet, to the patient, the movement seems perfectly plausible once its actions have been interpreted. Interestingly, this does not always happen instantly for the patient. Sometimes it takes the patient's left hemisphere as long to figure out what its left hand is doing as it would an outside observer. For example, in one session we presented the word phone to the right hemisphere of patient J.W. and asked him to verbalize what he saw. Of course, J.W. was speaking from his left hemisphere and his left hemisphere did not see the word 'phone', and his right hemisphere was mute. Therefore, he said he did not see anything. However, when we put a pen in his left hand and asked him to draw it, J.W. immediately started drawing a phone. For the outside observers who did not see the word 'phone' displayed, it took some time to make out what J.W. was drawing. J.W.'s left hemisphere was in the same boat. Fortunately for us, J.W. tends to articulate what he is thinking (a great trait for a research subject). He was quite confused by what he was drawing, and started making guesses about what he saw. It was not until the picture was almost complete that outside observers, including J.W.'s left hemisphere got what his left hand was drawing. At which point, J.W. exclaimed, 'Duh, it's a phone'. The communication between the hemispheres happened out on the paper and not within his head. In the meantime, his interpreter struggled to find an explanation for his actions. Usually, the interpreter's explanations come much more readily. For example, if we flash the command 'stand up' to J.W.'s right hemisphere, he will stand up. But if we ask him why he is standing up, he doesn't respond, 'well, you just told me to' because that command is not available to his left hemisphere. Instead, J.W. will say something like, 'I just felt like getting a coke'. His left hemisphere is compelled to concoct a story that provides an explanation, or interpretation, of his actions after they have already occurred.

The existence of a specialized system in the brain that is driven to interpret is adaptive on an evolutionary scale because it allows the individual to quickly adapt to a wide range of unexpected events in the environment. But the interpreter, and by extension consciousness, is only as good as the information available to it. Therefore, when the information is corrupted, the interpretation can be misguided. For example, Capgras syndrome patients, with a disconnection between the visual inputs and emotional responses, will instantly interpret the lack of emotional response to the sight of a loved one as the result of an imposter pretending to be their loved one [62]. In split-brain patients, this was nicely demonstrated in a memory study conducted by Liz Phelps. She showed both hemispheres of a split-brain patient a series of pictures that depicted a simple story, like a guy getting ready for work in the morning. Later, she showed both hemispheres some test pictures. Some of the pictures were included in the study, some were new pictures depicting an unrelated story, and some pictures were new pictures but fit with the story depicted in the study session. She found that while the right hemisphere was quite veridical in its recognition responses and rarely false alarmed to new but related pictures, the left hemisphere consistently false alarmed to the same pictures [46]. The left hemisphere made faulty interpretations based on the information available to it.

Another example of faulty interpretations due to faulty inputs is a study conducted by Alan Kingstone using a different kind of simultaneous concept task. In this study, he displayed a word to each hemisphere, like '10' to the right hemisphere and 'o'clock' to the left hemisphere. When the patient was asked to draw what he saw with one hand, he drew the face of a clock with the hands pointing to 10 o'clock. Previous researchers had concluded from similar results that subcortical transfer of higher-order information must have been occurring in these split-brain patients [63]. However, Kingstone modified the task to include two words that formed an emergent object, like 'toad' and 'stool'. If the information was being transferred subcortically, then the patient would draw a picture of a mushroom like anybody else. Indeed, when the two words were presented simultaneously to one hemisphere the patient drew the emergent concept. However, when the two words were presented to separate hemispheres, the patient drew a toad and a stool, but not a mushroom [64]. This occurred much more frequently with the left hand than the right (the right hemisphere would usually only draw the word that it saw) because the left hemisphere is able to exert some control of the ipsilateral hand, as we later confirmed [65]. The left hemisphere appears compelled to draw the word it saw after the right hemisphere draws the word it saw first, even though the final picture is not the normal representation of the two words together.

The function of the interpreter, faulty or not, extends to the realm of problem-solving as well. In most situations, the ability to make interpretations is a great problem-solving tool and very advantageous. If you can formulate a hypothesis about why a predator takes a particular route from day to day, then that hypothesis about the predator's movements can be used to predict future movements and keep you safe. However, when the sequence of events is purely random, then the drive to look for patterns and to formulate a hypothesis about the events can be suboptimal. Take the case of studies that utilize a probability-matching paradigm. In the typical paradigm, subjects try to guess which of two events will happen next: will it be a red light or a green light? Each event has a different probability of occurrence (e.g., the green light may appear on 70% of the trials while the red light appears on 30% of the trials) but the order of occurrence is entirely random. The subject may be presented hundreds of trials, and they are encouraged to guess as correctly as possible. Typically, subjects will guess a green and red light with the same probability in which they were presented (e.g., they will predict green light on 70% of the trials and red light on 30% of the trials) [66]. This is referred to as frequency matching, but it is a suboptimal strategy because the most trials they can correctly predict is 58%. The more optimal strategy is to choose the most frequent stimulus on 100% of the trials. This is referred to as maximizing, and it is the optimal strategy because you can correctly predict trials 70% of the time. However, humans do not tend to do this, but animals (including rats, pigeons, and crocodiles) do!! [67, 69]

Again, we blame our interpreter for this suboptimal behaviour. We are driven to form hypotheses and to look for patterns even when it's not warranted. Yellot [70] conducted a fascinating version of this task with human subjects in which he stopped the subjects at some point and asked them to explain what they were doing. The subjects often explained that they thought they figured out the pattern (providing elaborate sequences that ultimately failed), even though there was none and they were told at the beginning of the experiment that the trials were random. Randomness tends to be a very difficult concept for humans [71], and a particularly difficult phenomenon for the interpreter. Since the interpreter is specialized to the left hemisphere, we tested two split-brain patients with this paradigm. In both patients, we found that while the right hemisphere maximized in an optimal way like most animals, the left hemisphere frequency matched! [72]

The interpreter is a critical component of our conscious experience. It gives voice to our thoughts, emotions, and reactions, and it is driven to unify all those consciously emergent specialized processes throughout the brain into a coherent whole. Yet, as our studies with split-brain patients have demonstrated, the interpreter and our conscious experience will be limited by the inputs available to it. Even though the split-brain patient senses no difference after their surgery, the left hemisphere's conscious experience must be altered (albeit, maybe to a small degree) by the lack of specialized inputs from the right hemisphere. And for the right hemisphere, its conscious experience must be altered drastically.

IF THE RIGHT HEMISPHERE COULD TALK

What would the right hemisphere have to say if it could talk? If the right hemisphere had the language, problem-solving, and interpretive abilities of the left hemisphere then maybe split-brain patients would experience the conflicting, dual consciousness that early researchers worried about. But, in reality, the right hemisphere is much more impoverished than the left hemisphere and it certainly suffers much more from the disconnection than the left. While the right hemisphere's visual representations are much sharper and its perceptions of space are much keener than the left hemisphere's, the right hemisphere is probably, mute, autistic-like, and mentally impaired. So, does the right hemisphere despair at the sudden downgrade in its conscious experience? Of course, without a voice we can only speculate, but if the disconnected left hemisphere and other neurological patients are an accurate guide, than the answer is no.

With a muted and severely limited language ability, does the right hemisphere have the same unified conscious experience as the left hemisphere? We speculate that it does not have it to the same extent as the left hemisphere since the interpreter appears to be specialized to the left. However, recent work has suggested that the right hemisphere has some limited interpretative ability as well. Paul Corballis has postulated the existence of a 'right hemisphere interpreter' that is more 'visually intelligent' than the left and is dedicated to constructing a representation of the visual world [54]. Furthermore, we have found in probability-matching paradigms that utilize faces instead of other stimuli, that the right hemisphere will suddenly start to frequency match while the left hemisphere will respond randomly [73]. However, it is not clear whether that frequency-matching behaviour is really the result of hypothesis formation and actively seeking out a pattern. After all, goldfish can frequency match under the right conditions [67]. Of course, the true nature of the conscious experience of the right hemisphere is difficult to determine given the limited capacity to express itself, but our observations of the speaking left hemisphere and of other neurological patients leads us to believe that the right hemisphere's conscious experience is much more impoverished than the left hemisphere. No cause for alarm, though, since the right hemisphere knows no better.

SUMMARY

In our experience, the speaking left hemisphere of split-brain patients never complains about the shortcomings they may be experiencing due to the disconnection from the right. Some people may argue that the left hemisphere doesn't miss the right hemisphere because the right hemisphere contributes very little to the complexities of cognition. But, in the patients that we have tested, the right hemisphere is clearly better at part–whole relations [40], spatial relationships [41], apparent motion detection [42], mental rotation [43], spatial matching [44], mirror image discrimination [45], veridical memory recollections [46, 47], amodal completion [48], causal perception [49], and face processing [50–52, 73]. With an intact corpus callosum, these specialized processes in the right hemisphere must contribute to conscious experience in noticeable ways. Yet, we continue to observe in split-brain patients that the left hemisphere does not miss the right hemisphere. This simple observation is consistent with the idea that the contribution and availability of specialized neural circuits or brain modules constitute the entire conscious experience. The numerous modules localized in the right hemisphere are no longer available to the speaking left hemisphere and thus are not reflected when it reports out the nature of its conscious experience.

References

1. Gazzaniga, M.S. (1989) Organization of the human brain. *Science* 245:947–952.
2. Logothetis, N. (1998) Single units and conscious vision. *Philos Trans R Soc Lond B Biol Sci* 353:1801–1818.
3. Kanwisher, N. (2001) Neural events and perceptual awareness. *Cognition* 79:89–113.
4. Driver, J. and Vuilleumier, P. (2001) Perceptual awareness and its loss in unilateral neglect and extinction. *Cognition* 79:39–88.
5. Cooney, J.W. and Gazzaniga, M.S. (2003) Neurological disorders and the structure of human consciousness. *Trends Cogn Sci* 7 (4):161–165.
6. Funk, C.M., Putnam, M.C., & Gazzaniga, M.S. (in press) Consciousness. In Berntson, G.G. & Cacioppo, J.T. (Eds.), *Handbook of Neuroscience for the Behavioral Sciences*. Wiley & Sons: New York.
7. Ramachandran, V.S. (1995) Anosognosia in parietal lobe syndrome. *Conscious Cogn* 4:22–51.

8. Ramachandran, V.S. and Rogers-Ramachandran, D. (1996) Denial of disabilities in anosognosia. *Nature* 382:501–502.

9. Halligan, P.W. and Marshall, J.C. (1998) Neglect of awareness. *Conscious Cogn* 7:356–380.

10. O'Craven, K. and Kanwisher, N. (2000) Mental imagery of faces and places activates corresponding stimulus-specific brain regions. *J Cogn Neurosci* 12:1013–1023.

11. Kosslyn, S.M., *et al.* (2001) Neural foundations of imagery. *Nat Rev Neurosci* 2:635–642.

12. Bisiach, E. and Luzzatti, C. (1978) Unilateral neglect of representation space. *Cortex* 14:129–133.

13. Volpe, B.T., LeDoux, J.E. and Gazzaniga, M.S. (1979) Information-processing of visual-stimuli in an extinguished field. *Nature* 282 (5740):722–724.

14. Wessinger, C.M., Buonocore, M.H., Kussmaul, C.L. and Mangun, G.R. (1997) Tonotopy in human auditory cortex examined with functional magnetic resonance imaging. *Hum Brain Mapp* 5 (1):18–25.

15. Kanwisher, N., McDermott, J. and Chun, M.M. (1997) The fusiform face area: A module in human extrastriate cortex specialized for face perception. *J Neurosci* 17 (11):4302–4311.

16. Adolphs, R. (2002) Neural systems for recognizing emotion. *Curr Biol* 12 (2):169–177.

17. Decety, J. and Chaminade, T. (2003) Neural correlates of feeling sympathy. *Neuropsychologia* 41 (2):127–138.

18. Cosmides, L., Tooby, J., Fiddick, L. and Bryant, G.A. (2005) Detecting cheaters. *Trends Cogn Sci* 9 (11):505–506.

19. Breen, N., *et al.* (2000) Towards an understanding of delusions of misidentification: Four case studies. *Mind Lang* 15:74–110.

20. Gazzaniga, M.S. (2000) Cerebral specialization and interhemispheric communication: Does the corpus callosum enable the human condition? *Brain* 123:1293–1326.

21. Van Wagenen, W.P. and Herren, R.Y. (1940) Surgical division of commissural pathways in the corpus callosum: Relation to spread of an epileptic seizure. *Arch Neuro Psychiatr* 44:470–759.

22. Aboitiz, F., Scheibel, A.B., Fisher, R.S. and Zaidel, E. (1992) Fiber composition of the human corpus callosum. *Brain Res* 598:143–153.

23. Akelatis, A.J. (1941) Studies on the corpus callosum: Higher visual functions in each homonymous field following complete section of the corpus callosum. *Arch Neurol Psychiatr* 45:788.

24. Akelaitis, A.J. (1945) Studies of the corpus callosum IV. Diagnostic dyspraxia in epileptics following partial and complete section of the corpus callosum. *Am J Psychiatr* 101 (5):594–599.

25. Sperry, R.W. (1961) Cerebral organization and behavior – split brain behaves in many respects like 2 separate brains, providing new research possibilities. *Science* 133 (346):1749–1757.

26. Gazzainga, M.S., Bogen, J.E. and Sperry, R. (1962) Some functional effects of sectioning the cerebral commissures in man. *Proc Natl Acad Sci USA* 48:1756–1769.

27. Zaidel, E. (1991) Language functions in the two hemispheres following complete cerebral commissurotomy and hemispherectomy. In Boller, F. and Grafman, J. (eds.) *Handbook of Neuropsychology*, Vol. 4, pp. 115–150. Amsterdam: Elsevier.

28. Gazzaniga, M.S. (2005) Forty-five years of split-brain research and still going strong. *Nat Rev Neurosci* 6 (8):653–659.

29. Milner, B. (1962). In Mountcastle, V.B. (ed.) *Interhemispheric Relations and Cerebral Dominance*, pp. 177–198. Baltimore, Maryland: Johns Hopkins Press.

30. Zaidel, E. and Peters, A.M. (1981) Phonological encoding and ideographic reading by the disconnected right hemisphere: Two case studies. *Brain Lang* 14:205–234.

31. Zaidel, E. (1985) Benson, D.F. and Zaidel, E. *The Dual Brain*, pp. 205–231. New York: Guildford.

32. Baynes, K., Eliassen, J.C., L Lutsep, H. and Gazzaniga, M.S. (1998) Modular organization of cognitive systems masked by interhemispheric integration. *Science* 280:902–905.

33. Reuter-Lorenz, P.A. and Baynes, K. (1992) Modes of lexical access in the callosotomized brain. *J Cogn Neurosci* 4:155–164.

34. Baynes, K., Tramo, M.J. and Gazzaniga, M.S. (1992) Reading with a limited lexicon in the right hemisphere of a callosotomy patient. *Neuropsychologia* 30:187–200.

35. Gazzaniga, M.S., Nass, R., Reeves, A. and Roberts, D. (1984) Neurologic perspectives on right hemisphere language following surgical section of the corpus callosum. *Semin Neurol* 4:126–135.

36. Gazzaniga, M.S. and Miller, G.A. (1989) The recognition of antonymy by a language enriched right hemisphere. *J Cogn Neurosci* 1:187–193.

37. Gazzaniga, M.S. (1983) Right hemisphere language following brain bisection: A 20 year perspective. *Am Psychol* 38:525–537.

38. Kihlstrom, J.F. and Klein, S.B. (1997) Self-knowledge and self-awareness. In Snodgrass, J.D. and Thompson, R.L. (eds.) The Self Across Psychology: Self-Recognition, Self-Awareness, and the Self Concept. *Ann N Y Acad Sci*, 818, New York: New York Academy of Sciences, pp. 5–17.

39. Turk, D.J., Heatherton, T.F., Macrae, C.N., Kelley, W.M. and Gazzaniga, M.S. (2003) Out of contact, out of mind: The distributed nature of self. *Ann N Y Acad Sci* 1001:65–78.

40. Nebes, R. (1972) Superiority of the minor hemisphere in commissurotomized man on a test of figural unification. *Brain* 95:633–638.

41. Nebes, R. (1973) Perception of spatial relationships by the right and left hemispheres of a commissurotomized man. *Neuropsychologia* 7:333–349.

42. Forster, B.A., Corballis, P.M. and Corballis, M.C. (2000) Effect of luminance on successiveness discrimination in the absence of the corpus callosum. *Neuropsychologia* 38:441–450.

43. Corballis, M.C. and Sergent, J. (1988) Imagery in a commissurotomized patient. *Neuropsychologia* 26:13–26.

44. Corballis, P.M., Funnell, M.G. and Gazzaniga, M.S. (1999) A dissociation between spatial and identity matching in callosotomy patients. *Neuroreport* 10:2183–2187.

45. Funnell, M.G., Corballis, P.M. and Gazzaniga, M.S. (1999) A deficit in perceptual matching in the left hemisphere of a callosotomy patient. *Neuropsychologia* 38:441–450.

46. Phelps, E.A. and Gazzaniga, M.S. (1992) Hemispheric differences in mnemonic processing: The effects of left hemisphere interpretation. *Neuropsychologia* 30:293–297.

47. Metcalfe, J., Funnell, M. and Gazzaniga, M.S. (1995) Right-hemisphere memory superiority: Studies of a split-brain patient. *Psychol Sci* 6:157–164.

48. Corballis, P.M., Fendrich, R., Shapley, R. and Gazzaniga, M.S. (1999) Illusory contours and amodal completion: Evidence for a functional dissociation in callosotomy patients. *J Cogn Neurosci.* 11:459–466.

49. Roser, M.E., Fugelsang, J.A., Dunbar, K.N., Corballis, P.M. and Gazzaniga, M.S. (2005) Dissociating causal perception and causal inference in the brain. *Neuropsychology* 19:591–602.

50. Levy, J., Trevarthen, C. and Sperry, R.W. (1972) Reception of bilateral chimeric figures following hemispheric deconnexion. *Brain* 95:61–78.

51. Gazzaniga, M.S. and Smylie, C.S. (1983) Facial recognition and brain asymmetries: Clues to underlying mechanisms. *Ann Neurol* 13:536–540.

52. Miller, M.B., Kingstone, A. and Gazzaniga, M.S. (2002) Hemispheric encoding asymmetries are more apparent than real. *J Cogn Neurosci* 14 (5):702–708.

53. Gazzaniga, M.S. and Smylie, C.S. (1990) Hemispheric mechanisms controlling voluntary and spontaneous facial expressions. *J Cogn Neurosci* 2:239–245.

54. Corballis, P.M. (2003). Visuospatial processing and the right hemisphere interpreter, *Brain Cogn*, 53, 171–176, (eds.) Handbook of physiology. Sect. 1, Vol. 5, Pt. 2. (pp. 701–61). Bethesda (MD): American Physiological Society.

55. Tulving, E., Kapur, S., Craik, F.M., Moscovitch, M. and Houle, S. (1994) Hemispheric encoding/retrieval asymmetry in episodic memory: Positron emission tomography findings. *Proc Natl Acad Sci USA* 91:2016–2020.

56. Wig, G., Miller, M.B., Kingstone, A. and Kelley, W. (2004) Separable routes to human memory formation: Dissociating task and material contributions in prefrontal cortex. *J Cogn Neurosc* 16 (1):139–148.

57. Phelps, E.A., Hirst, W. and Gazzaniga, M.S. (1991) Deficits in recall following partial and complete commissurotomy. *Cereb Cortex* 1:492–498.

58. Nass, R.D. and Gazzaniga, M.S. (1987) Cerebral lateralization and specialization of human central nervous system. In Mountcastle, V.B., Plum, F. and Geiger, S.R. (eds.) *Handbook of Physiology*, Vol. 5, pp. 701–761. Bethesda (MD): American Physiological Society. Sect. 1, Pt. 2.

59. LeDoux, J.E., Risse, G.L., Springer, S.P., Wilson, D.H. and Gazzaniga, M.S. (1977) Cognition and commissurotomy. *Brain* 100:87–104.

60. Gazzaniga, M.S. (2008) *Human: The Science Behind What Makes Us Unique*, New York: HarperCollins.

61. Gazzaniga, M.S. and LeDoux, J.E. (1978) *The Integrated Mind*, New York: Plenum Press.

62. Ramachandran, V.S. (1998) Consciousness and body image: Lessons from phantom limbs, Capgras syndrome and pain asymbolia. *Philos Trans R Soc Lond B Biol Sci* 353 (1377):1851–1859.

63. Sergent, J. (1990) Furtive incursions into bicameral minds. *Brain* 113:537–568.

64. Kingstone, A. and Gazzaniga, M.S. (1995) Subcortical transfer of higher-order information – more illusory than real. *Neuropsychology* 9 (3):321–328.

65. Miller, M.B. and Kingstone, A. (2005) Taking the high road on subcortical transfer. *Brain Cogn* 57 (2):162–164.

66. Estes, W.K. (1961) A descriptive approach to the dynamics of choice behavior. *Behav Sci* 6:177–184.

67. Bitterman, M.E. (1965) The evolution of intelligence. *Sci Am* 212 (1):92–100.

68. Sergent, J. (1990) Furtive incursions into bicameral minds. *Brain* 113:537–568.

69. Hinson, J.M. and Staddon, J.E.R. (1983) Matching, maximizing and hillclimbing. *J Exp Anal Behav* 40:321–331.

70. Yellott, J.I.Jr (1969) Probability learning with noncontingent success. *J Math Psychol* 6:541–575.

71. Nickerson, R.S. (2002) The production and perception of randomness. *Psychol Rev* 109 (2):330–357.

72. Wolford, G., Miller, M.B. and Gazzaniga, M.S. (2000) The left hemisphere's role in hypothesis formation. *J Neurosci* 20:RC64.

73. Miller, M.B. and Valsangkar-Smyth, M. (2005) Probability matching in the right hemisphere. *Brain Cogn* 57 (2):165–167. New York: Guildford.

Visual Consciousness: An Updated Neurological Tour

Lionel Naccache

ABSTRACT

The scientific study of the cerebral substrate of consciousness has been marked by significant recent achievements, resulting partially from an interaction between the exploration of cognition in both brain-damaged patients and healthy subjects. Several neuropsychological syndromes contain marked dissociations which permit the identification of principles related to the neurophysiology of consciousness. The generality of these principles can then be evaluated in healthy subjects using a combination of experimental psychology paradigms, and functional brain-imaging tools. In this paper, I update[1] and extend a precedent review of the recent results relevant to visual phenomenal consciousness, which is the aspect of consciousness most frequently investigated in neuroscience. Through the exploration of neuropsychological syndromes such as 'blindsight', visual form agnosia, optic ataxia, visual hallucinations, neglect but also Capgras delusion and split-brain cognition, I highlight five general principles and explain how their generality has been demonstrated in healthy subjects using conditions such as visual illusions or subliminal perception. Finally, I describe the bases of a scientific model of consciousness, based on the concept of a 'global workspace', which takes into account the data reviewed.

---

[1] This article updates a previous paper addressing this issue [1].

INTRODUCTION

Scientific investigation of consciousness has recently stimulated experimental research in healthy human subjects, in neurological and psychiatric patients, and in some animal models. Although this major ongoing effort does not yet provide us with a detailed and explicit neural theory of this remarkable mental faculty, we already have access to a vast collection of results acting as a set of constraints on what should be a scientific model of consciousness. There are many ways to summarize and present this set of 'consciousness principles'. One may either use a chronological or a domain-specific strategy. Here, I deliberately adopt a narrative approach driven by a neurological perspective. This approach allows an emphasis of the crucial role played by the observation of brain-lesioned patients affected by neuropsychological syndromes. I argue that, as in other fields of cognitive neuroscience, clinical neuropsychology often offers profound and precious insights leading to the discovery of neural principles governing distinct aspects of the physiology of consciousness [2]. Most importantly, many of these principles also prove to be relevant and to generalize to the cognition of healthy human subjects. In a schematic manner, the 'borderline cases' provided by clinical neurology have the power to specifically illustrate a single property of consciousness by showing the consequences of its impairment. This magnifying effect makes it easier to isolate and delineate this property, and then to take it into account in more complex situations where it is functioning in concert with other processes.

I will focus our interest on a selected number of these properties, and will limit our investigation to visual phenomenal consciousness which is by far the most experimentally investigated aspect of consciousness.

CONSCIOUS REPORTABILITY

Following the psychologist Larry Weiskrantz [3] our criteria to establish subject's conscious perception of a stimulus will be the 'reportability' criteria: the ability to report explicitly to oneself or to somebody else the object of our perception: '*I see the word consciousness printed in black on this page*'. This criteria is fully operational, and can be easily confronted to other sources of information (external reality, functional brain-imaging data, …), therefore paving the way to an objective evaluation of subjective data, a scientific programme called 'heterophenomenology'

by Daniel Dennett [4]. It can be argued; however, that reportability might be a biased measure underestimating subjects' conscious state, and that forced-choice tasks using signal detection theory parameters (e.g., d-prime measure of objective discriminability) might be preferable [5]. However, discrediting reportability on these grounds in favour of purely objective measures is far from satisfying. Firstly, unconscious perception of a stimulus might have an impact on objective measures, as illustrated in many unconscious perception situations such as masked priming paradigms [6]. Secondly, to ignore subjective reports is somewhat of a counterproductive approach, because it may lead to simply giving up the original project of investigating consciousness. Finally, some authors contest the criteria of reportability by establishing differences between phenomenal consciousness and access consciousness, claiming that we are actually conscious of much more information than we can access and report [7]. The key problem with this definition of phenomenal consciousness lies in the way it can be established: How can we infer that subjects are phenomenally conscious of far more information than they can report? By taking at face value another of their conscious reports, namely their strong belief of visual completeness: 'I see everything present in the visual scene.' In other words, the problem with this definition of phenomenality is the incontrovertible need to rely on conscious reports to establish it: a form of logical circularity. If one wants to define phenomenal consciousness differently from conscious reportability, then one should resist the temptation to make use of subjects' reports to credit the existence of phenomenal consciousness. Note also that a conscious report is not a 'cut and paste' copy of a visual scene, but rather a conscious comment on an inner mental representation. This representation can originate from perceptual systems at multiple levels, but ultimately it results from their redescription by evaluative and interpretative systems. Valuably, conscious reports can be non-verbal and observable in disconnected right hemispheres of split-brain patients, in some aphasic patients or even become entirely covert, due to motor system impairments [8, 9].

Thus far, I have justified our adoption of the 'reportability' criteria to diagnose conscious perception in subjects. How then may we use it to specify a scientific programme to investigate systematically the neural basis of visual consciousness? By first recalling a basic but essential 'Kantian' statement: when we report being conscious of seeing an object, strictly speaking we are not conscious of this object belonging to external reality, rather we are conscious of some of the visual representations elaborated in our visual brain areas and participating to the flow of our visual phenomenal consciousness, as masterly expressed by the Belgian Surrealist Painter, René Magritte in his famous painting 'This is not a pipe' ('Ceci n'est pas une pipe' or 'La trahison des images', 1928–1929). This simple evocation of the concept of representation foreshadows the two fundamental stages in the search of the 'neural correlates of visual consciousness' [10]: (1) make a detailed inventory of the multiple representations of the visual world elaborated by different visual brain areas (from retina and lateral geniculate nuclei to ventral occipito-temporal and dorsal occipito-parietal pathways described by Ungerleider and Mishkin [11], in addition to superior colliculus mediated visual pathways); (2) identify among these different forms of visual coding which participate in visual phenomenal consciousness, and in these cases, specify the precise conditions governing the contribution of these representations to the flow of phenomenal consciousness. One may date the beginning of this scientific programme with the influential publication of Crick and Koch [12] who proposed, mainly on the basis of neuro-anatomical data, that neural activity in area V1 does not contribute to the content of our phenomenal consciousness.

BLINDSIGHT: HIGHLIGHTING THE ROLE OF VISUAL CORTEX

Some patients affected by visual scotoma secondary to primary visual cortex lesions display striking dissociations when presented with visual stimuli at the location of their scotoma. While claiming to have no conscious perception of these stimuli, they perform better than chance on forced-choice visual and visuomotor tasks such as stimulus discrimination, stimulus detection or orientation to stimulus spatial source by visual saccades. This phenomenon, discovered in the early 1970s [13–15], has been coined 'blindsight' by Weiskrantz. Compelling evidence supports the idea that such unconscious perceptual processes are subserved by the activity of subcortical visual pathways including the superior colliculus and by-passing primary visual cortex [16]. In a recent study, de Gelder and Weiskrantz enlarged the range of unconscious perceptual processes accessible to blindsight patients by showing that patient G.Y., whose fame is comparable to that of patient H.M. in the field of medial temporal lobe amnesia, was able to discriminate better than chance emotional facial expressions on forced-choice tasks [17]. This unconscious processing of fear faces in patient G.Y. was also found to interact with

the perception of conscious emotional faces and voices [18]. Taking advantage of this behavioural result, the authors used fMRI to demonstrate that this affective blindsight performance correlated with activity in an extra-geniculo-striate colliculo-thalamo-amygdala pathway independently of both the striate cortex and fusiform face area located in the ventral pathway [19]. In fact, this unconscious visual process discovered in blindsight subjects is also active in healthy human subjects free of any visual cortex lesions. One way to observe it consists of using paradigms of masked or 'subliminal' visual stimulation in which a stimulus is briefly flashed foveally for tens of milliseconds, then immediately followed by a second stimulus, suppressing conscious perception of the former. Whalen and colleagues used such a paradigm to mask a first fearful or neutral face presented during 33 ms by a second neutral face presented for a longer duration (167 ms). While subjects did not consciously perceive the first masked face, fMRI revealed an increase of neural activity in the amygdala on masked fearful face trials as compared to masked neutral face trials [20]. This interesting result has been replicated and enriched by a set of elegant studies conducted by Morris and colleagues [21, 22]. Recently however, Pessoa and colleagues challenged this view in normal controls by arguing that under strict conditions of unconscious processing, as assessed by objective discrimination measures, no residual activation of the amygdala could be observed [23]. The Pessoa et al. study capitalized on a previous experiment demonstrating that under conditions of high attentional load, a briefly presented fearful face did not activate the amygdala [24]. Beyond the risk of 'throwing the baby out with the bath water', frequently encountered in the area of subliminal perception, this set of criticisms certainly call for methodological improvements in the assessment of masked faces visibility. Such a methodological process occurred recently in the close area of masked word perception, driven by a seminal criticism of masked word visibility [5]. This work stimulated the use of more stringent masking conditions and led to the production of a rich literature describing perceptual, cognitive and motor processing of unconsciously perceived masked words (see [25] for a recent review).

The blindsight model and its extension in healthy subjects via visual masking procedures underlines the importance of the neocortex in conscious visual processing by revealing that a subcortical pathway is able to process visual information in the absence of phenomenal consciousness. In other words, these recent data are in close agreement with Hughlings Jackson's [26] hierarchical conception (formulated in particular in the 3rd and 4th principles of his 'Croonian lectures on the evolution and dissolution of the nervous system') attributing the more complex cognitive processes, including consciousness, to the activity of neocortex. Nevertheless, should we generalize the importance shown here for the primary visual cortex – the integrity of which seems to be a pre-requisite for visual consciousness – to the whole visual cortex?

VISUAL FORM AGNOSIA, OPTIC ATAXIA AND VISUAL HALLUCINATIONS: THE KEY ROLE OF THE VENTRAL PATHWAY

As a result of the seminal work of Ungerleider and Mishkin [11], visual cortex anatomy is considered to be composed of two parallel and interconnected pathways both supplied by primary visual cortex area V1: the occipito-temporal or 'ventral' pathway and the occipito-parietal or 'dorsal' pathway. The dorsal pathway mainly subserves visuo-motor transformations [27], while ventral pathway neurons represent information from low-level features to more and more abstract stages of identity processing, thus subserving object identification. This 'what pathway' is organized according to a posterior–anterior gradient of abstraction, the most anterior neurons located in infero-temporal cortex coding for object-based representations free from physical parameters such as retinal position, object size, or orientation [28–31]. Goodale and Milner reported a puzzling dissociation in patient D.F. suffering from severe visual form agnosia due to carbon monoxide poisoning [32]. As initially defined by Benson and Greenberg [33], this patient not only had great difficulties in recognizing and identifying common objects, but she was also unable to discriminate even simple geometric forms and line orientations. Anatomically, bilateral ventral visual pathways were extensively lesioned, while primary visual cortices and dorsal visual pathways were spared. Goodale and Milner presented this patient with a custom 'mail-box', the slot of which could be rotated in the vertical plane. When asked to report slot orientation verbally or manually patient D.F. performed at chance-level, thus confirming her persistent visual agnosia. However, when asked to post a letter into this slot she unexpectedly performed almost perfectly, while still being unable to report slot orientation consciously. This spectacular observation demonstrates how spared dorsal pathway involved in visuo-motor transformations was still processing visual information but without contributing to patient D.F.'s

phenomenal conscious content. This case suggests that some representations elaborated in this 'how pathway' are operating unconsciously while ventral pathway activity subserves our phenomenal visual consciousness. Since this influential paper, many studies have tested this hypothesis in healthy subjects using visual illusions [34–36]. For instance, Aglioti and colleagues engaged subjects in a Titchener-Ebbinghaus circles illusion task in which a given circle surrounded by larger circles appears smaller than the very same circle surrounded by smaller circles. While subjects consciously reported this cognitively impenetrable illusion, when asked to grip the central circle, online measures of their thumb–index distance showed that their visuo-motor response was free of the perceptual illusion and was adapted to the objective size of the circle[2].

An inverse dissociation supporting the same general principle was recently reported by Pisella and colleagues [40] who demonstrated the existence of an unconscious 'automatic pilot' located in the dorsal pathway. Their patient I.G. presented important stroke lesions affecting both dorsal pathways, while sparing primary visual cortices and ventral pathways. They designed a subtle task manipulating online motor corrections of pointing movements on a tactile screen on which visual targets appeared and could unexpectedly jump from one position to another. While normal subjects were capable of extremely fast and automatic visuo-motor corrections in this task, patient I.G. could only rely on very slow strategic and conscious corrections. Crucially, when tested in a more complex condition in which subjects had to inhibit an initiated pointing correction on some trials, patient I.G. committed far less errors than controls who were unable to inhibit very fast motor corrections and who reported being astonished by their own uncontrollable behaviour.

Taken together, these results are currently interpreted as dissociations between visuo-motor processes subserved by the activity of the dorsal visual pathway, the computations of which do not participate

---

[2] Since these first reports, Franz and colleagues [37, 38] challenged this interpretation by showing that when task difficulty was equated between perceptual and grasping tasks, action was not resisting to the illusion. However, recent studies taking into account these possible confounds reproduced the dissociation between perceptual and action performances (for a detailed review, see [39]).

[3] Area MT or V5, located within the dorsal pathway, is an important exception to this principle because: (1) its activity correlates directly with conscious reports of genuine or illusory visual motion [41]; (2) when lesioned [42] or transiently inactivated by trans-cranial magnetic stimulation [43] it results in akinetopsia (i.e., the inability to report visual motion); and (3) microstimulation within this area influences motion orientation discrimination in monkeys [44].

to our phenomenal consciousness[3], and other visual processes relying on ventral pathway activity which supplies our conscious perception. The strong version of this theoretical position is defended in particular by authors such as Goodale and Milner. The latter claims for instance that 'we have two (largely) separate visual systems. One of them is dedicated to the rapid and accurate guidance of our movements ..., and yet it lies outside the realm of our conscious visual awareness. The other seems to provide our perceptual phenomenology' [45]. Additional data originating from behavioural measures of subliminal priming, and functional brain-imaging data support this thesis [46, 47].

Lastly a recent functional brain-imaging study of consciously reportable visual hallucinations observed in patients with Charles-Bonnet syndrome[4] reinforces this conception, by revealing correlations between colour, face, texture and object hallucinations and increased levels of cerebral blood flow in the corresponding specialized visual areas located in the ventral visual pathway [48].

UNILATERAL SPATIAL NEGLECT: THE NECESSITY OF ATTENTIONAL ALLOCATION

The recent proposal of a cerebral substrate of visual consciousness through the distinction drawn between dorsal ('unconscious') and ventral ('conscious') pathways still bears some similarity to Jackson's conception since it relies on a similar anatomical partition between some sectors of the visual system which would supply the flow of our phenomenal consciousness, and other sectors which would process information out of our conscious awareness. However, we may posit a further question: Does visual information represented in the ventral pathway depends on some additional conditions to be consciously accessible and reportable? In other words, are we necessarily conscious of all visual information represented in the ventral pathway? A key answer to this question comes from unilateral spatial neglect (USN), a very frequent neuropsychological syndrome clinically characterized by the inability to perceive or respond to stimuli presented to the side contralateral to the site of lesion, despite the absence of significant sensory or

motor deficits. USN has two interesting characteristics: firstly, most USN patients display impaired visual phenomenal consciousness for objects located on their left side[5]. Some neglect patients even present a very pure symptom named 'visual extinction', and defined by the specific loss of phenomenal consciousness for left-sided stimuli presented in competition with right-sided stimuli, while the same left-sided stimuli presented in the absence of contralateral competing stimuli are available to conscious report. Secondly, USN syndrome is usually observed with lesions affecting the spatial attentional network – most often right parietal and/or superior temporal gyrus [50] cortices or fronto-parietal white matter pathways [51], but also right thalamic or right frontal lesions – sparing primary visual cortex and the whole ventral visual pathway. Recent behavioural and functional brain-imaging studies have reliably shown that this spared visual ventral pathway still represents the neglected visual information at multiple levels of processing culminating in highly abstract forms of coding [52–55]. For instance McGlinchey-Berroth and colleagues [56] demonstrated that left-sided neglected object pictures could be represented up to a semantic stage, as revealed by significant behavioural priming effects on the subsequent processing of consciously perceived semantically related words. More recently, Rees and colleagues [57] have shown that an unconsciously perceived extinguished visual stimulus still activates corresponding retinotopic regions of primary visual cortex and several extra-striate ventral pathway areas.

These results demonstrate that ventral pathway activation constitutes a necessary but not sufficient condition to perceive consciously visual stimuli. The additional mechanism, defective in USN patients and mandatory to conscious perception, seems to be the top-down attentional amplification supplied by the activity of the spatial attention network [58].

Recently we have been able to generalize this principle demonstrated by USN patients to healthy subjects, by investigating neural correlates of unconsciously perceived words using a visual masking procedure [59]. Using both fMRI and event related potential (ERP) recordings we observed significant activations of a left ventral pathway – the visual word form area, previously identified as the first non-retinotopic area responding to letter string stimuli [31] – by unconsciously perceived masked words. In a second

---

[4] This syndrome is characterized by vivid visual hallucinations in elderly patients with peripheral visual deficits. Charles Bonnet, a Swiss philosopher, first described this condition in the 1760s when he noticed his grandfather, who was blinded by cataract, described seeing birds and buildings which were not there.

[5] An exact definition of 'left side' remains the subject of many investigations, as visual neglect has been reliably observed at several distinct spatial frames of reference such as different subject-centered or 'egocentric' frames, and multiple environment or object-centered 'allocentric' frames [49].

experiment, we tested the specificity of these activations by using a masked priming paradigm: on each trial subjects consciously perceived a target word and classified it either as man-made or as a natural object. Subjects responded faster to visible words immediately preceded by that same masked word (e.g., table/table) than to different prime–target pairs (e.g., radio/table). This repetition priming effect was correlated to specific reductions of the BOLD signal in the visual word form area on repeated word trials as compared to non-repeated word trials. This repetition suppression effect is strongly suggestive of the activation of common neurons sharing the same response tuning properties by unconsciously perceived masked words and by unmasked words [60].

This work enabled us to compare brain activations elicited by briefly (29 ms) flashed words depending on whether it was consciously perceived or not. On masked trials a backward mask suppressed conscious perception of the word, while words flashed for the very same duration but not backward masked were consciously perceived and reported. When consciously perceiving a word, corresponding neural activity is hugely amplified and temporally sustained in ventral visual pathway by comparison with neural activity elicited by masked words. Moreover, conscious perception is systematically accompanied by the co-activation of a long-range distributed network, the epicentres of which involve prefrontal, anterior cingulate, and parietal cortices.

SOURCE AND EFFECTS OF TOP-DOWN ATTENTIONAL EFFECTS: ATTENTION IS NOT CONSCIOUSNESS

The crucial role of top-down attentional amplification on the perceptual fate of stimuli is likely to occur recursively at multiple stages of processing all along the ventral visual pathway, allowing large modulations of activation patterns elicited by the same stimulus according to the task being presently performed. The rich plasticity of visual representations observed in conscious strategical processing leads to the following question: Are unconscious visual representations impermeable to such top-down effects? Indeed, in most current theories of human cognition, unconscious processes are considered as automatic processes that do not require attention [61–63].

Kentridge et al. [64, 65] recently questioned this conception by testing the efficacy of several visual cues on the forced detection of targets in the hemianopic scotoma of the blindsight patient G.Y. They found that

a central, consciously perceived arrow pointing toward the region of the scotoma where the target would appear could enhance G.Y.'s performance, although the target remained inaccessible to conscious report[6]. In normal subjects, using a visual masking procedure [66], recently reported that unconscious repetition priming in a lexical decision task occurred only if the masked primes appeared at spatially attended locations.

We also investigated a similar issue related to the impact of temporal attention on visual masked priming effects [67]. In previous studies, we have shown that masked numerical primes can be processed all the way up to quantity coding [60, 68] and motor response stages [69]. When subjects had to compare target numbers to a fixed reference of 5, they were faster when the prime and target numbers fell on the same side of 5, and therefore called for the same motor response, than when they did not (i.e., response-congruity effect). They were also faster when the same number was repeated as prime and target (i.e., repetition priming effect). In three experiments manipulating target temporal expectancy, we were able to then demonstrate that the occurrence of unconscious priming in a number comparison task is determined by the allocation of temporal attention to the time window during which the prime–target pair is presented. Both response-congruity priming and physical repetition priming totally vanish when temporal attention is focused away from this time window. We proposed that when subjects focus their attention on the predicted time of appearance of the target, they open a temporal window of attention for a few hundreds of milliseconds. This temporal attention then benefits unconscious primes that are presented temporally close to the targets.

Taken together these findings are inconsistent with the concept of a purely automatic spreading of activation during masked priming and refute the view that unconscious cognitive processes are necessarily rigid and automatic. While several paradigms, such as inattentional blindness [70] or the attentional blink [71] suggest that conscious perception cannot occur without attention [72], our findings indicate that attention also has a determining impact on unconscious processing. Thus, attention cannot be identified with consciousness. One of the key criteria for automaticity

---

[6] This very elegant demonstration in patient G.Y. will require further investigations in additional blindsight patients, given that G.Y.'s residual vision has been recently interpreted in terms of low-level phenomenal vision through a set of subtle experiments manipulating visual presentations in both the spared visual field and within the scotoma [73].

is independence from top-down influences. However, these results suggest that, by this criterion, masked priming effects or unconscious blindsight effects cannot be considered as automatic. We propose that the definition of automaticity may have to be refined in order to separate the source of conscious strategic control from its effects. Processing of masked primes is automatic inasmuch as it cannot serve as a *source* of information for the subsequent definition of an explicit strategy (e.g., see [74]). However, this does not imply that it is impermeable to the *effects* of top-down strategic control, for example, originating from instructions and/or task context. As a matter of fact, I retrospectively found an explicit formulation of this principle 20 years ago by Daniel Kahneman and Anne Treisman [75]:

> … a dissociation between perception and consciousness is not necessarily equivalent to a dissociation between perception and attention. (…) To establish that the presentation is subliminal, the experimenter ensures that the subjective experience of a display that includes a word cannot be discriminated from the experience produced by the mask on its own. The mask, however, is focally attended. Any demonstration that an undetected aspect of an attended stimulus can be semantically encoded is theoretically important, but a proof of complete automaticity would require more. Specifically, the priming effects of a masked stimulus should be the same regardless of whether or not that stimulus is attended. (…). These predictions have yet to be tested.

This fundamental distinction drawn between attention and consciousness is also crucial for experimental investigations aiming at delineating the scope and limits of unconscious processing. Reconsidering the set of studies by Pessoa and colleagues refuting previous results of unconscious processing of masked faces (see above), their negative result could well be the consequence of two distinct factors: (1) the contamination of previous studies by some consciously visible faces, and (2) a stronger attentional engagement on masked faces in previous studies (reinforced if some faces were visible and could attract spatial and temporal attention to masked faces). If so, in order to maximize sensibility to detect genuine unconscious processing, faces have to be strongly masked but subject attention also has to be maximally engaged on those stimuli.

CONSCIOUSNESS IS A WORLD OF (NEURO) SCIENCE-FICTIONS

What is the subjective status of conscious perceptual representations? Are they more of less accurate 'cut and paste' copies of a visual scene, or could they be constructs marked by the systematic presence of interpretative processes, rationalizations, and beliefs? Beyond the broad range of philosophical traditions proposing distinct frameworks to theorize the links prevailing between external reality and mental representations, from Plato to Pyrrhon, Descartes, Spinoza, Husserl and Wittgenstein, clinical neuropsychology of vision offers unique sources of empirical knowledge to address this fundamental issue.

Consider for instance Capgras syndrome, a rare clinical situation during which a patient recognizes faces of familiar individuals, but elaborate an odd and very strong delusion inaccessible to criticism, claiming that the owner of this face is a look-alike imposter. When considered for a long time as an enigmatic psychotic phenomenon, cognitive neuroscience of vision recently offered a simple mechanistic scenario of this strange syndrome [76]. Capgras patients do explicitly and consciously recognize faces or other visual stimuli, in sharp contrast for instance with prosopagnosic patients. However, when looking at a familiar face patients affected by Capgras syndrome do not exhibit the emotional response normally observed such as autonomic skin conductance responses [77]. In other words, these patients are confronted with a strange dilemma: (1) they have a conscious access to the identity information of the face exemplar: 'This is the face of X', and (2) they lack the emotional reaction associated to familiarity. Far from adopting a purely logical posture and considering several possibilities able to provide a plausible account of this subjective dissociation, many patients produce an interpretation subtended by a strong belief: 'This individual looks like X but it's not X, this is a look-alike usurper!' In other terms, perceptual representations in these patients seem to incorporate interpretative processes or fictions. A fiction is not necessarily false, but a fiction is a belief and not a pure description of reality. This piece of evidence described here for Capgras patients is actually extremely frequent in several neuropsychological syndromes which do not exclusively concern visual perception: amnesic confabulations of Korsakov patients, reduplicative paramnesia, foreign-limb syndromes such as those observed in asomatognosic patients, or split-brain patients fictive interpretations. All these situations share a common principle: various conscious representations of these patients are characterized by a strong and obviously erroneous belief: false belief of remembrance, false belief of location, false belief of owns actions causality, false belief of limb ownership … The fiction and belief nature of these representations strikes us because of their obvious fallacy. However, beyond the fallacy present in several neuropsychological syndromes, I would argue that many aspects of conscious visual representations of the neurologically healthy subject share this general fictionalization property [78]. Indeed, one of the most powerful perceptual belief is the visual completeness illusion: when we open our eyes on a visual scene, we have the phenomenal sensation of seeing everything present in our visual field. Change or inattentional blindness paradigms demonstrated the fallacy of this belief: it is possible to change major components of an ecological visual scene (removing a building from a picture, inserting a gorilla crossing slowly a basket ball field in a short movie …) while the perceiver does not detect this change: we do not consciously access to every component of a visual scene [79, 80]. Another elegant illustration of this visual completeness illusion was provided by Rayner and Bertera [81]. They presented subjects with a window of readable text moving in synchrony with the eye, while parafoveal information was replaced by strings of X's. Subjective reports were characterized by the impression of seeing a whole page of text during the whole experiment. Visual iconic memory experiments also illustrate the fallacy nature of this visual completeness belief. The classical experiment by Sperling [82] demonstrates that when an array of 12 letters if briefly presented (~half a second), subject have the ability to consciously report only a subset of letters. However, they claim that they have a strong phenomenal sensation of having seen each of the letters.

Taken together, this set of apparently different clinical or experimental situations point toward a massive aspect of conscious vision: when consciously perceiving a visual scene, we do not merely build an 'objective' representation of it, but we systematically fill it with interpretations, significations, and beliefs. In a word, our conscious perception incorporates a process of fictionalization.

A THEORETICAL SKETCH OF CONSCIOUSNESS

Thus far, our non-exhaustive review has allowed us to isolate four general principles governing the physiology of visual consciousness. Firstly, a large number of processes coded in some sectors of the visual system – such as the subcortical colliculus mediated pathway, or some areas of the dorsal visual pathway – never participate in conscious visual representations. Secondly, a visual representation is reportable only if coded by the visual ventral pathway. Thirdly, this anatomical constraint is necessary but clearly not sufficient, as is nicely demonstrated in visual neglect. Top-down attentional amplification seems to be the additional and necessary condition for a visual representation coded in the

ventral pathway to reach conscious content. Finally, inspired by Posner's [83] distinctions between the *source* and the *effects* of a top-down attentional process, we propose that only conscious representations can be used as sources of strategic top-down attention, while some unconscious representations are highly sensitive to the effects of such attention. These principles help to better delineate the properties of conscious visual perceptions, and also argue for a distinction between two categories of non-conscious processes: those which never contribute to conscious content, and those which can potentially contribute to it.

These principles can be accounted for within the 'global neuronal workspace' theoretical framework developed by Dehaene, Changeux, Naccache and colleagues ([84–85], also see Baars this volume). This model, in part inspired from Bernard Baars' [87] theory, proposes that at any given time many modular cerebral networks are active in parallel and process information in an unconscious manner. Information becomes conscious; however, if the corresponding neural population is mobilized by top-down attentional amplification into a self-sustained brain-scale state of coherent activity that involves many neurons distributed throughout the brain. The long-distance connectivity of these 'workspace neurons' can, when they are active for a minimal duration, make the information available to a variety of processes including perceptual categorization, long-term memorization, evaluation, and intentional action. We postulate that this global availability of information through the workspace is what we subjectively experience as a conscious state. Neurophysiological, anatomical, and brain-imaging data strongly argue for a major role of prefrontal cortex, anterior cingulate, and the areas that connect to them, in creating the postulated brain-scale workspace.

Within this framework, the different unconscious visual processes reviewed in this paper can be distinguished and explained. The activity of subcortical visual processors such as the superior colliculus, which do not possess the reciprocal connections to this global neuronal workspace which are postulated to be necessary for top-down amplification, cannot access or contribute to our conscious content, as revealed by blindsight[7]. Moreover, the activity of other visual processors anatomically connected to this global workspace by reciprocal connections can still escape the content of consciousness due to top-down

_____

[7] Indeed neurons located in the superficial visual layers of superior colliculus receive direct input from parietal areas while projecting indirectly to intraparietal cortex through a thalamic synapse ([88, 89]).

attentional failure. This 'attentional failure' may result from a direct lesion of the attentional network (such as in USN), from stringent conditions of visual presentation (such as in visual masking), or even from the evanescence of some cortical visual representations too brief to allow top-down amplification processes (such as the parietal 'automatic pilot' revealed by optic ataxia patients[8]). This model also predicts that once a stream of processing is prepared consciously by the instructions and context, an unconscious stimulus may benefit from this conscious setting, and therefore show attentional amplification, such as in blindsight.

CONCLUSION

This theoretical sketch will of course necessitate further developments and revisions, but its set of predictions can already be submitted to experimentation. For instance, this model predicts that a piece of unconscious information cannot itself be used as a source of control to modify a choice of processing steps. Another prediction is to extend the sensitivity of some blindsight effects to top-down attention to other paradigms or relevant clinical syndromes, such as USN, attentional blink, or inattentional blindness.

Most notably, the fictionalization process inherent to conscious perception should stimulate intense theoretical efforts during the next decades. A potential track could be to incorporate and adapt in our models a concept proposed by Dennett in his 'multiple drafts' theory of consciousness [4]. Rather than being a pure broadcasting process of a locally coded unconscious representation, conscious access could also incorporate transcriptional and editing processes creating new versions of the representation. This introduces the possibility for biases, interpretations, and beliefs which are subtending this fictionalization dimension of conscious contents.

As a conclusion, I have tried in the present paper to describe how the observation of neurological patients has played a major role in the discovery of several important principles related to the neural bases of visual consciousness. However, this description is not written as a record of an heroic past era of brain sciences.

Clinical neuropsychologists and their patients are not dinosaurs, and we did not adopt here a 'paleontologist attitude'. On the contrary, this audacious neuropsychology of consciousness will provide us with exciting and unexpected observations, enabling us to tackle the most complex and enigmatic aspects of visual consciousness.

References

1. Naccache, L. (2005) Visual phenomenal consciousness: A neurological guided tour. *Prog Brain Res* 150C:185–195.
2. Ramachandran, V. and Blakeslee, S. (1998) *Phantoms in the Brain: Probing the Mysteries of the Human Mind*, New York: William Morrow and Company.
3. Weiskrantz, L. (1997) *Consciousness Lost and Found: A Neuropsychological Exploration*, New York: Oxford University Press.
4. Dennett, D.C. (1992) *Consciousness Explained*, London: Penguin.
5. Holender, D. (1986) Semantic activation without conscious identification in dichotic listening parafoveal vision and visual masking: A survey and appraisal. *Behav Brain Sci* 9:1–23.
6. Merikle, P.M., Smilek, D. and Eastwood, J.D. (2001) Perception without awareness: Perspectives from cognitive psychology. *Cognition* 79:115–134.
7. Block, N. (1995) On a confusion about the role of consciousness. *Behav Brain Sci* 18:227–287.
8. Gazzaniga, M.S., LeDoux, J.E. and Wilson, D.H. (1977) Language, praxis, and the right hemisphere: Clues to some mechanisms of consciousness. *Neurology* 27:1144–1147.
9. Laureys, S., Pellas, F., Van Eeckhout, P., Ghorbel, S., Schnakers, C., Perrin, F., Berre, J., Faymonville, M.E., Pantke, K.H., Damas, F., Lamy, M., Moonen, G. and Goldman, S. (2005) The locked-in syndrome: What is it like to be conscious but paralyzed and voiceless? *Prog Brain Res* 150:495–511.
10. Frith, C., Perry, R. and Lumer, E. (1999) The neural correlates of conscious experience: An experimental framework. *Trends Cogn Sci* 3:105–114.
11. Ungerleider, L.G. and Mishkin, M. (1982) Two cortical visual systems. In Ingle, D.J. Goodale, M.A. and Mansfield, R.J. (eds.) *Analysis of Visual Behavior*, pp. 549–586. Cambridge: MIT Press.
12. Crick, F. and Koch, C. (1995) Are we aware of neural activity in primary visual cortex? *Nature* 375:121–123.
13. Poppel, E., Held, R. and Frost, D. (1973) Residual visual function after brain wounds involving the central visual pathways in man. *Nature* 243:295–296.
14. Weiskrantz, L., Warrington, E.K., Sanders, M.D. and Marshall, J. (1974) Visual capacity in the hemianopic field following a restricted occipital ablation. *Brain* 97:709–728.
15. Perenin, M.T. and Jeannerod, M. (1975) Residual vision in cortically blind hemifields. *Neuropsychologia* 13:1–7.
16. Cowey, A. and Stoerig, P. (1991) The neurobiology of blindsight. *Trends Neurosci* 14:140–145.
17. de Gelder, B., Vroomen, J., Pourtois, G. and Weiskrantz, L. (1999) Non-conscious recognition of affect in the absence of striate cortex. *Neuroreport* 10:3759–3763.
18. de Gelder, B., Morris, J.S. and Dolan, R.J. (2005) Unconscious fear influences emotional awareness of faces and voices. *Proc Natl Acad Sci USA* 102:18682–18687.
19. Morris, J.S., DeGelder, B., Weiskrantz, L. and Dolan, R.J. (2001) Differential extrageniculostriate and amygdala responses to presentation of emotional faces in a cortically blind field. *Brain* 124:1241–1252.

---

[8] Within the global workspace model only explicit – or active – neural representations coded in the firing of one or several neuronal assemblies are able to reach conscious content. Therefore, a third class of unconscious processes can be described, those resulting from the neural architecture (fibre lengths and connections, synapses, synaptic weights) in which information is not explicitly coded. This type of unconscious information is also postulated to never participate to conscious content.

20. Whalen, P.J., Rauch, S.L., Etcoff, N.L., McInerney, S.C., Lee, M.B. and Jenike, M.A. (1998) Masked presentations of emotional facial expressions modulate amygdala activity without explicit knowledge. *J Neurosci* 18:411–418.

21. Morris, J.S., Ohman, A. and Dolan, R.J. (1999) A subcortical pathway to the right amygdala mediating 'unseen' fear. *Proc Natl Acad Sci USA* 96:1680–1685.

22. Morris, J.S., Öhman, A. and Dolan, R.J. (1998) Conscious and unconscious emotional learning in the human amygdala. *Nature* 393:467–470.

23. Pessoa, L., Japee, S., Sturman, D. and Ungerleider, L.G. (2006) Target visibility and visual awareness modulate amygdala responses to fearful faces. *Cereb Cortex* 16:366–375.

24. Pessoa, L., McKenna, M., Gutierrez, E. and Ungerleider, L.G. (2002) Neural processing of emotional faces requires attention. *Proc Natl Acad Sci USA* 99:11458–11463.

25. Kouider, S. and Dehaene, S. (2007) Levels of processing during non-conscious perception: A critical review of visual masking. *Philos Trans R Soc Lond B Biol Sci* 362:857–875.

26. Jackson, J.H. (1932) *Selected Writings of John Hughlings Jackson*, London: J. Taylor.

27. Andersen, R.A. (1997) Multimodal integration for the representation of space in the posterior parietal cortex. *Philos Trans R Soc Lond B Biol Sci* 352:1421–1428.

28. Lueschow, A., Miller, E.K. and Desimone, R. (1994) Inferior temporal mechanisms for invariant object recognition. *Cereb Cortex* 4:523–531.

29. Ito, M., Tamura, H., Fujita, I. and Tanaka, K. (1995) Size and position invariance of neuronal responses in monkey inferotemporal cortex. *J Neurophysiol* 73:218–226.

30. Grill-Spector, K., Kushnir, T., Edelman, S., Avidan, G., Itzchak, Y. and Malach, R. (1999) Differential processing of objects under various viewing conditions in the human lateral occipital complex. *Neuron* 24:187–203.

31. Cohen, L., Dehaene, S., Naccache, L., Lehericy, S., Dehaene-Lambertz, G., Henaff, M.A. and Michel, F. (2000) The visual word form area: Spatial and temporal characterization of an initial stage of reading in normal subjects and posterior split-brain patients. *Brain* 123 (Pt. 2):291–307.

32. Goodale, M.A., Milner, A.D., Jakobson, L.S. and Carey, D.P. (1991) A neurological dissociation between perceiving objects and grasping them. *Nature* 349:154–156.

33. Benson, D. and Greenberg, J. (1969) Visual form agnosia. A specific defect in visual discrimination. *Arch Neurol* 20:82–89.

34. Aglioti, S., DeSouza, J.F. and Goodale, M.A. (1995) Size-contrast illusions deceive the eye but not the hand. *Curr Biol* 5:679–685.

35. Gentilucci, M., Chieffi, S., Deprati, E., Saetti, M.C. and Toni, I. (1996) Visual illusion and action. *Neuropsychologia* 34:369–376.

36. Daprati, E. and Gentilucci, M. (1997) Grasping an illusion. *Neuropsychologia* 35:1577–1582.

37. Franz, V.H., Gegenfurtner, K.R., Bulthoff, H.H. and Fahle, M. (2000) Grasping visual illusions: No evidence for a dissociation between perception and action. *Psychol Sci* 11:20–25.

38. Franz, V.H. (2001) Action does not resist visual illusions. *Trends Cogn Sci* 5:457–459.

39. Kwok, R.M. and Braddick, O.J. (2003) When does the Titchener circles illusion exert an effect on grasping? Two- and three-dimensional targets. *Neuropsychologia* 41:932–940.

40. Pisella, L., Grea, H., Tilikete, C., Vighetto, A., Desmurget, M., Rode, G., Boisson, D. and Rossetti, Y. (2000) An 'automatic pilot' for the hand in human posterior parietal cortex: Toward reinterpreting optic ataxia. *Nat Neurosci* 3:729–736.

41. Tootell, R.B., Reppas, J.B., Dale, A.M., Look, R.B., Sereno, M.I., Malach, R., Brady, T.J. and Rosen, B.R. (1995) Visual motion aftereffect in human cortical area MT revealed by functional magnetic resonance imaging. *Nature* 375:139–141.

42. Zeki, S. (1991) Cerebral akinetopsia (visual motion blindness). A review. *Brain* 114 (Pt. 2):811–824.

43. Beckers, G. and Homberg, V. (1992) Cerebral visual motion blindness: Transitory akinetopsia induced by transcranial magnetic stimulation of human area V5. *Proc R Soc Lond B Biol Sci.* 249 (1325):173–178.

44. Salzman, C.D., Britten, K.H. and Newsome, W.T. (1990) Cortical microstimulation influences perceptual judgements of motion direction. *Nature* 346:174–177.

45. Milner, A. (1998) Streams and consciousness: Visual consciousness and the brain. *Trends Cogn Sci* 2 (1):25–30.

46. Bar, M. and Biederman, I. (1999) Localizing the cortical region mediating visual awareness of object identity. *Proc Natl Acad Sci USA* 96:1790–1793.

47. Bar, M., Tootell, R.B., Schacter, D.L., Greve, D.N., Fischl, B., Mendola, J.D., Rosen, B.R. and Dale, A.M. (2001) Cortical mechanisms specific to explicit visual object recognition. *Neuron* 29:529–535.

48. Ffytche, D.H., Howard, R.J., Brammer, M.J., David, A., Woodruff, P. and Williams, S. (1998) The anatomy of conscious vision: An fMRI study of visual hallucinations. *Nat Neurosci* 1:738–742.

49. Mesulam, M.M. (1999) Spatial attention and neglect: Parietal, frontal and cingulate contributions to the mental representation and attentional targeting of salient extrapersonal events. *Philos Trans R Soc Lond B Biol Sci* 354:1325–1346.

50. Karnath, H.O., Ferber, S. and Himmelbach, M. (2001) Spatial awareness is a function of the temporal not the posterior parietal lobe. *Nature* 411:950–953.

51. Thiebaut de Schotten, M., Urbanski, M., Duffau, H., Volle, E., Levy, R., Dubois, B. and Bartolomeo, P. (2005) Direct evidence for a parietal-frontal pathway subserving spatial awareness in humans. *Science* 309:2226–2228.

52. McGlinchey-Berroth, R. (1997) Visual information processing in hemispatial neglect. *Trends Cogn Sci* 1:91–97.

53. Driver, J. and Mattingley, J.B. (1998) Parietal neglect and visual awareness. *Nat Neurosci* 1:17–22.

54. Driver, J. and Vuilleumier, P. (2001) Perceptual awareness and its loss in unilateral neglect and extinction. *Cognition* 79:39–88.

55. Sackur, J., Naccache, L., Pradat-Diehl, P., Azouvi, P., Mazevet, D., Katz, R., Cohen, L. and Dehaene, S. (2008) Semantic processing of neglected numbers. *Cortex* 44:673–682.

56. McGlinchey-Berroth, R., Milberg, W.P., Verfaellie, M., Alexander, M. and Kilduff, P. (1993) Semantic priming in the neglected field: Evidence from a lexical decision task. *Cogn Neuropsychol* 10:79–108.

57. Rees, G., Wojciulik, E., Clarke, K., Husain, M., Frith, C. and Driver, J. (2000) Unconscious activation of visual cortex in the damaged right hemisphere of a parietal patient with extinction. *Brain* 123 (Pt. 8):1624–1633.

58. Mesulam, M.M. (1981) A cortical network for directed attention and unilateral neglect. *Ann Neurol* 10:309–315.

59. Dehaene, S., Naccache, L., Cohen, L., Bihan, D.L., Mangin, J.F., Poline, J.B. and Riviere, D. (2001) Cerebral mechanisms of word masking and unconscious repetition priming. *Nat Neurosci* 4:752–758.

60. Naccache, L. and Dehaene, S. (2001) Unconscious semantic priming extends to novel unseen stimuli. *Cognition* 80:223–237.

61. Posner, M.I. and Snyder, C.R.R. (1975) Attention and cognitive control. In Solso, R.L. (eds.) *Information Processing and Cognition: The Loyola Symposium*, Hillsdale: Erlbaum.

62. Schneider, W. and Shiffrin, R.M. (1977) Controlled and automatic human information processing: I. Detection, search and attention. *Psychological Review*, 84:1–66.

63. Eysenck, M. (1984) Attention and performance limitations. In Eysenck, M. (eds.) *A Handbook of Cognitive Psychology*, pp. 49–77. Hillsdale, NJ: L. Erlbaum Assoc.

64. Kentridge, R.W., Heywood, C.A. and Weiskrantz, L. (1999) Attention without awareness in blindsight. *Proc R Soc Lond B Biol Sci* 266:1805–1811.

65. Kentridge, R.W., Heywood, C.A. and Weiskrantz, L. (2004) Spatial attention speeds discrimination without awareness in blindsight. *Neuropsychologia* 42:831–835.

66. Lachter, J., Forster, K.I. and Ruthruff, E. (2004) Forty-five years after broadbent (1958): Still no identification without attention. *Psychol Rev.* 111: 880–913.

67. Naccache, L., Blandin, E. and Dehaene, S. (2002) Unconscious masked priming depends on temporal attention. *Psychol Sci* 13:416–424.

68. Naccache, L. and Dehaene, S. (2001) The priming method: Imaging unconscious repetition priming reveals an abstract representation of number in the parietal lobes. *Cereb Cortex* 11:966–974.

69. Dehaene, S., Naccache, L., Le Clec, H.G., Koechlin, E., Mueller, M., Dehaene-Lambertz, G., van de Moortele, P.F. and Le Bihan, D. (1998) Imaging unconscious semantic priming. *Nature* 395:597–600.

70. Mack, A. and Rock, I. (1998) *Inattentional Blindness*, Cambridge, Massachusetts: MIT Press.

71. Raymond, J.E., Shapiro, K.L. and Arnell, K.M. (1992) Temporary suppression of visual processing in an RSVP task: An attentional blink? *J Exp Psychol Hum Percept Perform* 18:849–860.

72. Posner, M.I. (1994) Attention: The mechanisms of consciousness. *Proc Nat Acad Sci USA* 91:7398–7403.

73. Stoerig, P. and Barth, E. (2001) Low-level phenomenal vision despite unilateral destruction of primary visual cortex. *Conscious Cogn.* 10 (4):574–587.

74. Merikle, P.M., Joordens, S. and Stolz, J.A. (1995) Measuring the relative magnitude of unconscious influences. *Conscious Cogn* 4:422–439.

75. Kahneman, D. and Treisman, A.M. (1984) Changing views of attention and automaticity. In Parasuraman, R., and Davies, R. (eds.) *Varieties of Attention*, pp. 29–61. New York: Academic Press.

76. Ellis, H.D. and Lewis, M.B. (2001) Capgras delusion: A window on face recognition. *Trends Cogn Sci* 5:149–156.

77. Ellis, H.D., Young, A.W., Quayle, A.H. and De Pauw, K.W. (1997) Reduced autonomic responses to faces in Capgras delusion. *Proc Biol Sci* 264:1085–1092.

78. Naccache, L. (2006) *Le Nouvel Inconscient. Freud, Christophe Colomb des neurosciences*, Paris: Odile Jacob,

79. O'Regan, J.K., Rensink, R.A. and Clark, J.J. (1999) Change-blindness as a result of 'mudsplashes'. *Nature* 398:34.

80. Simons, D.J. and Rensink, R.A. (2005) Change blindness: Past, present, and future. *Trends Cogn Sci* 9:16–20.

81. Rayner, K. and Bertera, J.H. (1979) Reading without a fovea. *Science* 206:468–469.

82. Sperling, G. (1960) The information available in brief visual presentation. *Psychol Monogr* 74:1–29.

83. Posner, M.I. (1994) Attention: The mechanisms of consciousness. *Proceedings of the National Academy of Sciences USA* 91:7398–7403.

84. Dehaene, S., Kerszberg, M. and Changeux, J.P. (1998) A neuronal model of a global workspace in effortful cognitive tasks. *Proc Nat Acad Sci USA* 95:14529–14534.

85. Dehaene, S. and Naccache, L. (2001) Towards a cognitive neuroscience of consciousness: Basic evidence and a workspace framework. *Cognition* 79:1–37.

86. Dehaene, S., Sergent, C. and Changeux, J. (2003) A neuronal network model linking subjective reports and objective physiological data during conscious perception. *Proc Natl Acad Sci USA* 100:8520–8525.

87. Baars, B.J. (1989) *A Cognitive Theory of Consciousness.* Cambridge, Massachusetts: Cambridge University Press.

88. Sparks, D.L. (1986) Translation of sensory signals into commands for control of saccadic eye movements: role of primate superior colliculus. *Physiol Rev.* 66 (1):118–171.

89. Clower, D.M., West, R.A., Lynch, J.C. and Strick, P.L. (2001) The inferior parietal lobule is the target of output from the superior colliculus, hippocampus, and cerebellum. *J Neurosci* 21 (16):6283–6291.

90. Stoerig, P. and Barth, E. (2001) Low-level phenomenal vision despite unilateral destruction of primary visual cortex. *Conscious Cogn.* 10(4):574–87.

91. Posner, M.I. (1994) Attention: The mechanisms of consciousness. *Proceedings of the National Academy of Sciences USA* 91:7398–7403.

92. Sparks, D.L. (1986) Translation of sensory signals into commands for control of saccadic eye movements: role of primate superior colliculus. *Physiol Rev.* 66(1):118–71.

The Neurophysiology of Self-Awareness Disorders in Conversion Hysteria

Patrik Vuilleumier

ABSTRACT

Conversion hysteria refers to neurological disorders at the borderline between neurology and psychiatry, characterized by impaired awareness of bodily or cognitive function (such as paralysis, anaesthesia, blindness, or amnesia) in patients who have no apparent organic lesion in the nervous system. Although it is assumed that conversion hysteria may result from a transformation of psychological trauma or emotional stress into physical symptoms, which can distort self-awareness for a particular neurological function in the patient, the exact mechanisms underlying this transformation remain largely unknown, in terms of both mental processes and neurocognitive substrates. In practice, therefore, the diagnosis is still often made by exclusion of organic brain diseases rather than by demonstration of a specific pattern of clinical signs. However, recent advances in functional neuroimaging techniques have begun to bring new insights into possible changes in brain activity associated with conversion disorders, and may potentially allow more direct diagnosis and better understanding of causal mechanisms in the future. Although neuroimaging results have provided partly conflicting results due to the heterogeneity of symptoms and small sample of patients studied so far, converging evidence points to a critical implication for a network of brain areas involved in motivational regulation and self-monitoring including orbitofrontal, anterior cingulate, and inferior lateral prefrontal cortex, which might in turn influence activity in other regions such as basal ganglia, thalamus, and sensori-motor cortices to induce specific functional impairments (e.g., paralysis or anaesthesia). These changes might reflect stereotyped patterns of adaptive responses to perceived threat, perhaps facilitated by previous associations or memories under the influence of stress factors. This article presents an overview of current issues and hypotheses concerning the neurobiological correlates of conversion hysteria, and proposes a general framework to integrate classic psychiatric models with recent data from functional brain imaging.

INTRODUCTION

Physicians as well as philosophers have been intrigued for more than 20 centuries by the presentation of patients who experience physical or intellectual disorders without any evidence for an underlying organic illness. Despite the tremendous improvements in medical knowledge and increasing sophistication of non-invasive diagnostic tools in recent years, such cases remain frequent and perplexing in clinical practice. Across different times and different theories, this condition has raised many questions on the relationships between mind and body, either when it is considered as an effect of obscure somatic anomalies on psychic functions or, vice versa, when it is conceived as the product of strong passions or ideas on bodily functions. Historically, scientific interests in such phenomena were closely related to the emergence of modern concepts of diseases in neurology and psychiatry, before these two disciplines diverged during the last 100 years.

This intriguing condition was initially called 'hysteria' by the ancient Egyptian and Greek physicians, who thought that it resulted from some dysfunction of the uterus in women (through its wandering in the body). In recent psychiatry classification systems, the term 'hysteria' has been replaced by 'conversion' disorder because of the recognition of important psychoemotional factors and the influence of psychoanalytical theories following Freud [1]. Yet, the psychological processes and the neurobiological underpinnings of this condition remain poorly understood by physicians and scientists alike, continuing to raise fundamental questions on mechanisms of self-consciousness, and still lying in a grey zone at the border between psychiatry and neurology. To acknowledge this historical legacy and the lack of a single explanatory framework, terms such as 'hysterical conversion' or 'conversion hysteria' are often used in practice, and will be employed interchangeably in this review.

According to the *Diagnostic and Statistical Manual for Mental Disorder, Fourth Edition* (DSM-IV) criteria, conversion hysteria is defined as a somatoform disorder characterized by a pseudo-neurological deficit (e.g., paralysis or anaesthesia) that is not explained by organic lesions and arises in relation to psychological stress or conflict, without a deliberate intention to feign the deficit (see Box 22.1)[1]. This deficit may involve a loss or distortion in elementary neurological functions, including not only motor or sensory symptoms, but also blindness or deafness, as well as gait problems, dystonia, aphonia, pseudo-seizures, or

---
[1]Cloninger in Halligan [2].

disturbances in higher-level functions such as amnesia or pseudo-dementia (Ganser syndrome). However, due to the lack of a coherent theoretical model, the current psychiatry classifications are somewhat inconsistent: hysterical memory loss is categorized as a form of dissociative disorder in DSM-IV, distinct from somatoform disorders, even though memory is clearly a neurological function. By contrast, both somatic conversion and hysterical amnesia are included among dissociative conditions in the ICD-10 classification. This discrepancy highlights the fact that current theories fail to capture all aspects of conversion hysteria satisfactorily [3]. Therefore, more empirical work combining psychological and biological perspectives may not only be useful to better understand the mechanisms by which psychological stressors or conflict can affect the conscious experience of movements, sensations, or memories, but also to clarify the possible commonalities between different kinds of conversion symptoms and their relationships to dissociative phenomena.

Recent advances in neuroimaging techniques provide new opportunities to investigate the changes in brain activity associated with psychiatric disorders, because they may offer useful hints about cognitive and affective processes implicated in conversion hysteria. However, to date, still relatively few imaging studies have attempted to identify specific neurobiological correlates for hysterical symptoms (for review see [4]). This stands in sharp contrast with abundant imaging research conducted in other psychiatric conditions such as depression, anxiety, or phobias. This also seems all the more striking given that the 'functional' deficits of conversion hysteria, without any visible organic lesions, would logically lend themselves to functional neurobiological investigations using brain imaging techniques. But over the last 10 years, only a handful of studies have used functional neuroimaging tools such as SPECT (single-photon emission computerized tomography), PET (positron emission tomography) or fMRI (functional magnetic resonance imaging) in order to investigate conversion disorders, always in small sample of patients. A few earlier attempts in the 1970s and 1980s have also employed other neurophysiological techniques, such as EEG (electroencephalography) or MEG (magnetoencephalography). The goal of the current review is to present a general summary of this imaging work, and discuss possible implications for neurobiological theories of conversion hysteria, focusing specifically on unexplained neurological symptoms in motor and sensory functions that are most common in neurology practice. Psychogenic memory loss may also occasionally arise [5] and will be only briefly mentioned here. Other 'positive' symptoms such as pseudo-seizures

[6, 7] or abnormal movements [8] will not be discussed, because little is known about their possible functional neural correlates. However, a complete model of conversion hysteria would eventually need to account for both negative and positive manifestations of this inherently proteiform condition. In any case, new findings from functional neuroimaging are not only likely to provide important constraints for future theories of conversion hysteria; but are also more generally apt to offer unique insights on the cerebral mechanisms of self-awareness.

CLINICAL PRESENTATION AND DIAGNOSIS

Conversion hysteria is a common and difficult problem in medical practice. Several studies conducted at different time periods in different countries converge to indicate an incidence of 5–10/100 000 in the general population, while it is thought to represent approximately 1% of consultations in a general hospital, and up to 4–9% of patients seen by neurologists or psychiatrists [9, 10]. However, the type of symptoms and clinical presentation may vary across different cultures and different medical settings. Poor socio-economic status and immigration conditions are common risk factors for the development and persistence of conversion symptoms.

A major issue is that, in practice, conversion hysteria is essentially diagnosed by exclusion, both in the standard definition criteria (see Box 22.1) and for clinical purposes [10]. Thus, in the clinic, this diagnosis is suspected when the symptoms and physical signs are not consistent with basic anatomical or physiological principles of the nervous system (e.g., sensory or motor losses that do not respect anatomical boundaries of normal innervation, paralysis with intact reflexes, etc.); when symptoms change or evolve erratically over time; and when radiological or electrophysiological tests show normal results. Typically, neurologists and psychiatrists first seek to exclude a wide range of organic lesions or dysfunctions by thorough medical exams (such as CT scan, MRI, EEG, EMG, or TMS), before making the diagnosis of conversion with sufficient certainty. However, such diagnosis by exclusion is necessarily fraught with problems and inconsistencies.

A number of 'positive' clinical signs have been described, but these are highly variable and unreliable. Furthermore, these signs usually depend on the particular symptoms presented by patients, rather than on specific features associated with conversion hysteria mechanisms per se. Following Babinski who

described his classic sign of toe extension to distinguish organic from hysterical hemiparesis, several other clinical manoeuvres may be used to bring out dissociation between subjective symptoms and objective motor functions [11]. For instance, in patients with hysterical paralysis, preserved strength in the affected limb can be observed during postural adjustment or locomotion while movements involving the same muscles are impossible to execute with voluntary commands [12]. Likewise, patients with hysterical blindness may fail to reach their own index finger with the other hand (which is easily done by truly blind persons using proprioception), or may still manifest normal stereoscopic vision despite an apparent monocular loss [13]. Nevertheless, although these clinical signs are useful indices of preserved neurological functions, it is worth recalling that striking dissociations between conscious subjective experience and actual objective performance can also be observed in some cases with clearly organic brain disorders such as blindsight, neglect, or amnesia [14, 15]. Conversely, some patients with brain damage may present with obvious neurological deficits, yet remain unaware of these and even deny them (a syndrome called 'anosognosia' [16]). Altogether, such phenomena suggest that the conscious experience associated with some behavioural abilities may dissociate from actual abilities themselves, and that such dissociation may result from either neurological brain lesions or certain psychological or emotional conditions. Moreover, these situations are also reminiscent of dissociative phenomena observed during hypnosis, a condition that has often been compared to hysteria since the time of Charcot (see [17, 18]) – although the classic relationships between hypnotic susceptibility and conversion is only relative [19] and still unclear [19, 20–22].

Another 'classic' positive sign described in conversion hysteria is 'la belle indifférence', which implies a lack of appropriate emotional response or no apparent worry for the deficit and its consequences [23]. However, this feature is also inconstant and unspecific. Moreover, a similar attitude may be seen in patients with organic neurological disorders and anosognosia (i.e., anosodiaphoria) [24]. Some authors have emphasized instead that conversion symptoms are often characterized by more affective expressions and more detailed descriptions, as compared with true organic symptoms [25], and thus seem to reflect a greater 'concern' rather than indifference from the patient.

More appropriate 'positive' signs may stem from the psychological causal factors underlying conversion hysteria. These are not only a key feature of the Freudian interpretations of conversion, but also constitute a major criterion for diagnosis according to DSM-IV (see Box 22.1). Yet, the role of specific stressors or

BOX 22.1

DIFFERENT DIAGNOSTIC CRITERIA FOR CONVERSION AND DISSOCIATION

The current definition of conversion disorder was historically derived from psychodynamic concepts according to which psychological conflicts are transformed and expressed by physical symptoms, leading to the internationally applied criteria of the DSM IV of the American Psychiatry Association:

1. One or more *symptoms* or deficits affecting voluntary motor or sensory function that suggest a neurological or other general medical condition.
2. Psychological factors are judged to be associated with the symptom or deficit because the initiation or exacerbation of the symptom or deficit is preceded by conflicts or other stressors.
3. The symptom or deficit is not intentionally produced or feigned (as in *Factitious Disorder* or *Malingering*).
4. The symptom or deficit cannot, after appropriate investigation, be fully explained by a general medical condition, or by the direct effects of a *substance*, or as a culturally sanctioned behaviour or experience.
5. The symptom or deficit causes clinically significant distress or impairment in social, occupational, or other important areas of functioning or warrants medical evaluation.
6. The symptom or deficit is not limited to pain or sexual dysfunction, does not occur exclusively during the course of *Somatization Disorder*, and is not better accounted for by another *mental disorder*.

The specific types of symptoms may involve motor, sensory, convulsion, or mixed presentations.

On the other hand, somatization disorders are classified as a broader category within the somatoform disorders, with the following criteria:

1. A history of many physical complaints beginning before age 30 years that occur over a period of several years and result in treatment being sought or significant impairment in social, occupational, or other important areas of functioning.
2. Each of the following criteria must have been met, with individual symptoms occurring at any time during the course of the disturbance:
   – four pain symptoms,
   – two gastrointestinal symptoms other than pain,

   – one sexual or reproductive symptom other than pain,
   – one pseudo-neurological symptom other than pain (conversion or dissociative symptoms such as amnesia).

By contrast, the International Classification of Diseases (ICD-10) of the World Health Organization includes conversion hysteria among dissociative disorders, and requires the following criteria:

1. No evidence of a physical disorder that can explain the symptoms that characterize the disorder (but physical disorders may be present that give rise to other symptoms).
2. Convincing associations in time between the symptoms of the disorder and stressful events, problems or needs.
3. In addition, for specific disorders:

Dissociative motor loss includes either (1) or (2):

1. Complete of partial loss of the ability to perform movements that are normally under voluntary control (including speech).
2. Various or variable degrees of in coordination or ataxia or inability to stand unaided.

Dissociative anaesthesia and sensory loss include either (1) or (2):

1. Partial or complete loss of any or all of the normal cutaneous sensations over part or all of the body (specify: touch, pin prick, vibration, heat, cold).
2. Partial or complete loss of vision, hearing, or smell.

Note that only disorders of physical functions normally under voluntary control and loss of sensations are included in these categories. Disorders involving pain and other complex physical sensations related to the autonomic nervous system or visceral functions are categorized under the somatization disorders. Moreover, the explicit incorporation of unconscious or non-intentional mechanisms in the diagnosis of conversion serves to differentiate such disorders from the willed and conscious production of symptoms, but also raises the question of how conscious awareness and will can be objectively defined in the patient.

conflicts for triggering hysterical symptoms is often problematic. Even though it is generally accepted that stressful situations or emotional factors are frequently preceding the onset of hysterical symptoms [26, 27], the importance of such factors and their relation to the symptoms often involve highly subjective judgments by the clinicians. It is not unusual that psychiatrists invoke a stressor that precedes the onset of symptoms by several years, whereas a more immediate effect of certain events or situations is noted in other patients. Their impact or even their existence may be difficult to ascertain. Moreover, in itself, the occurrence of 'psychological stress' or 'adverse life events' does not always seem sufficiently specific to distinguish conversion from other disorders such as somatization, malingering, or depression [10]. In addition, many patients with conversion hysteria do not report the occurrence of stressors, or perhaps do not easily reckon or admit these. Conversely, many patients with organic neurological diseases may also report stressful conditions preceding the initiation or exacerbation of their illness. For instance, an increased incidence of stress or adverse life events is commonly reported prior to the onset of truly neurological disorders such as stroke [28] or multiple sclerosis [29]. Among psychological stress factors associated with conversion, a history of sexual abuse is often mentioned, and particularly emphasized in early Freudian theories [1]. However, recent studies have shown that although this may be relevant in some patients [30], childhood trauma are by far not found in all cases [31]. Therefore, both the nature of the critical psychological stress responsible for conversion hysteria, and the temporal dynamics of its influences on behaviour, often remain elusive. It is likely that the type, context, or personal significance of these events is critical in determining conversion [27], but their exact characteristics, as well as their exact impact on mental, emotional, or physiological processes are still poorly defined.

More objective signs of stress can also be obtained. Early studies have described anomalies in the hypothalamic–pituitary–adrenal (HPA) axis that regulate neuroendocrine responses to stress, with impaired cortisol suppression test in patients with conversion hysteria [32]. Others studies have reported higher responses and reduced habituation in skin-conductance responses, indicative of higher autonomic sensitivity to novelty [33]. However, similar anomalies may be observed in other psychiatric disorders such as depression, anxiety, or post-traumatic stress disorder. Abnormal cortisol activity is also linked with chronic fatigue syndrome or burnout [34]. Hence, such anomalies are not specific to conversion disorders.

In addition, conversion hysteria is associated with an important comorbidity and overlaps with several other psychiatric conditions, including depression, fatigue, or somatization. In particular, many patients recovering from conversion symptoms eventually suffer from depression at a later stage [35, 36], and a history of depression is an important risk factor for poor prognosis and persistent conversion symptoms [37]. Such intricate relations raise a number of questions about the boundaries between these different diagnostic categories. In this perspective, it is likely that a better understanding of the functional neuroanatomy underlying conversion hysteria might also contribute to clarify its relationships with other psychiatry conditions.

CONVERSION HYSTERIA AND BRAIN DISEASES

Although by definition conversion hysteria reflects psychogenic symptoms without any organic medical cause, it may occasionally arise in patients suffering from a true cerebral disease. In such cases, conversion symptoms cannot be directly explained by the visible lesions alone, but may add to or modify the clinical complaints of the patient. Moreover, it was suggested by some neurologists more than a century ago that hysteria could sometimes constitute a 'complication' of organic brain disease [38, 39], and Shilder [40] wrote that brain dysfunction could sometimes induce 'organic neurotic attitudes' leading to stereotyped reactions and behaviours, including hysteria or anosognosia.

More recently, a study by Eames [41] reported that 'hysteria-like' behaviour was observed in 30% of patients seen in a rehabilitation ward after various types of brain injuries, as evaluated by systematic ratings of the caregivers. Such behaviours could include exaggeration, secondary gain expectancy, or non-organic patterns of the deficit. Interestingly, not all types of patients presented hysteria-like symptoms. Such behaviours were more frequent after diffuse brain lesions (e.g., closed injuries, anoxia, encephalitis) than after focal lesions (e.g., stroke), and after subcortical more than cortical lesions, suggesting a possible predisposition by dysfunctions affecting distributed brain networks. Similarly, Gould et al. [42] reported that 'atypical' deficits or signs suspected to have non-organic origin (such as fluctuating symptoms, patchy sensory loss, or 'give-away' weakness) were seen in 20% of patients who were admitted for an acute hemispheric stroke. Furthermore, a combination of both 'organic' and 'psychogenic' manifestations is sometimes observed in other diseases with diffuse brain anomalies, such as multiple sclerosis [43] and epilepsy [6]. In the latter cases, truly 'organic' manifestations (e.g., seizures) may be difficult to distinguish from non-organic manifestations (pseudo-seizures), and some patients may present with both types of phenomena.

Although these occasional associations between conversion hysteria and neurological diseases might occur purely by coincidence due to the high frequency of each kind of disorders, they challenge a too simple 'dichotomous' diagnostic strategy. Furthermore, they might provide valuable clues about the neurocognitive mechanisms underlying an impaired awareness of bodily functions in these patients. Indeed, some brain lesions might affect mental processes contributing to self-awareness or self-monitoring functions that are potentially also implicated in conversion hysteria. As such functions presumably rely on distributed brain networks, they might be more likely to be disrupted by diffuse or subcortical damage [41], and perhaps more likely to involve circuits that are not amenable to volitional conscious control [5, 6, 44].

On the other hand, a misdiagnosis of organic illness erroneously taken as conversion is a rare possibility. Although a few early studies suggested that patients with hysteria often developed a truly neurological disorder after several years of follow-up, more recent studies have clearly established that less than 5% of conversion symptoms are falsely diagnosed at the time of onset and then turn into an organic disease 5–10 years later [45, 46]. This misdiagnosis rate is similar to many other medical disorders. Yet, the lack of standard diagnostic tests and the absence of a universally accepted set of positive diagnostic criteria still constitute a major complication for clinical management of these patients, as well as for scientific approaches to the underlying neural and cognitive mechanisms.

NEUROBIOLOGICAL HYPOTHESES

In parallel to the dominant psychodynamic theory of conversion proposed by Freud and his successors, several neurobiological accounts have been put forward during the last two centuries. While Freudian theory assumed that affective conflicts or stress can be 'converted' into physical symptoms, it did not offer any precise mechanism to produce this conversion. By contrast, biological accounts have sought to elucidate the possible cerebral systems underlying the distortion of self-awareness in conversion patients; that is, how the mind may take control over the body. However, until recently, most of the neurobiological hypotheses have relied on speculations or analogies with various other conditions, rather than on empirical data about brain function in patients with hysteria (for detailed reviews see [4, 47]).

Prior to Freudian theory, some neurologists such as Charcot [48], Reynolds [38], or Babinski [49] suggested that strong ideas or strong emotions could somehow modify the functioning of neurological pathways and produce abnormal states leading to hysterical disorders (including negative effects like paralysis, as well as positive effects like convulsions). Consequently, Charcot classified hysteria among 'neuroses', that is, diseases characterized by functional disturbances in the nervous systems without structural disturbances (a category that also included epilepsy and Parkinson's disease, for which no visible substrate was known at the time). Babinski proposed replacing the term of hysteria by 'pithiatism' in order to emphasize the role of suggestion for inducing and reversing the symptoms, and he argued that emotion and individual predisposition were two important causal factors. At the same time, Janet insisted more on the internal psychological or cognitive mechanisms by suggesting that hysteria might involve a 'limitation of the field of consciousness' which precluded a full control on 'strong impressions' or 'strong ideas', so that the latter could then govern actions and thoughts of the individual through mechanisms operating a lower, unconscious level. This introduced an important notion of dissociation between conscious and unconscious domains in mental processes. But Janet offered no specific hints about the possible neural pathways by which such dissociation might arise, although he speculated that physiologically distinct systems might mediate conscious and unconscious functions (e.g., with selective dysfunction of higher attentive binocular visual centres, but sparing of lower reflexive monocular visual centres in cases with hysterical blindness).

Many of subsequent hypotheses have revisited the same issues, but invoked other concepts more directly derived from neuropsychology or neuroscience. Several different types of cerebral mechanisms have been considered to explain conversion hysteria, which emphasize different features of the disorder but are not mutually exclusive. Overall, the putative neurobiological mechanisms most commonly associated with the production of conversion symptoms include: inhibitory processes, attentional filtering, functional dissociation, interhemispheric disconnection, as well as phylogenetic reaction processes.

Inhibition theories derive from the psychodynamic notion of repression and generally postulate an active suppression of bodily function by inhibitory signals, imposed by cognitive or emotional processes on the affected system. Following Pavlov [50] who first proposed that such inhibition might be triggered in the cortex by overactivity in subcortical centres, several authors suggested that 'corticofugal inputs' could inhibit or gate sensory, motor, or memory function via the thalamus or brainstem reticular formation [51–53]. This inhibition has variably been ascribed to impaired attention or vigilance [51], motivation states [53], or particular kinds of stress or fears [52]. Early neurophysiology studies using somatosensory potentials provided indirect evidence for such inhibition [54]. More recently, inhibitory mechanisms mediated by ventromedial prefrontal cortex have also been suggested to account for reduced motor activation in a neuroimaging study of motor conversion [55]. However, there is still little direct evidence for active inhibition being a primary cause of hysterical deficits.

Likewise, attention theories propose that conversion hysteria might involve a selective filtering of sensory or motor information, preventing access to higher cortical processing stages associated with conscious awareness, while residual unconscious processing might still take place at lower stages. Such filtering by attention mechanisms has been suspected to arise not only at the level of subcortical nuclei [51] but also in anterior cingulate cortex (ACC) [17] or parietal cortex [56, 57]. However, although a lack of attention for the affected function (e.g., a left 'paralyzed' arm) may at first sight appear consistent with the deficits in awareness caused by neurological damage to attentional systems within the right hemisphere (i.e., neglect syndrome), it seems less consistent with clinical observations that a frequent characteristics of patients with conversion or somatization is their increased attention to physical symptoms or bodily sensations, rather than actual 'neglect' or 'unawareness' of affected body parts. Moreover, hysterical symptoms are often reduced by distraction or inattention, or sometimes even reversed by using 'narco-analysis'[58].

Dissociation theories partly overlap with attention and disconnection models of conversion, but refer to more complex cognitive architectures of information processing. These theories generally postulate that motor or perceptual representations formed in functional modules at low-level within the nervous system might become disconnected from the higher-level executive control or monitoring systems, which are presumably subserved by prefrontal cortical areas and responsible for conscious awareness [18, 59, 60]. Thus, motor or perceptual representations might fail to be represented or integrated with each other within consciousness [18], or they might be abnormally or incompletely represented in consciousness, incorporating some erroneous information that is distorted

by current state or retrieved from other sources, such as memory or past experiences [60]. Other theorists did not refer to dissociation within executive control systems, but similarly proposed that conversion symptoms might result from abnormal representations of body state, formed in higher somatosensory cortical areas (such as SII or insula) under the influence of certain attentional or emotional states [61, 62]. According to Damasio, 'somatic markers' are generated by the brain to anticipate the outcome of perceived or imagined events through the use of an 'as-if' loop, which simulates bodily states and feelings associated with these events or their consequence, prior to their occurrence. Thus, it might be possible that a false representation could be activated by this 'as-if system' in patients with conversion hysteria, somehow corrupting or parasitizing their internal body maps [47].

Disconnection theories emphasize more specific anatomical substrates by which motor or sensory information might fail to be normally transmitted between the two hemispheres [63, 64] or between different cortical regions [65, 66]. Thus, impaired transfer of inputs from the right hemisphere (involved in emotion and interoception) to the left hemisphere (involved in language and symbolic communication) might lead to distorted awareness for one hemibody and explain a more frequent occurrence of conversion symptoms on the left side [63]. However, this asymmetry was questioned by more recent systematic reviews [67, 68], and some conversion symptoms may affect both sides of the body (e.g., paraparesis). Impaired cross-talk between medial and lateral prefrontal areas has also been proposed to account for anomalies in intentional control of action or thoughts [66]. These disconnection hypotheses have not been supported by direct evidence so far, although some neuroimaging results are consistent with changes in functional connectivity between frontal and motor pathways (basal ganglia) during conversion symptoms [44].

Phylogenetic reaction theories do not directly refer to specific brain systems, but invoke evolutionary or ethological approaches to behaviour to propose that conversion hysteria may result from adaptive biological mechanisms that determine stereotyped responses to particular kinds of stress or threat [47, 69, 70]. Such responses might stem from partly hard-wired neural substrates inherited among various animal species including humans. For instance, Kretschmer [69] argued that two basic patterns of reflexive behaviour mediate instinctive reactions of self-preservation and potentially relate to conversion hysteria: motor immobilization (freezing) or motor agitation (flurry). Thus, hysterical paralysis might be viewed as instinctive reactions similar to those manifested by animals who simulate a broken limb or wing when exposed to danger (injury-feigning behaviour), or maintain prolonged immobility after stressful restraint (arrest behaviour). Likewise, hysterical convulsion might correspond to the frantic struggle of a pray to escape when attacked or captured. In humans, more complex aspects might also relate to social communication and illness behaviour (so-called 'sick role'), by which symptoms develop to call for attention and elicit care from others [71, 72].

Although the cerebral mechanisms for these instinctive behaviours are incompletely elucidated and their relation to conversion remains entirely speculative, phylogenetic models offer intriguing cues in order to explain not only defective (negative) but also excessive (positive) components of hysterical disorders. In addition, similar analogies have been drawn between animal self-preservation reactions to threat and some of the characteristics of other dissociative disorders [73], consistent with the presumed parallels between conversion and dissociation [3]. Furthermore, neural circuits responsible for stereotyped behavioural arrest responses to stress or threat have been related to dopaminergic networks in striatum, thalamus, and brainstem [74], whereas catatonic immobilization during certain emotional states is thought to involve a modulation of functional interactions between basal ganglia and prefrontal cortex [75, 76]. Interestingly, similar subcortical circuits have been implicated in some neuroimaging studies of hysterical paralysis [44, 77]. However, it remains to be determined whether such mechanisms may also apply to other types of conversion symptoms, such as hysterical blindness or amnesia. Moreover, phylogenetic or evolutionary perspectives are generally consistent with putative biological mechanisms related to inhibition, attention, or dissociation, as proposed by other theories mentioned above. After several decades during which these different accounts have rested on speculative grounds or indirect neuropsychological evidence, the recent development of functional brain imaging techniques can now provide new means to determine the role of specific neural mechanisms in the production of conversion hysteria, and to test more directly the hypotheses made by different theoretical accounts.

BRAIN IMAGING STUDIES OF CONVERSION

Several studies have used neurophysiology or neuroimaging methods to investigate the neural correlates of various types of conversion disorders, such as motor paralysis, anaesthesia, or blindness (for review see [4,

78, 79]). A better understanding of changes in brain function during such disorders would not only be useful to shed light on puzzling conditions of altered self-awareness, but also help the physicians to obtain new 'positive signs' of conversion. Ideally, this might ameliorate the management of these patients who typically reject a purely psychological diagnosis, by avoiding unnecessary 'exclusion' diagnostic tests whose negative results often exacerbate anxiety in patients and frustration in physicians. However, although neuroimaging approaches have already expanded our knowledge of conversion, the current data remain inconclusive due to a great heterogeneity of patients and symptoms, important differences in paradigms, and small samples of cases.

Many early studies employed EEG and event-related potentials (ERPs) to probe for neurophysiological anomalies associated with conversion. Most of these studies have typically reported a normal pattern of results for elementary sensory or motor components [80]. More recent MEG studies also reported normal activation of SI and SII by tactile stimulation in patients with hysterical anaesthesia [81]. Only a few studies using non-clinical protocols have described subtle changes in somatosensory ERPs, such as reduced responses to tactile stimuli close to detection threshold despite normal responses to supra-threshold stimuli [82]; slower rate of habituation to repeated stimuli [83]; or suppression of the P300 response to deviant stimuli within a continuous stream of touches on the affected limb [84]. Mild reductions of P300 responses were also reported for visual stimuli in hysterical blindness [85] and for auditory stimuli in hysterical deafness [86]. In the motor domain, some anomalies have been noted for the contingent negative variation (CNV) preceding movement execution [87] and for the N2 component elicited by responses with the affected hand in conflict/interference conditions [88], while TMS over motor cortex has shown either normal [89] or reduced [90] excitability. Taken together, these findings are consistent with intact activation of early stages of sensory or motor pathways, but point to some anomalies at higher stages involving attentional and cognitive control processes that presumably integrate sensory-motor functions with more complex representations related to goals, motivation, and self-relevance. However, most of these studies remain isolated and need further replication. Moreover, EEG and MEG methods have inherent limitations in anatomical resolution, precluding a more precise delineation of distributed neural networks that are presumably implicated in conversion disorders.

Other brain imaging studies have used hemodynamic or metabolic measures such as SPECT, PET, or fMRI (see summary in Table 22.1). A large majority of

TABLE 22.1   Summary of Functional Neuroimaging Studies in Conversion Hysteria

Authors	Patients	Symptoms	Duration	Other psychiatric symptoms	Method	Protocol	Neuroimaging findings
Motor loss Tiihonen, 1995	1 F	L hemiplegia and paresthesia	1 week	Panic attacks, major depression	SPECT	Left median nerve stim during symptoms and after recovery	↓R parietal + ↑R frontal during symptoms
Marshall, 1997	1 F	L leg paralysis	2.5 years	Major depression	PET	Preparation or execution of mvts with either leg	N activation in DLFC and cerebellum during preparation↓motor cx + ↑R ACC and OFC during attempted mvts
Yazici, 1998	3F, 2M	bilateral gait symptoms (astasia abasia)	1–24 weeks	N/A	SPECT	Resting state	↓in L temporal and parietal lobes
Spence, 2000	3 M patients 10 M healthy	2 L + 1 R arm weakness; 4 controls who feign paralysis 6 controls who move normally	6–15 months	Past depression in all patients	PET	Attempt to move joystick at fixed pace	↓L DLPFC in conversion;↓R ant MFG in feigners (irrespective of hand side)
Vuilleumier, 2001	6 F, 1 M	4 L + 3 R hemiparesis and paresthesia	<2 months	Mild depression in 5, personality disorder in 1	SPECT	Resting state + vibratory stim of both hands during and after symptoms	N activation of motor and somatosensory cx↓contra thalamus, putamen, caudate + coupling of basal ganglia with IFG + OFC
Burgmer, 2006	4 M patients 4 M, 3 F healthy	3 L, 1 R hemiparesis	1–8 months	Depression in 1	fMRI	Observation of movies showing L/R hand mvts and execution of L/R mvts	N (or↓) contra motor cx during execution + ↓contra motor cx during observation in patients
DeLange, 2007	5 F, 1 M	4 L, 4 R arm paresis	3–41 months	Depression in 1, anxiety and panic attack in 1	fMRI	Laterality decision on pictures of L/R hand	N contra motor cx and IPS for increasing mental rotation↑OFC, STG

Study	Subjects	Symptom	Duration	Comorbidity	Method	Task	Findings
Stone, 2007	3 F, 1 M patients 3 F, 1 M healthy	2 L + 2 R leg weakness 2 L + 2 R feigners	9–30 months	Depression and anxiety in 3 patients	fMRI	Mvts of ankle on either side	↓R MFG and OFC + ↑extent in motor cx + ↑ IFG, insula, putamen, SPL, and visual cx in patients↑SMA in feigners
Kanaan, 2007	1 F	R hemiparesis	15 months	Conduct disorder	fMRI	Cued recall of adverse life events and neutral personal events	↓L primary motor cx↑R amygdala, medial temporal cortex, IFG, ACC
Sensory loss Mailis-Gagnon, 2003	3 F, 1 M	1 L, 2 R, 1 bilat hypo / anesthesia and pain	1–9 years	Multiple (developmental or traumatic stress factors)	fMRI	Tactile (brush) and painful stim (von Frey probes)	↓SI, SII, thalamus, insula, inferior frontal, and posterior cingulate for all stim when non perceived↑rostral ACC to painful stim when unperceived
Ghaffar, 2007	3 F	2 L foot, 1 L hand numbness	4 months to 9 years	N/A	fMRI	L, R, or bilateral vibrotactile stim	↓activation SI contra to symptoms during unilateral stim + N activation SI during bilateral stim↓OFC, striatum, and thalamus in 2/3 during unilateral stim
Visual loss Werring, 2004	4 F, 1 M patients 4 F, 3M healthy controls	Reduced visual field or acuity	2–10 years	1 minor depression, 1 grief reaction	fMRI	Periodic visual stim (8 Hz), each eye separately	↓primary and secondary visual cx, bilateral↓ R ant cingulate↑L IFG, insula, striatum, thalamus, post cingulate, uncus

Abbreviations: ACC: anterior cingulate cortex, cx: cortex, F: female, IFG: inferior frontal gyrus, L: left, M: male, M1: primary motor cortex, MFG: middle frontal gyrus, mvts: movements, OFC: orbitofrontal cortex, R: right, SI: primary somatosensory cortex, SII: primary somatosensory cortex, SMA: supplementary motor area, STG: superior temporal gyrus, stim: stimulation. ↑=increase; ↓=decrease, N=normal activation.

IV. SEIZURES, SPLITS, NEGLECTS AND ASSORTED DISORDERS

these studies has focused on motor conversion disorders. A first pioneer study was carried by Tiihonen [91] who performed SPECT scans in a patient with left hemiparesis and numbness during sensory stimulation of the left arm, and reported relative decreases in right parietal lobe and increases in right frontal lobe, which returned to normal after recovery. Conversion symptoms were attributed to an inhibition of parietal areas due to frontal activation subsequent to stressful events. A similar interpretation was suggested in a later study by Marshall *et al.* [55], who used PET in a woman with left leg paralysis while she either prepared to move one leg or the other, moved her intact right leg, or attempted to move her left paralyzed leg. Although preparation to move activated dorsolateral frontal areas and cerebellum for both legs (suggesting preserved motor intention), attempted movements of the left leg did not activate contralateral motor areas (consistent with the absence of movement) but instead produced increases in the right ACC and orbitofrontal cortex (OFC) – unlike right leg movements that normally activated contralateral motor cortex only (Figure 22.1). These findings were taken to support the idea that motor volition and preparation were preserved but actively suppressed by cingulate and orbitofrontal areas, mediating unconscious affective or motivational control on willed actions. Two subsequent PET studies in healthy subjects who performed the same task but after hypnotic suggestion of unilateral paralysis also reported increases in ACC [92] or OFC [93] during movement attempts with the 'paralyzed' leg. However, activation of frontal and cingulate areas in this condition might potentially also reflect other cognitive processes such as effort [94], conflict [95], or increased self-monitoring and anxiety [88, 96].

A more recent fMRI by Stone *et al.* [97] also compared attempted movements with affected or normal leg in four patients with conversion, as well as in four controls who feigned weakness. But these authors found reduced activation in orbitofrontal and mediofrontal areas in patients during movements with the weak limb, together with bilateral increases in inferior frontal gyri and insula. In addition, motor cortex and basal ganglia showed more diffuse activation in conversion patients than in feigners (Figure 22.2). While these data suggest some impairment in motor control, perhaps reflecting effortful and uncoordinated movements with the affected limb, other changes in frontal and limbic regions also indicate anomalies in motivational and arousal functions. Moreover, regions in inferior frontal gyri showing increases in conversion patients are known to be engaged in monitoring and inhibition processes [98]. However, unlike previous results of Marshall *et al.* [55], here OFC was deactivated rather than hyperactivated.

In contrast to the proposal of an active inhibition by ACC or OFC on planned movements, other imaging findings suggest a dysfunction in motor preparation or intention. Spence *et al.* [99] found that patients with motor conversion activated less the left prefrontal cortex during paced movements made with the weak hand, relative to both feigners and healthy controls. This reduction was attributed to a disorder in motor generation processes that normally mediate willed action and selectively rely on the left frontal lobe [100].

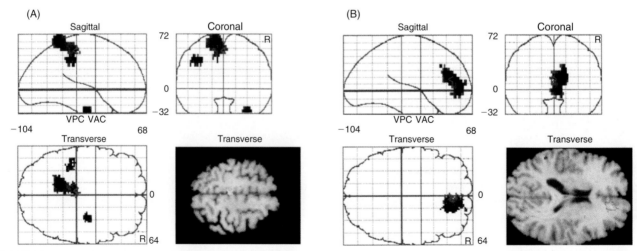

FIGURE 22.1   PET results in a patient with hysterical paralysis of the left leg, shown on a standard anatomical template in stereotactic space (*Source*: Adapted from [55]). (A) Activation during movement of the right (good) leg, compared to right motor preparation, showing increases centred in contralateral (left) primary motor and sensory cortex, plus left parietal and right inferior temporal cortex. (B) Activation during attempted movement of the left (affected) leg, compared to left motor preparation, showing no increases in contralateral sensorimotor areas, but selective activation of the right anterior cingulate and right OFC.

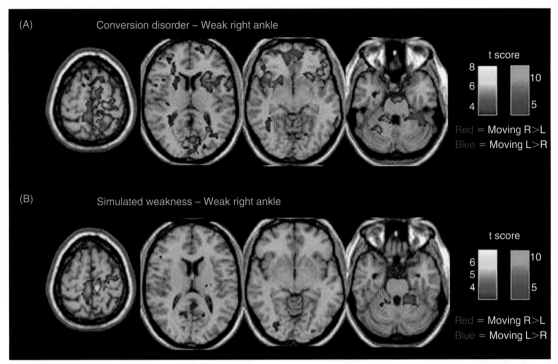

FIGURE 22.2   Functional MRI results in four patients with unilateral ankle weakness due to conversion hysteria and four healthy controls simulating unilateral weakness (group data), shown on transverse brain slices with images flipped to correspond with right-side ankle weakness (*Source*: Adapted from [98]). Red colours depict areas more active during right than left movements, whereas blue colours depict areas more active during left than right leg movements (left hemisphere shown on the right). (A) Conversion patients showed less strong and more diffuse activation in motor areas contralateral to the weak limb than in motor areas contralateral to the normal limb, together with additional activation in a wide network including bilateral basal ganglia, inferior frontal gyrus, left insula, and left visual cortex, while they showed relative deactivation in right middle frontal and orbitofrontal cortices. (B) Healthy controls simulating weakness activated primary motor areas contralateral to the moving limb, with additional activation in supplementary motor area only for the weak relative to the normal limb.

Unlike conversion patients, feigners showed less activation of the right prefrontal cortex in the same task. These data converge with other results to indicate that changes in brain activity in conversion hysteria differ from the pattern observed during conscious simulation [93, 97], although reduced activation in left frontal regions are also commonly associated with depression [101] and might potentially reflect non-specific comorbid anomalies in these patients. Non-specific changes in left frontal, temporal, and parietal regions have also been observed in other imaging studies of conversion patients [96, 102].

A more recent fMRI study provided further support to the notion of impaired generation of internal motor representations during motor conversion [103], by demonstrating that patients did not activate their motor cortex when they observed actions made by others with the same hand as their affected limb, unlike for the observation of actions involving the healthy hand (Figure 22.3). This lack of covert motor imitation was found despite a normal activation of the motor cortex during attempts to execute real movements with the affected hand. However, other studies reported

that primary motor cortex and parietal areas showed symmetrical increases during a motor imagery task requiring mental rotation of either right or left hand presented in pictures with different orientations [96], consistent with previous results of behavioural studies on covert motor planning [104, 105]. Altogether, the lack of motor activation in a passive condition of action observation [103] despite preserved activation of motor areas during explicit motor imagery tasks (or even real movements attempts) might suggest that internal motor plans can still be generated, but their initiation may fail or be abnormally modulated by motivational factors [88].

In keeping with this idea, motivational and emotional signals might also influence subcortical sites within motor pathways such as the basal ganglia, which control the initiation and execution of motor commands generated in cortex, and presumably integrate these motor commands with contextual factors coded in other brain regions. Reduced activation in the striatum (caudate and putamen) as well as the thalamus contralateral to motor symptoms was found by a SPECT study [44] in seven patients with unilateral weakness

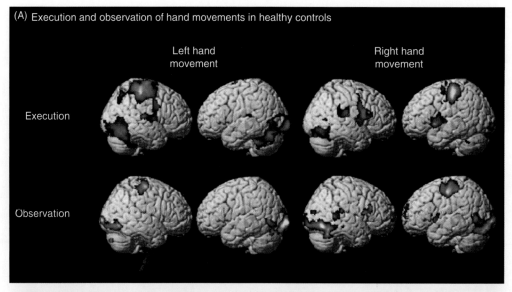

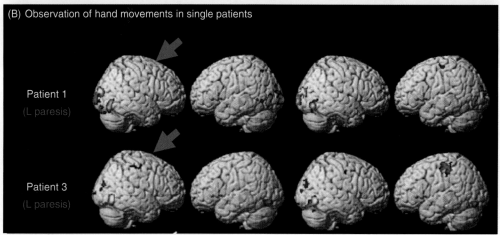

FIGURE 22.3   Functional MRI results during execution or observation of unilateral hand movements (Source: Adapted from [103]). (A) Activations in healthy subjects during execution and observation of movements made with either the right or the left hand (group data), showing an activation of contralateral motor cortex during both execution or observation. (B) Activations in two representative patients with left hysterical paresis during observation of left- or right-hand movements, showing normal increases contralateral to the intact (right) hand but no increases contralateral to the affected (left) hand. The arrows mark the expected localization of activation in the motor areas during observation of hand movements for the affected side.

and mild sensory symptoms, while they underwent passive stimulation by vibration of both limbs (affected and unaffected). Brain SPECT with bilateral stimulation was performed first during motor symptoms and then repeated a few months later after recovery. The asymmetry of activation in basal ganglia and thalamus disappeared after recovery (Figure 22.4A,B). Furthermore, the magnitude of hypoactivation in caudate nucleus observed at the time of symptoms predicted their duration until recovery. By contrast, activation of primary sensorimotor areas contralateral to the affected limb was enhanced during symptoms relative to the later recovery stage (Figure 22.4C). In addition, functional network analyses showed that functional decreases in

striato-thalamic circuits were correlated with concomitant changes in inferior and ventro-medial prefrontal areas (BA 44/45 and BA 11) in the same hemisphere, contralateral to the motor symptoms (Table 22.2). More recently, a volumetric MRI study also reported that patients with motor conversion disorders ($n = 10$) had generally smaller grey-matter density in right caudate and right thalamus as compared with a group of healthy individuals [77]. However, no information on the type and duration of symptoms was provided in this study.

Abnormal activation of striato-thalamic circuits typically occurs during Parkinson disease (i.e., decreases due to dopamine loss) or during Tourette syndrome

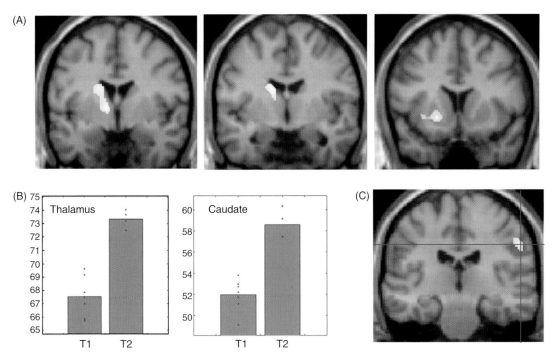

FIGURE 22.4   SPECT results in seven patients with unilateral weakness and hypoesthesia due to conversion hysteria (group data), during passive vibrotactile stimulation applied to both hands simultaneously (*Source*: Adapted from [44]). (A) Activation was increased in caudate, putamen, and thalamus contralateral to the symptoms when vibrotactile stimulation after recovery was compared to stimulation during symptoms. (B) Parameters of activity in thalamus and caudate during symptoms (T1) and after recovery (T2). (C) Conversely, activation was increased in somatosensory areas contralateral to the symptoms when vibrotactile stimulation during symptoms was compared to stimulation after recovery.

(i.e., increases due to probable genetic anomalies), which entail opposite dissociations between conscious volition and actual execution of movements. Thus, Parkinson patients experience a subjective blocking of actions despite their intention to move, whereas Tourette patients experience an irrepressible urge to move without purpose. These subcortical anomalies can variably reduce or enhance activation of motor cortical regions depending on experimental conditions [106]. Focal lesions in basal ganglia or thalamus (such as stroke) may also produce 'intentional neglect', characterized by a failure to use the contralesional limb despite normal motor strength [107]. The basal ganglia have a unique position within motor pathways in that their activity is strongly modulated by environmental context and motivational cues [108, 109], and such influences may operate without consciousness [110]. The caudate nucleus receives prominent limbic inputs from the amygdala and OFC, encoding emotional significance of events in relation to past experience, and may thus contribute to elicit or suppress specific patterns of motor behaviour in response to emotional states [108]. Inputs from amygdala and OFC may also act on thalamic nuclei to modulate activation of striato-cortical loops based on affective signals. Moreover, in animals, alert states with inhibition of motor

behaviour or protective limb immobility after injury are also known to implicate inhibitory processes mediated by striatal and thalamic pathways [74, 111]. A role of these subcortical regulatory circuits in motor conversion would therefore accord with phylogenetic theories that suggest a 'primitive' psychobiological adaptive role of hysteria behaviour, with self-preservation value in the context of perceived threats [69–71]. Hysterical paralysis could thus involve a suppression of motor readiness or initiation through a modulation of specific basal ganglia and thalamo-cortical systems, under the influence of emotional signals from limbic brain regions such as the amygdala, OFC, and/or anterior cingulate gyrus [44]. This neural network might enable some emotional states or experiences to affect motor, sensory, or even cognitive processing, perhaps also partly owing to previous experiences and particular attentional states of the individual [18, 47, 60]. Such changes might in turn modulate the degree of activation of primary motor cortex during initiation or preparation of movements, producing either decreases [55, 103], increases [44, 97], or no changes [112] depending on the task conditions.

Indirect evidence in support of emotional influences on motor processes in conversion was recently provided by an ingenious fMRI study that compared

TABLE 22.2   Network Analysis of Activation Changes During Motor Conversion Using Scaled Subprofile Model (SSM)

	Factor 1	Factor 2	Factor 3
Eigenvalue	5.46	2.24	2.14
Variance explained (%)	45.5	18.6	17.9
(A) Brain areas:			
BA 4	0.84		
BA 6	0.90		
BA 8		0.88	
BA 9–44		−0.65	
BA 44–45		−0.58	0.66
BA 46			
BA 10	−0.75		
BA 11			0.66
ACC		0.70	
BA 1-2-3	0.87		
BA 5–7	0.97		
BA 39–40	0.57	0.68	
BA 37	−0.53	0.76	
BA17–18			
BA 22		−0.72	
BA 20–21	−0.75		
BA 38	−0.55	−0.82	
Caudate			0.68
Lenticular	−0.92		
Thalamus			0.72
(B) Scan acquisitions:			
T1 – contra	0.43	−0.06	**0.58**
T1 – ipsi	**0.59**	**0.37**	0.21
T2 – contra	**0.77**	−0.07	−0.24
T2 – ipsi	**0.80**	−0.11	−0.26

SSM is a modified principal component analysis used to identify networks of regions that form significant covarying patterns (topographic profiles) associated with a specific state (see Alexander and Moeller, 1994; *Hum Brain Mapp* 1994; 2: 79–94). SSM was performed on 20 anatomically defined regions of interest (ROIs) in the SPECT study of Vuilleumier et al. (2001), for both hemispheres contralateral and ipsilateral to motor symptoms, with bilateral vibrotactile stimulation during symptoms (T1) and after recovery (T2). Factors indicate overlapping functional networks of brain areas whose activity was found to covary across subjects and scans. Coefficients indicate the degree to which brain regions (A) and individual hemispheres (B) contribute to (or 'weigh' in) each topographical profile. For clarity, factor loadings <0.5 in topographical profiles are not shown. The first 2 factors reveal a network of sensorimotor cortical areas (factor 1) and attentional areas (factor 2), which were activated by vibro-tactile stimulation during both T1 and T2, but with reduced expression in the hemisphere contralateral to symptoms when these are present (factor 1 at T1). Factor 3 reveal a network of subcortical & frontal areas, including ventral-orbital regions (BA11 and BA 44/45), which were associated with the presence of symptoms and expressed in the hemisphere contralateral to symptoms when these are present (T1).

brain activation to short auditory narratives probing memory for either stressful or neutral events, in a patient with unilateral hysterical paralysis [113]. Narratives concerning the critical stressful events that supposedly triggered conversion symptoms in this patient did only enhance activation of the right peri-hippocampal regions, right amygdala, right inferior frontal cortex, and anterior cingulate, but also decreased activity in left motor cortex contralaterally to the (right-sided) symptoms. This motor 'deactivation' was observed even though no movement was required, and similar responses were made with the left hand to both emotional and neutral events in the recognition memory task. However, no changes were reported for OFC, basal ganglia, or thalamus. Further studies using a similar induction procedure would be interesting to perform in other patients and during different conversion symptoms.

Fewer imaging investigations have been performed in patients with somatosensory hysterical symptoms, such as hemi-anaesthesia or functional pain disorders. Ghaffar et al. [114] compared brain activation to vibrotactile stimulation applied unilaterally or bilaterally in three patients with hysterical anaesthesia of one limb. Results showed a reduced activation of the primary (and to a lesser extent secondary) areas of somatosensory cortex only during unilateral stimulation of the affected limb, while bilateral stimulation produced symmetrical activations in both hemispheres. A similar pattern was found in OFC for all three patients, as well as in the striatum and thalamus for two patients. These different responses to unilateral and bilateral stimulation were attributed to a reversible functional suppression of sensory processing due to attentional mechanisms. Another more detailed fMRI study [115] reported a complex pattern of changes in four patients with chronic sensory loss and pain in one or more limbs. Blocks of either non-noxious or noxious tactile stimulation were applied to the affected and unaffected limbs. Four different patterns of responses were found in different brain areas. First, unlike stimulation on the normal side (which were always perceived and reported), noxious and non-noxious stimulation on the affected limb (which were not perceived or not reported) did not activate the thalamus, insula, inferior frontal, and posterior cingulate regions. Second, some areas activated by perceived stimuli on the intact limb were deactivated during stimulation on the affected limb (relative to a baseline without any stimulation), including contralateral SI and SII, as well as bilateral prefrontal areas. It is unclear whether such deactivation by stimulation may reflect inhibitory effects, or greater activation in the baseline condition. Third, ACC showed selective increases during unperceived/unreported stimulation on the affected limb than during perceived stimulation on the unaffected side. Fourth, several regions in prefrontal and parietal cortex (including a part of SI) were similarly activated by unperceived and perceived stimuli, although the commonalities of these responses was not directly tested. These complex changes across a wide brain network were interpreted as the result of attentional and emotional processes triggered by stressful or painful conditions, perhaps

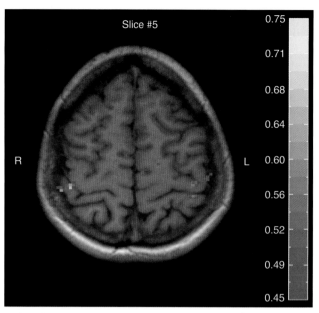

FIGURE 22.5　Functional MRI results in a patient (19-year-old right-handed woman) with left hemi-anaesthesia due to conversion hysteria (normal MRI of the brain and spine, and normal sensory and motor evoked potentials), following a minor car accident (Vuilleumier & Assal, unpublished data). Activation during blocks of bilateral tactile stimulation showed bilateral increases in somatosensory cortex, but stronger in the contralateral than ipsilateral hemisphere.

exacerbated by individual predispositions or developmental factors [115]. Although results may not generalize due to the small sample and heterogeneity of patients in this study, it is notable that increased activity arose in the anterior and rostral cingulate regions during stimulation of the affected limb (while more dorsal regions in ACC were activated by stimulation of the normal limb), in keeping with similar activation during attempted movements in some studies of motor conversion [55, 97]. Moreover, EEG and MEG findings in patients with hysterical anaesthesia also suggest that early neural responses in SI and SII are normal, while later responses associated with cognitive or affective processes might be disturbed [81, 84]. Other unpublished fMRI results from our group also showed preserved (and even enhanced) responses to tactile stimuli in a patient with hemi-anaesthesia due to conversion (Figure 22.5).

Only a single imaging study investigated hysterical visual loss [116]. Neural responses to visual stimulation by whole-field colour flickers were reduced in visual cortex, and accompanied by decreased (rather than increased) activation in ACC. On the other hand, increased activity was found in several regions including posterior cingulate, insula, temporal poles, as well as the thalamus and striatum on both sides. This pattern was again interpreted as an effect of inhibitory modulation by limbic areas on sensory visual processing, consistent with previous findings in motor conversion [55].

Finally, psychogenic amnesia is another type of hysterical deficit without organic cause that has been increasingly investigated by neuropsychological and neuroimaging approaches in recent years [5]. Although a detailed review of this syndrome is beyond the scope of this paper, and it is considered as a separate category of dissociative disorders in DSM-IV classification, it is noteworthy that psychogenic amnesia shares some clinical features with conversion reactions, including its frequent occurrence after stressful situations and occasional

mixture with organic factors such as mild brain injury (concussion). While functional neuroimaging studies also point to anomalies in frontal and limbic regions potentially associated with emotion and self-attribution processes, together with changes in medial temporal lobe regions associated with memory, it remains to be determined whether the 'mnestic blockade' of psychogenic amnesia involves neural processes regulating awareness of memory function that are at least partly common to neural processes regulating awareness of motor or sensory functions (see Box 22.2). Further studies elucidating the commonalities and differences

---

BOX 22.2

PSYCHOGENIC AMNESIA AND DISSOCIATION

Some patients may present with memory impairments without a discernable neurological cause, typically after one or more stressful life events. This type of 'psychogenic' or 'dissociative' amnesia differs from the classic amnesic syndromes caused by brain lesions in that autobiographic retrograde memory is predominantly affected with no or more variable problems in memory for new information.[1] This may be accompanied by other dissociative or depersonalization phenomena, such as fugue disorders. The dissociative disorders were once classified together with other conversion disorders as forms of hysteria, but are now considered separately despite some commonalities. Cognitive and brain imaging research has begun to reveal some of the cerebral mechanisms underlying psychogenic amnesia, borrowing from the well-known architecture of memory systems. Single-case studies have shown decreases in activation of medial temporal lobe and basal forebrain region during such episodes,[2,3] while some regions in right amygdala and right anterior temporal lobe may still respond more to familiar than unfamiliar material despite a lack of explicit recognition. Abnormal activations in anterior cingulate, prefrontal areas, and caudate have also been found.[3,4]

Markowitsch[5] proposed that such memory deficits may result from a functional suppression or disconnection between frontal and temporal areas within the right hemisphere, triggered by intense environmental stress or psychological trauma, and/or brain injuries in some cases, leading to a subsequent inability to retrieve affectively laden information that is stored with personal autobiographical memories. This, in turn, would disrupt the subjective experience of selfhood in memory retrieval. By contrast, semantic information stored in left hemisphere might remain more accessible and allow preserved anterograde learning. Furthermore, it was proposed that this 'mnestic blockade' might be facilitated by the release of steroids (cortisol) due to stress or depression, which can exert suppressive effects on hippocampal function and memory.[6] Although it is unclear how such hormonal factors could affect limbic circuits in the right hemisphere more than in the left hemisphere, right hemisphere predominance would also be consistent with other asymmetries associated with sensorimotor conversion[7] and pseudo-seizure disorders.[8]

1. Kopelman, M.D. and Kapur, N. (2001). The loss of episodic memories in retrograde amnesia: Single-case and group studies. *Philos Trans R Soc Lond B Biol Sci* 356 (1413), 1409–1421.
2. Markowitsch, H.J. *et al.* (1998). Psychic trauma causing grossly reduced brain metabolism and cognitive deterioration. *Neuropsychologia* 36 (1), 77–82.
3. Yasuno, F. *et al.* (2000). Functional anatomical study of psychogenic amnesia. *Psychiatry Res* 99 (1), 43–57.
4. Glisky, E.L. *et al.* (2004). A case of psychogenic fugue: I understand, aber ich verstehe nichts. *Neuropsychologia* 42 (8), 1132–1147.

5. Markowitsch, H.J. (2003). Psychogenic amnesia. *Neuroimage* 20 Suppl 1, S132–S138.
6. Markowitsch, H.J. (1999). Functional neuroimaging correlates of functional amnesia. *Memory* 7 (5–6), 561–583.
7. Stern, D.B. (1983). Psychogenic somatic symptoms on the left side: Review and interpretation. In: Myslobodsky, M.S. (ed.) *Hemisyndromes: Psychobiology, Neurology, Psychiatry.* pp. 415–445, New York: Academic Press.
8. Devinsky, O. *et al.* (2001). Nondominant hemisphere lesions and conversion nonepileptic seizures. *J Neuropsychiatr Clin Neurosci* 13 (3), 367–373.

between the functional neuroanatomy of these different types of psychogenic reactions might contribute to better understand the relationships between conversion and dissociation disorders [3].

CONCLUSIONS

In spite of decades of interest in conversion hysteria, a number of important aspects concerning its causal factors and clinical manifestations still remain to be clarified; and recent attempts to identify specific cerebral correlates for conversion symptoms by using neurophysiology or neuroimaging techniques still remain conflicting. However, several progresses have been made in recent years and may now begin to provide new clues about the possible biological and cognitive underpinnings of these disorders. Despite some divergence in specific findings between studies, and despite a large heterogeneity between patients and symptoms, the results obtained from functional neuroimaging have contributed to delineate a network of brain areas including orbitofrontal and inferior frontal cortex, anterior cingulate, basal ganglia, thalamus, as well as sensory or motor regions (depending on actual symptoms), which all appear to be critically implicated in conversion hysteria. On the one hand, most fMRI and PET studies have found changes in activity arising within brain regions involved in the affected, motor, sensory, or mnemonic functions (e.g., during motor, somatic, or amnesic symptoms, respectively), typically with concomitant changes in limbic regions associated with emotional and motivational regulation such as orbitofrontal and medial prefrontal areas (exhibiting either increases [55, 115], decreases [97], or changed coupling [44] of activity), as well as other subcortical regions such as amygdala or striatum. On the other hand, most neurophysiology studies using EEG or MEG have found normal activation of primary motor or sensory cortical areas, with occasional anomalies in later components such as P300, consistent with a lack of damage to low-level sensorimotor pathways but more complex anomalies in higher-level modulatory or integrative processes.

Whether observed changes in the activity of these brain areas reflect causes, consequences, comorbidity markers, or compensatory mechanisms is however still unclear at present. Studies testing brain responses directly related to impaired function (e.g., movement attempts during hysterical paralysis [55, 97, 100]) may disclose activation reflecting not only this function alone but also vary as a function of actual performance (failure, attempt, or reduced), and in addition yield a mixture of other activations related to intentional, emotional, executive, and/or monitoring processes that might be engaged by the task and the context. Alternative approaches testing brain responses to more passive stimulation in order to elicit covert activation of cognitive or emotional pathways [96, 103, 113] might provide useful information to characterize functional neural changes associated with conversion hysteria across different types or degrees of clinical deficits. However, these approaches may require a precise model of the tested function and of the normal effects of such indirect paradigms in order to interpret the findings in an informative manner. For instance, the role of specific mechanisms putatively involved in the generation of conversion symptoms (e.g., inhibition, attention, or disconnection) might be tested using paradigms borrowed from current neurobiological models of sensorimotor, emotion, or memory processing.

A key role of orbitofrontal and medial prefrontal areas in hysteria conversion, as suggested by imaging studies, would be consistent with a major function of these areas in integrating the emotional significance of external events with past experiences and self-representations, and in forming expectancies about the outcome associated with these events. OFC is particularly critical for the generation of sensory and mnemonic aspects of expectancies associated with certain affective cues or states [117], and it is likely to be activated in response to stressful situations that trigger conversion hysteria, perhaps under the influence of other limbic regions such as the amygdala. Such activation of OFC might then promote the generation of abnormal functional states in motor or sensory networks, involving either a stereotyped adaptive mode of response (e.g., to perceived threat, as postulated by phylogenetic theories) or some reinstatement of past associations or memories (e.g., acquired by personal experience or observations, as proposed by some dissociation theories). Whether these functional changes involve an inhibition of normal processing or an impairment in normal readiness or responsiveness of specific neural pathways still remains to be determined, but these different neural mechanisms may not necessarily be exclusive. Moreover, because emotional responses in limbic areas and their influences on connected brain regions can arise without awareness (and even without any direct emotional experience) [118], such effects might generate conversion behaviour without intentional control and thus enter awareness of the patient as a distorted experience of motor will or self-perception. Chronic or acute stress may further contribute to promote the retrieval of representations and behaviours mediated by limbic circuits such as amygdala, while reducing those mediated by cortical and hippocampal regions [119]. Likewise, a disruption in the dynamic integration between awareness of agency and immediate sensation, and the control of bodily function or memory retrieval, might also underlie some aspects of other dissociative disorders subsequent to emotional stressors.

Finally, it is essential that modern neuroimaging approaches to conversion hysteria should not constitute a simple return to neurogenic models that preceded Freudian psychodynamic accounts, but rather yield more testable predictions about both psychological and neurobiological mechanisms underlying the clinical concept of 'conversion' in hysteria. A better understanding of these common but still enigmatic disorders will not only offer precious insights on cerebral processes mediating self-awareness, but also help refine the clinical diagnosis and management of patients. Just like conversion hysteria has too often been seen as a disease of imagination, neurobiological accounts have too often rested on pure speculations, without sufficient positive evidence to support them. However, thanks to the development of functional neuroimaging and current advances in cognitive and affective neurosciences, the time seems now ripe to gain a much deeper knowledge in one of the most ancient and most physical reaction of the human mind to perceived stress and distress.

References

1. Freud, S. and Breuer, J. (1895) *Studies on Hysteria*, New York: Basic Books/Hogarth Press. 1955.
2. Cloninger, C.R. (2001) The origins of DSM and ICD criteria for conversion and somatization disorders. In *Contemporary approaches to the study of hysteria: Clinical and theoretical perspectives*. P.W. Halligan, C. Bass, and J.C. Marshall (eds.) Oxford: UK: Oxford University Press. pp. 49–62.
3. Brown, R.J., *et al.* (2007) Should conversion disorder be reclassified as a dissociative disorder in DSM V? *Psychosomatics* 48 (5):369–378.
4. Vuilleumier, P. (2005) Hysterical conversion and brain function. *Prog Brain Res* 150:309–329.
5. Markowitsch, H.J. (2003) Psychogenic amnesia. *Neuroimage* 20 (Suppl 1):S132–138.
6. Devinsky, O., *et al.* (2001) Nondominant hemisphere lesions and conversion nonepileptic seizures. *J Neuropsychiatr Clin Neurosci* 13 (3):367–373.
7. Reuber, M. and Elger, C.E. (2003) Psychogenic nonepileptic seizures: Review and update. *Epilepsy Behav* 4 (3):205–216.
8. Reich, S.G. (2006) Psychogenic movement disorders. *Semin Neurol* 26 (3):289–296.
9. Carson, A.J., *et al.* (2000) Do medically unexplained symptoms matter? A prospective cohort study of 300 new referrals to neurology outpatient clinics. *J Neurol Neurosurg Psychiatry* 68 (2):207–210.
10. Krem, M.M. (2004) Motor conversion disorders reviewed from a neuropsychiatric perspective. *J Clin Psychiatry* 65 (6):783–790.
11. Okun, M.S. and Koehler, P.J. (2004) Babinski's clinical differentiation of organic paralysis from hysterical paralysis: effect on US neurology. *Arch Neurol* 61 (5):778–783.
12. Karnik, A.M. and Hussain, M.S. (2000) Paraplegia diagnosed by a new physical sign. *South Med J* 93 (7):724–725.
13. Chen, C.S., *et al.* (2007) Practical clinical approaches to functional visual loss. *J Clin Neurosci* 14 (1):1–7.
14. Weiskrantz, L. (1986) *Blindsight: A Case Study and Implications*, Oxford: Clarendon Press.
15. Driver, J. and Vuilleumier, P. (2001) Perceptual awareness and its loss in unilateral neglect and extinction. *Cognition* 79 (1–2):39–88.
16. Vuilleumier, P. (2004) Anosognosia: The neurology of beliefs and uncertainties. *Cortex* 40 (1):9–17.
17. Spiegel, D. (1991) Neurophysiological correlates of hypnosis and dissociation. *J Neuropsychiatr Clin Neurosci* 3:440–445.
18. Oakley, D.A. (1999) Hypnosis and conversion hysteria: A unifying model. *Cog Neuropsychiatr* 4:3.
19. Roelofs, K., *et al.* (2002) Hypnotic susceptibility in patients with conversion disorder. *J Abnorm Psychol* 111 (2):390–395.
20. Van Dyck, R. and Hoogduin, K. (1989) Hypnosis and conversion disorders. *Am J Psychother* 43 (4):480–493.
21. Foong, J., *et al.* (1997) Interrogative suggestibility in patients with conversion disorders. *J Psychosom Res* 43 (3):317–321.
22. Persinger, M.A. (1994) Seizure suggestibility may not be an exclusive differential indicator between psychogenic and partial complex seizures: The presence of a third factor. *Seizure* 3 (3):215–219.
23. Stone, J., *et al.* (2006) La belle indifference in conversion symptoms and hysteria: systematic review. *Br J Psychiatr* 188:204–209.
24. Vuilleumier, P. (2000) Anosognosia. In Bogousslavsky, J. and Cummings, J.L. (eds.) *Disorders of Behavior and Mood in Focal Brain Lesions*, pp. 465–519, Cambridge University Press.
25. Schuepbach, W.M., *et al.* (2002) Accuracy of the clinical diagnosis of 'psychogenic disorders' in the presence of physical symptoms suggesting a general medical condition: A 5-year follow-up in 162 patients. *Psychother Psychosom* 71 (1):11–17.
26. Binzer, M., *et al.* (1997) Clinical characteristics of patients with motor disability due to conversion disorder: A prospective control group study. *J Neurol, Neurosurg Psychiatr* 63:83–88.
27. Roelofs, K., *et al.* (2005) The impact of early trauma and recent life-events on symptom severity in patients with conversion disorder. *J Nerv Ment Dis* 193 (8):508–514.
28. House, A., *et al.* (1990) Life events and difficulties preceding stroke. *J Neurol Neurosurg Psychiatr* 53 (12):1024–1028.
29. Mohr, D.C., *et al.* (2004) Association between stressful life events and exacerbation in multiple sclerosis: A meta-analysis. *BMJ* 328 (7442):731.
30. Roelofs, K., *et al.* (2002) Childhood abuse in patients with conversion disorder. *Am J Psychiatr* 159 (11):1908–1913.
31. Binzer, M. and Eisemann, M. (1998) Childhood experiences and personality traits in patients with motor conversion symptoms. *Acta Psychiatr Scand* 98 (4):288–295.
32. Tunca, Z., *et al.* (1996) Is conversion disorder biologically related with depression? A DST study. *Biol Psychiatr* 39 (3):216–219.
33. Horvath, T., *et al.* (1980) Attention in hysteria: A study of Janet's hypothesis by means of habituation and arousal measures. *Am J Psychiatr* 137 (2):217–220.
34. Pruessner, J.C., *et al.* (1999) Burnout, perceived stress, and cortisol responses to awakening. *Psychosom Med* 61 (2):197–204.
35. Binzer, M. and Kullgren, G. (1998) Motor conversion disorder: A prospective 2- to 5-year follow-up study. *Psychosomatics* 39 (6):519–527.
36. Crimlisk, H.L., *et al.* (1998) Slater revisited: 6 year follow up study of patients with medically unexplained motor symptoms. *Brit Med J* 316:582–586.

37. Carson, A.J., *et al.* (2003) The outcome of neurology outpatients with medically unexplained symptoms: A prospective cohort study. *J Neurol Neurosurg Psychiatry* 74 (7):897–900.

38. Reynolds, J. (1869) Paralysis, and other disorders of motion and sensation, dependent on idea. *BMJ* 2:483–485.

39. Gowers, W.R. (1893). *A manual of diseases of the nervous system.*

40. Schilder, P. (1935) *The image and appearance of the human body*, London: Kegan, Paul, Trench, Trubner, and Company.

41. Eames, P. (1992) Hysteria following brain injury. *J Neurol Neurosurg Psychiatr* 55 (11):1046–1053.

42. Gould, R., *et al.* (1986) The validity of hysterical signs and symptoms. *J Nerv Ment Dis* 174:593–597.

43. Nicolson, R. and Feinstein, A. (1994) Conversion, dissociation, and multiple sclerosis. *J Nerv Ment Dis* 182 (11):668–669.

44. Vuilleumier, P., *et al.* (2001) Functional neuroanatomical correlates of hysterical sensorimotor loss. *Brain* 124 (Pt 6):1077–1090.

45. Stone, J., *et al.* (2003) The 12 year prognosis of unilateral functional weakness and sensory disturbance. *J Neurol Neurosurg Psychiatr* 74 (5):591–596.

46. Stone, J., *et al.* (2005) Systematic review of misdiagnosis of conversion symptoms and "hysteria'. *BMJ* 331 (7523):989.

47. Kozlowska, K. (2005) Healing the disembodied mind: contemporary models of conversion disorder. *Harv Rev Psychiatry* 13 (1):1–13.

48. Charcot, J.M. (1892) *Leçons du Mardi à la Salpêtrière (1887–1888)*, Bureau du Progrès Médical.

49. Babinski, J. and Dagnan-Bouveret, J. (1912) Emotion et hystérie. *Journal de Psychologie* 9 (2):97–146.

50. Pavlov, I.P. (1941) *Lectures on Conditioned Reflexes. Vol. 2: Conditioned Reflexes and Psychiatry*, New York: International Publishers.

51. Whitlock, F.A. (1967) The aetiology of hysteria. *Acta Psychiat Scand* 43:144–162.

52. Ludwig, A.M. (1972) Hysteria: A neurobiological theory. *Arch Gen Psychiatr* 27:771–777.

53. Sackeim, H.A., *et al.* (1979) A model of hysterical and hypnotic blindness: Cognition, motivation, and awareness. *J Abnorm Psychol* 88 (5):474–489.

54. Hernandez Peon, R., *et al.* (1963) Somatic evoked potentials in one case of hysterical anaesthesia. *Electroencephalogr Clin Neurophysiol* 15:889–892.

55. Marshall, J.C., *et al.* (1997) The functional anatomy of a hysterical paralysis. *Cognition* 64:B1–bB8.

56. Sierra, M. and Berrios, G.E. (1999) Towards a neuropsychiatry of conversive hysteria. In Halligan, P.W. and David, A.S (eds.) *Conversion Hysteria: Towards a Cognitive Neuropsychological Account (Special Issue of the Journal Cognitive Neuropsychiatry)* pp. 267–287. Hove, UK: Psychology Press Publication.

57. Ramasubbu, R. (2002) Conversion sensory symptoms associated with parietal lobe infarct: Case report, diagnostic issues and brain mechanisms. *J Psychiatry Neurosci* 27 (2):118–122.

58. Hurwitz, T.A. (2004) Somatization and conversion disorder. *Can J Psychiatr* 49 (3):172–178.

59. Kihlstrom, J.F. (1994) One hundred years of hysteria. In Steven Jay Lynn, E.J.W.R. *et al.*, (eds.) *Dissociation: Clinical and Theoretical Perspectives*, pp. 365–394. New York: Guilford Press.

60. Brown, R.J. (2004) Psychological mechanisms of medically unexplained symptoms: An integrative conceptual model. *Psychol Bull* 130 (5):793–812.

61. Miller, L. (1984) Neuropsychological concepts of somatoform disorders. *Int J Psychiatr Med* 14 (1):31–46.

62. Damasio, A.R. (2003) *Looking for Spinoza: Joy, Sorrow and the Feeling Brain*, New York: Harcourt.

63. Galin, D., *et al.* (1977) Lateralization of conversion symptoms: More frequent on the left. *Am J Psychiatry* 134:578–580.

64. Stern, D.B. (1983) Psychogenic somatic symptoms on the left side: Review and interpretation. In Myslobodsky, M.S. (ed.) *Hemisyndromes: Psychobiology, Neurology, psychiatry,* pp. 415–445. New York: Academic Press.

65. Flor-Henry, P., *et al.* (1981) A neuropsychological study of the stable syndrome of hysteria. *Biol Psychiatr* 16:601–616.

66. Ballmaier, M. and Schmidt, R. (2005) Conversion disorder revisited. *Funct Neurol* 20 (3):105–113.

67. Roelofs, K., *et al.* (2000) The question of symptom lateralization in conversion disorder. *J Psychosom Res* 49 (1):21–25.

68. Stone, J., *et al.* (2002) Are functional motor and sensory symptoms really more frequent on the left? A systematic review. *J Neurol Neurosurg Psychiatr* 73 (5):578–581.

69. Kretschmer, E. (1948) *Hysteria: Reflex and instinct*, London: Peter Owen.

70. Demaret, A. (1994) Origine phylogénétique des symptômes en psychopathologie. L'exemple de l'hystérie. *Acta psychiatrica Belgica* 94:280–298.

71. Miller, E. (1987) Hysteria: Its nature and explanation. *Br J Clin Psychol* 26 (Pt 3):163–173.

72. Merskey, H. (1995) *The analysis of hysteria: Understanding conversion and dissociation*, London: Gaskell/Royal College of Psychiatrists.

73. Nijenhuis, E.R., *et al.* (1998) Animal defensive reactions as a model for trauma-induced dissociative reactions. *J Trauma Stress* 11 (2):243–260.

74. Klemm, W.R. (2001) Behavioral arrest: In search of the neural control system. *Prog Neurobiol* 65 (5):453–471.

75. Northoff, G. (2002) What catatonia can tell us about 'top-down modulation': A neuropsychiatric hypothesis. *Behav Brain Sci* 25 (5):555–577. discussion 578–604

76. Moskowitz, A.K. (2004) 'Scared stiff': Catatonia as an evolutionary-based fear response. *Psychol Rev* 111 (4):984–1002.

77. Atmaca, M., *et al.* (2006) Volumetric investigation of brain regions in patients with conversion disorder. *Prog Neuropsychopharmacol Biol Psychiatr* 30 (4):708–713.

78. Black, D.N., *et al.* (2004) Conversion hysteria: Lessons from functional imaging. *J Neuropsychiatr Clin Neurosci* 16 (3):245–251.

79. Broome, M.R. (2004) A neuroscience of hysteria. *Curr Opin Psychiatr* 17:465–469.

80. Howard, J.E. and Dorfman, L.J. (1986) Evoked potentials in hysteria and malingering. *J Clin Neurophysiol* 3:39–50.

81. Hoechstetter, K., *et al.* (2002) Psychogenic sensory loss: Magnetic source imaging reveals normal tactile evoked activity of the human primary and secondary somatosensory cortex. *Neurosci Lett* 323 (2):137–140.

82. Levy, R. and Mushin, J. (1973) The somatosensory evoked response in patients with hysterical anaesthesia. *J Psychosom Res* 17 (2):81–84.

83. Moldofsky, H. and England, R.S. (1975) Facilitation of somatosensory average-evoked potentials in hysterical anesthesia and pain. *Arch Gen Psychiatr* 32 (2):193–197.

84. Lorenz, J., *et al.* (1998) Differentiation of conversive sensory loss and malingering by P300 in a modified oddball task. *Neuroreport* 9:187–191.

85. Towle, V.L., *et al.* (1985) Diagnosing functional visual deficits with the P300 component of the visual evoked potential. *Arch Ophthalmol* 103 (1):47–50.

86. Fukuda, M., *et al.* (1996) Event-related potential correlates of functional hearing loss: Reduced P3 amplitude with preserved N1 and N2 components in a unilateral case. *Psychiatr Clin Neurosci* 50 (2):85–87.

87. Drake, M.E. (1990) Clinical utility of event-related potentials in neurology and psychiatry. *Sem Neurol* 10:196–203.

88. Roelofs, K., *et al.* (2006) Hyperactive action monitoring during motor-initiation in conversion paralysis: An event-related potential study. *Biol Psychol* 71 (3):316–325.

89. Meyer, B.U., *et al.* (1992) Motor responses evoked by magnetic brain stimulation in psychogenic limb weakness: Diagnostic value and limitations. *J Neurol* 239:251–255.

90. Foong, J., *et al.* (1997) Corticospinal function in conversion disorder. *J Neuropsychiatr Clin Neurosci* 9 (2):302–303.

91. Tiihonen, J., *et al.* (1995) Altered cerebral blood flow during hysterical paresthesia. *Biol Psychiatr* 37 (2):134–135.

92. Halligan, P.W., *et al.* (2000) Imaging hypnotic paralysis: Implications for conversion hysteria. *Lancet* 355 (9208):986–987.

93. Ward, N.S., *et al.* (2003) Differential brain activations during intentionally simulated and subjectively experienced paralysis. *Cognit Neuropsychiatr* 8 (4):295–312.

94. Paus, T., *et al.* (1998) Regional differences in the effects of task difficulty and motor output on blood flow response in the human anterior cingulate cortex: A review of 107 PET activation studies. *Neuroreport* 9 (9):37–47.

95. Badre, D. and Wagner, A.D. (2004) Selection, integration, and conflict monitoring; assessing the nature and generality of prefrontal cognitive control mechanisms. *Neuron* 41 (3):473–487.

96. de Lange, F.P., *et al.* (2007) Increased self-monitoring during imagined movements in conversion paralysis. *Neuropsychologia* 45 (9):2051–2058.

97. Stone, J., *et al.* (2007) fMRI in Patients with Motor Conversion Symptoms and Controls with Simulated Weakness. *Psychosom Med.*

98. Robbins, T.W. (2007) Shifting and stopping: fronto-striatal substrates, neurochemical modulation and clinical implications. *Philos Trans R Soc Lond B Biol Sci* 362 (1481):917–932.

99. Spence, S.A. (1999) Hysterical paralyses as disorders of action. In Halligan, P.W. and David, A.S. (eds.) *Conversion Hysteria: Towards a Cognitive Neuropsychological Account (Special Issue of the Journal Cognitive Neuropsychiatry)* pp. 203–226. Hove, UK: Psychology Press Publication.

100. Spence, S.A., *et al.* (2000) Discrete neurophysiological correlates in prefrontal cortex during hysterical and feigned disorder of movement. *Lancet* 355:1243–1244.

101. Drevets, W.C. (2000) Functional anatomical abnormalities in limbic and prefrontal cortical structures in major depression. *Prog Brain Res* 126:413–431.

102. Yazici, K.M. and Kostakoglu, L. (1998) Cerebral blood flow changes in patients with conversion disorder. *Psychiatr Res: Neuroimag* 83:163–168.

103. Burgmer, M., *et al.* (2006) Abnormal brain activation during movement observation in patients with conversion paralysis. *Neuroimage* 29 (4):1336–1343.

104. Maruff, P. and Velakoulis, D. (2000) The voluntary control of motor imagery. Imagined movements in individuals with feigned motor impairment and conversion disorder. *Neuropsychologia* 38 (9):1251–1260.

105. Roelofs, K., *et al.* (2002) Motor initiation and execution in patients with conversion paralysis. *Acta Psychol (Amst)* 110 (1):21–34.

106. Dagher, A. and Nagano-Saito, A. (2007) Functional and anatomical magnetic resonance imaging in Parkinson's disease. *Mol Imaging Biol* 9 (4):234–242.

107. von Giesen, H., *et al.* (1994) Cerebral network underlying unilateral motor neglect: Evidence from positron emission tomography. *J Neurol Sci* 125:129–138.

108. Mogenson, G.J. and Yang, C.R. (1991) The contribution of basal forebrain to limbic-motor integration and the mediation of motivation to action. *Adv Exp Med Biol* 295:267–290.

109. Delgado, M.R., *et al.* (2004) Motivation-dependent responses in the human caudate nucleus. *Cereb Cortex* 14 (9):1022–1030.

110. Pessiglione, M., *et al.* (2007) How the brain translates money into force: A neuroimaging study of subliminal motivation. *Science* 316 (5826):904–906.

111. De Ceballos, M.L., *et al.* (1986) Do enkephalins in basal ganglia mediate a physiological motor rest mechanism? *Movement Disord* 1:223–333.

112. Defayolle, M., *et al.* (1963) ['Critical' Study on the Use of the Rorschach with Multiple Choice.] *J Med Lyon* 44:1205–1212.

113. Kanaan, R.A., *et al.* (2007) Imaging repressed memories in motor conversion disorder. *Psychosom Med* 69 (2):202–205.

114. Ghaffar, O., *et al.* (2006) Unexplained neurologic symptoms: An fMRI study of sensory conversion disorder. *Neurology* 67 (11):2036–2038.

115. Mailis-Gagnon, A., *et al.* (2003) Altered central somatosensory processing in chronic pain patients with 'hysterical' anesthesia. *Neurology* 60 (9):1501–1507.

116. Werring, D.J., *et al.* (2004) Functional magnetic resonance imaging of the cerebral response to visual stimulation in medically unexplained visual loss. *Psychol Med* 34 (4):583–589.

117. Roesch, M. and Schoenbaum, G. (2006) From associations to expectancies: Orbitofrontal cortex as gateway between the limbic system and representational memory. In Zald, D. and Rauch, S.L., (eds.) *The Orbitofrontal Cortex*, Oxford: Oxford University Press.

118. Dolan, R.J. and Vuilleumier, P. (2003) Amygdala automaticity in emotional processing. *Ann N Y Acad Sci* 985:348–355.

119. Tsoory, M.M., *et al.* (2007) Amygdala modulation of memory-related processes in the hippocampus: potential relevance to PTSD. *Prog Brain Res* 167:35–51.

Leaving Body and Life Behind: Out-of-Body and Near-Death Experience

Olaf Blanke and Sebastian Dieguez

ABSTRACT

Out-of-body experiences (OBEs) and near-death experiences (NDEs) are complex phenomena that have fascinated mankind from time immemorial. OBEs are defined as experiences in which a person seems to be awake and sees his body and the world from a disembodied location outside his physical body. Recent neurological and neuroscientific research suggests that OBEs are the result of disturbed bodily multisensory integration, primarily in right temporo-parietal cortex. NDEs are more loosely defined, and refer to a set of subjective phenomena, often including an OBE, that are triggered by a life-threatening situation. Although a number of different theories have been proposed about the putative brain processes underlying NDEs, neurologists and cognitive neuroscientists have, so far, paid little attention to these phenomena. This might be understandable but is unfortunate, because the neuroscientific study of NDEs could provide insights into the functional and neural mechanisms of beliefs, concepts, personality, spirituality, magical thinking, and the self. Based on previous medical and psychological research in cardiac arrest patients with NDEs, we sketch a neurological framework for the study of so-called NDEs.

Out-of-body experiences (OBEs) and near-death experiences (NDEs) have accompanied and fascinated humanity since times immemorial and have long been the province of circles interested in the occult. Many authors have even argued that these experience provide evidence for mind-brain independence or even the persistence of life after death. The neurology of OBEs and NDEs takes a different stance and proposes to study the brain mechanisms that are associated with these experiences. Accordingly, OBEs have been studied by neurologists and cognitive scientists, as they allow to investigate the functional and neural mechanisms of bodily awareness and self-consciousness in specific brain regions. In the present paper we will review these recent neuroscientific data on OBEs. The situation is quite different for NDEs. Although many different theories have been proposed about putative underlying brain processes, neurologists and cognitive neuroscientists have paid little attention to these experiences. This is unfortunate, because the scientific study of NDEs could provide insights into the functional and neural mechanisms of many facets of human experience such as beliefs, concepts, personality, spirituality, magical thinking, and the self. Moreover, as we will review, there is a frequent confusion between OBEs and NDEs (e.g., [1–2]). This is probably due to the fact that OBEs are often associated with NDE, if not one of the NDE key feature [3–5]. In the following, we will describe OBEs and NDEs, providing definitions, incidences, key phenomenological features, and reviewing some relevant psychological and neurocognitive mechanisms.

OBES

Definition

In an OBE, people seem to be awake and feel that their 'self', or centre of experience, is located outside of the physical body. They report seeing their body and the world from an elevated extracorporeal location [6–10]. The subject's reported perceptions are organized in such a way as to be consistent with this elevated visuo-spatial perspective. The following example from Irwin ([11], case 1) illustrates what individuals commonly experience during an OBE: 'I was in bed and about to fall asleep when I had the distinct impression that "I" was at the ceiling level looking down at my body in the bed. I was very startled and frightened; immediately [afterwards] I felt that I was consciously back in the bed again'.

We have defined an OBE by the presence of the following three phenomenological features: the feeling of being outside of one's physical body (disembodiment); the perceived location of the self at a distanced and elevated visuo-spatial perspective (perspective); and the experience of seeing one's own body (autoscopy)

from this elevated perspective [10]. In other proposed definitions of OBEs it suffices to experience disembodiment. For example, Alvarado defined OBEs as 'experiences in which the sense of self or the centre of awareness is felt to be located outside of the physical body' ([12], p. 331; see also [13]) and Irwin as experiences in which 'the centre of consciousness appears to the experient to occupy temporarily a position which is spatially remote from his/her body' [11]. Brugger's definition requires disembodiment and a distanced visuo-spatial perspective: 'the feeling of a spatial separation of the observing self from the body' [8]. OBEs therefore seem to constitute a challenge to the experienced spatial unity of self and body under normal conditions, that is, the feeling that there is a 'real me' that resides in my body and is both the subject and agent of my experiences [14–15]. Probably for this reason, OBEs have attracted the attention of philosophers [16–17], psychologists [6, 11, 18], and neurologists [7, 19–21] alike, and many have conceptualized OBEs as an extreme example of deviant bodily self-consciousness arising from abnormal brain processes that code for the feeling of embodiment under normal conditions.

Incidence

How common are OBEs in the general population? This question is still difficult to answer for the following reasons: (1) different investigators have asked quite different questions about the presence of an OBE; (2) have used different methods (mail, phone or personal interviews); and (3) most studies have been carried out in populations of college students, mostly from anglo-saxon psychology departments. Depending on the questions asked, how they are asked, who the samples include and how an OBE is defined, the results are very likely to differ. Accordingly, it is not surprising that questionnaire studies have estimated the OBE incidence in the general population as ranging from 8% to 34% (reviewed in [6]). Also the two key features (autoscopy and distanced visuo-spatial perspective), as used in recent neurobiologically motivated studies by Brugger and Blanke, were not considered as necessary OBE-features in most of these surveys. We thus agree with Blackmore [6] that incidences above 10% are very likely overestimates and we conservatively suggest that ~5% of the general population have experienced an OBE. From a cross-cultural point of view OBEs seem to occur and be part of folklore in many parts of the world, although to date very few studies have investigated this interesting issue [22].

Phenomenology

OBEs have to be distinguished from two other phenomena that also involve autoscopy: autoscopic hallucinations and heautoscopy. Whereas there is no disembodiment in autoscopic hallucinations and always disembodiment in OBEs, many subjects with heautoscopy generally do not report clear disembodiment, but are not able to localize their self unambiguously (self location may alternate between an embodied location and an extracorporeal one, or they might feel 'localized' at both positions at the same time). Accordingly, the visuo-spatial perspective is body-centred in autoscopic hallucinations, extracorporeal in the OBE, and at different extracorporeal and corporeal positions in heautoscopy, with the impression of seeing one's own body (autoscopy) present in all three forms of autoscopic phenomena (Figure 23.1; for further details, see [7–8, 20, 23–24]).

OBEs have been the province of esoteric circles for much of its history. From this literature one may nevertheless find abundant phenomenological details and varieties of OBEs (e.g., [25–27]; for review see [6]). In addition, subjects with repeated OBEs (so-called 'astral travellers') have not just given detailed accounts about their OBEs, but also proposed several procedures to induce OBEs that might be approached more systematically by researchers. These authors also reported about the phenomenological characteristics of the disembodied body, its location with respect to the physical body, the appearance of the autoscopic body, and the vestibular and bodily sensations associated with the experience (see [7]). Yet, only a small minority of subjects with OBEs experience more than one or two in a lifetime. OBEs are therefore difficult to study because they generally are of short duration, happen only once or twice in a lifetime [6, 9] and occur under a wide variety of circumstances that will be reviewed in the following.

Precipitating Factors

Several precipitating factors of OBEs have been identified. We review findings from neurology, psychiatry, drugs, and general anaesthesia. OBEs will also be discussed in the section on the phenomenology of NDEs.

Neurology

Only few neurological cases with OBEs have been reported in the last 50 years. Early reports were by Lippman ([28], case 1 and 2), Hécaen and Green ([29], case 3), Daly ([30] case 5), and Lunn ([31], case 1). More recently, Devinsky et al. ([19], case 1, 2, 3, 6, and 10), Maillard et al. ([32], case 1), and Blanke et al. ([7], case 1, 2a, and 3) reported further cases. OBEs have been observed predominantly in patients with epilepsy and migraine. Thus, Lippman reported two migraine patients with OBEs [28] and Green reported that 11%

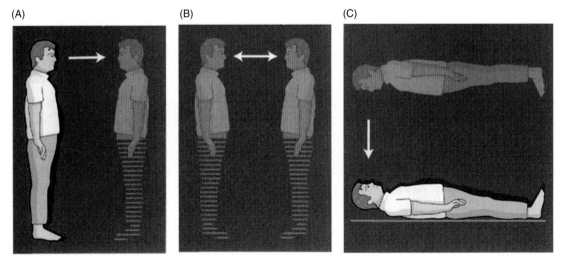

(A)   (B)   (C)

FIGURE 23.1 Illustration of three types of autoscopic phenomena (from Blanke and Mohr [23]). In this figure the phenomenology of (A): autoscopic hallucination (AH), (B) heautoscopy (HAS), and (C) out-of-body experience (OBE) is represented schematically. The experienced position and posture of the physical body for each autoscopic phenomenon is indicated by full lines and the experienced position and posture of the disembodied body (OBE) or autoscopic body (AH, HAS) in blurred lines. The finding that AH and HAS were mainly reported from a sitting/standing position and OBE in a supine position is integrated into the figure. The experienced visuo-spatial perspective during the autoscopic phenomenon is indicated by the arrow pointing away from the location in space from which the patient has the impression to see (AH: from the physical body; OBE: from a disembodied body or location; HAS: alternating or simultaneously from either the fashion between physical and/or the autoscopic body). *Source*: Modified from Blanke et al. [7], with permission from Oxford University Press.

of the OBE-subjects that participated in her survey suffered from migraine headaches [9]. Devinsky *et al.* [19] reported the largest study of neurological OBE-patients and described patients whose OBE was associated with non-lesional epilepsy (cases 6 and 10), with epilepsy due to an arteriovenous malformation (cases 2 and 3), or associated to post-traumatic brain damage (case 1). In Blanke *et al.*'s study [7], OBEs were due to a dysembryoplastic tumour (cases 1 and 2a) and in one patient was induced by focal electrical stimulation (case 3). Maillard *et al.* reported epileptic OBEs in a patient with focal cortical dysplasia ([32], case 1).

Grüsser and Landis [21] proposed that a paroxysmal vestibular dysfunction might be an important mechanism for the generation of OBEs. Devinsky *et al.* [19] observed the frequent association of vestibular sensations and OBEs and in Blanke *et al.*'s [7] study, the importance of vestibular dysfunction in OBEs was underlined by their presence in all patients with OBEs and by the fact that vestibular sensations were evoked in a patient at the same cortical site where higher currents induced an OBE [33]. In more detail, it has been suggested that OBEs are associated with specific vestibular sensations, namely graviceptive and otolithic sensations [7, 34–35]. Otolithic sensations are characterized by a variety of sensations including feelings of elevation and floating, as well as 180° inversions of one's body and visuo-spatial perspective in extrapersonal space. They may be associated with brain damage [36–37], but also occur in healthy subjects during orbital and parabolic flight during space missions or the microgravity phase of parabolic flights [38–39]. Interestingly, responses to microgravity may either be experienced as an inversion of the subject's body and visuo-spatial perspective in extrapersonal space (body inversion illusion) or as an inversion of the entire extrapersonal visual space that seems inverted by 180° to the stable observer (room-tilt illusion; [38–39]). Based on these functional similarities Blanke *et al.* [7] suggested that an otolithic dysfunction might not only be an important causal factor for room tilt and body inversion illusions, but also for OBEs (for further details, see [34–35]).

In addition to vestibular disturbances, it has been reported that OBE-patients may also experience paroxysmal visual body-part illusions such as phantom limbs, supernumerary phantom limbs, and illusory limb transformations either during the OBE or during other periods related to epilepsy or migraine [7, 19, 31, 33, 40]. Blanke *et al.* [33] reported a patient in whom OBEs and visual body-part illusions were induced by electrical stimulation at the right temporo-parietal junction (TPJ). In this patient an OBE was induced repetitively by electrical stimulation whenever the patient looked straight ahead (without fixation of any specific object). If she fixated her outstretched arms or legs she had the impression that the inspected body part was transformed, and had an illusory, but very realistic, visual impression of limb shortening and of illusory limb movement whenever the limbs were bent at the elbow or knee. Finally, with closed eyes the patient did have neither an OBE nor a visual body-part illusion, but perceived her upper body as moving towards her legs [33]. These data suggest that visual illusions of body parts and visual illusions of the entire body (such as autoscopic phenomena) might depend on similar neural structures, as argued by previous authors [20, 40]. They also show that visual body-part illusions and OBEs are influenced differently by the behavioural state of the subject (body posture and eye closure).

Another functional link between OBE and disturbed own body perception is suggested by the fact that OBEs and autoscopic hallucinations (and heautoscopy) depend differently on the patient's position prior to the experience. This suggests that proprioceptive and tactile mechanisms influence both phenomena differently [34]. Thus, during neurological OBEs patients are in supine position [7, 23], an observation also made by Green [9] in 75% of OBEs in healthy subjects. Interestingly, most techniques that are used to deliberately induce OBEs recommend a supine and relaxed position [6–11]. This contrasts with the observation that subjects with autoscopic hallucination or heautoscopy are either standing or sitting at the time of their experience [7, 23, 41]. It thus seems that OBEs depend on the subject's position prior or during the experience and that these differential proprioceptive, vestibular, and tactile mechanisms differentiate them from other types of autoscopic phenomena (see 'Summary' below). The observation of OBEs during general anaesthesia and sleep (see 'General anaesthesia' and [10]) also corroborates the notion that OBEs are facilitated by the sensory signals predominating in supine body position. Moreover, rapid bodily localizational changes such as brutal accelerations and decelerations have been associated with OBEs. This has been reported for a long time by mountain climbers who unexpectedly fell [42–46], as well as in car accidents [19, 25] and in the so-called 'break-off phenomenon' experienced by airplane pilots [47]. In this last case, a pilot might initially fail to sense correctly the position, motion, or tilt of the aircraft as well as his own body position with respect to the surface of the earth and the gravitational 'earth-vertical'. These feelings can lead to several experiences grouped under the term 'break-off phenomenon' that are characterized by feelings of physical separation from the earth, lightness, and an altered sense of the pilot's own orientation with respect to the ground and the aircraft [47–49]. Some pilots have even described a feeling of detachment, isolation, and remoteness from their immediate surroundings which they sometimes describe as an OBE with disembodiment, elevated visuo-spatial perspective, and autoscopy [47, 50]. At one extreme, pilots feel being all of a sudden *outside* the aircraft watching themselves while flying, and being 'broken off from reality' [47]. These OBEs are most often experienced by jet aviators flying alone, especially at high altitudes (above 10 000 m), although helicopter pilots can experience this phenomenon already at an altitude of 1500–3000 m [47, 50]. They seem facilitated by mental absorption (the pilot is unoccupied with flight details) and by the length and visual monotony of the mission [48].

With respect to the underlying neuroanatomy, as mentioned above, we can only rely on a few neurological OBE-patients with circumscribed brain damage. In some of Devinsky *et al.*'s [19] patients with OBEs the seizure focus was estimated only by electroencephalographic (EEG) recordings and localized to the temporal lobe or posterior temporal region (standard MRI (magnetic resonance imaging) or computer tomography was normal in most patients). Yet, in one patient the lesion was found in the temporal lobe and in another patient in the frontal and temporal lobes [19]. Lunn [31] described an OBE-patient with post-traumatic brain damage in the parietal lobe and Daly [30] an OBE-patient with damage to the temporal lobe. More recent lesion analysis based on MRI revealed a predominant involvement of the right TPJ in patients with OBEs [7, 23, 32]. Moreover, in the case already described, Blanke *et al.* [33] have shown that OBEs can be induced by electrical stimulation of the TPJ pointing to the importance of this region in the generation of OBEs (Figure 23.2).

Psychiatry

While reports of autoscopic hallucinations and heautoscopy are not rare in patients suffering from schizophrenia, depression and personality disorders [7, 19–20, 40, 51–52], Bünning and Blanke [10] found only two cases of OBE in psychiatric patients. One had severe depression [29] and the other patient was undiagnosed [53]. Two questionnaire surveys have investigated OBEs in schizophrenia [54–55] and found a similar incidence and phenomenology as in healthy subjects. A study in psychiatric patients suffering from post-traumatic stress disorder found a four-fold increase in prevalence as compared to healthy subjects [56]. Moreover, the personality measure of schizotypy is positively correlated with OBEs in healthy subjects

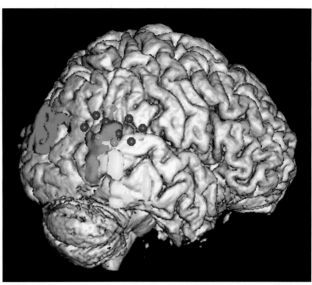

FIGURE 23.2 Lesion analysis of patients with documented brain anomalies and OBE. Mean lesion-overlap analysis of five neurological patients with OBE in whom a lesion could be defined (Patients 1, 2, 3, 5, and 6 from [7]). The MRI of all patients was transformed into Talairach space and projected on the MRI of one patient. Each colour represents a different OBE patient. Mean overlap analysis centred on the TPJ. For details, see [7] and [24]. *Source*: Modified from Blanke *et al.* [7], reproduced with permission from Oxford University Press.

[57–58] and has also been shown to relate behaviourally and neurally (at the TPJ) to OBEs [59–60]. As this trait reflects a continuum between healthy subjects and schizophrenic patients, these data suggest that OBEs might be more frequent in schizophrenic patients than currently thought. Finally, other personality traits such as individuals' somatoform [61–62] (but not general dissociative [60]) tendencies, body dissatisfaction [62], or dissociative alterations in one's body image during a mirror-gazing task [63] have also been linked to OBEs.

Drugs

The administration of different pharmacological substances has presumably been used since immemorial times in ritual practices to induce abnormal experiences including OBEs [22]. These include marijuana, opium, heroin, mescaline, ketamine, and lysergic acid diethylamide (LSD) [6, 21, 52, 64–65]. Concerning marijuana, Tart [64] found that OBE occurred in 44% of a sample of 150 college students who used this drug (see also [10]), that is, a much higher frequency than in the general population. However, a majority of the subjects with OBEs of this study frequently used other drugs such as LSD. It is thus not known whether the higher frequency of OBEs is due to marijuana consumption or the consumption of other drugs. Experiences related to OBEs such as a feeling of floating or of being dissociated from one's body, have also been induced under controlled conditions by marijuana administration compared with placebo administration [66], although similar data with respect to OBEs or other autoscopic phenomena are lacking.

General Anaesthesia

It has long been known that conscious perceptions may occur under general anaesthesia. As Spitellie *et al.* [67] put it: 'Awareness during anaesthesia is as old as the specialty itself'. Insufficient levels of anaesthesia combined with the application of muscle relaxants seem to be the main cause of this preserved awareness. Another pathophysiological factor might be related to haemodynamic cerebral deficits, most notably in anaesthesized patients undergoing cardiac and post-traumatic surgery [68–69]. OBEs in association with general anaesthesia have been described in retrospective case collections by Muldoon and Carrington [25] and Crookall [70], but also in more recent patient studies ([71] patient 3; [72] 4 of 187 patients). A patient from Cobcroft and Forsdick [72] reports: 'I had the strangest [...] sensation of coming out of my self; of being up at the ceiling looking down on the proceedings [of the operation]. After the initial realization that I couldn't communicate at all, came the feeling of acceptance ... of being aware of having one hell of an experience'. Several of the patients reported by Osterman *et al.* [73] said that they 'left their body during the operation at some point'. Although it seems that OBEs are quite rare during general anaesthesia, this is probably linked to the relative infrequency of visual awareness during this state, and the much higher frequency of auditory perceptions (89%), sensations of paralysis (85%), motor illusions and bodily transformations (30–40%), and pain (39%). Visual perceptions were reported in only 27% of patients ([74]; see also [72]). Yet, among patients with visual perceptions, many reported disembodiment and seeing the surgeon and other people and/or surroundings of the operating theatre during the actual operation. Thus, if analyzed only with respect to the presence of visual awareness and experiences in the context of general anaesthesia, OBEs and OB-like experiences are not so rare. This is of special interest because paralysis, complex own body perceptions, and supine position are not only frequent during general anaesthesia with preserved awareness, but also key features in subjects with OBEs of spontaneous or neurological origin [6–7, 23, 75]. Concerning haemodynamic cerebral deficits that have been shown to be associated with an increased incidence of awareness during anaesthesia (see review in [10]), it is interesting to note that they may lead to rather selective and initially focal decreases in cerebral blood flow and as a consequence induce transient or manifest brain infarctions that frequently include the TPJ [76], suggesting that OBEs under general anaesthesia might be related to the functional and anatomical pathomechanisms described in neurological patients with epilepsy, migraine, and cerebrovascular disease. We will return to effects of general anaesthesia in the section on NDEs.

Summary

The reviewed data point to an important involvement of the right TPJ in OBEs of neurological origin. The observation that electrical stimulation of this area may induce OBEs and other abnormal own body perceptions further suggests that during OBEs the integration of proprioceptive, tactile, visual, and vestibular information of one's body fails, due to discrepant central own body representations. We have suggested [7, 23] that autoscopic phenomena (including OBEs) result from a failure to integrate multisensory bodily information and proposed that they result from a disintegration in bodily or personal space (due to conflicting tactile, proprioceptive, kinaesthetic, and visual signals) and a second disintegration between personal and extrapersonal space (due to conflicting visual and vestibular signals caused by a vestibular otolithic dysfunction). While disintegration in personal space was present in all three forms of autoscopic phenomena, differences between the different forms of autoscopic phenomena were mainly due to differences in strength and type of the vestibular dysfunction. Following this model, OBEs were associated with a strong otolithic vestibular disturbance, whereas heautoscopy was associated with a moderate and more variable vestibular disturbance, and autoscopic hallucinations were devoid of any vestibular disturbance. Neuroimaging studies have revealed the important role of the TPJ in vestibular processing, multisensory integration as well as the perception of human bodies or body parts and the self (see [10, 24]). This has recently been studied in healthy subjects. Blanke *et al.* [77], performed an evoked potential study and a transcranial magnetic stimulation study with healthy participants as well as intracranial electrode recordings in a patient with OBEs due to epilepsy. The evoked potential study showed the selective activation of the TPJ at 330–400 ms after stimulus onset (see also [60]) when healthy volunteers imagined themselves in the position and visual perspective that is generally reported by people experiencing spontaneous OBEs. The transcranial magnetic stimulation study showed that magnetic interference with the TPJ during this same time period impaired performance in this task, as opposed to stimulation over a control site at the intraparietal sulcus. No such interference was observed for imagined spatial transformations of external objects, suggesting the selective implication of the TPJ in mental imagery of one's own body and OBEs. Moreover, in an epileptic patient with OBEs due to seizure activity at the TPJ, performing the own body imagery task, while evoked potentials were recorded from intracranial electrodes, we found task-specific activation at the TPJ. Together, these results by Blanke *et al.* [77] (see also [60, 78]) suggest that the TPJ is a crucial structure for the conscious experience of the spatial unity of self and body (for detailed reviews, see [10, 23, 34–35, 79]) and that the associated brain processing is disturbed in OBEs. We now turn to NDEs, which as we will see offer more insights into the mechanisms involved in OBEs.

NDEs

Definition

In different life-threatening situations, people can sometimes experience vivid illusions and hallucinations as well as strong mystical and emotional feelings often grouped under the term of near-death experiences (NDEs). These medical situations seem to involve cardiac arrest, perioperative or post-partum complications, septic or anaphylactic shock, electrocution, coma resulting from traumatic brain damage, intracerebral haemorrhage or cerebral infarction, hypoglycaemia, asphyxia, and apnoea. To this date, systematic studies on the incidence of NDEs in verified medical conditions only exist for cardiac arrest patients [80–83]. Other situations that are merely *experienced* as life-threatening have also been reported to be associated with NDEs, although they often are not objectively life-threatening (mild or not life-endangering diseases, depression, minor accidents, falls, and other circumstances [80]).

Several definitions have been attempted for NDEs. Moody [3], who coined the term NDE, defined it as 'any conscious perceptual experience which takes place during … an event in which a person could very easily die or be killed […] but nonetheless survives' ([84], p. 124). Irwin [85] defined NDEs as 'a transcendental experience precipitated by a confrontation with death' and Nelson *et al.* [86] state that 'NDEs are responses to life-threatening crises characterized by a combination of dissociation from the physical body, euphoria, and transcendental or mystical elements'. Greyson [87] proposed that NDEs are 'profound subjective experiences with transcendental or mystical elements, in which persons close to death may believe

they have left their physical bodies and transcended the boundaries of the ego and the confines of space and time'. Many more such broad definitions of the NDE have been given [88–89] rendering their scientific study difficult. They seem to include a large variety of phenomena and not all researchers may agree that the investigated phenomenon (or assembly of phenomena) of a given study, may actually concern NDEs or typical NDEs. Below, we have reviewed the most frequent and characteristic perceptual and cognitive features of NDEs (see 'Phenomenology'). To complicate matters NDEs (just like OBEs) are difficult to study as their occurrence is generally unpredictable and they are usually not reported at their moment of occurrence, but days, months or even years later.

Incidence

Early studies of NDEs among survivors of cardiac arrest, traumatic accidents, suicide attempts, and other life-threatening situations estimated an incidence of 48% [4] or 42% [5]. Greyson [90] suggested that this rate is probably too high as these studies were retrospective, often carried out many years after the NDE occurred, were using self-selected populations, and lacked appropriate control populations. He rather estimated the incidence of NDEs between 9% and 18%. More recent and better controlled prospective studies focussed on cardiac arrest patients and confirmed lower estimations, with values ranging between 6% and 12%. Parnia *et al.* [81] found an incidence of 6.3%, Greyson [83] of 10%, and Van Lommel *et al.* [80] of 12%. Yet, as is the case for OBEs, in the absence of a clear and widely accepted definition of NDEs, it will remain difficult to define the exact incidence of NDEs [87–90]. In order to avoid this problem most recent studies have used a score above a certain value on Greyson's scale ([91], see below).

Early studies failed to find demographic correlates of the NDE. Neither age, nor gender, race, occupational status, marital status or religiosity seemed to predict the probability to experience a NDE [4–5]. More recently, both Van Lommel *et al.* [80] and Greyson [83] found that young age is associated with a higher probability of NDEs in cardiac arrest patients, although this finding might be confounded by increased medical recovery rates in younger cardiac arrest patients [80, 83]. Another finding is that women tend to have more intense NDEs than men [4, 80] an observation that might partly be related to Moody's [3] suggestion that women might be less afraid to report NDEs or the fact that women have been found to score generally higher on anomalous-perception questionnaires than male subjects [59]. It is possible that having had a NDE facilitates the reoccurrence of such experiences, as 10% of subjects reported multiple NDEs [80]. NDEs have been described in many different cultures and times. Although some consistency can be found in cross-cultural reports, the specific phenomenology (i.e., the structure and the contents of the experience) may nevertheless vary [92–96].

Phenomenology

Moody [3, 84] initially listed 15 key features in NDEs (see Table 23.1). Yet, not one single NDE in his study included all 15 NDE features. Moreover, none of these 15 NDE features was present in all reported NDEs, and no invariable temporal sequence of features could be established. Due to these difficulties, standardized questionnaires have subsequently been developed to identify and measure more precisely the occurrence of NDEs and their intensity (or depth). Ring [4] developed the Weighted Core Experience Index on the basis of structured interviews of 102 persons who found themselves "near-death". The scale is based on 10 features that he gathered from the literature as well as interviews with people with NDEs. His 10 features were: the subjective feeling of being dead, feelings of peace, bodily separation, entering a dark region, encountering a presence or hearing a voice, experiencing a life review, seeing or being enveloped in light, seeing beautiful colours, entering into the light, and encountering visible spirits. According to the presence or absence of each of these features, the score ranges between 0 and 29. This scale has been criticized because it is largely based on arbitrary selected and weighted features, and seemed to contain several uncommon features of NDEs as estimated by other authors. Ring [4] also elaborated a sequence of 5 NDE-stages, the presence of which he considered to be representative of the 'core NDE' (see Table 23.1). To address the aforementioned limitations, Greyson [91] developed a NDE scale that has been used by many recent investigators. He began by selecting 80 features from the existing literature on NDEs and subsequently reduced these to 33 features. He further arrived at a final 16-item scale with a maximum score of 32. This questionnaire has been shown to have several advantages as compared to other questionnaires, especially good test–retest reliability (even for a follow-up at 20 years; [97]) and item score consistency [98]. In his original study, Greyson [91] defined four components of a NDE – cognitive, affective, paranormal, and transcendental – which he later reduced to a classification of three main types of NDEs, according to the specific dominance of the phenomenological components: cognitive, affective, and

transcendental types [99]. See Table 23.1 for these and other classifications of the NDE. In the following we describe the main phenomena that characterize NDEs.

OBEs

OBE are considered a key feature of NDEs, although their frequency was found to vary greatly between different studies. Ring [4] found that 37% of subjects with a NDE experienced disembodiment ('being detached from their body') of whom about half also experienced autoscopy (no detailed data were reported on elevation or visuo-spatial perspective). Greyson and Stevenson [102] found an incidence of 75% of disembodiment (without detailing the presence of autoscopy or elevated visuo-spatial perspective). Sabom [5] reported a 'sense of bodily separation' in 99%, a number in stark contrast with the figure of 24% found by Van Lommel et al. [80]. Disembodiment during NDEs has been reported to be accompanied by auditory and somatosensory sensations [85]. NDE subjects with OBEs characterized by disembodiment and elevated visuo-spatial perspective often report seeing the scene of the accident or operating room. Greyson [103] mentions the example of an NDE in a 26-year-old patient with pulmonary embolism: 'I (the real me, the soul, the spirit, or whatever) drifted out of the body and hovered near the ceiling. I viewed the activity in the room from this vantage point. The hospital room was to my right and below me. It confused me that the doctors and nurses in the room were so concerned about the body they had lifted to the bed. I looked at my body and it meant nothing to me. I tried to tell them I was not in the body (p. 393)'. Future studies on OBEs during NDEs should characterize OBEs with respect to recently defined phenomenological characteristics and enquire systematically about the associated sensations as done in neurological patients (such as visual, auditory, bodily, or vestibular sensations) as well as the presence of disembodiment, autoscopy, elevated perspective permitting to distinguish between autoscopic hallucination, heautoscopy, and OBE. This will allow describing the phenomenology of OBEs during NDEs in more detail and allow relating these data to recent neurological and neurobiological observations on OBEs. Not much is currently known about whether OBEs that are associated with NDEs differ from OBEs without NDE features or whether NDEs with or without OBEs differ. Alvarado [104] found that OBEs in subjects who believed to be close to death were phenomenologically richer than those who did not, with more feelings of passing through a tunnel, hearing unusual sounds, and seeing spiritual entities. Two additional features reached

TABLE 23.1 Phenomenological Features of NDEs According to Several Authors

Moody [3]	Ring [4]	Greyson [91]
Identified 15 common elements in NDEs based on a sample of 150 reports. No statistics were provided.	Identified five stages of a 'core experience', based on structured interviews and a measurement scale (WCEI: weighted core experience index) administered to 102 individuals who have been near death, 48% of whom reported a NDE. These stages tended to appear in sequence, with the earlier ones being more frequent and the latter ones indicating the "depth" of the experience.	Devised a typology of NDEs based on his development of the 16-item NDE scale. On the basis of cluster analysis, he arrived at ones four categories of NDEs each comprising four features.

1. Ineffability
2. Hearing oneself pronounced dead
3. Feelings of peace and quiet
4. Hearing unusual noises
5. Seeing a dark tunnel
6. Being 'out of the body'
7. Meeting 'spiritual beings'
8. Experiencing a bright light as a 'being of light'
9. Panoramic life review
10. Experiencing a realm in which all knowledge exists
11. Experiencing cities of light
12. Experiencing a realm of bewildered spirits
13. Experiencing a 'supernatural rescue'
14. Sensing a boarder or limit
15. Coming back 'into the body'
	1. Peace and well-being, reported by 60%.
	2. Separation from the physical body (OBE), reported by 37% (half of whom had an autoscopic OBE)
	3. Entering a tunnel-like region of darkness, reported by 25%
	4. Seeing a brilliant light, reported by 16%
	5. Through the light, entering another realm, reported in 10%
		1. Cognitive features
		   – time distortion
		   – thought acceleration
		   – life review
		   – revelation
		2. Affective
		   – peace
		   – joy
		   – cosmic unity
		   – encounter with light
		3. Paranormal
		   – vivid sensory events
		   – apparent extrasensory perception
		   – precognitive visions
		   – OBEs
		4. Transcendental
		   – sense of an 'otherworldly' environment
		   – sense of a mystical entity
		   – sense of deceased/religious spirits
		   – sense of border/point of no return'

Sabom [5]	Noyes and Slymen [100]	Lundahl [101]
Proposed from his investigation of 48 subjects with NDE three main types of experiences.	Conducted a factor analysis of questionnaire responses from 189 victims of life-threatening accidents, and found the following three factors of subjective effects that accounted for 41% of the variance.	Summarized the NDE literature and extracted what he saw as the 10 main stages.
1. 'autoscopic' (i.e., the NDE is essentially an OBE) 2. transcendental (apparently entering another 'dimension' through a tunnel and meeting a personified light) 3. combined (involving an OBE and transcendental features)	1. Depersonalization (loss of emotion, separation from the body and feelings of strangeness or unreality) 2. Hyperalertness (vivid and rapid thoughts, sharper vision and hearing) 3. Mystical consciousness (feeling of great understanding, vivid images, life review)	1. peace 2. bodily separation 3. sense of being dead 4. entering the darkness 5. seeing the light 6. entering another world 7. meeting others 8. life review 9. deciding to or being told to return to life 10. returning to the body

statistical significance, namely seeing one's physical body and seeing lights (see also [105]). Of course, it might be the case that due to the very presence of these features these subjects *believed* they had been close to death (there were no medical data available in this study). Owens *et al.* [106] compared the phenomenology of NDEs in subjects being medically close to death with NDEs where subjects only *believed* to be close to death (as established from medical records). They found that former patients tended to report more often seen lights and enhanced cognition than the latter group [106]. There were no significant differences between both groups in seeing a tunnel (see below), having an OBE and a life review (see below). Finally, Nelson *et al.* [107] found that 76% of subjects with NDEs also experienced an OBE. ~40% of these patients had their OBE only as part of the NDE episode, ~33% also had OBEs in other circumstances, and ~26% had an OBE only in other circumstances, that is, not associated with the NDE. This last number was significantly higher than non-NDE-related OBEs in an age-matched control group of healthy subjects [107]. Further links might exist between rare, so-called supernaturalistic OBEs [11], and OBEs during NDEs. Collectively, these data suggest that OBEs and NDEs may share some functional and brain mechanisms, but also point towards the involvement of distinct mechanisms.

The Tunnel and the Light

Experiencing a passage through some darkness or a tunnel is experienced by ~25% of subjects with NDEs [4–5, 80]. This may be associated with the sensation of movement of one's own body such as forward vection, flying or falling, at varying speeds. Drab [108] and Owens *et al.* [106] suggest that the experience of a tunnel is associated with the presence of severe medical conditions (such as cardiac arrest, drowning, trauma, profuse blood loss), as opposed to mild injuries, fear, or fatigue. Woerlee [109] provides the following example: 'After I had floated close to the ceiling for a short time, I was sucked into a tunnel … It was black and dark around me, somewhat frightening, but this did not last long: at the end of the tunnel I saw a clear light towards which I travelled.' (p. 211). The tunnel experience or darkness may thus be associated with the subsequent experience of an intense light. Drab [108] found this to be the case in half of the subjects with NDEs who reported the experience of a tunnel. Ring [4] and Sabom [5] found that 30% and Van Lommel *et al.* [80] that 23% of subjects with NDE reported seeing a light, but did not specify if this was associated with the experience of a tunnel. The light is usually white or yellow, very bright, but not experienced as painful.

It seems to cover a larger area in the visual field when subjects experience vection [108].

The Life Review

The life review has been defined as the perception of 'unusually vivid, almost instantaneous visual images of either the person's whole life or a few selected highlights of it' ([85], p. 204). Heim [42] reports the following life review during a mountain fall: '… I saw my whole past-life take places in many images, as though on a stage at some distance from me. I saw myself as the chief character in the performance. Everything was transfigured as though by a heavenly light and everything was beautiful without grief, without anxiety, and without pain.' Life reviews were found in 13–30% of subjects with NDEs [4, 80, 91, 100, 110]. Stevenson and Cook [111] analysed 122 subjects with NDEs and reported that the number of distinct life memories may range from a few images (one or two) to the impression of a rapid flow of countless images depicting their entire life. Some subjects reported that the life review unfolds with an infinite number of images, simultaneously ('all at once'). It is usually experienced very vividly, associated with bright colours and can occur as moving in chronological order or in the opposite order (i.e., ending or starting with childhood; [96]). It can also purportedly involve elements of the future [112]. Two studies speculated that life reviews are especially frequent in drowning victims, as compared to other situations [110, 113]. Conversely, it seems that suicide survivors [114] and children with NDEs [115–116] rarely report life reviews.

Meeting of Spirits

People often report seeing or feeling different entities or people during NDEs. Greyson [117] gives the following example from the report of a man admitted to the hospital due to cardiac disease: '… he experienced an apparent encounter with his deceased mother and brother-in-law, who communicated to him, without speaking, that he should return to his body' (p. 315). The encounters are sometimes identified as supreme beings, pure energy, spiritual guides, angels, helpers, or familiar people, but also as demons or tormentors [118–120]. These encounters are reported frequently during NDEs (40% of the subjects in Ring's study [4]; 52% in Greyson's study ([83]: 'sense of deceased/religious spirits', see Table 23.1). Sometimes subjects report to feel (rather than see) the presence of an unfamiliar person, a mystical, or a supreme entity (reported by 26% of NDE subjects in Greyson [83]).

The seen or felt person may also be familiar, but is most often a deceased relative or friend. Ring [4] and Kelly [120] found that 8% (13%) of seen or felt persons were dead relatives, whereas Fenwick and Fenwick ([121], 39%) and Van Lommel et al. ([80], 32%) found this more frequently. Kelly [120] analyzed this feature further by comparing 74 people with NDEs who reported to have perceived one or more deceased relatives with 200 people with NDE who did not. She found that deceased relatives are more frequently reported than deceased friends or children (in this study only 4% of people with NDEs reported seeing persons that were alive at the time of the NDE [120]). Encounters of dead relatives have long been reported in the occult literature as 'apparitions' and are supposed to be frequent in so-called 'deathbed visions' [92, 122]. Sometimes verbal or thought communication (often described as 'telepathic') has been reported to take place between the subject and the encounters. Physical interactions such as touch or embraces are sometimes described as well [117]. Some of these features have also been reported in neurological patients with heautoscopy [23].

Positive and Negative Emotions

NDE reports often consist of feelings of peace and calm (and sometimes ecstasy), despite the experienced severity of the situation. Whereas Ring [4] found that 60% of subjects with a NDE reported feelings of peace (56% in [80]), Sabom [5] noted such feelings in all of his subjects with NDE. Greyson [83] analyzed the feelings of peace and joy separately and found 85% for peace and 67% for joy. A related feature might be the loss of pain sensations as subjects with NDE often report to be relieved from the unbearable pain they were enduring minutes earlier. Heim [42] reports his own experience when falling from a cliff: 'There was no anxiety, no trace of despair, nor pain; but rather calm seriousness, profound acceptance, and a dominant mental quickness and sense of surety ...' Many subjects also report feelings of absolute love, all encompassing acceptation, often by a supreme entity which is associated with a radiant light. Nevertheless, NDEs may also be associated with negative emotions, 'hell'-like features, encounters with tormentors or frightfully devoid of any meaning [123]. The exact incidence of such negative NDEs is not known, but is assumed to be rather low [117].

Other Features

In this section we have listed other NDE features about which less is known concerning their phenomenology, frequency, and association with other features. These features are realness, mental clarity, sense of time, mystical features, and the experience of border and return.

Realness and mental clarity: Although NDEs are often described as highly realistic sensations, we were not able to find detailed estimates. In the literature we found reports that NDEs are often experienced as 'real' or 'realer than real' [124]. Some authors have argued that NDEs are qualitatively different from dreams or drug-induced hallucinations (e.g., [3]). As one subject wrote: 'For many years, it was the most real thing that ever happened to me. Yes, far more real and vivid than any real-life incident. It was so real, detailed and so vivid and consistent ...; in fact, so totally un-dream-like!' ([96], p. 137). Thus, many subjects with NDEs believe them to involve *actual* disembodiment, meeting of spirits, seeing of lights, or being in the afterworld rather than mere *experiences* thereof. These subjects are often reluctant to refer to NDEs in psychological or neurophysiological terms [82]. Realness is sometimes also reported as mental clarity or cognitive enhancement. Owens et al. [106] found that the report of clear experience, perception, and cognition was more frequent in subjects who suffered serious life-threatening conditions than those who only thought themselves in great biological danger. Greyson [83] found that 44% of NDE subjects reported accelerated thought with their NDE. Heim [42] also refers to this aspect during his mountain fall: 'All my thoughts and ideas were coherent and very clear, and in no way susceptible, as are dreams, to obliteration ... The relationship of events and their probable outcomes were viewed with objective clarity, no confusion entered at all'.

Sense of time: A distorted sense of time is a frequent feature of NDEs, but has not been described in detail in statistical and phenomenological terms. Heim [42] reported that 'time became greatly expanded' during his fall. Greyson [83] found that 67% of NDE subjects reported an alteration of the sense of time, whereas this was much less frequent in a control group of subjects without NDEs (4%). Based on the reviewed phenomenology we suggest that the presence of a distorted sense of time, mental clarity, and life review might co-occur in subjects with NDEs.

Mystical and transcendental features. A feeling of 'oneness' with the universe or of 'cosmic unity' was present in 52% of subjects with NDEs in Greyson's study [83]. Twenty per cent of Ring's [4] subjects and 54% of Sabom's [5] subjects with NDEs reported the 'visit' of a supernaturalistic environment. This value is considerably smaller in people reporting OBEs (~1%; [11]), but more frequent in subjects who report multiple OBEs. Descriptions here vary considerably, but most often seem to involve the experience of seeing pleasant sights like cities of light, green and flowered meadows, and vivid colours. Sometimes, images reminiscent of religious iconography are perceived [125].

Border and Return. A symbolic or concretely perceived limit or border is sometimes reported by subjects with NDEs. Greyson [83] found this in 41% and Van Lommel *et al.* [80] in 8%. NDEs (and OBEs) are often reported to end abruptly without the experience of intentional control [85]. A patient, resuscitated by electrical defibrillation after an anterior myocardial infarction, reported: 'It appeared to me … that I had a choice to re-enter my body and take the chances of them [the medical staff] bringing me around or I could just go ahead and die, if I wasn't already dead. I knew I was going to be perfectly safe, whether my body died or not. They thumped me a second time. I re-entered my body just like that' ([126], p. 65). The immediate aftermath is frequently the return of pain and the realization that one is alive (similar observations have also been reported in neurological patients with OBEs and related experiences such as heautoscopy; see below and [7] case 4).

Folk-psychological Accounts and Psychological Aspects

Following psychoanalytic theory, several researchers consider NDEs as a defence mechanism unfolding in a hopeless, life-threatening situation. Noyes and Kletti [110, 127] were influential with their suggestion that the experience during a NDE may reflect a form of depersonalization, whereby the endangered subject 'separates' from the body and the current events in order to be 'dissociated' from the unsupportable consequences of death and pain. Pfister [128] was perhaps the first to propose a psychoanalytic theory of NDEs. Following Heim's [42] accounts of NDEs in fall survivors, he suggested that 'persons faced with potentially inescapable danger attempt to exclude this unpleasant reality from consciousness and "replace" it with pleasurable fantasies which protect them from being paralysed by emotional shock' ([129], p. 613). By this process, it was then argued that subjects 'split' into an observing self and a body. The OBE component of many NDEs, in particular, has been seen as the prototypic experiential correlate of this detachment [1, 130]. However, this psychoanalytic account has been criticized on several grounds, mostly because of the lack of empirical evidence for it and the differences between the symptoms of dissociation in psychiatric populations and the reports of NDE subjects (for more details, see [131–132]), as well as many

methodological and scientific concerns about psychoanalysis itself. Other psychological authors suggested that NDEs are the consequence of a human tendency to deny death [1, 130], the release of archetypical concepts of death [133], or the (symbolic or literal) regression to the experience of coming to life ([134–135]; but see [96]). These approaches of NDEs suffer from the same methodological and scientific concerns as psychoanalytical propositions.

More quantitative approaches have proposed to analyze psychological variables of people with NDEs, as estimated by interviews and questionnaire surveys. Yet, as with OBEs, no clear psychopathological features have been found [117, 131] and subjects with NDEs and without NDEs do not differ with respect to measures of intelligence, extraversion, neuroticism, or anxiety. Unfortunately, only a small number of subjects with NDEs have been studied in this systematic manner [136–137]. People with NDEs were also found to report more often so-called paranormal experiences prior to their NDE [83, 112], as well as other complex experiences such as OBEs, feelings of being united with the universe, feeling the presence of God and otherworldly entities, or having past-life memories [102]. Kohr [138] found similar tendencies in people with NDEs: they reported repeated OBEs and higher interest in dreams, past-lives, and meditation. This suggests that subjects with NDEs might differ from other subjects in being more open to unusual experiences (and also willing to report these) and being attentive to the so-called inner-states [129]. It might also be that this personality trait is linked to the larger concept of 'magical thinking', which has been shown to depend on right hemispheric activity and affinity to 'paranormal' thought [139]. People with NDEs as well as people with OBEs [11] also score higher than control subjects on absorption (a measure that refers to the tendency to immerse in imagination and internal states) and the related trait of fantasy proneness (a tendency to have vivid hallucinations, blurred distinction between reality and imagination, enhanced sensory experiences and heightened visual imagery) [117, 137]. The fact that this personality factor is shared among subjects with OBEs and NDEs again suggests common predisposing factors. On a related note, Ring [140] suggested that subjects with NDEs are more likely to have suffered abuse, stress, illness, and social problems during childhood than a control group (see also [132]). Measures of dissociation (and depersonalization) have also been associated with NDEs. Subjects with NDEs scored higher than controls, but were below the range of pathological conditions on this measure [141]. Britton and Bootzin [142] also found significantly higher scores in their group of NDE subjects on the Dissociative Experiences Scale (DES) than in their control group (again these scores were different between both groups, but within the normal range).

Neurology of NDEs

Although several authors have speculated on the neurology of NDEs, there is an almost complete absence of neurological data. Medical and neurological conditions that have been associated with NDEs and that are associated with brain interference or brain damage are cardiac arrest, general anaesthesia, temporal lobe epilepsy, electrical brain stimulation, and sleep abnormalities (e.g., REM intrusions). As more systematic studies have focussed on the investigation of the frequency and intensity of NDEs in cardiac arrest patients [80–83] we will start by reviewing these studies with respect to potential neurological mechanisms (see also [143]).

Brain Anoxia in Cardiac Arrest Patients

The data reported in the large prospective study by Van Lommel et al. [80] describes several clinical characteristics of patients that are likely to report a NDE after cardiac arrest. In most of these patients cardiac arrest occurred in the hospital ($n = 234$; 68%) and resuscitation was initiated within 2 minutes after cardiac arrest ($n = 190$; 81%). Loss of consciousness lasted less than 5 minutes ($n = 187$; 80%). Yet, loss of consciousness was diagnosed independently of a neurological or electroencephalographic examination and estimated only by electrocardiogram records. We therefore do not have detailed neurological and EEG data about brain function in the critical clinical period that is frequently assumed to be associated with NDEs. This is likely due to the medical emergency situation and the lack of time to evaluate neurological function during resuscitation. Nevertheless, Van Lommel et al. [80] 'defined clinical death (independent of neurological data) as a period of unconsciousness caused by insufficient blood supply to the brain because of inadequate blood circulation, breathing, or both.' The remaining patients were resuscitated outside the hospital ($n = 101$; 29%) and probably suffered from longer periods of cardiac arrest ($n = 88$; 80%) and probably unconsciousness for more than 10 minutes ($n = 62$; 56%) as estimated by the authors. 36% ($n = 123$) of all investigated patients were unconscious, as defined above, for over an estimated period of 60 minutes.

Twelve per cent of the total of 344 patients investigated in that study [80] reported an NDE. The data showed that younger patients with a first myocardial infarction and with a previous NDE reported NDEs more frequently, while prolonged reanimation was associated with less frequent NDEs. Moreover, male patients and patients who were reanimated outside the hospital reported less NDE features. Van Lommel et al. [80] argue that the diminished frequency of NDEs in patients with prolonged reanimation might be due to memory loss or deficient short-term memory in these patients. This statement seems premature since no quantitative and detailed neurological or neuropsychological assessment on short- or long-term memory was carried out or reported in the acute or later phases of the study. Furthermore, no EEG records and neuroimaging examinations (MRI or computer tomography) were studied and compared between cardiac arrest patients with and without NDEs. We believe that neurological and neuropsychological data as well as EEG and neuroimaging data in cardiac arrest patients with NDEs will be crucial in describing eventually some of the neurocognitive mechanisms of NDEs. Several recent studies have reported neurological data about brain function and brain damage in patients suffering from more serious consequences of cardiac arrest such as prolonged loss of consciousness in coma, vegetative state, minimally conscious state, as well as milder associated neurological conditions (see Chapter 3). Unfortunately, we were not able to find similar studies reporting such data for cardiac arrest patients with NDEs, who are most often considered to have maintained pre-morbid brain functions (although this has never been confirmed by neuropsychological testing). Given the common aetiological origin, we suggest that patients with NDEs following cardiac arrest may suffer from brain damage that is milder, but anatomically similar, to the brain damage reported in patients with mild forms of post-anoxic brain damage of cardiac or pulmonary origin, as for example, reported by Ammermann et al. [144]. This study showed that brain damage in such patients is symmetrical and predominantly affects grey and white matter in several cortical and subcortical regions without affecting the brainstem (Figure 23.3). These regions include the frontal and occipital cortex (including the optic radiation) as well as the hippocampus, the basal ganglia, and the thalamus confirming earlier results that have also revealed damage to watershed regions such as the TPJ [145–147]. Importantly, damage or interference with these regions may be linked to several key features of NDEs (see below).

In the same year than Van Lommel et al.'s publication, a smaller prospective study on NDEs in cardiac arrest survivors was reported [81], but again did not present any neuroimaging data or results of neurological,

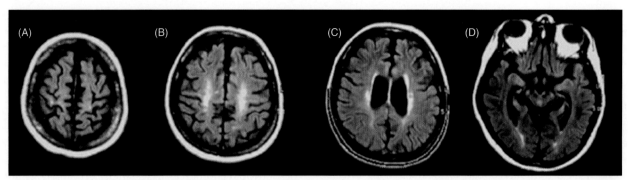

FIGURE 23.3 MRI of the brain of a cardiac arrest patient with excellent recovery. MRI reveals a distinct pattern of brain damage including white matter damage in three brain areas: In proximity of the primary motor and premotor cortex (A and B), periventricular white matter lesions (C), and in proximity of primary visual cortex including the optic radiation (D). *Source*: Modified from Ammermann *et al.* [144] reproduced with permission from Elsevier.

neuropsychological, or EEG examinations. We reiterate that EEG records during or immediately after the cardiac arrest period will be important, as well as multichannel EEG recordings during later periods that would allow detecting or excluding subtle potential abnormalities and correlating them with potential neurological, neuropsychological, and neuroimaging abnormalities. In addition, the patient sample was small [81] and only four cardiac arrest patients (6%) reported NDEs (as defined by the Greyson's scale [91]). A third study [82] found that NDEs occurred with a frequency of 23% in the same clinical population, but also did not report neurological, neuropsychological, EEG, or neuroimaging data. Finally, Greyson [83] found a frequency of 10% and found no differences in cognitive functions between cardiac arrest patients with and without NDEs. For the cognitive examination the investigators applied the mini-mental status that is often used for brief clinical pre-evaluations of patients with dementia [148]. Although, the latter test revealed normal performance in cardiac arrest patients with and without NDEs (score of ~27) this examination does not permit detailed testing of memory, language, spatial thought, visual, auditory, attention, and executive functions as is done with standard neuropsychological examinations. Despite the variability in frequency estimations of NDEs in cardiac arrest survivors in these four studies, the two larger ones seem to agree on 10–12%, but unfortunately do not provide any empirical data on the neurology of NDEs.

Other MRI-based techniques might allow describing potential brain damage in cardiac arrest patients with NDEs. Thus, diffusion-weighted MRI allows the detection of focal cerebral infarctions in the acute phase [149–150], due to its sensitivity for ischaemia-induced changes in water diffusion [151]. Els *et al.* [152] have shown that diffusion-weighted MRI may

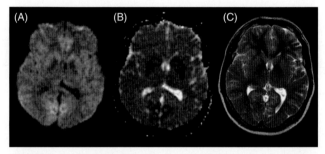

FIGURE 23.4 MRI of the brain of a cardiac arrest patient with excellent recovery. Whereas standard T2-weighted MRI (Figure 23.4C; compare to Figure 23.3) did not reveal any abnormalities, diffusion-weighted MRI in the acute phase (15 hours after resuscitation) revealed MRI abnormalities that are compatible with bilateral brain damage. These are shown in Figure 23.4A and consist of bilateral hyperintense damage in proximity to primary visual cortex and the optic radiation (compare also with Figure 23.3D). In addition, the apparent diffusion coefficient (ADC; Figure 23.4B) maps showed prominent signal decrease in the same locations as DWI, compatible with ischemic brain damage. *Source*: Modified from Els *et al.* [152] with permission from Blackwell Publishing.

allow to reveal correlates of cerebral anoxia in cardiac arrest patients independent of severity of anoxia, that is, even in patients who recover very well (Figure 23.4). Moreover, standard T1 and T2 weighted MRI may not always reveal brain damage in these patients. It thus seems that different techniques of MRI in the acute as well as the chronic phase in such patients will be necessary to reveal potential functional and structural lesions causing distinct features of NDEs.

Several authors have argued that brain anoxia may account for the auditory, visual, and memory aspects of NDEs (heard noises, perceived lights and tunnels, life review, encounters). The mechanisms involved have been proposed to occur as a cascade of events, beginning by a neuronal desinhibition in early visual cortex, spreading to other cortical areas and leading to NDE-features such as tunnel vision and lights [96,109,153–154]. However, the actual sequence of NDE features remains an unexplored area. Based on the reviewed data, it seems clinically plausible that cardiac arrest patients with NDEs may suffer from acute and/or chronic damage or interference with a subset of widespread cortical and subcortical areas, including grey and white matter, that have been described in cardiac arrest patients. Especially, damage to bilateral occipital cortex and the optic radiation (Figure 23.3D and 4C) may lead to the visual features of NDEs such as seeing the tunnel or surrounding darkness (i.e., bilateral peripheral visual field loss) and lights (damage to the optic radiation is often associated with macular sparing and hence centrally preserved vision), whereas interference with the hippocampus may lead to heightened emotional experiences and experiential phenomena due to epileptogenic interference, including memory flashbacks and the life review (see below). Moreover, interference with the right TPJ may lead to OBEs [7, 23, 33] whereas interference with the left TPJ may cause the feeling of a presence, the meeting of spirits, and heautoscopy [155–156]. This proposition extends previous post-anoxic accounts of NDEs by linking the different features to different brain regions that may be damaged in cardiac arrest patients with rapid recovery of consciousness and neuropsychological functioning. These speculations have to be regarded with caution, as to date, no neurological, neuropsychological, EEG, and neuroimaging data exist to corroborate this claim empirically. We also note that models only based on the pathophysiology of brain anoxia do not account for NDEs occurring in situations that are not related to cardiac arrest such as polytraumatism, general anaesthesia, and hypoglycaemia. Nor do they account for NDEs occurring during mountain falls as well as other fearful situations leading to NDEs [96,129]. As stated by Blackmore [96], brain anoxia is probably one of several, related, mechanisms that lead to NDEs.

Experimental Brain Hypoxia in Healthy Subjects

Lempert et al. [157] have experimentally induced syncopes in 42 healthy subjects using cardiovascular manipulations (hyperventilation, orthostasis, Valsalva manoeuvres) with the aim of investigating the symptoms of transient cerebral hypoxia. They found that many of their subjects reported NDE-like sensations. Thus, 16% had OBEs, 35% feelings of peace and painlessness, 17% saw lights, 47% reported entering another world, 20% encountered unfamiliar beings,

and 8% had a tunnel experience. Two subjects were even reminded of previous spontaneous NDEs. These data suggest that NDEs may be approached experimentally in healthy subjects (although anxiety, vagal effects, as well as other non-hypoxia-related mechanisms may also play an important role [157]).

General Anaesthesia

NDEs may also occur during general anaesthesia. Thus, Cobcroft and Forsdick [72] have reported patients who during general anaesthesia experienced OBEs (see 'General anaesthesia' in the OBE section) as well as sensations of moving in a tunnel, seeing people and operating theatre details, seeing bright lights and surrounding whiteness. This was found in 4% of a large sample of patients having undergone general anaesthesia [72] and was confirmed by other investigators [73–74]. There is also a report of a NDE in a 12-year-old boy (known for mild cerebral palsy) who underwent general anaesthesia for elective uncomplicated surgery [158]. Monitoring during general anaesthesia did not reveal any signs of awakening, hypoxia, ischaemia, or hypoglycaemia. Yet, this young patient, who did not know about NDEs, reported the following 'strange dream': 'I was sleeping and suddenly I felt awake and had the impression that I was leaving my body … I could see from above my whole body lying on the back on the operating table … and surrounded by many doctors … I felt as being above my physical body … I was like a spirit … and I was floating under the ceiling of the room. … but then I had a sensation of lightness … and I felt relaxed and comfortable … I had the impression that everything was real … I then saw a dark tunnel in front of me … and I felt attracted to it … I passed through the tunnel very fast and at its end I saw … a bright light … I heard noises … [and] voices … [158]'. Interestingly, anaesthetic agents such as propofol (as applied in this patient) are known to have neuroexcitatory effects [159] inducing in some patients seizure-like activity and decreased metabolism in the dorsolateral pre-frontal cortex, posterior parietal cortex (including the TPJ), and temporal lobe [160]. Lopez et al. [158] speculated accordingly that interferences of anaesthetic agents in these areas may lead to the induction of some features of NDE, such as OBEs, seeing lights, being dragged through a tunnel and peace of mind.

Independent of general anaesthesia, substances such as Ketamine, LSD and cannabinoids, as well as many others [161–163] may also lead to experiences resembling some of the NDE features, like the feelings of joy and bliss, visual hallucinations (including tunnels, lights and people), transcendental features

[163–164], and OBEs [10–64]. Feelings that the experience is veridical are not rare when using such substances, as well as the impression of 'mental clarity' and enhanced cognition [163]. Other authors, however, argued that drug administration, instead of facilitating NDEs, may also diminish their frequency [4–5] or have no effect on the frequency of NDEs (in cardiac arrest patients; [80, 83]).

Epilepsy and Brain Stimulation

Many observations link NDEs to epilepsy and especially to complex partial seizures. This evidence includes (i) interictal EEG signs (spikes and spike-waves) in subjects with NDEs; (ii) interictal manifestations such as the interictal temporal lobe syndrome; (iii) similarity of NDEs with several known sensory and cognitive ictal symptoms; (iv) experimental induction of some of these symptoms by electrical cortical stimulation in awake humans; (v) and frequent damage to the hippocampus, a major epileptogenic region, in cardiac arrest patients.

Whereas the neurological examination is frequently normal in patients with temporal lobe epilepsy, neuropsychological examinations often reveal mild to moderate memory impairments characterized by deficits in learning, recognition, delayed recall, or fluency tasks either for verbal or visuo-spatial material [165–166]. Moreover, these distinct memory deficits have been correlated with hippocampal sclerosis, decreased volume, and metabolic changes of this structure, as shown by functional MRI, magnetic resonance volumetry, and magnetic resonance spectroscopy [167–168]. Such examinations in cardiac arrest patients with NDEs might thus reveal similar circumscribed deficits and brain damage, at least in some of these patients.

Britton and Bootzin [142] performed EEG recordings via 19 scalp electrodes in healthy subjects who have reported a previous NDE. They were able to demonstrate the presence of abnormal epileptic interictal EEG activity over the left mid-temporal region in 22% of these subjects (one subject had bilateral abnormal activity). No epileptic seizures were recorded in or reported by any of the subjects. Abnormal activity was most prominent over mid-temporal regions and characterized by spikes and spike-waves, as well as sharp waves (Figure 23.5). The authors added that subjects with NDE also reported more often than the control group several temporal lobe symptoms (TLS) (Figure 23.6) compatible with the interictal temporal lobe syndrome [169]. These include deepened emotionality, nascent religious interest, enhanced philosophical preoccupation, moralism, sense of personal destiny, as well as others (although patients with temporal lobe epilepsy

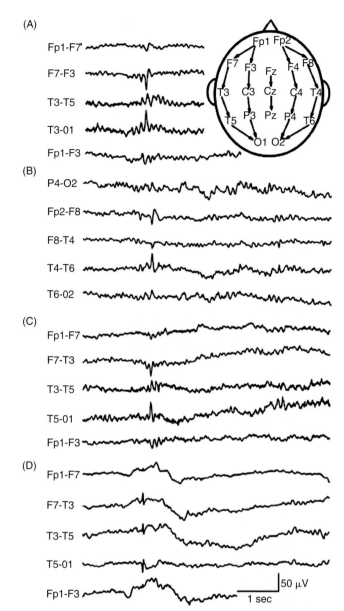

FIGURE 23.5 Examples of interictal epileptiform discharges in the temporal lobe of subjects with NDE. (A), (B), and (C) Stage 2 sleep; (D) REM sleep. The illustration of the head shows the placement of the electrodes in the 10–20 system with an anterior–posterior bipolar reference scheme. Each tracing shows the localized brain activity from the area of the two electrodes indicated. *Source*: From Britton and Bootzin [142]; with permission from Blackwell Publishing.

may not always show these signs [170–172]). Finally, Britton and Bootzin [142] report that abnormal epileptic activity in subjects with previous NDEs was correlated with their score on an NDE scale [91], but not with trauma-related measures such as post-traumatic stress disorder, dissociation, or previous head trauma.

Many features of the NDE have been described as symptoms of epileptic seizures and have also been

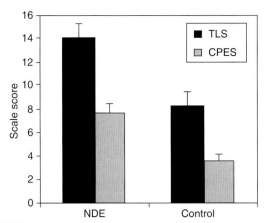

FIGURE 23.6 Symptoms evocative of interictal and ictal temporal lobe syndrome in subjects with NDE. Scores on the temporal lobe symptoms (TLS) and complex partial epileptic signs (CPES) subscales of the Personal Philosophy Inventory [197] in subjects with NDE and a control group of age- and gender-matched participants with no history of life-threatening event. Items include experiences of sleepwalking, olfactory hypersensitivity, hypergraphia, feelings of intense personal significance and unusual perceptions. *Source*: From Britton and Bootzin [142]; with permission from Blackwell Publishing.

induced in a controlled setting by electrical cortical stimulation. Thus, direct electrical cortical stimulation [33, 173] and focal epileptic activity at the TPJ [7, 19] may induce OBEs as well as vestibular sensations [7, 33, 173–174]. Memory flashbacks and life reviews have long been known to occur as a symptom of temporal lobe epilepsy and are generally referred to as experiential phenomena [175–180]. Experiential phenomena have also been induced by electrical cortical stimulation of the temporal lobe, the hippocampus, and the amygdala [177–180], as well as the frontal and the parietal cortex [181–183]. One of Hughlings Jackson's [175] patients with temporal lobe epilepsy describes an ictal life review: 'The past is as if present, a blending of past ideas with present … a peculiar train of ideas of the reminiscence of a former life, or rather, perhaps, of a former psychologic state.' ([184], p. 1741). Recently, Vignal *et al.* [185] re-investigated memory flashbacks and life reviews in patients with pharmacoresistant epilepsy during spontaneous seizures and by electrical cortical stimulation with intracranial electrodes. Among a population of 180 subjects, they found 17 patients that described 55 memory flashbacks. These were quite variable, but could be repeatedly evoked in a given subject by the electrical stimulation of specific areas. Within the temporal cortex, Vignal *et al.* [185] evoked memory flashbacks and life reviews by electrical stimulation of the amygdala, the hippocampus, and the parahippocampal gyrus. One evoked memory flashback was: '… it is always thoughts from

childhood, it is always visual, it is a place behind the house, the field were my father put his car, near a lake … Yes, it is pleasant because we were going to get the car from behind the house, it is a happy memory, it is never unpleasant' ([185], p. 92). Similar observations have been reported earlier by Penfield and Jaspers [176] by electrical stimulation of the lateral temporal cortex. This suggests that both the stimulation of the medial and the lateral temporal structures can be at the origin of experiential phenomena, including memory flashbacks and life review. Another feature of the NDE that can be observed in epileptic seizures and by electrical cortical stimulation is the feeling of a presence, namely the experience of feeling and believing that someone is nearby, without being able to see this person [155, 186–189]. Arzy *et al.* [156] were able to induce the feeling of a presence by electrical cortical stimulation in a patient with pharmacoresistant epilepsy undergoing pre-surgical epilepsy evaluation. The patient reported an 'illusory shadow', who mimicked her body position and posture when her left TPJ was stimulated. She also reported a negative feeling about the experience, sensing hostile intentions from this unfamiliar 'shadow'. The feeling of a presence (in neurological or psychiatric patients) may also be quite elaborated and the felt person may be identified or interpreted as a mystical or supreme entity, or guardian angel ([7] (case 5), [31, 155]). The seen double during heautoscopy has also been linked to the left TPJ [23] and may also be experienced as a mystical or supreme entity ([7] (case 4), [23]). The experience of such a heautoscopic double may be of great emotional and personal relevance [8, 155]. Also, heautoscopy is often associated with the experience of sharing of thoughts, words, or actions with the double or other people. Thus, patients with heautoscopy (but not OBEs) experience to hear the autoscopic body talk to them [190] or experience that they communicate with the illusory body by thought ([7], case 5), a finding reminiscent of people reporting about the meeting of spirits during NDEs. Other patients with heautoscopy stated that the autoscopic body is performing the actions they were supposed to do ([19], case 9) or fights with other people that could be of potential danger to the patient ([7], case 5).

To summarize, many NDE features (OBE, feeling of presence, meeting with spirits, memory flashbacks, and life review) are known symptoms of epileptic discharge or electrical stimulation of hippocampus, amygdala, and parahippocampal gyrus as well as more lateral, neocortical temporal areas including the TPJ. The most common cause of temporal lobe epilepsy is hippocampal dysplasia and sclerosis following brain anoxia, as the hippocampus is one of the most anoxia-sensitive brain regions in humans, and is damaged in almost all patients with cardiac arrest (as well as the TPJ which is a classical watershed region). Although more empirical investigations on this issue are clearly needed, interference and damage to hippocampus and TPJ and consequent clinical and subclinical manifestations of partial epileptic seizures thus seem likely candidates as major pathomechanisms of NDEs.

Sleep Abnormalities and Brainstem Mechanisms

Recently it has been suggested that subjects with NDEs report more frequently symptoms that might be associated with a sleep disorder associated with REM intrusions (or rapid eye movement intrusions) as compared to age-matched control subjects without NDEs [86, 107] (see chapter 8 for more details on REM sleep). This was especially the case in subjects who had NDEs with OBEs (whether as part of their NDE or occurring at a different time [107]). REM intrusions were estimated based on questions such as 'Just before falling asleep or just after awakening, have you ever seen things, objects or people that others cannot see?' and 'Have you ever awakened and found that you were unable to move or felt paralyzed?'. Both items were reported significantly more often in subjects with NDEs. Visual and auditory hallucinations were also reported to be more frequent in subjects with OBEs during NDEs. Nelson et al. [86, 107] suggest that NDEs and OBEs may be related to muscular atonia during REM intrusions due to abnormal brainstem processing. REM intrusions are relatively frequent in the normal population and associated with sleep paralysis (a temporary paralysis of the body during sleep–wake transitions) in about 6% of the population. Symptoms similar to NDEs are also found in other medical conditions involving sleep or brainstem disturbances such as narcolepsy (a disorder involving excessive daytime sleepiness; [191]), peduncular hallucinations [192], hypnagogic and hypnopompic hallucinations [193], as well as sleep paralysis [194]. Finally, patients with Guillain-Barré syndrome (an acute autoimmune disturbance of the peripheral nervous system leading in some cases to severe peripheral sensorimotor deficits that may require intensive care) have also been reported to have OBEs as well as NDE-like features [195]. In a series of 139 such patients, mental disturbances have been found in 31% and included vivid and unusual dreams, visual illusions and hallucinations, as well as paranoid delusions. Interestingly, REM sleep was highly abnormal in these particular patients. The investigators did not inquire about OBEs directly, but some patients reported relevant phenomena such as vivid or dreamlike sensations of losing the sense of one's body, meeting people, hovering or floating weightlessly over their body, or having the impression to have left one's body. Moreover, patients with the Guillain-Barré syndrome also reported complex own body illusions that have been linked functionally to OBEs such as illusory body-part dislocations, the inversion-illusion, and room-tilt illusion [7, 34–35].

COGNITIVE NEUROSCIENCE OF NDE PHENOMENA

The reviewed data suggest that many functional and neural mechanisms are involved in the generation of the wide range of phenomena grouped under the term NDE. These mechanisms include mainly visual, vestibular, multisensory, memory, and motor mechanisms. Concerning brain regions the reviewed studies suggest damage to and/or interference with different cortical, subcortical, and brainstem mechanisms, as well as the peripheral nervous system. Interference with the functioning of this extended network also seems to occur in situations characterized by stress, physical exhaustion, rapid accelerations or decelerations, and deliberate relaxation. Although the neural mechanisms of many illusions and hallucinations have been described in detail, there are – at this stage – not even preliminary data on the neurology of the different phenomena associated with NDEs. Systematic neurological research is needed to fill this gap as has already been done for related experiences (such as the OBE) or related medical conditions in cardiac arrest patients (coma, vegetative state, minimally conscious states). Although abnormalities in brainstem and peripheral nervous system may lead to NDE phenomena, we argue that major insights into these experiences will be gained by applying research techniques from cognitive neurology and cognitive neuroscience to NDE phenomena in order to reveal their cortical and subcortical mechanisms. We have reviewed evidence that suggests that some NDE phenomena can be linked to distinct brain mechanisms. This was shown for the OBE (damage to right TPJ), tunnel vision and seeing of foveal lights (bilateral occipital damage including the optic radiation with macular sparing and/or foveal hallucinations), feeling of a presence and meeting of spirits (damage to left TPJ), as well as memory flashbacks, life review, and enhanced emotions (hippocampal and amygdala damage). All structures have been shown to be frequently damaged in those cardiac arrest patients that show excellent recovery and who are so far the best studied patient group with NDE phenomena.

Based on the selective sites of brain damage in cardiac arrest patients (with excellent recovery) and the associations of key NDE phenomena to some of these same areas we would like to suggest that two main types of NDEs exist, depending on the predominantly affected hemisphere. We propose that type 1 NDEs are due to bilateral frontal and occipital, but predominantly right hemispheric brain damage affecting the right TPJ and characterized by OBEs, altered sense of time, sensations of flying, lightness, vection, and silence. Type 2 NDEs are also due to bilateral frontal and occipital, but predominantly left hemispheric brain damage affecting the left TPJ and characterized by feeling of a presence, meeting of and communication with spirits, seeing of glowing bodies, as well as voices, sounds, and music without vection. We expect emotions and life review (damage to unilateral or bilateral temporal lobe structures such as the hippocampus and amygdala) as well as lights and tunnel vision (damage to bilateral occipital cortex) to be associated with type 1 and type 2 NDEs. Unfortunately, the few existing empirical studies on NDEs in patients with well-defined medical conditions lack neurological, neuropsychological, neuroimaging, and EEG data and to our knowledge no phenomenological analysis of case collections has tried to differentiate the two different types of NDEs in the way we are proposing here. Our proposition remains therefore speculative. We are confident that future neuroscientific studies in cardiac arrest patients with NDEs are likely to reveal the functional neuroanatomy of several NDE phenomena, likely implicating distributed bilateral cortical and subcortical brain mechanisms. There are also the promising experimental results by Britton and Bootzin [142] and previous earlier suggestions by Persinger [196] that link NDE phenomena to symptoms of temporal lobe epilepsy. We therefore also expect additional insights into the neural mechanisms of NDE phenomena through studies investigating the incidence of NDE phenomena (by carrying out detailed interviews and questionnaires) and neuropsychology in patients with focal epilepsies as well as other neurological patients suffering from focal brain damage.

CONCLUSION

The present review has summarized findings on the functional and neural mechanisms of OBEs and NDEs. Whereas OBEs and their underlying brain mechanisms are currently investigated by several research groups and point to the importance of bodily multisensory integration at the right TPJ, the data on the neural mechanisms of NDEs are extremely sparse or altogether absent. We have argued above that the investigation of NDEs in cardiac arrest patients as well as neurological patients may be one possibility to start investigating the functional and neural mechanisms of NDEs. We agree with French [143] who suggested that 'given the heterogenous nature of the NDE … [t]here is no reason to assume that a single comprehensive theory will explain the entire phenomenon'. We add that there is also no reason to assume that an NDE is just one phenomenon, as opposed to a group of loosely associated experiences due to interference with different brain functions and brain mechanisms. Yet, after countless studies and speculations that have focussed on 'life after life' and 'survival of bodily death' in 'survivors' of life-threatening situations, we propose that future studies on NDEs may want to focus on the functional and neural mechanisms of NDE phenomena in patient populations as well as healthy subjects. We speculate that this might eventually lead to the demystification of NDEs, just as that of OBEs is well under way. More importantly, the scientific study of these varied complex experiences may allow studying the functional and neural mechanisms of beliefs, personality, spirituality, and the self, that have and will continue to intrigue scientists, scholars, and laymen alike.

References

1. Menz, R.L. (1984) The denial of death and the out-of-the-body experience. *J Relig Health* 23:317–329.
2. Blackmore, S.J. (1994) Out-of-body experiences and confusionism: A response to Woodhouse. *New Ideas Psychol* 12:27–30.
3. Moody, R.A. (1975) *Life after Life*, Covington, GA: Mockingbird Books.
4. Ring, K. (1980) *Life at Death: A Scientific Investigation of the Near-Death Experience*, New York: Conward, McCann & Geoghegan.
5. Sabom, M.B. (1982) *Recollections of Death: A Medical Investigation*, New York: Harper & Row.
6. Blackmore, S. (1982) *Beyond the Body: An Investigation of Out-of-Body Experiences*, London: Heinemann.
7. Blanke, O., et al. (2004) Out-of-body experiences and autoscopy of neurological origin. *Brain* 127:243–258.
8. Brugger, P. (2002) Reflective mirrors: Perspective taking in autoscopic phenomena. *Cogn Neuropsychiatr* 7:179–194.
9. Green, C.E. (1968) *Out-of-the-Body Experiences*, London: Hamish Hamilton.
10. Bünning, S. and Blanke, O. (2005) The out-of-body experience: Precipitating factors and neural correlates. *Prog Brain Res* 150:331–350.
11. Irwin, H.J. (1985) *Flight of Mind: A Psychological Study of the Out-of-Body Experience*, Metuchen, NJ: The Scarecrow Press Inc.
12. Alvarado, C.S. (2001) Features of out-of-body experiences in relation to perceived closeness to death. *J Nerv Ment Dis* 189:331–332.
13. Alvarado, C.S. (2000) Out-of-body experiences. In Cardeña, E. et al., (eds.) *Varieties of Anomalous Experiences*, pp. 183–218 Washington, DC: American Psychological Association.

14. Blackmore, S. (2003) *Consciousness: An Introduction*, Oxford: Oxford University Press.

15. Zahavi, D. (2005) *Subjectivity and Selfhood: Investigating the First-Person Perspective*, Cambridge: MIT Press.

16. Metzinger, T. (2003) *Being No One*, Cambridge: MIT Press.

17. Metzinger, T. (2005) Out-of-body experiences as the origin of the concept of a 'soul'. *Mind Matter* 3:57–84.

18. Palmer, J. (1978) The out-of-body experiences: A psychological theory. *Parapsychol Rev* 9:19–22.

19. Devinsky, O., *et al.* (1989) Autoscopic phenomena with seizures. *Arch Neurol* 46:1080–1088.

20. Brugger, P., *et al.* (1997) Illusory reduplication of one's own body: Phenomenology and classification of autoscopic phenomena. *Cogn Neuropsychiatr* 2:19–38.

21. Grüsser, O.J. and Landis, T. (1991) The splitting of 'I' and 'me': Heautoscopy and related phenomena. In Grüsser, O.J. and Landis, T. (eds.) *Visual Agnosias and Other Disturbances of Visual Perception and Cognition*, pp. 297–303. Amsterdam: Macmillan.

22. Sheils, D. (1978) A cross-cultural study of beliefs in out-of-the-body experiences, waking and sleeping. *J Soc Psychol Res* 49:697–741.

23. Blanke, O. and Mohr, C. (2005) Out-of-body experience, heautoscopy, and autoscopic hallucination of neurological origin: Implications for neurocognitive mechanisms of corporeal awareness and self consciousness. *Brain Res Rev* 50:184–199.

24. Blanke, O. and Arzy, S. (2005) The out-of-body experience: Disturbed self-processing at the temporo-parietal junction. *Neuroscientist* 11:16–24.

25. Muldoon, S. and Carrington, H. (1951) *The Phenomena of Astral Projection*, London: Rider & Co.

26. Yram. (1972) *Practical Astral Projection*, New York: Samuel Weiser.

27. Monroe, R.A. (1974) *Journeys Out of the Body*, London: Corgi.

28. Lippman, C.W. (1953) Hallucinations of physical duality in migraine. *J Nerv Ment Dis* 117:345–350.

29. Hécaen, H. and Green, A. (1957) Sur l'héautoscopie. *Encéphale* 46:581–594.

30. Daly, D.D. (1958) Ictal affect. *Am J Psychiatr* 115:171–181.

31. Lunn, V. (1970) Autoscopic phenomena. *Acta Psychiatr Scand* 46 (Suppl. 219):118–125.

32. Maillard, L., *et al.* (2004) Semiologic value of ictal autoscopy. *Epilepsia* 45:391–394.

33. Blanke, O., *et al.* (2002) Stimulating illusory own body perceptions. *Nature* 419:269–270.

34. Lopez, C. and Blanke, O. (2007) Neuropsychology and neurophysiology of self-consciousness: Multisensory and vestibular mechanisms. In Holderegger, A. *et al.* (eds.) *Hirnforschung und Menschenbild. Beiträge zur interdisziplinären Verständingung.* pp. 183–206. Academic Press, Fribourg and Schwabe, Basel.

35. Lopez, C., *et al.* (2007) Body ownership and embodiment: Vestibular and multisensory mechanisms. *Neurophysiol Clin.* 38:149–161.

36. Smith, B.H. (1960) Vestibular disturbances in epilepsy. *Neurology* 10:465–469.

37. Brandt, T. (1999) Central vestibular disorders. In Brandt, T. (ed.) *Vertigo: Its Multisensory Syndromes*, 2nd Edition. pp. 167–246. London: Springer.

38. Lackner, J.R. (1992) Sense of body position in parabolic flight. *Ann NY Acad Sci* 656:329–339.

39. Mittelstaedt, H. and Glasauer, S. (1993) Illusions of verticality in weightlessness. *Clin Investig* 71:732–739.

40. Hécaen, H. and de Ajuriaguerra, J. (1952) *Méconnaissances et Hallucinations Corporelles*, Paris: Masson.

41. Dening, T.R. and Berrios, G.E. (1994) Autoscopic phenomena. *Br J Psychiatr* 165:808–817.

42. Heim, A. (1892) Notizen über den Tod durch Absturz. *Jahrbuch des Schweizer Alpenklub* 27:327–337.

43. Ravenhill, T.H. (1913) Some experiences of mountain sickness in the Andes. *J Trop Med Hyg* 16:313–320.

44. Habeler, P. (1979) *The Lonely Victory*, New York: Simon and Shuster, pp. 166–176.

45. Brugger, P., *et al.* (1999) Hallucinatory experiences in extreme-altitude climbers. *Neuropsychi Neuropsy Behav Neurol* 12:67–71.

46. Firth, P.G. and Bolay, H. (2004) Transient high altitude neurological dysfunction: An origin in the temporoparietal cortex. *High Alt Med Biol* 5:71–75.

47. Benson, A.J. (1999) Spatial disorientation: Common illusions. In Ernsting, J. *et al.*, (eds.) *Aviation Medicine*, 3rd Edition. pp. 437–454. Oxford: Butterworth & Heinmann.

48. Clark, B. and Graybiel, A. (1957) The break-off phenomenon: A feeling of separation from the earth experienced by pilots at high altitude. *J Aviat Med* 28:121–126.

49. Sours, J.A. (1965) The 'break-off' phenomenon: A precipitant of anxiety in jet aviators. *Arch Gen Psychiatr* 13:447–456.

50. Tormes, F.R. and Guedry, F.E. (1975) Disorientation phenomena in naval helicopters pilots. *Aviat Space Environ Med* 46:387–393.

51. Menninger-Lerchenthal, E. (1935) *Das Truggebilde der eigenen Gestalt (Heautoskopie, Doppelgänger)*, Berlin: Kärger.

52. Lhermitte, J. (1939) *L'Image de Notre Corps*, Paris: L'Harmattan.

53. Zutt, J. (1953) 'Aussersichsein' und 'auf sich selbst Zurückblicken' als Ausnahmezustand: Zur Psychopathologie des Raumerlebens. *Nervenarzt* 24:24–31.

54. Blackmore, S. (1986) Out-of-body experiences in schizophrenia: A questionnaire survey. *J Nerv Ment Dis* 174:615–619.

55. Röhricht, F. and Priebe, S. (1997) Disturbances of body experience in schizophrenic patients. *Fortschr Neurol Psychiatr* 65:323–336.

56. Reynolds, M. and Brewin, C.R. (1999) Intrusive memory in depression and posttraumatic stress disorder. *Behav Res Ther* 37:201–215.

57. McCreery, C. and Claridge, G. (1995) Out-of-the-body experiences and personality. *J Soc Psych Res* 60:129–148.

58. McCreery, C. and Claridge, G. (2002) Healthy schizotypy: The case of out-of-the-body experiences. *Pers Indiv Differ* 32: 141–154.

59. Mohr, C., *et al.* (2006) Perceptual aberrations impair mental own-body transformations. *Behav Neurosci* 120:528–534.

60. Arzy, S., *et al.* (2007) Duration and not strength of activation in temporo-parietal cortex positively correlates with schizotypy. *Neuroimage* 35:326–333.

61. Murray, C.D. and Fox, J. (2005) Dissociational body experiences: Differences between respondents with and without prior out-of-body-experiences. *Br J Psychol* 96:441–456.

62. Murray, C.D. and Fox, J. (2005) The out-of-body experience and body image: Differences between experients and nonexperients. *J Nerv Ment Dis* 193:70–72.

63. Terhune, D.B. (2006) Dissociative alterations in body image among individuals reporting out-of-body experiences: A conceptual replication. *Perc Motor Skills* 103:76–80.

64. Tart, C. (1971) *On Being Stoned: A Psychological Study of Marijuana Intoxication*, Palo Alto: Science and Behaviour Books.

65. Aizenberg, D. and Modai, I. (1985) Autoscopic and drug induced perceptual disturbances: A case report. *Psychopathology* 18:97–111.

66. Siegel, R.K. (1977) Hallucinations. *Sci Am* 237:132–140.

67. Spitellie, P.H., *et al.* (2002) Awareness during anesthesia. *Anesthesiol Clin N Am* 20:555–570.

68. Sandin, R.H. (2003) Awareness 1960–2002, explicit recall of events during general anesthesia. *Adv Exp Med Biol* 523:135–147.

69. Sandin, R.H., *et al.* (2000) Awareness during anesthesia: A prospective case study. *Lancet* 355:707–711.

70. Crookall, R. (1964) *More Astral Projections: Analyses of Case Histories*, London: Aquarian Press.

71. Ranta, S.O.V., *et al.* (1998) Awareness with recall during general anesthesia: Incidence and risk factors. *Anesth Analg* 86:1084–1089.

72. Cobcroft, M.D. and Forsdick, C. (1993) Awareness under anesthesia: the patients' point of view. *Anaesth Intens Care* 21:837–843.

73. Ostermann, J.E., *et al.* (2001) Awareness under anesthesia and the development of post traumatic stress disorder. *Gen Hosp Psychiatr* 23:193–204.

74. Moermann, N., *et al.* (1993) Awareness and recall during general anesthesia. *Anesthesiology* 79:454–464.

75. Irwin, H.J. (1999) Out-of-body experiences. In Irwin, H.J. (ed.) *An Introduction to Parapsychology*, 3rd Edition. pp. 219–241. Jefferson, NC: McFarland.

76. Ringelstein, E.B. and Zunker, P. (1998) Low-flow infarction. In Ginsberg, M. and Bogousslavsky, J. (eds.) *Cerebrovascular Disease: Pathophysiology, Diagnosis and Management*, Vol. 2, pp. 1075–1089. Cambridge: Blackwell Science Inc.

77. Blanke, O., *et al.* (2005) Linking out-of-body experience and self processing to mental own-body imagery at the temporoparietal junction. *J Neurosci* 25:550–557.

78. Arzy, S., *et al.* (2006) Neural basis of embodiment: Distinct contributions of temporoparietal junction and extrastriate body area. *J Neurosci* 26:8074–8081.

79. Lenggenhager, B., *et al.* (2006) Functional and neural mechanisms of embodiment: Importance of the vestibular system and the temporal parietal junction. *Rev Neurosci* 17:643–657.

80. Van Lommel, P., *et al.* (2001) Near-death experience in survivors of cardiac arrest: A prospective study in the Netherlands. *Lancet* 358:2039–2045.

81. Parnia, S., *et al.* (2001) A qualitative and quantitative study of the incidence features and aetiology of near-death experiences in cardiac arrest survivors. *Resuscitation* 48:149–156.

82. Schwaninger, J., *et al.* (2002) A prospective analysis of near-death experiences in cardiac arrest patients. *J Near Death Stud* 20:215–232.

83. Greyson, B. (2003) Incidence and correlates of near-death experiences in a cardiac care unit. *Gen Hosp Psychiatr* 25:269–276.

84. Moody, R.A. (1977) *Reflections on Life After Life*, St. Simon's Island, GA: Mockingbird Books.

85. Irwin, H.J. (1999) Near-death experiences. In Irwin, H.J. (ed.) *An Introduction to Parapsychology*, 3rd Edition. pp. 199–217. Jefferson, NC: McFarland.

86. Nelson, K.R., *et al.* (2006) Does the arousal system contribute to near death experience? *Neurology* 66:1003–1009.

87. Greyson, B. (2005) 'False positive' claims of near-death experiences and 'false negative' denials of near-death experiences. *Death Stud* 29:145–155.

88. Smith, R.P. (1991) The examination of labels – a beginning. *J Near Death Stud* 9:205–209.

89. Greyson, B. (1999) Defining near-death experiences. *Mortality* 4:7–19.

90. Greyson, B. (1998) The incidence of near-death experiences. *Med Psychiatr* 1:92–99.

91. Greyson, B. (1983) The near-death experience scale: Construction, reliability, and validity. *J Nerv Ment Dis* 185:327–334.

92. Osis, K. and Harraldsson, E. (1977) *At the Hour of Death*, New York: Avon.

93. Zaleski, C. (1988) *Otherworld Journeys: Accounts of near-death experience in medieval and modern times*, Oxford: Oxford University Press.

94. Walker, B.A. and Serdahely, W.J. (1990) Historical perspectives on near-death phenomena. *J Near Death Stud* 9:105–121.

95. Groth-Marnat, G. (1994) Cross-cultural perspectives on the near-death experience. *Aust Parapsychol Rev* 19:7–11.

96. Blackmore, S. (1993) *Dying to Live: Near-Death Experiences*, Buffalo, NY: Prometheus Books.

97. Greyson, B. (2007) Consistency of near-death experience accounts over two decades: Are reports embellished over time? *Resuscitation* 73:407–411.

98. Lange, R., *et al.* (2004) A Rasch scaling validation of a 'core' near-death experience. *Br J Psychol* 95:161–177.

99. Greyson, B. (1985) A typology of near-death experiences. *Am J Psychiatr* 142:967–969.

100. Noyes, R. and Slymen, D. (1978–1979) The subjective response to life-threatening danger. *Omega* 9:313–321.

101. Lundahl, C.R. (1993) The near-death experience: A theoretical summarization. *J Near Death Stud* 12:105–118.

102. Greyson, B. and Stevenson, I. (1980) The phenomenology of near-death experiences. *Am J Psychiatr* 137:1193–1196.

103. Greyson, B. (1993) Varieties of near-death experiences. *Psychiatry* 56:390–399.

104. Alvarado, C.S. (2001) Features of out-of-body experiences in relation to perceived closeness to death. *J Nerv Ment Dis* 189:331–332.

105. Gabbard, G.O., *et al.* (1981) Do 'near-death experiences' occur only near death? *J Nerv Ment Dis* 169:374–377.

106. Owens, J.E., *et al.* (1990) Features of 'near-death experience' in relation to whether or not patients were near death. *Lancet* 336:1175–1177.

107. Nelson, K.R., *et al.* (2007) Out-of-body experience and arousal. *Neurology* 68:794–795.

108. Drab, K. (1981) The tunnel experience: Reality or hallucination? *Anabiosis* 1:126–152.

109. Woerlee, G.M. (2005) *Mortal Minds: The Biology of Near-Death Experiences*, Amherst, NY: Prometheus Books.

110. Noyes, R. and Kletti, R. (1977) Depersonalisation in response to life-threatening danger. *Comprehen Psychiatr* 18:375–384.

111. Stevenson, I. and Cook, E.W. (1995) Involuntary memories during severe physical illness or injury. *J Nerv Ment Dis* 183:452–458.

112. Groth-Marnat, G. (1989) Paranormal phenomena and the near-death experience. In Zollschan, G.Z. *et al.*, (eds.) *Exploring the Paranormal: Perspectives on Belief Experience*, pp. 105–116. Sturminster Newton: Prism Press.

113. Dlin, B.M. (1980) The experience of surviving almost certain death. *Adv Psychosom Med* 10:111–118.

114. Rosen, D.H. (1975) Suicide survivors. *West J Med* 122:289–294.

115. Morse, M., *et al.* (1986) Childhood near-death experiences. *Am J Dis Child* 140:1110–1114.

116. Serdahely, W.J. (1990) Pediatric near-death experiences. *J Near Death Stud* 9:33–39.

117. Greyson, B. (2000) Near-death experiences. In Cardeña, E. *et al.* (eds.) *Varieties of Anomalous Experiences*, pp. 315–352. Washington, DC: American Psychological Association.

118. Judson, I.R. and Wiltshaw, E. (1983) A near-death experience. *Lancet* 2:561–562.

119. Lundahl, C.R. (1992) Angels in near-death experiences. *J Near Death Stud* 11:49–56.

120. Kelly, E.W. (2001) Near-death experiences with reports of meeting deceased people. *Death Stud* 25:229–249.

121. Fenwick, P. and Fenwick, E. (1996) *The Truth in the Light: An Investigation of over 300 Near-Death Experiences*, New York: Penguin.

122. Barrett, W. (1926) *Death-bed Visions*, London: Methuen.

123. Greyson, B. and Bush, N.E. (1992) Distressing near-death experiences. *Psychiatry* 55:95–110.
124. Potts, M. (2002) The evidential value of near-death experiences for belief in life after death. *J Near Death Stud* 20:233–258.
125. Irwin, H.J. (1987) Images of heaven. *Parapsychol Rev* 18:1–4.
126. Rogo, S. (1986) *Life after Death: The Case for Survival of Bodily Death*, London: Guild Publishing.
127. Noyes, R. and Kletti, R. (1976) Depersonalization in the face of life-threatening danger: A description. *Psychiatry* 39:19–27.
128. Pfister, O. (1930) Shockdenken und Shock-Phantasien bei Höchster Todesgefahr. *International Zeitung Psychoanalysis* 16:430–455.
129. Roberts, G. and Owen, J. (1988) The near-death experience. *Br J Psychiatr* 153:607–617.
130. Ehrenwald, J. (1974) Out-of-the-body experiences and the denial of death. *J Nerv Ment Dis* 159:227–233.
131. Gabbard, G.O. and Twemlow, S.W. (1984) *With the eyes of the mind: An empirical analysis of out-of-body states*, New York: Praeger.
132. Irwin, H.J. (1993) The near-death experience as a dissociative phenomenon: An empirical assessment. *J Near Death Stud* 12:95–103.
133. Grosso, M. (1983) Jung, parapsychology, and the near-death experience: Toward a transpersonal paradigm. *Anabiosis* 3:3–38.
134. Grof, S. and Halifax, J. (1977) *The Human Encounter with Death*, New York: Dutton.
135. Sagan, C. (1979) *Broca's Brain: Reflections on the Romance of Science*, New York: Random House.
136. Locke, T.P. and Shontz, F.C. (1983) Personality correlates of the near-death experience: A preliminary study. *J Am Soc Psychical Res* 77:311–318.
137. Twemlow, S.W. and Gabbard, G.O. (1984) The influence of demographic/psychological factors and pre-existing conditions on the near-death experience. *Omega* 15:223–235.
138. Kohr, R.L. (1983) Near-death experiences, altered states, and psi sensitivity. *J Near Death Stud* 3:157–176.
139. Brugger, P. and Taylor, K.I. (2003) ESP: Extrasensory perception or effect of subjective probability? *J Consc Stud* 6–7:221–246.
140. Ring, K. (1992) *The Omega Project: Near-Death Experiences, UFO Encounters, and Mind at Large*, New York: Morrow.
141. Greyson, B. (2000) Dissociation in people who have near-death experiences: Out of their bodies or out of their minds? *Lancet* 355:460–463.
142. Britton, W.B. and Bootzin, R.R. (2004) Near-death experiences and the temporal lobe. *Psychol Sci* 15:254–258.
143. French, C.C. (2005) Near-death experiences in cardiac arrest survivors. *Prog Brain Res* 150:351–367.
144. Ammermann, H., *et al.* (2007) MRI brain lesion pattern in patients in anoxia-induced vegetative state. *J Neurol Sci* . doi: 10.10.16/j.jns.2007.03.026
145. Adams, J.H., *et al.* (2000) The neuropathology of the vegetative state after an acute brain insult. *Brain* 123:1327–1338.
146. Chalela, J.A., *et al.* (2001) MRI identification of early white matter injury in anoxic-ischemic encephalopathy. *Neurology* 56:481–485.
147. Kinney, H.C. and Samuels, M.A. (1994) Neuropathology of the persistent vegetative state: A review. *J Neuropathol Exp Neurol* 53:548–558.
148. Folstein, M.F., *et al.* (1975) 'Mini-mental state': A practical method for grading the cognitive state of patients for the clinician. *J Psychiatr Res* 12:189–198.
149. Moseley, M.E., *et al.* (1990) Diffusion-weighted MR imaging of anisotropic water diffusion in cat central nervous system. *Radiology* 176:439–445.
150. Rother, J., *et al.* (1996) MR detection of cortical spreading depression immediately after focal ischemia in the rat. *J Cereb Blood Flow Metab* 16:214–220.
151. Fiehler, J., *et al.* (1992) Diffusion-weighted imaging in acute stroke: A tool of uncertain value? *Cerebrovasc Dis* 14:187–196.
152. Els, T., *et al.* (2004) Diffusion-weighted MRI during early global cerebral hypoxia: A predictor for clinical outcome? *Acta Neurol Scand* 110:361–367.
153. Rodin, E.A. (1980) The reality of death experiences: A personal perspective. *J Nerv Ment Dis* 168:259–263.
154. Greyson, B. (1998) Biological aspects of near-death experiences. *Persp Biol Med* 42:14–32.
155. Brugger, P., *et al.* (1996) Unilaterally felt 'presences': The neuropsychiatry of one's invisible *Doppelgänger*. *Neuropsychi Neuropsychol Behav Neurol* 9:114–122.
156. Arzy, S., *et al.* (2006) Induction of an illusory shadow person. *Nature* 443:287 .
157. Lempert, T., *et al.* (1994) Syncope and near-death experience. *Lancet* 344:829–830.
158. Lopez, U., *et al.* (2006) Near-death experience in a boy undergoing uneventful elective surgery under general anesthesia. *Pediatr Anesth* 16:85–88.
159. Walder, B., *et al.* (2002) Seizure-like phenomena and propofol: A systematic review. *Neurology* 58:1327–1332.
160. Veselis, R.A., *et al.* (2002) A neuroanatomical construct for the amnesic effects of propofol. *Anesthesiology* 97:329–337.
161. Carr, D. (1982) Pathophysiology of stress-induced limbic lobe dysfunction: A hypothesis for NDEs. *J Near Death Stud* 2:75–89.
162. Saavedra-Aguilar, J.C. and Gomez-Jeria, J.S. (1989) A neurobiological model for near-death experiences. *J Near Death Stud* 7:205–222.
163. Jansen, K.L.R. (1997) The Ketamine model of the near-death experience: A central role for the *N*-methyl-*D*-aspartate receptor. *J Near Death Stud* 16:5–26.
164. Siegel, R. (1980) The psychology of life after death. *Am Psychol* 35:911–931.
165. Pegna, A.J., *et al.* (1998) Comprehensive postictal neuropsychology improves focus localization in epilepsy. *Eur Neurol* 40:207–211.
166. Flügel, D., *et al.* (2006) A neuropsychological study of patients with temporal lobe epilepsy and chronic interictal psychosis. *Epilepsy Res* 71:117–128.
167. Pegna, A.J., *et al.* (2002) Is the right amygdale involved in visuospatial memory? Evidence from MRI volumetric measures. *Eur Neurol* 47:148–155.
168. Zubler, F., *et al.* (2003) Contralateral medial temporal lobe damage in right but not left temporal lobe epilepsy: A (1)H magnetic resonance spectroscopy study. *J Neurol Neurosurg Psychiatr* 74:1240–1244.
169. Waxman, S.G. and Geschwind, N. (1975) The interictal behavior syndrome of temporal lobe epilepsy. *Arch Gen Psychiatr* 32:1580–1586.
170. Blumer, D. (1999) Evidence supporting the temporal lobe epilepsy personality syndrome. *Neurology* 53 (5 Suppl 2):S9–S12.
171. Schomer, D.L., *et al.* (2000) Temporolimbic epilepsy and behaviour. In Mesulam, M.M. (ed.) *Principles of Behavioural and Cognitive Neurology*, 2nd Edition. pp. 373–405. Oxford: Oxford University Press.
172. Trimble, M. and Freeman, A. (2006) An investigation of religiosity and the Gastaut-Geschwind syndrome in patients with temporal lobe epilepsy. *Epilepsy Behav* 9:407–414.
173. Penfield, W. (1955) The role of the temporal cortex in certain psychical phenomena. *J Ment Sci* 101:451–465.

174. Kahane, P., *et al.* (2003) Reappraisal of the human vestibular cortex by cortical electrical stimulation study. *Ann Neurol* 54:615–624.

175. Jackson, J.H. (1888) On a particular variety of epilepsy ('intellectual aura'): One case with symptoms of organic brain disease. *Brain* 11:179–207.

176. Penfield, W. and Jasper, H. (1954) *Epilepsy and the functional anatomy of the human brain*, Boston, MA: Little, Brown and Co.

177. Gloor, P. (1990) Experiential phenomena of temporal lobe epilepsy: Facts and hypotheses. *Brain* 113:1673–1694.

178. Gloor, P., *et al.* (1982) The role of the limbic system in experiential phenomena of temporal lobe epilepsy. *Ann Neurol* 12:129–144.

179. Bancaud, J., *et al.* (1994) Anatomical origin of deja vu and vivid 'memories' in human temporal lobe epilepsy. *Brain* 117:71–90.

180. Halgren, E., *et al.* (1978) Mental phenomena evoked by electrical stimulation of the human hippocampal formation and amygdale. *Brain* 101:83–117.

181. Bancaud, J. and Talairach, J. (1992) Clinical semiology of frontal lobe seizures. *Adv Neurol* 57:3–58.

182. Chauvel, P., *et al.* (1995) The clinical signs and symptoms of frontal lobe seizures: Phenomenology and classification. *Adv Neurol* 66:115–125.

183. Blanke, O., *et al.* (2000) Simple and complex vestibular responses induced by electrical cortical stimulation of the parietal cortex in humans. *J Neurol Neurosurg Psychiatr* 69:553–556.

184. Hogan, E.R. (2003) The 'dreamy state': John Hughlings-Jackson's ideas of epilepsy and consciousness. *Am J Psychiatr* 160:1740–1747.

185. Vignal, J.P., *et al.* (2007) The dreamy state: Hallucinations of autobiographic memory evoked by temporal lobe stimulations and seizures. *Brain* 130:88–99.

186. Jaspers, K. (1913) Über leibhafte Bewusstheiten (Bewusstheits täuschungen), ein psychopathologisches Elementarsymptom. *Z Pathopsychol* 2:150–161.

187. Lhermitte, J. (1951) The visual hallucination of the self. *BMJ* 1:431–444.

188. Critchley, M. (1955) *The Divine Banquet of the Brain and Other Essays*, New York: Raven Press.

189. Blanke, O., *et al.* (2003) Hearing of a presence. *Neurocase* 9:329–339.

190. Brugger, P., *et al.* (1994) Heautoscopy, epilepsy, and suicide. *J Neurol Neurosurg Psychiatr* 57:838–839.

191. Overeem, S., *et al.* (2001) Narcolepsy: Clinical features, new pathophysiologic insights, and future perspectives. *J Clin Neurophysiol* 18:78–105.

192. Manford, M. and Andermann, F. (1998) Complex visual hallucinations: Clinical and neurobiological insights. *Brain* 121:1819–1840.

193. Takata, K., *et al.* (1998) Night-time hypnopompic visual hallucinations related to REM sleep disorder. *Psychiatr Clin Neurosci* 52:207–209.

194. Cheyne, J.A. (2005) Sleep paralysis episode frequency and number, types, and structure of associated hallucinations. *J Sleep Res* 14:319–324.

195. Cochen, V., *et al.* (2005) Vivid dreams, hallucinations, psychosis and REM sleep in Guillain-Barré syndrome. *Brain* 128:2535–2545.

196. Persinger, M.A. (1994) Near-death experiences: Determining the neuroanatomical pathways by experiential patterns and stimulation in experimental settings. In Bessette, L. (ed.) *Healing: Beyond Suffering or Death*, pp. 277–286. Québec: Chabanel.

197. Persinger, M.A. (1983) Religious and mystical experience as artifacts of temporal lobe functioning: A general hypothesis. *Perc Motor Skills* 57:1257–1262.

The Hippocampus, Memory, and Consciousness

Bradley R. Postle

ABSTRACT

This chapter reviews the cognitive and neurological profile of medial temporal-lobe (MTL) amnesia as relates to conscious phenomenology. Topics include the selectivity of the memory deficit vis-à-vis other cognitive functions; the selectivity of the deficit, within the myriad abilities that can be called mnemonic, to the conscious accessing of information acquired post trauma; the seeming normalcy of many aspects of the patient's conscious experience; and the severe constraints that damage to the MTL places on the candidate information and qualia that can make up the contents of consciousness. Particularly relevant to the latter are relatively recent, still controversial ideas that ascribe to the hippocampus important functions that extend beyond its traditionally accepted role in memory encoding – retrieval of autobiographical episodic memory, relational binding, and imagining new experiences.

PROLOGUE: ROAD TRIP

One of the privileges afforded graduate students at MIT's Behavioural Neuroscience Laboratory has been the opportunity to transport the renowned amnesic

patient H.M. from and to his home, a handful of hours distant, for his roughly semiannual research visits[1]. His renown derived from the profound influence that the study of his global amnesia, first described by Scoville and Milner in 1957 [2], had had on the neuroscience and psychology of memory. For example, it had provided the impetus for lesion studies of the role of the hippocampus and adjacent structures in learning and memory in rodents, nonhuman primates,

---

[1] Anecdotes relating to H.M.'s life as a celebrated patient can be found in [1].

and humans [3], for electrophysiological studies of long-term potentiation (LTP) [4, 5], for the idea of the hippocampus as a cognitive map [6], and for many theoretical models of learning and memory [7].

The convention for H.M.'s transport was for the designated graduate student to travel with a companion, and there was never a shortage of volunteers (typically a fellow student or a postdoc) eager to take a 'road trip' with this famous patient. On one such trip the two scientists-in-training and their charge sought to pass the time by playing a game in which each player selects a colour – on this occasion, green, blue, and white – and accumulates points for each car painted in his or her colour that passes in the opposite direction on the highway. Each player counts aloud, and the gaps between passing cars are typically filled with cheering and good-natured banter. H.M. participated fully in the game, selecting his colour, accurately keeping track of his running total, and participating in the debate about whether a teal-coloured car should be scored as blue, green, or neither. Indeed, on this occasion H.M. won, accruing a score of 20 first. A round of congratulations was exchanged, followed by a lull as the car rolled through the undulating central Massachusetts countryside. A few minutes later, the guest traveller, eager to maximize his once-in-a-lifetime opportunity to gain first-hand insight from this famous patient, asked 'H___, what are you thinking about right now?' H.M. replied that his count of white cars had now increased to 36.

The driver and guest were both impressed that this patient, famously incapable of remembering virtually anything that had occurred in his life since his 1953 surgery, had accurately maintained and updated a running count of arbitrarily selected 'target stimuli' across a span of several minutes, with no evident source of external support or reinforcement. The three travellers commented on this before the guest traveller redirected the conversation to a line of questions that was typical of these trips: *Do you know what today's date is? Do you know who the current President is? Do you know who we are; where we're going today?* H.M. complied with good-natured responses, as always, clearly enjoying the interaction with and attention from these young, engaged travelling companions. Very quickly, however, H.M. initiated another typical element in the driving-with-H.M. script, by steering the conversation towards a reminiscence from his youth, the portion of his life still mentally accessible after his surgery. (The story, about riding the Silver Meteor passenger train on a multi-day trip to visit an Aunt in Florida, had already been told several times at that point in the trip, a product of the teller not remembering the previous tellings.)

At that point, sensing a 'teachable moment', the driver of the car interjected with a question of his own:

'H_____, do you remember what game we were playing a few minutes ago?'

No, he didn't.

'It involved counting cars of different colours; do you remember what your colour was?'

No.

'The three colours were green, blue, and white; do you remember which was yours?'

No, the cues didn't help.

'Do you remember who won the game?'

No recollection even of the triumph that had, only a few minutes before, produced in H.M. a modest chuckle and satisfied smile.

This vignette illustrates several points about the cognitive profile and conscious phenomenology of medial temporal-lobe (MTL) amnesia that will be taken up in this chapter: the selectivity of the memory deficit vis-à-vis other cognitive functions; the selectivity of the deficit, within the myriad abilities that can be called mnemonic, to the conscious accessing of information acquired post trauma; the seeming normalcy of many aspects of the patient's conscious experience; and the severe constraints that damage to the MTL places on the candidate information and qualia that can make up the contents of consciousness.

BACKGROUND

The study of patients with anterograde amnesia resulting from damage to the hippocampus and adjacent structures of the MTL has contributed enormously to our understanding of the organization of memory, of its relation to other aspects of cognition and behaviour, and of its neural bases. Perhaps the most important principle to derive from the study of anterograde amnesia is that it is inaccurate to depict *memory* as a unitary domain of cognition, in the way that one might characterize *vision* or *language*. Indeed, a hallmark of a 'pure' case of anterograde amnesia is the inability to encode (or learn) new information, despite relatively intact abilities to retrieve premorbid memories[2], to remember a small amount of information, such as a phone number, for tens of seconds or

---

[2] As we shall see, although there is ongoing controversy about the quality of some types of premorbid memories in these patients, neurologists find it 'clinically useful to describe amnesia as a failure to learn new information, which is distinct from a retrieval deficit' [8] p. 41.

even longer, and to demonstrate the improvements that accompany repeated performance of routine behaviours or repeated exposure to stimuli. Also spared in anterograde amnesia is every other major domain of cognition – sensory perception, language comprehension and production, motor control, intelligence, and so on. Because this condition produces so circumscribed a deficit of cognition, it provides an interesting case with which to examine the relation of consciousness to memory vs. other domains of cognition. The analysis in this chapter will begin with a review of the neurological exam and its implications, followed by the anatomical and physiological profile of the amnesic brain, followed by considerations of cognitive effects of damage to the MTL. It will end with a consideration of phenomenology (Box 24.1).

THE NEUROLOGICAL EXAM AND ITS IMPLICATIONS FOR CONSCIOUSNESS

Anterograde amnesia is diagnosed when a neurological exam and neuropsychological testing reveal a specific deficit in the ability to learn new information, as assessed by poor performance on subsequent tests of memory for this new information. In a case described by Mega [8], for example, the patient had a normal general medical exam. She could, upon hearing a spoken list of digits, correctly recite lists of six in the forward order, and lists of five when instructed to recall them in reverse order. On the Mini Mental State Exam (MMSE), a dementia screen that evaluates knowledge of where one is and when it is (year, season, month, date, day of the week) at the time of testing, counting backward from 100 by sevens, and following simple instructions, she responded correctly to 28 out of 30 questions, missing only two that required recall of information provided earlier in the exam. Her vocabulary was intact, as assessed by the ability to name 59 of 60 black-and-white drawings of objects from the Boston Naming Test. When asked to name as many animals as possible within a minute, an index of retrieval from semantic memory and, particularly, the control of this retrieval, she named 19. Executive function was intact, as assessed by tests evaluating the ability to perform mental arithmetic, to change strategy after covert changes of the rule in the Wisconsin Card-Sorting Test, and to withhold responses on a speeded responding test. Finally, and perhaps most striking for one not familiar with such cases, her full-scale intelligence quotient (IQ) as assessed by the Wechsler Adult Intelligence Scale-Revised (WAIS-R) was within the normal range.

Against this backdrop of normal functioning, however, the patient exhibited marked impairment on several formal tests of recall and recognition. For example, she demonstrated marked impairments on tests requiring recall of a list of 16 words several minutes after she had heard them (California Verbal Learning Test, CVLT), requiring recall of the content

---

BOX 24.1

ANTEROGRADE VS. RETROGRADE MEMORY

Although the severity of anterograde amnesia can differ across patients as a function of the nature and size of the lesion, it remains stable within a patient for the remainder of his or her life. This is illustrated by case H.M., who has been tested numerous times, across a span of greater than 25 years, on his ability to identify from photographs people who were famous during specific decades (e.g., Oliver North from the 1980s, John L. Lewis from the 1940s, Warren G. Harding from the 1920s, and so on). On each occasion that he was tested on this Famous Faces test [9] – in 1974, 1977, 1980, 1988, 1989, 1990, 1994, 1997, and 2000 – his performance never varied between 0% and 20% correct for photos taken after the onset of his amnesia (i.e., portraying people from 1950s to 1980s). For stimuli assessing premorbid knowledge, in contrast, H.M.'s performance never varied between 50% and 75% correct for photos from the 1940s and 1930s, and it dropped off to between 15% and 50% for photos from the 1920s, the decade in which he was born. By contrast, the mean performance of 19 age- and education-matched control subjects starts high and declines steadily, and nearly monotonically, from approximately 75% correct for the 1980s to 30% for the 1920s [10]. (It is interesting to note that, for items from the 1940s and 1930s, H.M.'s performance exceeds the control group's mean performance of approximately 40% correct. This is perhaps because the remote memories of the neurologically healthy group have endured more interference over the years than have those of H.M.) A more detailed consideration of retrograde amnesia is provided in Box 24.4.

of two short stories 30 minutes after they had been read aloud (Wechsler Memory Scale (WMS) delayed paragraph recall), and requiring recall of a complex nonsense figure 30 minutes after she had first seen it and successfully copied it (Rey-Osterrieth complex figure recall).[3] One concise (if overly simplistic) way to summarize this patient's clinical profile, which is characteristic of anterograde amnesia, is that she displayed a normal full-scale IQ but an abnormally low *memory quotient* (as assessed by the WMS). Another important distinction revealed here is between long-term memory (LTM) and short-term memory (STM). Although these terms can have different meanings in different contexts, to the cognitive neuroscientist the former refers to memory for information that has not been in conscious awareness for at least several tens of seconds (but possibly for as long as several decades) prior to its retrieval, whereas the latter refers to the temporary retention of a limited amount of information beginning the moment that this information is no longer accessible to the senses. (Thus, for example, your memory for what time you woke up today is an example of LTM, not STM. Sceptics of this convention need only consider the penultimate vignette that concludes this chapter.)

From this profile we see that many domains of mental function remain intact after the onset of anterograde amnesia. One can infer from these results that this patient can, when prompted, call into conscious awareness much of the impressively vast amount of knowledge that she (like most typically developing humans) has acquired during her life (such as the names of a plethora of different kinds of animals and common objects, facts about political history, knowledge about numbers and their mathematical manipulation, etc.); consciously recite to herself lists of digits and think about how to reverse their order; consciously reason about what the rules of a novel card-sorting game might be, come to the realization that the rules have changed, and think about what the new rule might be; and so on. As an interim conclusion, then, we might infer that many aspects of consciousness are largely unaffected by anterograde amnesia. This conclusion is also consistent with the impression that one might draw from the vignette that opened this chapter. Next we will consider how the evidence about the damage sustained by the amnesic brain, as well as the effects of this damage on the brain's functioning,

informs our understanding of the conscious phenomenology of the anterograde amnesic patient.

THE IMPLICATIONS OF MTL DAMAGE FOR NEUROANATOMICAL AND NEUROPHYSIOLOGICAL CORRELATES OF CONSCIOUSNESS

Patients demonstrating the classic neuropsychological profile of a pure anterograde amnesia, such as the patient profiled in the preceding section, invariably have sustained damage that is largely confined to one or more elements of the *medial temporal lobe-diencephalic memory system*, which comprises the hippocampal complex (dentate gyrus, cornu Ammonus (a.k.a., the hippocampus proper), and subiculum), and adjacent structures of the MTL – the parahippocampal, perirhinal, and entorhinal cortices – and two closely anatomically linked structures – the mammillary bodies of the hypothalamus and the anterior thalamic nuclei. Also important to the MTL memory system is the fornix, a bundle of fibers leaving the hippocampal complex that synapse on the mammillary bodies and on neurons of the basal forebrain. A postmortem examination of the brain of Mega's patient revealed bilateral hippocampal sclerosis – cell loss in the CA1 fields of the hippocampus accompanied by gliotic change – and an absence of pathological changes in cortex. Importantly, there was no evidence of the widespread cortical damage that is associated with such neurodegenerative disorders as dementia of the Alzheimer's type[4] [8]. The possible aetiology of this damage was not considered. (In contrast, a retrieval deficit, as considered in Box 24.2, would be associated with damage to the dorsolateral prefrontal cortex (PFC) [8]).

The bilateral damage to H.M.'s MTL, produced by surgical aspiration intended to treat his intractable epilepsy [2], was considerably more extensive. Detailed structural imaging with magnetic resonance imaging (MRI) indicates that H.M.'s lesion is bilaterally symmetrical, and includes the medial temporal polar cortex, most of the amygdaloid complex, most of the entorhinal cortex, and the rostral half of the hippocampus proper. The caudal half of the hippocampus (approximately 2 cm in length), although intact, is atrophic. The mammillary nuclei are shrunken. In addition, the cerebellum

---

[3] Details about the testing procedures for each of the tests listed here, as well as the brain systems and mental abilities that they are intended to measure, can be found in [11].

[4] *Dementia* is distinguished from *amnesia* by the clinical presentation, along with a memory impairment, of marked impairment of one or more nonmnemonic domains of behaviour, including perception, receptive or productive language, executive control, and motor control.

BOX 24.2

LOST FOREVER OR TEMPORARILY MISPLACED?[5]

The presence of anterograde amnesia, alone, does not permit one to distinguish between a 'consolidation block' (i.e., impaired encoding) account vs. disordered storage or disordered retrieval accounts of hippocampal function. In the years following the report of case H.M. [2], which launched the modern study of the MTL and of amnesia, the emphasis was on 'the central role of the learning impairment' [12] (p. 233). By the late 1960s, however, accumulating evidence that many kinds of learning could be spared in amnesic patients ([12, 13]) led to the alternative proposal that the amnesic syndrome was best characterized not as a disorder of encoding, but rather as one of storage or retrieval [14]. For example, when Warrington and Weiskrantz [15] tested amnesic subjects and neurologically healthy control subjects 10 minutes after reading 16 words, the patients performed as well as control subjects on what the authors termed a 'cued recall' task, but were markedly impaired on a test of Yes/No recognition. (The cued recall task from [15] used a procedure that came to be known as word-stem completion, in which the first three letters of a studied word were presented and the subject was 'required to identify the stimulus word' (p. 420). It will be revisited in Box 24.3.) These results, together with evidence of disproportionate sensitivity to interference from items

presented prior to or after the critical information, were taken as evidence for 'altered control of information in storage' (p. 419) in amnesia, and against the consolidation block account.

These early studies illustrated that the study of amnesia could provide powerful insight into the organization of human memory, and the 1970s witnessed an explosion of LTM research, in both memory-impaired and normal populations. One result of this development was increased understanding of the differences between anterograde and retrograde memory (Box 24.1), which led to a convincing refutation of strong versions of storage- and retrieval-based accounts of anterograde amnesia [9, 16].

The ambiguity of whether the patient's deficit is one of encoding vs. one of retrieval also has implications for the clinic, in that, for example, evidence of impaired recall of recently presented information, alone, cannot distinguish an isolated deficit in *learning* new information from a deficit in *retrieving* it. To differentially diagnose anterograde amnesia from a retrieval deficit, it is important to follow up a finding of poor 10-minute recall with retrieval cues. If the availability of cues produces a marked improvement in performance, the diagnosis of a retrieval deficit is indicated [8].

---

demonstrates marked atrophy (a finding assumed to have resulted not from the surgery, but rather from the patient's decades-long history of taking anticonvulsant medication [17]). Importantly, the lateral temporal, frontal, parietal, and occipital lobe cortices appeared normal for a 66-year-old individual [18].

When we contrast the lesions of these two patients, one quite circumscribed and the other considerably more extensive, we see that they do not invade the brain regions whose function is implicated in waking consciousness. The brain regions whose level of activation differentiates conscious from unconscious mental states include lateral and medial frontal and parietal cortex, and thalamus (for more detail, see Chapter 15, and [19–21]). Similarly, the lesions of these MTL amnesic patients largely spare the territories of the so-called 'default network' of cortical regions that

display elevated levels of activity when subjects are at rest: medial posterior cingulate and dorso- and ventromedial frontal cortex; lateral inferior parietal cortex; and medial and lateral aspects of temporal polar cortex. (Portions of this latter area were resected during H.M.'s surgery.) Ideas about functional significance of activity in this network include 'unconstrained, spontaneous cognition – [e.g.,] daydreams', maintaining balance within neural networks and systems, and 'instantiat[ing] the maintenance of information for interpreting, responding to, and even predicting environmental demands' [22] (pp. 1249–1250).

Turning to the functioning of the brain of MTL amnesics, there is a surprising paucity of published information on this topic (this despite an abundance of data for patients with, for example, mild cognitive impairment and with Alzheimer's disease). H.M. has undergone a brain scan with single photon emission computed tomography (SPECT), a method that can measure blood flow in tissue. In comparison to the scan of a healthy, age- and education-matched control

---

[5]A more thorough treatment of this question can be found in [16], from which the title of this box was appropriated.

subject, H.M.'s thalamus and cortical mantle appear to show normal levels of blood flow, with the exception of the MTL, from which no signal is detected [23]. Other evidence for normal cortical functioning in H.M. comes from a functional MRI (fMRI) scan acquired while he performed a novel picture encoding task. This scan revealed task-related activity in a portion of caudal MTL that was spared by the surgeon, an effect that was comparable to what was seen in control subjects [17]. This rather thin set of observations from the human is supplemented, however, by controlled studies in experimental animals. In baboons with surgically produced neurotoxic lesions of entorhinal and perirhinal cortex, positron emission tomography (PET) scans revealed pre-to-postoperative hypometabolic changes in several brain regions, including inferior parietal, posterior cingulate, sensorimotor, posterior temporal, and rostral occipital regions, as well as in thalamus. No differences were observed in lateral prefrontal, anterior cingulate, anterior temporal, or insular cortex [24]. (These rhinal cortex lesions produced significant impairment of recognition memory [25].) A study in rats that used a similar procedure found significant hypometabolism (as measured by PET) in bilateral frontal, parietal, and temporal regions four days after unilateral chemical lesion of entorhinal cortex, an effect that persisted 4 weeks later only in temporal cortex [26].

This summary of the structural damage associated with relatively pure cases of anterograde amnesia, and its physiological sequelae, leaves equivocal the question of whether the lesions that are sufficient to produce anterograde amnesia would be expected to affect directly the phenomenological consciousness of these patients. Considering data from amnesic patients themselves, it is clear that their lesions do not directly invade brain regions known to be necessary for conscious awareness. Additionally, the scant amount of information available from case H.M. does not show any obvious alterations in the physiology of consciousness-related regions. In the baboon, however, bilateral damage to entorhinal cortex produced lasting alterations in many cortical and subcortical regions, some of which may correspond to regions that, in the human, contribute importantly to conscious awareness. An analogous effect may be more transient in rats, although the lesion in this case was unilateral. Finally, it is worth noting that the lesions in the animal studies, although targeting portions of the MTL memory system, spared the hippocampus proper. Thus, at this point in our exploration we have found, at best, only indirect hints that conscious awareness may be altered in patients with MTL amnesia. We shall see in the next section, however, that targeted evaluation of specific cognitive functions in these patients uncovers deficits that are not readily evident from standard clinical and neuroradiological exams.

THE EFFECTS OF MTL DAMAGE ON VARIOUS MENTAL FUNCTIONS AND THEIR IMPLICATIONS FOR CONSCIOUSNESS

LTM

By far, the most influential framework for thinking of the relations between consciousness and memory has been Tulving's distinction between *autonoetic*, *noetic*, and *anoetic* states of awareness with respect to memory retrieval [27]. Derived from a Greek word appropriated by philosophers to refer to 'mind' or 'intellect,' the term 'noetic' in this context roughly corresponds to 'knowing'. Thus autonoetic (or 'self-knowing') awareness refers to an instance of memory retrieval that 'is not only an objective account of what has happened or what has been seen or heard … [but also] necessarily involves the feeling that the present recollection is a reexperience of something that has happened before' [28] (p. 597). 'At the core of autonoetic memory', writes Moscovitch [29], 'is a sense of personal self and the subjective experiences associated with that self or ascribed to it' (p. 611). In relation to the structure of memory, autonoetic awareness is the defining feature of episodic memory, the subcategory of declarative memory corresponding to events that one has personally experienced. Noetic ('knowing') awareness, in contrast, 'occurs when one thinks about something that one knows, such as a mathematical, geographical, or even personal fact, without reexperiencing or reliving the past in which that knowledge was acquired' [29] (p. 611). Noetic awareness characterizes the phenomenology associated with retrieving information from semantic memory, the other subcategory of declarative memory. Finally the concept of anoetic ('not knowing') awareness captures the fact that nondeclarative memory can be expressed without the individual's awareness that his or her performance is being influenced by a prior experience (see Box 24.3). For example, when H.M.'s performance on the completion of three-letter word stems or on the identification of briefly flashed words displays a robust level of influence of a prior study session [30], it does so despite an apparent lack of awareness on the part of the patient that there even was a study session 5 minutes prior to the test, let alone that his performance reflects the influence of that session. (Thus, perhaps 'anoetic performance' would be a better term.) There exists a large and complex literature, extending back even

BOX 24.3

'MEMORY WITHOUT AWARENESS'

A second major focus of memory research beginning in the 1970s was what came to be known as *implicit* or *nondeclarative* memory (for reviews, see [31, 32]). The consequent development of theoretical and methodological sophistication in this domain led to a more nuanced interpretation of some of the earlier reports of intact performance by amnesic subjects. With word-stem completion, for example, it was shown that the performance of amnesic subjects relative to age- and education-matched control subjects depended on the precise phrasing of instructions about how to process the three-letter stem: When subjects were instructed to complete the three-letter stem to 'the first word that comes to mind,' and no reference was made to the prior study episode, amnesic patients often generated target words at a level that was comparable to that of control subjects (i.e., they exhibited intact *repetition priming*); when, in contrast, they were instructed to use the three-letter stem as a cue with which to retrieve an item from the studied list, amnesic patients were typically impaired ([33]). (The former procedure, which most closely resembles that from ref. [15], came to be known

as word-stem completion *priming*, the latter as word-stem *cued recall*.) Thus, the intact performance of amnesic patients in [15] came to be reinterpreted as an early demonstration of intact performance by amnesic subjects on a priming task, a phenomenon that fell under the rubric of *nondeclarative memory*.

In parallel to this research in nondeclarative memory, by the late 1980s, the dominant neuropsychologically inspired view was that memory was organized into distinct systems, with the principal distinction being between MTL-dependent declarative memory and MTL-independent nondeclarative memory[6]. From this perspective, the function of the *MTL memory system* was one of encoding information that is active in the subjective present (e.g., the products of the visual and auditory perception of an event, together with the emotions that they engendered) and effecting its 'transition from perception to memory' [34] (p. 1384) by binding together its anatomically discrete representations (in our example, visual, auditory, and affective). Only by undergoing this process of MTL-mediated *consolidation* could a memory later be called back into conscious awareness via volitional retrieval processes.

---

before Tulving's seminal paper [27], that grapples with the question of how to determine precisely the level of awareness that accompanies performance on different memory tasks. This literature is reviewed comprehensively elsewhere [29, 35], and the remainder of this section will draw on it only to the extent that it addresses directly the goals of this chapter.

The standard neuropsychological model of the MTL memory system, the development of which is sketched in Boxes 24.2, 24.3, and 24.4, includes two important tenets that we will examine in detail. One is the time-limited role for MTL-mediated consolidation, a feature necessitated by the temporal gradient that typifies retrograde amnesia following damage to the MTL (Box 24.4, [36]). The second is the hierarchical arrangement of the elements in the MTL memory system, with memory formation depending on the funnelling of activity from nonmnemonic cortical regions first into perirhinal or parahippocampal cortex, then into entorhinal cortex, and finally 'up' to hippocampus ('up' in the sense of the apex of the hierarchy) [37]. Recently, questions have been raised about both of these tenets of the standard

neuropsychological model that have important implications for the neurobiology of consciousness.

A challenge to the idea of a time-limited role for the hippocampus in memory consolidation has come in the form of the *multiple trace theory* (MTT) of hippocampal function [38]. MTT posits that each instance of memory retrieval also prompts the encoding by the hippocampus of a new memory trace, such that over time a single memory comes to be stored as multiple traces. To the extent that elements of these traces overlap, this process leads to the development of semantic knowledge that is independent of the episodes in which the information was learned. So, for example, if learning about

---

[6] In parallel with the development of memory-systems models were transfer appropriate-processing models, which appealed to the overlap of mental processes engaged at study vs. test as the critical factor in determining memory performance. However, because this development emerged largely via the study of neurological healthy individuals, its application to the amnesic syndrome has been only indirect. A comprehensive overview of recent theoretical developments in human memory research can be found in [7].

BOX 24.4

RETROGRADE MEMORY AND CONSOLIDATION

Retrograde memory refers to memory for information encountered prior to the insult to the MTL. Were one to start from a strict assumption that the hippocampus is an engine of encoding, one might expect that memory for an event that occurred the day before the MTL insult would be as strong as (if not stronger than) memory for an event that occurred years earlier. However, no such cases of anterograde amnesia accompanied by the absence of any retrograde memory impairment have ever been reported. Instead, irreversible damage to the MTL invariably also produces some retrograde memory loss. However, there are marked differences in the effects of MTL damage on anterograde vs. retrograde memory. Whereas the former is stable across time, the latter is more variable, perhaps, as we shall see below, in systematic ways.

The strength and duration of retrograde amnesia can be sensitive to the amount of tissue damaged (particularly cortical tissue outside the MTL), the patient's age at the time of MTL trauma, and other factors [39]. For case H.M., his retrograde memory has been estimated to extend back to 11 years prior to his surgery [40]. Unlike anterograde amnesia, however, many studies suggest that retrograde amnesia can be characterized by a temporal gradient, such that memory for events that occurred shortly prior to the MTL trauma is worse than is memory for events that occurred several years earlier. Quantitative studies of this phenomenon, carried out in amnesic patients [41], in psychiatric patients undergoing electroconvulsive therapy [42], in a variety of animal preparations [36], and in formal computational modelling [43], indicate that this gradient takes the form of a monotonic function. Such a replicable, systematic pattern of results requires an explanation at the level of memory processing, and the explanation that has made its way into the textbooks is *consolidation*. More a description than a detailed account of a process, the concept of consolidation captures the logic that the MTL must continue to play a role in memory processing after the initial encoding of information, but that this role is time limited. Thus, memory for information that was encoded shortly before MTL damage was incurred is vulnerable to disruption, because consolidation of that memory is still underway. Memory for information that was encoded long before the trauma, in contrast, is more likely to be preserved, because the 'process' of consolidation had been completed. (A thorough summary of recent developments in the study of retrograde memory, including an intriguing phenomenon known as 'reconsolidation,' can be found in a special section of the journal *Learning Memory* (2006, 13(5)) that is devoted to this topic.)

US Presidents in primary school and taking a family trip to Washington DC both create traces representing the proposition that 'Thomas Jefferson was the third President of the United States,' repeated iterations of this process create a representation that can be retrieved independently of any reference to any one of the contexts in which this information was encountered. In this way, the memory that *Thomas Jefferson was the third President of the United States* becomes a *semantic* memory. Should damage to the hippocampus be sustained several years after the learning took place, the patient would nonetheless be able to retrieve this knowledge. On this prediction, the MTT and the standard neuropsychological model are in accord. The specific memory of the visit to the Jefferson Memorial during the family trip to Washington DC, however, remains an *autobiographical episodic* memory that is dependent on the hippocampus for the remainder of the subject's life. Thus, MTT would predict that access to this autobiographical episodic memory would be severely impoverished, if not completely impossible, after extensive damage to the MTL (particularly to the hippocampus). The standard neuropsychological model, in contrast, would hold that autonoetic awareness for remote autobiographical episodic memories can be comparable to that experienced by neurologically intact individuals when recalling a memory of the same vintage. At the time of this writing, this debate is far from being resolved [44, 39].

A second debate currently underway in the memory community relates to the retrieval of episodic memory, and can be thought of, for our present purposes, as a debate as to whether there are distinct processes corresponding to the autonoetic vs. noetic awareness that can accompany memory retrieval. No one disputes that recognition can either be accompanied by an autonoetic sense that 'yes, I've seen this person before and I recall distinctly when and where it was that I first encountered her' or by a noetic 'feeling of familiarity' such that '*I know that I've seen this person before, but I don't recall who she is, or where or when it was that I have previously encountered her.*' What is contentious, however, is whether there exist two processes – *recollection* and *familiarity* – that underlie these two phenomenological experiences. The alternative is simply that memories of different strengths can give rise to different phenomenological experiences, in this case autonoetic vs. noetic awareness, but that the actual underlying process of memory retrieval is the same in both cases. The details of this debate in the cognitive psychology community ([45, 46]) are beyond the scope of this chapter. What is relevant to our current interest, however, are reports that these two putative processes may be neurobiologically dissociable.

Results from fMRI in humans [47] and lesion studies in humans [48–51] and rats [52], have been interpreted as evidence that recollection is differentially supported by the hippocampus, whereas familiarity is supported by nonhippocampal elements of the MTL memory system, of which the perirhinal cortex is particularly emphasized [53]. An implication of this 'dual processes' account is that autonoetic awareness at the time of retrieval may depend on the hippocampus proper, whereas noetic awareness may be supported by nonhippocampal elements of the MTL. In contrast, the standard neuropsychological model would hold that any differences in retrieval-related phenomenology associated with damage to different elements of MTL memory system would be quantitative, rather than qualitative, because it denies the possibility that different elements of this system differentially support discrete memory-related processes. (Indeed, one recent account of this view aligns itself with 'single process' theories from cognitive psychology that deny a fundamental difference between recollection and familiarity [54]). As is the case with the differing views of the time-limited consolidation model vs. the MTT, satisfactory resolution of the question of one vs. two retrieval-related processes is probably several years off.

STM

STM can be thought of as the retention in conscious awareness of information that is no longer accessible to the senses. As we shall see here, it represents yet another case in which received wisdom about the mnemonic functions of the hippocampus has come under reappraisal. In this instance, however, a function previously believed to be independent of the integrity of the hippocampus is now being shown, under some conditions, to depend on it. As we saw in the earlier section on the neurological exam, anterograde amnesia

is characterized by a preserved ability to prehend a spoken list of items (in this case, digits) and to recite it back to the speaker. Formal demonstrations of this [55–58] contributed to the development of cognitive models specifying a fundamental distinction between STM and LTM [59], as well as to the idea that STM is independent of the MTL memory system. (To be thoroughly precise, therefore, this name would need to be expanded to 'MTL declarative LTM system'.)

The recent reconsideration of the dependence of STM on the MTL has its roots in a detailed theory of what might be the specific operations performed by the hippocampus that give it its privileged function with respect to the formation of LTM. In brief, this theory holds that the hippocampus effects the operation of representing and learning the relationships between items in the environment. This might include the arbitrary rule for written English of '*i* before *e*, except after *c*,' or the concrete spatial content of 'Zidane struck the free kick from the left side of the field, lofting the ball over the heads of the Brazilian defenders and into the right side of the goal box, where Henry, running in unmarked, volleyed it into the back of the net'. (Incidentally, Eichenbaum [60] has argued that the demonstration of a necessary role for the hippocampus for nondeclarative memory for the relationships between stimuli (e.g., learning cue–context relationships embedded in a visual search task [61]) rules out the view that the hippocampus 'could be a "gateway" for awareness to enter into memory' (p. 775).) Motivated by this 'relational binding' model, recent studies have demonstrated that patients with hippocampal damage are impaired on tests of STM, with lags as short as 1 second, for spatial relationships between items in a display [62, 63]. This suggests that one qualitative effect of hippocampal damage on phenomenological consciousness is to disrupt the ability to represent the relationships between discrete objects.[7] Whether this is also true for the real-time perception and experience of complex scenes, or only for instances when a mental image of the relationship between no-longer-perceivable items must be retained, will require additional research. A suggestion of what the answer might be, however, has already appeared in the form of the study to which we now turn.

---

[7] Another recent study has described a deficit in MTL patients in 4-second delayed recognition of visually presented stimuli that impose no explicit relational binding requirements (location of squares, face identity, color identity [64]). However, in view of the small number of amnesic subjects tested (three) and the heterogeneity of their lesions, it would be premature to draw strong conclusions about the implications of this one study for our understanding of the role of the MTL in STM.

Imagining New Experiences

The debates summarized at the beginning of this section relate to whether the hippocampus is necessary for autonoetic awareness during memory retrieval. But what about thinking about experiences that have never actually occurred, such as might happen when one daydreams, or when one thinks about what might happen at an upcoming event? One group has reasoned that because these phenomenological experiences would seem to draw on many of the same psychological processes required for autonoetic awareness of an episodic memory (e.g., mental imagery, a sense of 'being there', maintenance of a narrative structure), the ability to imagine new experiences might also be dependent on the hippocampus. (This line of reasoning depends on many precepts of the MTT.) In their experiment they asked patients with bilateral hippocampal damage to construct new imagined experiences, such as 'Imagine you are lying on a white sandy beach in a beautiful tropical bay' and 'Imagine that you are sitting in the main hall of a museum containing many exhibits'. Their results indicated that the imagined experiences of the patients contained markedly less experiential richness than did those of healthy control subjects. A more detailed analysis also revealed lower 'spatial coherence' (a measure of the contiguousness and spatial integrity of an imagined scene) in the performance of the patients, and the authors speculated that this might be at the root of the overall poor performance of the patients [65]. Although these results and their interpretation are also likely to be met with scepticism from some circles, they raise the possibility that the constraints on conscious phenomenology imposed by damage to the hippocampus are not limited to memory retrieval, but may also extend to prospective thought.

To summarize this section, many recent developments in memory research, although some of them are still controversial, point to the possibility that the contributions of the hippocampus to phenomenological consciousness may extend beyond the processing of the present so that the events of the present can later be revisited. They suggest that the hippocampus may also be necessary for rich autonoetic awareness, as well as for spatially coherent thinking about the very recent past, the present, and even the future.

WHAT IT IS LIKE TO BE AMNESIC?

Despite the currently unsettled state of the domains of contemporary memory research that were summarized in the preceding section, the first two analytic sections of this chapter established that many quantitatively measurable correlates of the conscious experience of the MTL amnesic patient are not appreciably changed from what they must have been prior to the neurological insult. This might justify what is arguably the most direct approach to investigating the phenomenal consciousness that is characteristic of MTL amnesia – interrogating patients. Before embarking on this exercise, however, a brief review of a few concepts from the philosophy of consciousness will prove to be useful. Within the tradition of phenomenology, the *stream of consciousness* is held to provide coherence and continuity to conscious experience. As summarized by Thompson and Zahavi [66], 'Phenomenological analyses point to the 'width' or 'depth' of the 'living present' of consciousness: our experience of temporal[ly] enduring objects and events, as well as our experience of change and succession, would be impossible were we conscious only of that which is given in a punctual now and were our stream of consciousness composed of a series of isolated now points, like a string of pearls. According to Husserl [67], the basic unit of temporality is not a "knife-edge" present, but a "duration block" ...' (p. 77). The relevance of this concept to anterograde amnesia is clear, and is further bolstered by empirical evidence that relates to H.M.'s perception of the passage of time. In his experiment, Richards [68] asked 'Without the normal recall for events, how fast does time pass for H.M.? Does one hour, one day or one year seem just as long to this unique individual as to us?' (p. 279). The results indicated that whereas time reproduction (and thus, by inference, the experienced passage of time) was normal for intervals less than 20 second, it was grossly distorted for longer intervals. In answer to his passage-of-time question, Richards concluded by extrapolating from the data that 'one hour to us is like 3 minutes to H.M.; one day is like 15 minutes; and one year is equivalent to 3 hours for H.M.' (p. 281). Thus, for H.M., the width of his 'living present' may, in fact, be best characterized as a knife-edge.

A second concept from philosophy that is germane to our pursuit is that of *fringe consciousness* [65], summarized by Seager [69] as 'the background of awareness which sets the context for experience ... [a]n example is our sense of orientation or rightness in a familiar environment' (p. 10). Fringe consciousness situates a person, preventing the feeling that one has simply popped into the world at that moment.

Moving on, then, to the interrogation, self-report from H.M. suggests that one phenomenological quality of anterograde amnesia is a pervasive anxiety about what may have happened just beyond the edge of the truncated duration block of the living present:

'Right now, I'm wondering, have I done or said anything amiss? You see, at this moment everything looks clear to me, but what happened just before? … It's like waking from a dream; I just don't remember … Every day is alone, in itself. Whatever enjoyment I've had, whatever sorrow I've had.' [1] (p. 138).

On another occasion, during an exchange between H.M. and researcher William Marslen-Wilson (relayed by Hilts [1]) the patient confessed to worrying about giving the wrong answer, whether during formal testing or just in conversation.

'It is a constant effort, H____ said. You must always "wonder how is it going to affect others? Is that the way to do it? Is it the right way?" … Asked if he worried about these things a lot, struggled with his thought to get right answers, he said yes, all the time. "But why?" "I don't know," said H____.' (p. 140)

The experience of disordered fringe consciousness is evident in amnesic patient Clive Wearing, a distinguished British musicologist, conductor, and keyboardist whose amnesia resulted from herpes encephalitis, a condition that can produce severe damage to the hippocampus while leaving the rest of the brain relatively unscathed. Wearing has been featured in several television documentaries, one of which, at the time of this writing, can be viewed on the World Wide Web[8]. The video clip opens with the camera panning in on Wearing and his wife sitting in a city park.

Wife: 'Do you know how we got here?
'Wearing: 'No.'
Wife: 'You don't remember sitting down?'
Wearing: 'No.'
Wife: 'I reckon we've been here about 10 minutes at least.'
Wearing: 'Well, I've no knowledge of it. My eyes only started working now …'
Wife: 'And do you feel absolutely normal?'
Wearing: 'Not absolutely normal, no. I'm completely confused.
Wife: 'Confused?'
Wearing (agitatedly): 'Yes. If you've never eaten anything, never tasted anything, never touched anything, never smelled something, what right have you to assume you're alive?'
Wife: 'Hmm. But you are.'
Wearing: 'Apparently, yes. But I'd like to know what the hell's been going on!'

(In making these pronouncements about his senses, it is clear that Wearing is speaking figuratively, not literally.) Thus, for Wearing, too, each waking moment feels as though he is just waking up from sleep. The journal

that he keeps is filled with multiple entries that all contain variants of the same message. For example, directly under the entry '10:49 am I Am Totally Awake – First time', which appears on the first line of a page, is a second entry '11:05 am I Am Perfectly Awake – First time', and so on. When left alone in his room, the patient fills entire pages in this way with entries made at intervals ranging from 5 to 45 minutes.

These anecdotes capture an essential quality of the conscious phenomenology of the MTL amnesic patient, the near-continual experience of just having awakened from unconscious sleep. The plight of the MTL amnesic patient, then, is to be fully cognizant of, if not preoccupied by, the fact that one is not cognizant of the daily events of one's life.

CONCLUSIONS

The MTL's contributions to conscious awareness are at once minimal and profound. They are minimal in that they would seem to contribute little to the ongoing operations that comprise the contents of our moment-to-moment conscious awareness – perception, retrieval and contemplation of semantic knowledge, language processing (receptive and productive), social interactions, and so on. They are undeniably profound, however, in that they underlie the width of the stream of consciousness and the integrity of fringe consciousness. This chapter has highlighted several important questions that remain to be resolved. Physiologically, what are the contributions of the MTL to the quality and quantity of activity in the main complex of brain structures whose activity underlies awareness [20, 70]? Psychologically, what explains the phenomenological difference between autonoetic and noetic awareness? Empirically, are the recent findings that suggest a necessary role for the MTL in some kinds of STM and in the ability to imagine new experiences replicable and generalizeable?

EPILOGUE: A FINAL WORD

'"What happened to you? …' asked researcher Marslen-Wilson. 'Well,' said H____, 'I think of an operation. I have an argument with myself right there – did the knife slip a little? Or was it a thing that's naturally caused when you have this kind of operation?' 'That caused what?' Marslen-Wilson asked. 'The loss of memory, but not of reality', H_____ said." [1] (pp. 139–140)

[8] http://www.youtube.com/watch?v = OmkiMlvLKto&mode = related&search =

ACKNOWLEDGEMENTS

The author thanks Suzanne Corkin, William Jagust, Sterling Johnson, and Elizabeth Kensinger for helpful replies to queries, Lawrence Shapiro for comments on an earlier draft, and Morris Moscovitch for sharing selected advance galleys of the *Cambridge Handbook of Consciousness*. B.R.P. received support from NIH MH064498.

References

1. Hilts, P.J. (1995) *Memory's Ghost*, New York: Simon & Schuster.
2. Scoville, W.B. and Milner, B. (1957) Loss of recent memory after bilateral hippocampal lesions. *J Neurol, Neurosurg Psychiatr* 20:11–21.
3. Squire, L.R. (1987) *Memory and Brain*, New York: Oxford University Press.
4. Bliss, T. and Lomo, T. (1973) Long-lasting potentiation of synaptic transmission in the dentate area of the anesthetized rabbit following stimulation of the perforant path. *J Physiol* 232:331–341.
5. Bliss, T.P.V., Collingridge, G.L. and Morris, R.G.M. (2003) Introduction to 'long-term potentiation: Enhancing neuroscience for 30 years'. *Philos Transac: Biol Sci* 358.
6. O'Keefe, J. and Nadel, L. (1978) *The Hippocampus as a Cognitive Map*, London, England: Oxford University Press.
7. Tulving, E. and Craik, F.I.M. (2000) *The Oxford Handbook of Memory*, New York: Oxford University Press.
8. Mega, M.S. (2003) Amnesia: A disorder of episodic memory. In D'Esposito, M. (ed.) *Neurological Foundations of Cognitive Neuroscience*, pp. 41–66. Cambridge, MA: MIT Press.
9. Marslen-Wilson, W.D. and Teuber, H.-L. (1975). Memory for remote events in anterograde amnesia: Recognition of public figures from news photographs. 13: 353–364.
10. Kensinger, E.A. and Corkin, S. (2000) Retrograde memory in amnesia: A famous faces study with the amnesic patient H.M. *Poster presented at the annual meeting of the Society for Neuroscience* 26:1241.
11. Lezak, M.D. (1995) *Neuropsychological Assessment*, 3rd Edition. New York: Oxford University Press.
12. Milner, B., Corkin, S. and Teuber, H.-L. (1968) Further analysis of the hippocampal amnesic syndrome: 14 year follow-up study of H.M. *Neuropsychologia* 6:215–234.
13. Warrington, E.K. and Weiskrantz, L. (1968) A new method of testing long-term retention with special reference to amnesic patients. *Nature* 217:972–974.
14. Warrington, E.K. and Weiskrantz, L. (1970) The amnesic syndrome: Consolidation or retrieval? *Nature* 228:628–630.
15. Warrington, E.K. and Weiskrantz, L. (1974) The effect of prior learning on subsequent retention in amnesic patients. *Neuropsychologia* 12:419–428.
16. Squire, L.R. (2006) Lost forever or temporarily misplaced? The long debate about the nature of memory impairment. *Learn Memory* 13:522–529.
17. Corkin, S. (2002) What's new with the amnesic patient H.M.? *Nat Rev Neurosci* 3:153–160.
18. Corkin, S., Amaral, D.G., Gonzalez, R.G., Johnson, K.A. and Hyman, B.T. (1997) H.M.'s medial temporal-lobe lesion: Findings from MRI. *J Neurosci* 17:3964–3979.
19. Fiset, P., Paus, T., Daloze, T., Plourde, G., Meuret, P., Bonhomme, V., Hajj-Ali, N., Backman, S.B. and Evans, A.C. (1999) Brain mechanisms of propofol-induced loss of consciousness in humans: A positron emission tomographic study. *J Neurosci* 19:5506–5513.
20. Laureys, S. (2005) The neural correlate of (un)awareness: Lessons from the vegetative state. *Trend Cognit Sci* 9:556–559.
21. Maquet, P. (2000) Functional neuroimaging of normal human sleep by positron emission tomography. *J Sleep Res* 9:207–231.
22. Raichle, M.E. (2006) The brain's dark energy. *Science* 314:1249–1250.
23. Corkin, S. (personal communication).
24. Meguro, K., Blaizot, X., Kohdoh, Y., Le Mestric, C., Baron, J.C. and Chavoix, C. (1999) Neocortical and hippocampal glucose hypometabolism following neurotoxic lesions of the entorhinal and perirhinal cortices in the nonhuman primate as shown by PET: Implications for Alzheimer's disease. *Brain* 122:1519–1531.
25. Chavoix, C., Blaizot, X., Meguro, K., Landeau, B. and Baron, J.C. (2002) Excitotoxic lesions of the rhinal cortex in the baboon differentially affect visual recognition memory, habit memory, spatial executive functions. *Eur J Neurosci* 15:1225–1236.
26. Hayashi, T., Fukuyama, H., Katsumi, Y., Hanakawa, T., Nagahama, Y., Yamauchi, H., Tsukada, H. and Shibasaki., H. (1999) Cerebral glucose metabolism in unilateral entorhinal cortex-lesioned rats: An animal PET study. *Neuroreport* 10:2113–2118.
27. Tulving, E. (1985) Memory and consciousness. *Can Psychol* 26:1–12.
28. Wheeler, M.A. (2000) Episodic memory and autonoetic awareness. In Tulving, E. and Craik, F.I.M (eds.) *The Oxford Handbook of Memory*, pp. 597–608. New York: Oxford University Press.
29. Moscovitch, M. (2000) Theories of memory and consciousness. In Tulving, E. and Craik, F.I.M (eds.)*The Oxford Handbook of Memory* pp. 609–625 New York: Oxford University Press.
30. Postle, B.R. and Corkin, S. (1998) Impaired word-stem completion priming but intact perceptual identification priming with novel words: evidence from the amnesic patient H.M.. *Neuropsychologia* 36:421–440.
31. Schacter, D.L. (1987) Implicit memory: History and current status. *J Exp Psychol: Lear, Mem Cognit* 13:501–518.
32. Squire, L.R., Knowlton, B. and Musen, G. (1993) The structure and organization of memory. *Ann Rev Psychol* 44:453–495.
33. Gabrieli, J.D.E., Keane, M.M., Stanger, B.Z., Kjelgaard, M.M., Corkin, S. and Growdon, J.H. (1994) Dissociations among structural-perceptual, lexical-semantic, and event-fact memory systems in amnesia, Alzheimer's disease, and normal subjects. *Cortex* 30:75–103.
34. Squire, L.R. and Zola-Morgan, S. (1991) The medial temporal lobe memory system. *Science* 253:1380–1386.
35. Roediger, H.L.I., Rajaram, S. and Geraci, L. (2007) Three forms of consciousness in retrieving memories. In Zelazo, P.D. Moscovitch, M. and Thompson, E. (eds.) *The Cambridge Handbook of Consciousness.* pp. 251–288. Cambridge, UK: Cambridge University Press.
36. Squire, L.R. (1992) Memory and the hippocampus: A synthesis from findings with rats, monkeys, and humans. *Psychologic Rev* 99:195–231.
37. Broadbent, N.J., Clark, R.E., Zola, S. and Squire, L.R. (2002) The medial temporal lobe and memory. In Squire, L.R. and Schacter, D.L (eds.) *Neuropsychology of Memory*, 3rd Edition. pp. 3–23. New York: The Guilford Press.
38. Nadel, L. and Moscovitch, M. (1997) Memory consolidation, retrograde amnesia and the hippocampal complex. *Curr Opin Neurobiol* 7:217–227.
39. Squire, L.R. and Bayley, P.J. (2007) The neuroscience of remote memory. *Curr Opin Neurobiol* 17:185–196.
40. Sagar, J.H., Cohen, N.J., Corkin, S. and Growdon, J.H. (1985) Dissociations among processes in remote memory. In Olton, D.S.,

Gamzu, E., and Corkin, S. (eds.) *Memory Dysfunctions: An Integration of Animal and Human Research From Preclinical and Clinical Perspectives*, pp. 533–535. New York: Annals of the New York Academy of Sciences.

41. Squire, L.R., Haist, F. and Shimamura, A.P. (1989) The neurology of memory: Quantitative assessment of retrograde amnesia in two groups of amnesic patients. *J Neurosci* 9:828–839.

42. Squire, L.R., Slater, P.C. and Chace, P.M. (1975) Retrograde amnesia: temporal gradient in very long-term memory following electroconvulsive therapy. *Science* 187:77–79.

43. Alvarez, P. and Squire, L.R. (1994) Memory consolidation and the medial temporal lobe: A simple network model. *Proc Natl Acad Sci USA* 91:7041–7045.

44. Moscovitch, M., Nadel, L., Winocur, G., Gilboa, A. and Rosenbaum, R.S. (2006) The cognitive neuroscience of remote episodic, semantic and spatial memory. *Curr Opin Neurobiol* 16:179–190.

45. Wixted, J.T. and Stretch, V. (2004) In defense of the signal detection interpretation of remember/know judgments. *Psychonomic Bulletin & Review* 11:616–641.

46. Yonelinas, A.P. (2002) The nature of recollection and familiarity: a review of 30 years of research. *J Mem Lang* 46:441–517.

47. Yonelinas, A.P., Otten, L.J., Shaw, K.N. and Rugg, M.D. (2005) Separating the brain regions involved in recollection and familiarity in recognition memory. *J Neurosci* 25:3002–3008.

48. Aggleton, J.P., Vann, S.D., Denby, C., Dix, S., Mayes, A.R., Roberts, N. and Yonelinas, A.P. (2005) Sparing of the familiarity component of recognition memory in a patient with hippocampal pathology. *Neuropsychologia* 43:1810–1823.

49. Bastin, C., Van der Linden, M., Charnallet, A., Denby, C., Montaldi, D., Roberts, N. and Mayes, A.R. (2004) Dissociation between recall, recognition memory performance in an amnesic patient with hippocampal damage following carbon monoxide poisoning. *Neurocase* 10:330–344.

50. Yonelinas, A., Kroll, N.E., Quamme, J.R., Lazzara, M.M., Sauve, M.J., Widaman, K.F. and Knight, R.T. (2002) Effects of extensive temporal lobe damage or mild hypoxia on recollection and familiarity. *Nat Neurosci* 5:1236–1241.

51. Yonelinas, A., Kroll, N.E.A., Dobbins, I., Lazzara, M. and Knight, R.T. (1998) Recollection and familiarity deficits in amnesia: Convergence of remember/know, process dissociation and receiver operating characteristic data. *Neuropsychology* 12:323–339.

52. Fortin, N., Wright, S. and Eichenbaum, H. (2004) Recollection-like memory retrieval in rats is dependent on the hippocampus. *Nature* 431:188–191.

53. Brown, M.W. and Aggleton, J.P. (2001) Recognition memory: What are the roles of the perirhinal cortex, hippocampus? *Nat Rev Neurosci* 2:51–61.

54. Wais, P.E., Wixted, J.T., Hopkins, R.O. and Squire., L.R. (2006) The hippocampus supports both the recollection and the familiarity components of recognition memory. *Neuron* 49:459–466.

55. Baddeley, A.D. and Warrington, E.K. (1970) Amnesia, the distinction between long-and short-term memory. *J Verb Learn Verb Behav* 14:575–589.

56. Drachman, D.A. and Stahl, S. (1966) Memory and the hippocampal complex. *Arch Neurol* 15:52–61.

57. Teuber, H.-L., Milner, B. and Vaughan, H.G.Jr. (1968) Persistent anterograde amnesia after stabwound of the basal brain. *Neuropsychologia* 6:279–282.

58. Wickelgren, W.A. (1968) Sparing of short-term memory in an amnesic patient: implications for strength theory of memory. *Neuropsychologia* 6:235–244.

59. Baddeley, A.D. and Hitch, G. (1970) Working memory: Past, present … and future? In Osaka, N., Logie, R.H. and D'Esposito, M. (eds.) *The Cognitive Neuroscience of Working Memory*, pp. 1–20. Oxford, UK: Oxford University Press.

60. Eichenbaum, H. (1999) Conscious awareness, memory and the hippocampus. *Nat Neurosci* 2:775–776.

61. Chun, M.M. and Phelps, E.A. (1999) Memory deficits for implicit contextual information in amnesic subjects with hippocampal damage. *Nat Neurosci* 2:844–847.

62. Hannula, D.E., Tranel, D. and Cohen., N.J. (2006) The long and the short of it: Relational memory impairments in amnesia, even at short lags. *J Neurosci* 26:8352–8359.

63. Olson, I.R., Page, K., Moore, K.S., Chatterjee, A. and Verfaellie, M. (2006) Working memory for conjunctions relies on the medial temporal lobe. *J Neurosci* 26:4596–4601.

64. Olson, I.R., Moore, K.S., Stark, M. and Chatterjee, A. (2006) Visual working memory is impaired when the medial temporal lobe is damaged. *J Cognit Neurosci* 18:1087–1097.

65. Hassabis, D., Kumaran, D., Vann, S.D. and Maguire., E.A. (2007) Patients with hippocampal amnesia cannot imagine new experiences. *Proc Natl Acad Sci USA* 104:1726–1731.

66. Thompson, E. and Zahavi, D. (2007) Philosophical Issues: Phenomenology. In Zelazo, P.D., Moscovitch, M. and Thompson, E. (eds.) *The Cambridge Handbook of Consciousness*, pp. 67–88. Cambridge, UK: Cambridge University Press.

67. Husserl, E. (1991) *On the Phenomenology of the Consciousness of Internal Time (1893–1917)*, Dordrecht: Kluwer Academic Publishers. (J.B. Brough, Trans.)

68. Richards, W.A. (1973) Time reproductions by H.M. *Acta Psychologica* 37:279–282.

69. Seager, (2007) A brief history of the philosophical problem of consciousness. In Zelazo, P.D., Moscovitch, M. and Thompson, E. (eds.) *The Cambridge Handbook of Consciousness*, pp. 9–33. Cambridge, UK: Cambridge University Press.

70. Tononi, G. (2004) An information integration theory of consciousness. *BMC Neurosci* 5:42.

Syndromes of Transient Amnesia

Chris Butler and Adam Zeman

ABSTRACT

An isolated and self-limiting impairment of conscious memory can occur in a variety of clinical contexts including transient global amnesia (TGA), transient epileptic amnesia (TEA) and psychogenic amnesia. Understanding of the pathophysiological mechanisms and neuropsychological profiles of these fascinating syndromes is growing. In this chapter, we describe each in turn, highlighting recent advances in the field, and explore some questions that transient amnesia raises about the relation between consciousness and memory.

For most of us, transient lapses of memory are a minor and, at worst, irritating feature of everyday life. They are usually brief, item specific and alleviated by a pertinent cue. Occasionally, we find ourselves with no recollection for longer periods of activity. Some such experiences raise intriguing questions about the relation between consciousness and memory. When

the long distance truck driver suddenly 'comes to', realizing that he remembers nothing of the last 10 miles driven, has he merely failed to form long-term memories during that period, or was his consciousness in some way impaired throughout?

Clinical syndromes of transient amnesia are more dramatic. The patient typically presents with a story of sudden onset but self-limiting memory impairment, during which he was unable to retain new information (anterograde amnesia) or remember past events (retrograde amnesia). Despite this, he was able to carry out complex, purposeful actions and engage in conversation. He appeared, in other words, despite his memory loss, to be fully 'conscious', at least in the neurosurgical sense of the term – able to respond to events in the well-integrated fashion most of us can manage while awake. But what of the contents of his consciousness? In some sense, his awareness and self-awareness were undoubtedly affected by his amnesia during the attack. How does memory loss impact on our experience?

In this chapter, we first describe features of the principle clinical syndromes of transient amnesia – transient global amnesia (TGA), transient epileptic amnesia (TEA) and psychogenic amnesia – and then discuss several interactions between amnesia and consciousness: (i) the effect of transient amnesia on consciousness in its key senses of wakefulness and awareness, (ii) its effect, specifically, on the consciousness of self, (iii) the distinction between conscious but unremembered behaviour and the complex 'unconscious' behaviours known as automatisms.

TRANSIENT GLOBAL AMNESIA

TGA is a striking clinical syndrome, characterized by the abrupt onset of a profound but transient anterograde amnesia, together with a variable degree of retrograde amnesia. The name was coined in 1964 by Fisher and Adams in a paper describing the clinical features of 17 patients [1], although several authors published accounts of similar cases using different terminology at around the same time [2–5]. It has been suggested [6] that, prior to this period, the syndrome remained buried within the literature on psychogenic, or hysterical amnesia.

> A 63-year-old, recently retired teacher was brought to the Accident and Emergency department by her husband. One hour earlier, she had telephoned him from the local gym where she had just finished her daily workout and said: 'I don't know where I am. What's happening? Where am I?' Despite his reassurances, she had continued to repeat the same questions. On examination, she was disoriented in time and place, had no recollection for events of the previous week and was unable to retain new information – including the identity of the attending doctor. Besides the amnesia, there were no other neurological signs or symptoms. A CT scan of the head was normal. Over the following 6 hours, her memory deficit gradually resolved although she was left with a dense 'gap' for the episode of transient amnesia itself and for the preceding trip to the gym.

Clinical Features

The most widely accepted diagnostic criteria for TGA were introduced by Hodges and Warlow [7]:

1. Attacks must be witnessed and information available from a capable observer who was present for most of the attack.
2. There must be a clear-cut anterograde amnesia during the attack.
3. Clouding of consciousness and loss of personal identity must be absent, and the cognitive deficit must be limited to amnesia (i.e., no aphasia, apraxia, etc.).
4. There should be no accompanying focal neurological symptoms during the attack and no significant neurological signs afterwards.
5. Epileptic features must be absent.
6. Attacks must resolve within 24 hours.
7. Patients with recent head injury or active epilepsy (i.e., remaining on medication or one seizure in the past 2 years) are excluded.

TGA is a relatively infrequent occurrence, having an annual incidence of between 3 and 10 per 100 000 [6]. Nonetheless, it has attracted considerable attention in the scientific literature and circa 1500 cases have been described [8]. The mean age of onset is 62 years [6] and the condition occurs almost exclusively in individuals between the ages of 40 and 80. In younger people, a similar phenomenon may occur following head injury [9], but such attacks are usually excluded from the rubric of TGA. A recent review of all literature cases [8] failed to find any significant difference in frequency between the sexes.

Ever since the early reports, it has been noticed that TGA is often preceded by a period of intense emotional or physical stress. Frequently reported triggers include immersion in cold water, sexual intercourse, receipt of distressing news or a heated argument. The onset of anterograde amnesia is betrayed by repetitive questioning, often related to attempts at self-orientation such as 'What day is it?' or 'What am I doing here?' Although a small amount of information can be retained for a few seconds, it is rapidly lost when the patient's attention shifts. The retrograde amnesia may cover a few hours prior to the attack onset or be much more extensive. Witnesses usually describe the patient as 'confused', but careful examination reveals that there is no impairment of conscious level or of other cognitive functions such as attention, language or perception. In contrast to psychogenic forms of amnesia, knowledge of personal identity is always retained. Non-specific symptoms such as headache, nausea or dizziness may be present, but there are no focal neurological deficits. Symptoms usually resolve gradually over 4–10 hours, with recovery of retrograde memory occurring more rapidly than anterograde memory [10]. The majority of patients, therefore, do not present to a neurologist in the acute phase. After recovery, a dense amnesic gap for the attack itself persists. There is no clinically significant, long-term cognitive impairment, although more subtle deficits have been reported. Recurrence is rare and occurs at a rate of around 3–5% per year.

Aetiology

Ever since the first descriptions of TGA, there has been considerable debate about its aetiology and this debate remains unresolved. TGA-like attacks have been reported in association with brain tumours, sodium amobarbital injection, high altitude, herpes simplex encephalitis and the use of marijuana. This suggests that TGA could be a 'final common pathway' with numerous potential triggers.

Epilepsy

Fisher and Adams believed that the most likely explanation for TGA was cerebral seizure activity and several other early authors also maintained this position [11–17]. This idea has now largely fallen out of favour for a number of reasons. Epilepsy is, by definition, a recurrent condition whereas patients usually experience only a single episode of TGA in their lifetime. The duration of most TGA attacks is also uncharacteristically long for epileptic seizures. Other common features of generalized or partial epilepsy are absent during the attack. Finally, electroencephalography (EEG) recordings during or after a TGA attack are almost invariably normal or show only minor non-specific abnormalities [18, 19]. In a series of 114 patients followed up over a mean of 34 months following TGA, Hodges and Warlow identified a small subset (7%) that subsequently developed epilepsy [20]. These patients, in keeping with more recent descriptions of TEA (see below), typically had briefer and recurrent amnesic episodes.

Migraine

Several authors have proposed a causal link between migraine and TGA [21–24]. A past history of migraine has been reported to be present in up to 30% of patients with TGA [7], a significantly higher proportion than in controls, and migrainous features, particularly headache and nausea, accompany about 20% of TGA attacks [6]. Olesen and Jorgensen suggested

that the underlying pathological mechanism behind both TGA and migraine might be the experimentally observed phenomenon of spreading depression [25]. A range of stimuli, applied directly to the cortex, may induce a wave of depolarization that spreads at a rate of 3–5 mm/minute and reduces cerebral blood flow for a period of about 1 hour. Spreading depression can be elicited in the hippocampus of experimental animals, in which it provokes a transient period of amnesia. According to the migraine hypothesis, emotional or physical stressors lead to the release of glutamate in the hippocampus triggering spreading depression and hippocampal dysfunction. Critics argue that the migraine hypothesis does not readily account for the age range of TGA or its low recurrence rate.

Arterial

Permanent amnesia can result from stroke, most frequently when involving the thalamus bilaterally [26]. It is, therefore, reasonable to ask whether TGA is a form of transient ischaemic attack (TIA). A number of studies have, however, shown that patients with TGA have fewer vascular risk factors than control subjects with TIA and a more favourable prognosis in terms of mortality and cerebrovascular events [7, 8]. Recent imaging studies (below) have shown changes in the hippocampus in the days following attacks but the features are not typical of standard ischaemic stroke.

Venous

A more recent theory is that originated by Lewis [27], which postulates that the well-recognized triggers of TGA lead to an increase in central venous pressure. In susceptible individuals, this should cause venous ischaemia in medial temporal and diencephalic brain regions. Support for this idea comes from reports of jugular valve insufficiency leading to retrograde venous flow during a Valsalva-like manoeuvre in 73.4% of TGA patients compared with 35.7% of controls [28].

Psychological

Emotional stress as a trigger for TGA is well recognized. It has been reported that TGA patients are more likely to have phobic personality traits [29] and a past history and family history of psychiatric disease [30] than normal control subjects and patients with TIAs. These authors propose that, in such individuals, hyperventilation in response to a stressful situation leads to a reduction of cerebral blood flow in medial temporal regions and consequent transient amnesia [31].

Neuroimaging

For many years, structural brain imaging was thought to be entirely normal in the majority of TGA cases. Recently, however, a number of studies have shown that, in the period immediately following a TGA attack (within 24–72 hours of onset), diffusion weighted magnetic resonance imaging (MRI) can detect small (1–2 mm), punctate hippocampal lesions, indicating areas of restricted diffusion, in about 70% of patients [32]. These lesions are most frequently found in the CA1 subfield of the hippocampus, a region known to be particularly sensitive to hypoxic injury, and may be unilateral or bilateral (see Figure 25.1). At repeat scanning 4–6 months later, the lesions are no longer detectable and memory function has returned to normal. The pathophysiology of these abnormalities remains unclear, although they have been used to support hypotheses of both arterial and venous aetiologies [28, 33].

Neuropsychology

Formal neuropsychological testing during a TGA attack bears out the clinical impression. The patient is able to hold and manipulate information normally in working memory as tested, for example, by backwards digit span [34]. However, on tests of long-term anterograde memory, such as, delayed recall of a word list, story or complex figure performance is at floor [6]. Interestingly, despite having no recollection of stimuli encountered during the attack, patients nonetheless demonstrate perceptual priming [35] suggesting that, as with more permanent amnesia from medial temporal lobe or diencephalic damage, implicit memory remains intact.

During the episode, patients also lose access to memories acquired prior to the onset of the attack (retrograde amnesia) to some degree. The initial acquisition of such memories is, of course, beyond the reach of experimental manipulation so assessment of retrograde

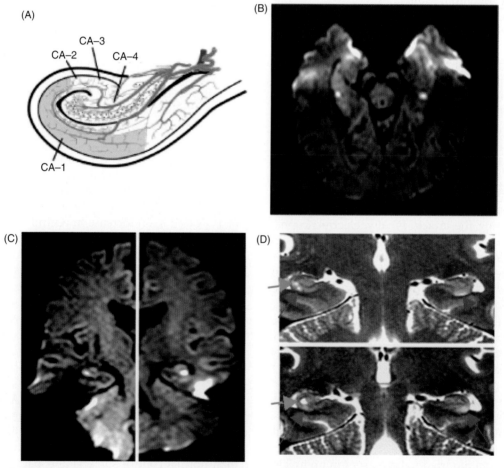

FIGURE 25.1   Magnetic resonance imaging in TGA. (A) Hippocampal subfields, (B)–(D) Typical lesions seen in the hippocampus within 48 hours after onset on axial and coronal diffusion-weighted and T_2-weighted sequences, respectively. Note in this case the bilateral T_2 lesions in the CA-1 sector of the cornu ammonis (red arrow) extending over 4–5 mm (slice thickness 2 mm), which are clearly separated from the cavity of the pre-existing vestigial hippocampal sulcus (green arrow) located in deeper subcortical layers in the vicinity of the gyrus dentatus [32]. (Reproduced with permission of Oxford University Press.)

amnesia can be difficult. In the acute and recovery phase of TGA, tests probing memory for both personal and public facts and events have revealed variable patterns of impairment across individuals. In general, accounts of personally experienced episodes are 'curiously empty and lacking in colour, as if reduced to the bare bones of memory' [36]. They lack what has been called 'autonoetic consciousness' – the feeling of having experienced the past episode oneself [37]. Retrograde amnesia may affect memories from across the lifespan [38] or from a more limited time period prior to the attack [39].

During the recovery phase, retrograde memory improves more rapidly than anterograde memory. In some cases, memories are recovered in chronological order whereas in others more salient, detailed memories return first no matter what age they are [10, 38]. Anterograde memory impairment lasts much longer than is clinically apparent. Deficits, particularly in story recall, can be demonstrated several days and, in some cases, several months later. Following recovery from TGA, patients are left with complete amnesia for events that occurred during the attack. There is also usually a short, permanent retrograde amnesia for events that occurred in the 1–2 hours leading up to the attack [6].

TRANSIENT EPILEPTIC AMNESIA

Amnesia is a cardinal feature of the majority of epileptic seizures, particularly generalized and complex partial seizures. This amnesia is usually only one manifestation of a wide disruption of cerebral function that results in loss or alteration of consciousness during the ictus. However, it has been recognized for over a century that, occasionally, memory impairment may be the sole feature of epileptic seizures. In 1888, the renowned British neurologist Hughlings-Jackson described the case of Dr Z, a medical practitioner who suffered from an unusual variety of epilepsy [40]. During seizures, he retained consciousness and was able to engage in complex, purposeful behaviour for which he was later amnesic. On one occasion he felt the onset of a seizure whilst examining a patient. During this attack, he correctly diagnosed pneumonia, prescribed treatment and wrote in the patient's notes, but later had no recollection of having done so.

When Fisher and Adams first described the syndrome of TGA [1], they concluded that it was most likely due to cerebral seizure activity. It is now clear that this is not true for the majority of TGA attacks (see above). However, despite using stringent diagnostic criteria for

TGA, Hodges and Warlow discovered that a significant minority (7%) of the patients in their series went on to develop complex partial seizures [7]. This observation, together with a steady trickle of case reports in the literature, has led to increasing interest in the syndrome of TEA – a term, introduced by Kapur [41], which not only emphasizes the similarity to, but also the differences from TGA.

A 58-year-old carpet fitter experienced 28 episodes of transient amnesia over 18 months. All occurred upon waking in the night and lasted about 20 minutes. He repetitively questioned his wife, but was responsive and coherent throughout. During one attack he was unable to recall the death of his brother a few days earlier. Routine EEG and MRI were normal. Lamotrigine abolished the attacks but they briefly returned, with associated olfactory hallucinations, during a period of non-compliance, and ceased again when he restarted the medication. At interview, he described rapid forgetting of recently acquired memories, patchy loss of salient autobiographical memories from the past 30 years, such as his wife's abdominal surgery and the wedding of his son, and significant new difficulties navigating around his local area.

The diagnosis of TEA is made when a patient meets the following diagnostic criteria [42, 43]:

1. a history of recurrent witnessed episodes of transient amnesia;
2. cognitive functions other than memory judged to be intact during typical episodes by a reliable witness;
3. evidence for a diagnosis of epilepsy based on one or more of the following:
   - a epileptiform abnormalities on EEG,
   - the concurrent onset of other clinical features of epilepsy (e.g., lip-smacking, olfactory hallucinations),
   - a clear-cut response to anticonvulsant therapy.

Clinical Features

Review of the literature [42] and our recent, detailed study of 50 cases [43], reveal TEA to have many consistent features. As with TGA, TEA typically begins in late middle to old age (mean 62 years). Why this age group should be particularly susceptible to both conditions remains uncertain. The amnestic attacks are characterized by a mixed anterograde and retrograde amnesia. In comparison with TGA, there is considerable variation in the relative extent of these two components. Some patients, for example, have incomplete anterograde amnesia and are later able to 'remember not having been able to remember'. Other patients have minimal or no obvious retrograde amnesia and only realize that they have had an attack when they are later unable to recall part of their day. The preservation of other cognitive functions such as attention, perception, language and executive function is revealed by the patient's continued ability to respond appropriately to conversation and act in a purposeful manner. In our series, there were reports of patients driving, winning a hand at bridge, sight-reading piano pieces and translating text from French into English. Certain additional features may accompany the amnesia. Most commonly (in almost half the cases in our series), patients experience hallucinations of smell or taste which are usually unpleasant – 'like burning rubber', 'metallic', 'rotten'. The attack typically lasts around 30 minutes to 1 hour. However, much longer episodes, even persisting for several days, have been reported and may reflect non-convulsive status epilepticus [44, 45]. Whereas TGA is usually a one-off event, patients with TEA experience recurrent attacks of memory loss, with an average frequency of around 13 per year [43].

There is a close and intriguing relationship between TEA and sleep. Approximately three-quarters of patients will have at least one amnesic attack upon waking and one-quarter only ever experience amnesia in this context [43]. Some have described such attacks as very similar to, only more persistent than, the disorientation many of us have briefly felt upon waking in an unfamiliar place. One patient noted in his journal: 'Woke up at 3.30 a.m. – had no idea where I was. After stumbling around to find a light switch, found that I was in a small room in the P ... Hotel in Milan. Initially had no idea why I was here. Found documents in room with my itinerary ... Gradually began to recall that I was on a trip to attend meetings in Milan and Lugano.' The reason for the relationship between sleep and TEA is not yet clear. It may be that the transition from sleep to waking acts as a trigger to an epileptogenic area in memory-related brain regions. Alternatively, amnesia upon waking may reflect persistent post-ictal dysfunction of such brain regions following a seizure during sleep. In one case, for example, morning amnesia was always preceded by a brief arousal at around 2 a.m. when the patient sat up in bed, staring and said 'Oh, the smell, the smell' before going straight back to sleep.

Given the apparent similarity between TEA attacks and the amnesia observed in TGA and other forms of medial temporal lobe amnesia, it can expected that TEA results from disruption of function in the hippocampus and related structures. Certain clinical features, including the frequent co-occurrence of olfactory hallucinosis and the predominance of temporal lobe epileptiform abnormalities on the EEG, would support this hypothesis. One patient, who was admitted to hospital during a very prolonged episode of epileptic amnesia, underwent ictal FDG-PET scanning which revealed focal hypermetabolism in the left anterior hippocampus (see Figure 25.2). One month later, this abnormality had resolved.

In common with other forms of late-onset epilepsy, TEA generally responds well to a low dose of anticonvulsant medication. However, despite complete

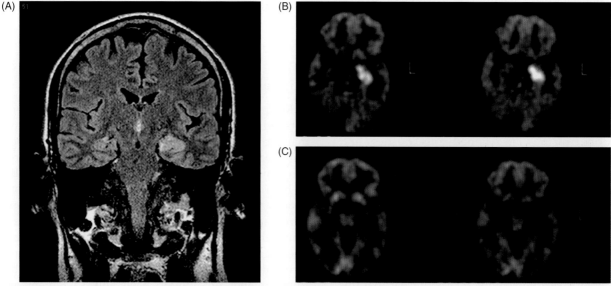

FIGURE 25.2   Neuroimaging during a prolonged episode of TEA. (A) FLAIR MRI scanning during a prolonged episode of TEA revealed hyperintensity in the left hippocampus, (B) FDG-PET scanning during the same episode showed hypermetabolism localized to the left anterior hippocampus, (C) This region had returned to normal 1 month later.

cessation of acute amnesic attacks, the patient often complains of ongoing memory difficulties. Two problems are particularly common.

Accelerated Long-Term Forgetting

About 50% of patients with TEA report that, although they are able to retain new information over the short term, these memories seem to evaporate over a few days or weeks. For example, immediately after returning from holiday in the Rhineland, a patient gave an intricately narrated slide presentation to his family. However, 2 months later he had no recollection of his trip to Germany or of the slideshow. This problem can be extremely debilitating, and led to the early retirement of a number of patients in our series. However, it falls under the radar of standard neuropsychological tests, which typically assess retention of information over a period of less than 1 hour. Since TEA patients usually perform very well on such tests, their difficulties are sometimes mislabelled as 'psychological'.

However, if memory for a story, a list of words or a series of designs is tested at longer intervals – up to 3 weeks – a clear difference emerges between TEA patients and neurologically normal control subjects (see Figure 25.3) [43]. The cause of Accelerated Long-term Forgetting (ALF) is not yet known. It may be related to seizure activity (presumably sub-clinical, since frank seizures were no longer present in the patients tested) or to underlying structural pathology in memory-related brain areas. With regard to current models of memory, ALF has been interpreted as representing a deficit in long-term 'systems' consolidation, a hypothetical

process by which memory traces are reorganized in the brain over time and thus become more resistant to disruption. The relationship between TEA attacks and waking therefore becomes particularly intriguing given recent interest in the possibility that memory consolidation processes are most active during sleep [46–48].

Autobiographical Memory Loss

Even more common amongst TEA patients is the complaint, in about 70%, of a patchy loss of remote, salient autobiographical memories, often extending back over many decades of their life. They frequently report, for example, being unable to remember family holidays or weddings from the past 20 to 30 years, even when prompted with photographs. As mentioned above, autobiographical memory is difficult to assess formally since the original encoding episode is beyond the control of the experimenter. This problem is enhanced in TEA by the patchy nature of the memory loss. However, using a semi-structured interview in which subjects are requested to provide detailed episodic memories relating to a particular topic (e.g., moving house) for each decade of their lives, we exposed significant differences between patients and controls (see Figure 25.4) [43].

Remote memory loss in the absence of significant impairment of anterograde memory has been termed 'focal retrograde amnesia'. Some authorities have questioned whether this can ever be caused by purely 'organic' brain disease [49], and its pathophysiological basis is still far from clear. However, the phenomenon has potential to reveal much about the brain processes behind autobiographical recollection.

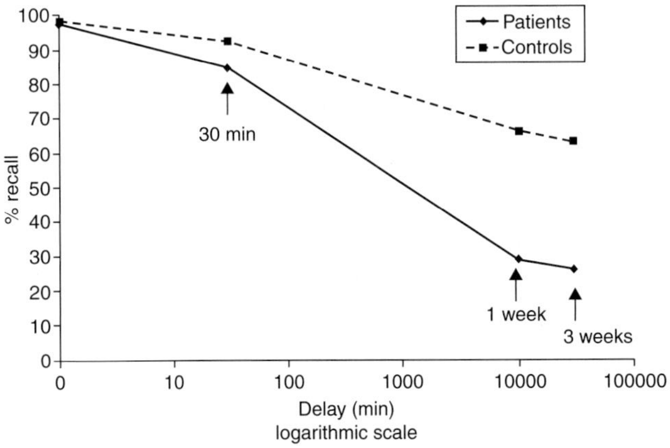

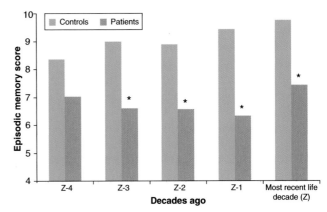

FIGURE 25.3 ALF in TEA 24 patients with TEA and 24 normal controls learnt a list of 15 words. Despite normal learning and initial recall, patients showed accelerated forgetting over 3 weeks [43]. (Reproduced with permission from John Wiley and Sons Inc.)

FIGURE 25.4 Autobiographical memory impairment in TEA Mean scores of TEA patients ($n = 22$) and matched control subjects ($n = 18$) on the episodic memory component of the Modified Autobiographical Memory Interview (*$P < 0.001$) [43]. (Reproduced with permission from John Wiley and Sons Inc.)

A third interictal problem occurs in some patients. In our recent series, 18/50 patients complained of impairment of topographical memory – difficulty in recognizing familiar landmarks and in navigating previously familiar routes.

PSYCHOGENIC AMNESIA

Cases of transient amnesia straddle the border between psychiatry and neurology, and highlight just how artificial and misleading the traditional distinction between these two disciplines can be. As discussed above, TGA, generally thought of as a 'neurological' condition with hints of 'organic pathology' in the medial temporal lobes, can be triggered by psychological stressors and may even be more common amongst people with certain personality traits. Other instances of transient amnesia, in which there is no obvious neuropathological explanation, may be more easily explained in purely psychological terms. Such cases, variably termed 'psychogenic amnesia', 'functional amnesia', 'dissociative amnesia' or 'hysterical amnesia', are characterized by:

'a memory loss that is attributable to an instigating event or process that does not result in insult, injury or disease affecting brain tissue, but that produces more forgetting than would normally occur in the absence of that instigating event or process' [50].

Psychogenic amnesia may be divided into two main subtypes after Kopelman [51]: situation-specific psychogenic amnesia and global psychogenic amnesia. In the former, there is a temporally circumscribed amnesia for a specific and usually emotionally charged event such as a criminal offence. The degree of amnesia is proportional to the violence of the offence, and up to 30% of convicted homicide cases have amnesia claimed at trial [52]. Rates are higher in so-called 'crimes of passion', where a murder is unpremeditated and associated with extreme emotional arousal, and if alcohol or drug intoxication is involved. Although the mechanism of this type of amnesia is unclear, it is unlikely to be due to malingering, or 'putting it on', and in many legal systems, amnesia does not in itself constitute a defence. On occasions, the defendant may claim decreased responsibility for a crime on account of an 'intrinsic' brain disorder such as epilepsy, sleepwalking or hypoglycaemia. Although such conditions are only very rarely implicated in violent crime, they can result in amnesia and pose considerable diagnostic challenges.

Global psychogenic amnesia is not restricted to a single event but involves memory loss for a large swathe of the patient's life.

A 43-year-old construction worker was brought to hospital by colleagues. That morning, he had suffered a minor head injury when his forklift truck collided, at low speed, with an earth bank. Since then, he had a 'complete loss of memory', with no recollection of any past events. He was unable to remember his own name and failed to recognize his colleagues or, when she arrived, his recently estranged wife. Despite this, there was no apparent difficulty in learning new information – he could recount in detail the events following his arrival at hospital. MRI of the brain was normal. It later emerged that, since an acrimonious separation from his wife, he had been showing signs of depression and drinking heavily. He had suffered a period of concussion following a motorcycle accident in his 20's.

The onset typically follows a stressful experience, such as a marital or financial crisis, and there is often a background of depression or alcohol abuse [53]. It is thought that psychogenic amnesia is commonly associated with a history of 'organic' transient amnesia [54]. Knowledge of personal identity is often impaired: this is not a feature of organic amnesia. There may be a period of wandering, 'psychogenic fugue' that typically lasts for a few hours or days. There is usually a relative preservation of anterograde memory, so that patients are able to 'relearn' about themselves, although they may complain that such memories lack the experiential aspect, or 'autonoetic consciousness', that defines true episodic memory. Recovery is frequently protracted and incomplete. The brain mechanisms responsible for psychogenic amnesia are unknown. It has been proposed that there is a functional disconnection between memory storage and retrieval mechanisms in the frontal and temporal lobes [55] and functional neuroimaging studies have revealed decreased brain metabolism, at baseline and during attempted memory retrieval, in the right frontal cortex [56].

HEAD INJURY

Following closed head injury, there is often a period of posttraumatic amnesia (PTA) during which new learning is grossly impaired and there is retrograde memory loss for events leading up to the head injury. This can occur even in mild injuries which produce no coma. The retrograde amnesia gradually shrinks until the patient can recall all but the brief instant preceding the head injury. The duration of the anterograde amnesia is predictive of the final neuropsychological outcome [57]. The memory deficits are usually accompanied by a variety of other cognitive and behavioural problems including impaired attention, agitation, lethargy and disinhibited behaviour. The pathological mechanisms underlying PTA may be a combination of focal contusions, characteristically in the frontal or temporal lobes, diffuse axonal injury and secondary effects of hypoxia or ischemia. Sometimes, a mild head injury such as sustained during sport, may trigger an episode of typical TGA with repetitive questioning. This tends to occur in people below the usual age range for TGA, and may be recurrent [9].

DRUGS

A period of transient memory impairment can also result from administration of several types of drug including benzodiazepines, anticholinergics, ketamine (an N-methyl-D-Aspartate (NMDA) receptor antagonist) and alcohol. Benzodiazepines, particularly midazolam, are widely used in clinical practice as an adjunct to or even replacement of anaesthesia. The resultant, short lived and predominantly anterograde amnesia is thought to result from specific impairment of memory encoding, not just a generalized reduction in alertness [58]. Retrograde memory is unaffected. Benzodiazepines act as agonists at inhibitory $GABA_A$ receptors and the specificity of the cognitive deficit may be partially due to the abundance of these receptors in the hippocampal complex. Declarative, conscious memories appear to be specifically targeted: certain types of procedural memory and perceptual priming have been shown to remain intact [59, 60].

TRANSIENT AMNESIA AND CONSCIOUSNESS

The amnesic syndrome, in both its permanent and transient forms, offers insights into the relationships between memory and consciousness. In this closing section, we will explore these with regard to transient amnesia. Neither 'memory' nor 'consciousness' are straightforward, unitary concepts so an initial clarification of terms is required [61]. We will then consider three aspects of their relationships: (i) the effect of transient amnesia on consciousness, in the senses of 'wakefulness' and 'awareness'; (ii) the effect of transient amnesia on the consciousness of self; (iii) the distinction between conscious but unremembered behaviour and 'automatism'.

The syndromes we have described in this chapter affect the ability to form or retrieve long-term declarative memories, but leave the following kinds of memory intact: working or 'short-term' memory (the ability to hold information 'in mind' and to manipulate

it mentally); perceptual memory (underlying the processes of perceptual classification that allow us, for example, to identify glimpses of the same object from different views); semantic memory (our database of explicit knowledge about language and the world) and procedural memory (a collective term used to refer to memories that guide behaviour without requirement for explicit recollection – like memories for motor skills and conditioned responses). The key senses of 'consciousness' we need to consider here are wakefulness, a conscious *state*, and 'awareness' or 'experience', the current *contents* of consciousness.

The Effect of Transient Amnesia on Consciousness

Consciousness in the sense of 'wakefulness' is unaffected by transient amnesia of the kinds we have discussed in this chapter. Correspondingly, the abilities, normally on line during ordinary wakefulness, to perform complex, goal-directed actions and to monitor their execution, are also unaffected, at least over short periods. We have seen that patients with transient amnesia are able to walk, use objects, talk and drive; during episodes of TGA patients have been reported variously to persevere with carpentry, put together the alternator of a car, row a small dingy to the seashore, perform a complex bell ringing routine, and engage in ballroom dancing [6]. Patients with TEA whom we have studied recently have managed, during attacks, to sight read piano pieces, translate between languages and win a hand of cards. Of course, their performance is liable to falter if they forget what they are meant to be doing: presumably in the cases just noted the activity itself provided a continuing series of cues that kept the performer on task.

What of these patients' awareness, the contents of their experience, during attacks? To judge by their own reports, patients are indeed aware of themselves and their surroundings during episodes of transient amnesia, but this awareness is altered in various ways. Thus, sufferers usually recognize and are perplexed by their inability to remember events from a few minutes ago, if anterograde memory is disabled, or from the more distant past, if retrograde memory is affected. The quality of recollection, more generally, may be altered in patients with an associated impairment of 'autonoetic consciousness', whose remote memories lose their colour and detail. It is possible, though this has not so far been investigated, that during episodes of transient amnesia there is a subtle but pervasive alteration of experience of the present, if this depends to some extent on the operation of structures in the limbic system involved in memory formation and retrieval [62].

The Effect of Transient Amnesia on the Consciousness of Self

Patients sometimes become distressed during episodes of transient amnesia because of their inability to situate their current experience in a coherent context. Failing to recognize his son or his new bungalow during an episode of TEA, our patient RG was found in tears by his wife. He explained: 'I can't remember anything, it feels horrible'.

The abilities to contextualize our experience, to interpret it through a personal narrative and incorporate it in our autobiography, are important elements in our consciousness of self. Antonio Damasio has contrasted this 'extended consciousness' to the 'core consciousness' that normally confers '… a consciousness of oneself as an immediate subject of experience, unextended in time' [63]: it is '… a transient entity, ceaselessly recreated for each and every object with which the brain interacts' [64]. In transient amnesia the core self is intact: sufferers are in no doubt about the ownership of their experiences, but the extended self, rooted in the past and reaching towards the future, is imperilled by the loss of access to personally significant memories. The theme of the interdependence of the self and autobiographical memory is echoed in other contemporary theories of self-knowledge [65].

In TEA, specifically, the temporary loss of access to remote memories that occurs during the attack is accompanied, between attacks, by a persistent, patchy, but dense loss of memories for some salient autobiographical events, often extending back for several decades. Like the transient loss of access, this depletion of autobiographical memory is sometimes distressing. Its tempo and mechanism, its impact on the sense of self and the role of anticonvulsant drugs in preventing its progression are all uncertain at present.

The Distinction between Conscious but Unremembered Behaviour and 'Automatism'

The diagnosis of TGA or TEA requires evidence from a witness that the patient was 'conscious' at the time of the episode – that is to say, able to behave normally in all respects other than those governed by the memory dysfunction. Sometimes, however, there is no witness to clarify this point. We may then be left in a quandary as to whether awareness itself, or merely memory, was impaired at the time. This important,

but potentially problematic, distinction was underlined by Dr Z, Hughlings-Jackson's physician–patient with epileptic amnesia, who wrote in his diary, on the occasion mentioned earlier in this chapter, of his 'unconscious – or perhaps I should say unremembered – diagnosis'. In this case, Dr Z's preserved abilities to converse with his patient, examine him and record the correct diagnosis demonstrate that he was conscious at the time, beyond all reasonable doubt, even if he was amnesic for the process afterwards. But what of those occasions, familiar to most of us, when we have no recollection of an episode of apparently well integrated but relatively simple behaviour – for example of a 20 minute drive down a familiar road – in the absence of a witness? Are episodes like these due to transient amnesia without impairment of awareness at the time? Or might awareness be disengaged as well as memory? These questions raise a further fascinating, fundamental, issue: how complex must behaviour be to provide clear evidence for awareness? Although this draws us away from the main subject of the chapter, we shall address the question briefly.

In general, we tend to regard behaviour that is clearly purposeful, and that demonstrates flexible selection of means appropriate to an agent's ends, as evidence for awareness. The ability to converse intelligently and responsively, for example, is normally taken to be conclusive evidence for awareness as it involves just this kind of cognitive flexibility. Automatisms – complex behaviours in the absence of conscious awareness and/or volitional intent – provide test cases for our understanding of the role of awareness in action. The most familiar examples come from realms of sleep and epilepsy.

Sleepwalkers navigate around their surroundings with some, but often insufficient, care, running a real risk of inadvertent injury. They are usually unable to give an account of themselves and remember little or nothing about episodes afterwards. They are thought to be 'unconscious' during episodes – both asleep and unaware – and, indeed, they do not normally exhibit the capacity for flexible and appropriate selection of means to ends. But there are difficult intermediate cases. Sleepwalking is occasionally associated with quite elaborate, and apparently goal-directed behaviour that is nevertheless entirely or largely unremembered afterwards and unintended by the perpetrator in his normal waking state. In a well-known Canadian case, for example, a man was acquitted of the murder of his mother-in-law, an act he had committed after driving 12 km to his in-laws' home, on the grounds that he was sleepwalking [66]. The intuitive notion that the brains of people who sleepwalk are in a twilight state between sleep and waking has been borne out by a recent imaging study demonstrating activity at waking levels in regions of the brain controlling movement while activity in other regions of the cortex, particularly frontal cortex, remains at sleeping levels [67].

Hughlings-Jackson referred to 'all kinds of doings after epileptic fits' under the rubric of automatisms. Contemporary epileptologists recognize five categories of epileptic automatism, 'more or less coordinated adapted epileptic activity occurring during the state of clouding of consciousness ... and usually followed by amnesia for the event': (i) oropharyngeal, for example lip-smacking or chewing movements; (ii) expression of emotion, most often fear; (iii) gestural, such as tapping, rubbing, fidgeting or flag-waving movements; (iv) ambulatory, including walking, running or bicycling movements; (v) verbal, usually single words or short phrases [68]. As a rule, patients are unaware of these behaviours, in the sense that they cannot interact with others or report their behaviour at the time, though this is not always the case even for the types of automatism just listed.

In TEA, as we have seen, patients can interact normally and describe their experiences during attacks despite their subsequent amnesia: for these reasons we would not regard these episodes – like Dr Z's during his unremembered consultation – as automatisms. However, the observation that epileptic activity can disable some but not other psychological capacities complicates the understanding of automatisms: for example, a focal frontal lobe seizure might selectively impair decision-making capacities, interfering with 'volitional intent' but not with perception or memory. Whether a resulting crime is the result of an automatism may be a question for lawyers rather than for scientists.

Finally what of that drive along a familiar road of which we cannot recall a single detail? The cause of the amnesia in such cases is open to investigation, at least in principle. It could be that we had normal awareness of events throughout, but failed to lay down a permanent record of them because they were so mundane. If so, reaction times and accuracy of response should be normal at the time. It could be that the subsequent amnesia reflects a redirection of attention – towards the music on the radio, an internal dialogue, a daydream. If so, questioning at such times should allow report of the current focus of attention; reaction times and accuracy measures are likely to reflect our relative absorption in matters other than driving. If – and this seems highly unlikely – the amnesia is the result of true loss of awareness, probing should once again be revealing, and potentially life-saving!

CONCLUSION

The syndromes of transient amnesia are characterized by a temporary loss of conscious access to knowledge of the past and an inability to lay down new, consciously accessible memories. TGA, TEA and psychogenic amnesia have distinct clinical and neuropsychological features, which are summarized in Table 25.1. These

TABLE 25.1 Distinguishing Clinical Features of the Transient Amnesic Syndromes

	Transient global amnesia	Transient epileptic amnesia	Psychogenic amnesia
Typical age	50–70 years	50–70 years	Also younger
Past medical history	Migraine	Nil	'Organic' transient amnesia, substance abuse, psychiatric illness
Precipitants	Cold water, physical exertion, psychological stress	Waking	Minor head injury, stress, depression
Ictal memory profile	Profound anterograde amnesia with repetitive questioning; variable retrograde amnesia; non-declarative memory intact	Variable anterograde and retrograde amnesia (may later partially recall attack); retrograde procedural memory intact	Highly variable: often profound retrograde amnesia with loss of personal identity; relatively preserved anterograde memory; procedural memory may be impaired
Other features	Headache/nausea may be present	Sometimes: olfactory hallucinations; oroalimentary automatisms; brief loss of responsiveness	Focal 'neurological' symptoms or signs, e.g. hemiparesis may be present
Duration	Typically 4–10 hours	Usually < 1 hour but may last much longer (days)	Days or months
Recurrence	Rare	Mean frequency = 13/year	Rare
Postictal/interictal memory	Grossly intact, but subtle deficits may persist for months	Accelerated forgetting, remote autobiographical memory loss and topographical amnesia	Variable: may 'relearn' the past causing memories to lack 'autonoetic consciousness'

syndromes raise interesting questions about the relationship between memory and consciousness, and provide an arena in which to investigate them further. Patients with transient amnesia are able to act as their own control subjects, and thus eliminate some of the interindividual variation that plagues many lesion studies. Future work should address the status of perceptual experience during transient amnesia, and examine whether implicit memory is truly spared – to test, for example, the recent hypothesis that the hallmark of the deficit in amnesia is not so much conscious access to memory but relational processing [69, 70]. In addition, the persistent autobiographical memory deficits in patients with TEA offer an ideal opportunity to investigate the contentious issue of focal retrograde amnesia, and examine its effect upon that philosophically slippery creature – the self.

References

1. Fisher, C.M. and Adams, R.D. (1964). *Transient global amnesia.* Acta Neurol Scand, 40 (Suppl-83).
2. Bender, M.B. (1960) Single episode of confusion with amnesia. *Bull NY Acad Med* 36:197–207.
3. Poser, C.M. and Ziegler, D.K. (1960) Temporary amnesia as a manifestation of cerebrovascular insufficiency. *Trans Am Neurol Assoc* 85:221–223.
4. Guyotat, J. and Courjon, J. (1956) Les ictus amnésiques. *J Med Lyon* 37:697–701.
5. Evans, J.H. (1966) Transient loss of memory, an organic mental syndrome. *Brain* 89 (3):539–548.
6. Hodges, J.R. (1991) *Transient Amnesia*, London: WB Saunders.
7. Hodges, J.R. and Warlow, C.P. (1990) The aetiology of transient global amnesia. A case–control study of 114 cases with prospective follow-up. *Brain* 113 (Pt 3):639–657.
8. Quinette, P., *et al.* (2006) What does transient global amnesia really mean? Review of the literature and thorough study of 142 cases. *Brain* 129 (Pt 7):1640–1658.
9. Haas, D.C. and Ross, G.S. (1986) Transient global amnesia triggered by mild head trauma. *Brain* 109 (Pt 2):251–257.
10. Kapur, N., *et al.* (1998) Recovery of function processes in human amnesia: evidence from transient global amnesia. *Neuropsychologia* 36 (1):99–107.
11. Godlewski, S. (1968) Amnesic episodes (transient global amnesia). (Clinical study based on 33 unpublished cases). *Sem Hop* 44 (9):553–577.
12. Lou, H. (1968) Repeated episodes of transient global amnesia. *Acta Neurol Scand* 44 (5):612–618.
13. Tharp, B.R. (1969) The electroencephalogram in transient global amnesia. *Electroencephalogr Clin Neurophysiol* 26 (1):96–99.
14. Cantor, F.C. (1971) *Transient global amnesia and temporal lobe seizures*, AAN presentation.
15. Gilbert, G.J. (1978) Transient global amnesia: manifestation of medial temporal lobe epilepsy. *Clin Electroencephalogr* 9:147–152.
16. Rowan, A.J. and Protass, L.M. (1979) Transient global amnesia: clinical and electroencephalographic findings in 10 cases. *Neurology* 29 (6):869–872.
17. Deisenhammer, E. (1981) Transient global amnesia as an epileptic manifestation. *J Neurol* 225 (4):289–292.
18. Miller, J.W., *et al.* (1987) Transient global amnesia and epilepsy. Electroencephalographic distinction. *Arch Neurol* 44 (6):629–633.
19. Jacome, D.E. (1989) EEG features in transient global amnesia. *Clin Electroencephalogr* 20 (3):183–192.
20. Hodges, J.R. and Warlow, C.P. (1989) Syndromes of transient amnesia: towards a classification. A study of 153 cases. *J Neurol, Neurosurg Psychiatr* 53 (10):834–843.
21. Gilbert, J.J. and Benson, D.F. (1972) Transient global amnesia: report of two cases with definite etiologies. *J Nerv Ment Dis* 154 (6):461–464.
22. Laplane, D. and Truelle, J.L. (1974) The mechanism of transient global amnesia. Apropos of some unusual cases. *Nouv Presse Med* 3 (12):721–725.
23. Olivarius, B.D. and Jensen, T.S. (1979) Transient global amnesia in migraine. *Headache* 19 (6):335–338.
24. Caplan, L. (1981) Transient global amnesia and migraine. *Neurology* 31 (9):1167–1170.
25. Olesen, J. and Jorgensen, M.B. (1986) Leao's spreading depression in the hippocampus explains transient global amnesia. A hypothesis. *Acta Neurol Scand* 73 (2):219–220.
26. Schmahmann, J.D. (2003) Vascular syndromes of the thalamus. *Stroke* 34 (9):2264–2278.
27. Lewis, S.L. (1998) Aetiology of transient global amnesia. *Lancet* 352 (9125):397–399.
28. Sander, K. and Sander, D. (2005) New insights into transient global amnesia: Recent imaging and clinical findings. *Lancet Neurol* 4 (7):437–444.
29. Inzitari, D., *et al.* (1997) Emotional arousal and phobia in transient global amnesia. *Arch Neurol* 54 (7):866–873.
30. Pantoni, L., *et al.* (2005) Clinical features, risk factors, and prognosis in transient global amnesia: A follow-up study. *Eur J Neurol* 12 (5):350–356.
31. Pantoni, L., Lamassa, M. and Inzitari, D. (2000) Transient global amnesia: A review emphasizing pathogenic aspects. *Acta Neurol Scand* 102 (5):275–283.
32. Bartsch, T., *et al.* (2006) Selective affection of hippocampal CA-1 neurons in patients with transient global amnesia without long-term sequelae. *Brain* 129 (Pt 11):2874–2884.
33. Winbeck, K., *et al.* (2005) DWI in transient global amnesia and TIA: Proposal for an ischaemic origin of TGA. *J Neurol, Neurosurg Psychiatr* 76 (3):438–441.
34. Quinette, P., *et al.* (2003) Working memory and executive functions in transient global amnesia. *Brain* 126 (Pt 9):1917–1934.
35. Kapur, N., *et al.* (1996) Long-term perceptual priming in transient global amnesia. *Brain Cogn* 31 (1):63–74.
36. Hodges, J.R. and Ward, C.D. (1989) Observations during transient global amnesia. A behavioural and neuropsychological study of five cases. *Brain* 112 (Pt 3):595–620.
37. Wheeler, M.A., Stuss, D.T. and Tulving, E. (1997) Toward a theory of episodic memory: The frontal lobes and autonoetic consciousness. *Psychol Bull* 121 (3):331–354.
38. Guillery-Girard, B., *et al.* (2004) The dynamic time course of memory recovery in transient global amnesia. *J Neurol Neurosurg Psychiatry* 75 (11):1532–1540.
39. Kritchevsky, M. (1997) Transient global amnesia and functional retrograde amnesia: Contrasting examples of episodic memory loss. *Philos Transac Royal Soc B: Biol Sci* 352 (1362):1747–1754.
40. Hughlings-Jackson, J. (1888) On a particular variety of epilepsy (intellectual aura), one case with symptoms of organic brain disease. *Brain* 11:179–207.
41. Kapur, N. and Markowitsch, H.J. (1990) Transient epileptic amnesia: A clinically distinct form of neurological memory disorder. In *Transient Global Amnesia and Related Disorders*, pp. 140–151 New York: Hogrefe and Huber.
42. Zeman, A.Z.J., Boniface, S.J. and Hodges, J.R. (1998) Transient epileptic amnesia: A description of the clinical and

neuropsychological features in 10 cases and a review of the literature. *J Neurol, Neurosurg Psychiatr* 64 (4):435–443.

43. Butler, C.R., *et al.* (2007) The syndrome of transient epileptic amnesia. *Ann Neurol* 61 (6):587–598.

44. Lee, B.I., *et al.* (1992) Prolonged ictal amnesia with transient focal abnormalities on magnetic resonance imaging. *Epilepsia* 33 (6):1042–1046.

45. Vuilleumier, P., Despland, P.A. and Regli, F. (1996) Failure to recall (but not to remember): Pure transient amnesia during nonconvulsive status epilepticus. *Neurology* 46 (4):1036–1039.

46. Walker, M.P. and Stickgold, R. (2006) Sleep, memory, and plasticity. *Annu Rev Psychol* 57:139–166.

47. Walker, M.P. (2005) A refined model of sleep and the time course of memory formation. *Behav Brain Sci* 28 (01):51–64.

48. Ellenbogen, J.M., *et al.* (2006) Interfering with theories of sleep and memory: Sleep, declarative memory, and associative interference. *Curr Biol* 16 (13):1290–1294.

49. Kopelman, M.D. (2000) Focal retrograde amnesia and the attribution of causality: An exceptionally critical review. *Cogn Neuropsychol* 17 (7):585–621.

50. Schacter, D.L. and Kihlstrom, J.F. (1989) Functional amnesia. *Handbook Neuropsychol* 3:209–231.

51. Kopelman, M.D., *et al.* (2002) Psychogenic amnesia *The Handbook of Memory Disorders* Chichester: John Wiley & Sons Ltd pp. 451–471.

52. Pyszora, N.M., Barker, A.F. and Kopelman, M.D. (2003) Amnesia for criminal offences: A study of life sentence prisoners. *J Forensic Psychiatr Psychol* 14 (3):475–490.

53. Kritchevsky, M., Chang, J. and Squire, L.R. (2004) Functional amnesia: Clinical description and neuropsychological profile of 10 cases. *Learn Mem* 11 (2):213–226.

54. Berrington, W.P., Liddell, D.W. and Foulds, G.A. (1956) A re-evaluation of the fugue. *J Ment Sci* 102 (427):280–286.

55. Markowitsch, H.J. (2003) Psychogenic amnesia. *Neuroimage* 20 (1):S132–S138.

56. Markowitsch, H.J. (1999) Functional neuroimaging correlates of functional amnesia. *Memory* 7 (5):561–584.

57. Levin, H.S., O'Donnell, V.M. and Grossman, R.G. (1979) The Galveston orientation and amnesia test. A practical scale to assess cognition after head injury. *J Nerv Ment Dis* 167 (11):675–684.

58. Curran, H.V. and Birch, B. (1991) Differentiating the sedative, psychomotor and amnesic effects of benzodiazepines: A study with midazolam and the benzodiazepine antagonist, flumazenil. *Psychopharmacology* 103 (4):519–523.

59. Thomas-Antérion, C., *et al.* (1999) Midazolam effects on implicit and explicit memory processes in healthy subjects. *Psychopharmacology* 145 (2):139–143.

60. Arndt, J., Passannante, A. and Hirshman, E. (2004) The effect of midazolam on implicit and explicit memory in category exemplar production and category cued recall. *Memory* 12 (2):158–173.

61. Zeman, A. (2002) *Consciousness: A user's guide*, Yale University Press.

62. Lee, A.C., *et al.* (2005) Perceptual deficits in amnesia: Challenging the medial temporal lobe 'mnemonic' view. *Neuropsychologia* 43 (1):1–11.

63. Gallagher, S. (2000) Philosophical conceptions of the self: Implications for cognitive science. *Trend Cogn Sci* 4 (1):14–21.

64. Damasio, A.R. (1999) *The Feeling of What Happens*, New York: Harcourt Brace.

65. Conway, M.A. (2005) Memory and the self. *J Mem Lang* 53 (4):594–628.

66. Broughton, R., *et al.* (1994) Homicidal somnambulism: A case report. *Sleep* 17 (3):253–264.

67. Bassetti, C., *et al.* (2000) SPECT during sleepwalking. *The Lancet* 356 (9228):484–485.

68. Oxbury, J., Polkey, C.E. and Duchowny, M. (2000) *Intractable Focal Epilepsy*, London: WB Saunders.

69. Ryan, J.D., *et al.* (2000) Amnesia is a deficit in relational memory. *Psychol Sci* 11 (6):454–461.

70. Eichenbaum, H. and Cohen, N.J. (2001) *From Conditioning to Conscious Recollection: Memory Systems of the Brain*, New York: Oxford University Press.

Consciousness and Aphasia

Paolo Nichelli

ABSTRACT

Different language impairments allow us to investigate how much the use of language can influence the content of conscious awareness and therefore of thinking and reasoning. Pure anarthria (differently form mutism) and verbal short-term memory deficits are associated with an impairment of the effect of covert speech on the content of working memory. Dynamic aphasia impairs the processes involved in the transition between thinking and speaking. However, even the most severe agrammatic patients can retain reasoning about others' beliefs that according to some theories can only take place in explicit sentences of a natural language.

Error monitoring is also impaired in many aphasic patients and in some of them is associated with complete lack of error awareness (anosognosia for aphasia).

INTRODUCTION

One aspect of consciousness [1] refers to the availability of mental representations for use in other cognitive processes. Mental states are conscious if they can be reported, reasoned about, voluntary acted on, or recollected. Block [2] describes such states and their content as access-conscious, that is other cognitive processes have access to them. This chapter will deal with this aspect of consciousness.

In a clinical setting one can be said to be conscious or aware of something whenever a verbal or a nonverbal description can be provided of the object of that awareness. Aphasic patients can hardly provide precise verbal descriptions of what they see, feel, want, and think. Furthermore, they might have altered comprehension or associated cognitive deficits severe enough to impair their ability with nonverbal descriptions. In order not to underestimate the mental representations they have access to (the 'content' of their consciousness) one has to look carefully for alternative means to obtain controlled responses or indirect evidence of what the aphasic patient is aware of.

In this chapter I will explore the issue of the mental representation available to aphasic patients by using the Baddeley's model of working memory [3]. Within this framework I will analyse the relationships between inner speech, working memory, and different aphasic syndromes. Related to the question of mental representations available to aphasic patients is the question of the relationship between thinking and aphasia. According to some authors certain forms of reasoning can only take place in explicit (i.e., conscious) sentences of a natural language: I will examine this issue by analysing the special case of retained 'Theory of Mind' (ToM) understanding in patients with severe agrammatism. Lastly, I will consider consciousness in its monitoring component and review the topics of language output monitoring and anosognosia of aphasia.

CONSCIOUSNESS AND WORKING MEMORY

The concept of working memory refers to a limited capacity system allowing the temporary storage and manipulation of information necessary for complex tasks as comprehension learning and reasoning. Baddeley's initial model [4] proposed the existence of three functional components of working memory: an attentional control system (the 'central executive'), aided by two subsidiary slave systems, the 'phonological loop', and the 'visuospatial sketchpad'. The two slave systems are assumed to hold respectively phonological and visuospatial information. A fourth component, the 'episodic buffer', was added more recently [5] on the basis of a number of empirical findings. The episodic buffer is assumed to be a limited capacity store that is capable of multidimensional coding. It allows the binding of information to create integrated episodes and it provides a temporary interface between the slave systems and long-term memory (LTM). It is controlled by the central executive, which is responsible for binding information from a number of sources into coherent episodes. Retrieval of

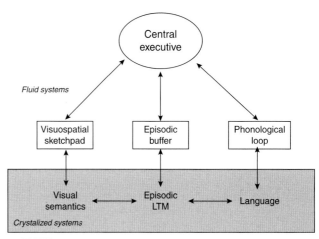

FIGURE 26.1 The current version of Baddeley's multicomponent working memory model. The episodic buffer is assumed to form a temporary storage that allows information from the subsystem to be combined with data from long-term memory into integrated chunks. This system is assumed to form a basis for conscious awareness. *Source*: Based on Baddeley [6].

such episodes is based on conscious awareness. Figure 26.1 shows the four components of the 'fluid' working memory model (subserving attention and temporary storage) and their proposed relations to 'crystallized' cognitive systems (shaded area), capable of accumulating long-term knowledge.

It is argued that some components of the model have a modular organization [7]. However, this would not be the case for the biological mechanism of the episodic buffer (the binding), for which the process of synchronous firing [8] is assumed to be the most promising hypothesis [5].

Within the working memory model, short-term storage and manipulation of verbal material is accomplished by the 'slave system' called the 'phonological loop' [9]. In turn, the phonological loop is conceived as a modular system. The main characteristic of this system is the distinction of two separate components: a phonological non-articulatory short-term store [10] and an articulatory rehearsal mechanism [11]. The phonological store consists of auditory memory traces that are subject to rapid decay. The articulatory rehearsal mechanism is an active process that can refresh the content of the phonological store, thus preventing trace decay. Auditory material is registered directly in the phonological store while visually presented verbal information is transformed into phonological code by silent articulation and thereby encoded into the phonological store.

The notion of such a model (Figure 26.2) is supported by the following findings:

1. *The phonological similarity effect*: Immediate memory is poorer for phonologically similar items (e.g., P, T,

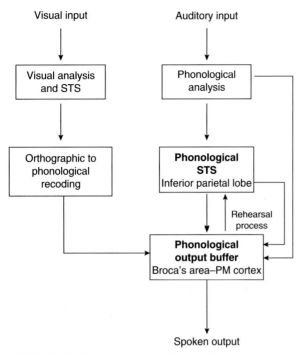

Visual input　　　　Auditory input

Visual analysis and STS

Phonological analysis

Orthographic to phonological recoding

Phonological STS
Inferior parietal lobe

Rehearsal process

Phonological output buffer
Broca's area–PM cortex

Spoken output

FIGURE 26.2　The proposed model for the phonological loop. Auditory information is analysed and fed into a phonological short-term store. From this system, information can either pass into the phonological output buffer or be rehearsed, both overtly and subvocally. Visually presented stimuli are transferred from an orthographic to a phonological code and thereby registered within the phonological output buffer. STM: short-term store; PM: premotor. *Source:* Based on Baddeley [6].

C, V, B) as compared with dissimilar items (e.g., R, W, Y, Z, Q). Semantic similarity has comparatively little effect [12].

2. *The word length effect*: Immediate memory span is better with short than with long words. This is explained by the fact that short words can be articulated faster, so that more words can be silently articulated before they decay [13].

3. *The effect of articulatory suppression*: Memory for verbal material is impaired when people are asked to say something irrelevant aloud. This is assumed to block the articulatory rehearsal process, thereby leaving memory traces in the phonological loop to decay. With visually presented items the information is transferred from a visual to an auditory code. Articulatory suppression prevents this transfer, and in that case the phonological similarity effect disappears. On the contrary, with auditory presentation concurrent articulation suppresses the word length effect but not the phonological similarity effect [14]. It is therefore assumed that the word length effect is due to the articulatory rehearsal mechanism, while the phonological similarity effect reflects the

process going on within the phonological store, which directly receives auditory information but needs the mediation of the articulatory rehearsal mechanism to be fed by visual information.

WHAT IS 'INNER SPEECH'

The term 'inner speech' has been used in many ways. First, it refers to the subjective phenomenon of talking to oneself, of developing an auditory–articulatory image of speech without uttering a sound. Second, it refers to the objectively measurable ability to appreciate the auditory–articulatory structure of speech irrespective of its meaning [15]. Third, it refers to any measurable effect of covert speech on the content of verbal short-term memory.

INNER SPEECH AND ANARTHRIA

Pure anarthria is a rare disorder commonly defined as a total inability to articulate speech in the absence of any deficit both of auditory comprehension and of written language. It can follow either cortical, subcortical, and brain stem lesions. Anarthria should be kept separate from mutism (inability or unwillingness to speak in the absence of any brain lesion capable to affect the articulatory planning), as well as from dysarthria (a speech disorder due to weakness or incoordination of speech muscles).

Some anarthric patients (see for instance the patient described by Levine *et al.* [15]) subjectively report that they do not speak silently. Yet, several authors have claimed that anarthria does not affect covert articulation: they based this assumption on the finding that anarthric patients perform short-term memory tasks differently from normal subjects who are prevented from articulating [16–18]. However Cubelli and Nichelli [19] showed that anarthric patients perform short-term memory tasks differently also from normal subjects who are allowed to subvocally rehearse.

Furthermore, anarthric patients' performance demonstrates dissociation between patients with pontine lesions and patients with frontal opercular lesions. Pontine patients (i.e., patients with 'locked-in' syndrome) do not show a word length effect with both auditory and visual stimuli but they do show a phonological similarity effect with visual stimuli. On the other hand, patients with fronto-opercular anarthria do show a word length effect with auditory but not with visual stimuli. In a further study Cubelli *et al.* [20] demonstrated that anarthric patients score in the lower bounds of the performance of normal subjects suppressing articulation at a task of subvocal counting (e.g., when they are requested to count the number of items a stimulus appears in the centre of a computer screen). These results have been interpreted as due to the impaired functioning of a circuit dependent on supplementary motor area in the case of the locked-in syndrome and to the impairment of multiple afferent and efferent connection of the lateral premotor system in the case of cortical anarthria. In conclusion, anarthric patients' performance with tasks involving subvocal rehearsal demonstrates that they are not simply 'mute', as their inability on overt articulation is associated with a more subtle impairment of covert articulation. It appears therefore that 'inner speech' (in this case the 'inner voice') is dependent for its operation on brain mechanisms involved in 'outer' speech.

INNER SPEECH IN CONDUCTION APHASIA

Conduction aphasia is a language disorder characterized by selective defect of oral repetition of words or sentences in the presence of relative preservation of auditory comprehension. The general level of articulation, rate of speech, and use of grammatical elements is fluent, but speech output is usually disrupted by phonemic paraphasias and anomias.

Kurt Goldstein [21] suggested that conduction aphasia is a disturbance of 'inner speech', a central language process mediating between nonverbal thought and external speech. Fienberg et al. [22] hypothesized that if that assumption were correct patients with conduction aphasia should fail on tasks requiring the generation of phonological representation of words even when no overt speech is required. They tested this hypothesis in five patients who had conduction aphasia with similar speech disturbances. The patients were presented with pictures and were required to perform, without overt vocalization, comparisons of word length and homophonic and rhyming matches. Four patients successfully performed such judgements on words they could not vocalize, but one patient could not. The findings provided evidence for heterogeneity within the class of conduction aphasia and suggested that 'inner speech' might be impaired only in a subgroup of conduction aphasics.

Further studies [23] have demonstrated that a majority of patients with conduction aphasia also shows a selective deficit in verbal short-term memory. One Italian patient, P.V., with a very pure and specific deficit in auditory short-term memory, was extensively tested to determine whether her deficit could be explained within the working memory framework [11]. She appeared to be intellectually entirely normal, with a high level of verbal and performance I.Q., and excellent LTM [24]. Her immediate memory span was no more than 2 items with auditory presentation and about 3–4 items with visual presentation. Her performance was affected by phonological similarity with spoken but not with visual presentation, as if she had a phonological store but was not using the articulatory rehearsal process to feed it. That this was indeed the case was also confirmed by lack of the usual deleterious effect of articulatory suppression on the span of visually presented items. However, she also showed a defective phonological store, as demonstrated by the progressive impairment at a task of shadowing spoken words by presenting them at various rates. While she was able to perform this task at slow rates, her performance fell behind that of controls as speed increased and phonological store was needed as a buffer to avoid temporary overload [9].

A particularly interesting observation concerns P.V.'s ability at learning: while she was very good at learning lists of meaningful words Baddeley et al. [25] demonstrated that she could not learn unfamiliar words, such as the vocabulary of a foreign language. Within the framework of the Baddeley's working memory model such a deficit of the phonological loop prevented the episodic buffer to build associations between new words and semantic nodes to be stored in LTM.

INNER SPEECH AND DYNAMIC APHASIA

In 1885 Lichtheim [26] reported a patient with a striking dissociation between his inability to talk or write spontaneously and his ability to name objects, repeat words and phrases, read and write under dictation. This pattern of speech disturbance was termed 'transcortical motor aphasia' and subsequently subdivided in two types, both sharing the common characteristic of preserved word repetition. One type is characterized by effortful non-fluent spontaneous speech in which phonemic paraphasic errors were common. The second type, named by Luria [27] 'dynamic aphasia' is characterized by sparsely produced but normally articulated spontaneous speech. Luria and Tsvetkova [28] provided the first analytic investigation of dynamic aphasia. They hypothesized that 'inner speech with its predicative function which takes part in forming the structure or scheme of a sentence is disturbed in cases of dynamic aphasia'. In this framework 'inner speech' is defined as 'a mechanism used by the subjects for the transition from a preliminary idea to the extended verbal proposition' and provides the so-called linear schema of the sentence.

Costello and Warrington [29] reported a patient, who, after a left frontal lobe tumour, manifested a selective speech disorder with all the hallmarks of a dynamic aphasia. His speech was very sparse, with long response latencies and, on many occasions, with a complete absence of response. At the same time there was no evidence of impaired comprehension or naming difficulties. His repetition was excellent and his literacy skill (reading and spelling) satisfactory. On the few occasions that he did use speech spontaneously there was no evidence of paraphasic errors and his speech it was grammatically correct, with normal articulation and prosody. His ability to generate sentences was significantly better given a pictorial context than a verbal context. Although he could order a sequence of pictures, he had the greatest difficulty in ordering the constituent words of a sentence. Based on these findings Luria's hypothesis that dynamic aphasia was due to an impairment of inner speech which provides 'the linear scheme of a sentence' was disconfirmed. It was concluded that dynamic aphasia does not reflect a deficit of language processing but rather the selective impairment of verbal planning.

In a more recent case report and review of dynamic aphasia literature Robinson *et al.* [30] suggested there are two subtypes of dynamic aphasia. The first subtype is characterized by a propositional language impairment resulting in inability to generate a single response on word and sentence level. This deficit is specific to language production and is associated with left posterior frontal damage (Brodman area 45). On the basis of a computational model of prefrontal cortex functioning, Robinson *et al.* [31] proposed that this type of dynamic aphasia might be the result of damage to a 'context' module containing units responsible for selection of verbal response options. The second subtype, associated with bilateral frontal and subcortical involvement, is characterized by a propositional language impairment resulting in inability to *generate a fluent sequence of novel thought* on discourse level generation tasks in the context of preserved ability to generate a single response on word and sentence level generation tasks.

In his influential theoretical model of speech production, Levelt [32] proposed that *conceptual preparation* processes are responsible for the generation of new conceptual structures or messages that is subsequently realized in over speech. Several linguistic theories [33–35]

highlighted the importance of *focusing* and *attention* as key properties of discourse structure, whereby 'focusing' is defined as a process of directing attention to a particular set of concepts or topic in conversation. According to Robinson *et al.* [30] dynamic aphasia patients of the first type might be impaired at one of the mechanisms involved at the stage of conceptual preparation (selecting a single response option among competitors), while patients of the second type might be impaired in generating multiple potential messages that are intended to be communicated and in focusing attention on a specific message to be expressed.

While speaking is fluent one is not aware of antecedent 'inner speech', probably because it so quickly becomes overt. Dynamic aphasia offers a window to explore the interface between thought and language. Careful neuropsychological investigation of patients with dynamic aphasia is just beginning to disentangle the processes that are involved in the transition between thinking and speaking.

TOM IN AGRAMMATISM

The thoughts that precede language are generally not conscious. However, upon introspection, we sometimes seem to think and to reason in the language we speak. According to some theories [36, 37] certain forms of reasoning can only take place in explicit sentences of a natural language. Other investigators [38] have proposed that propositions support thinking by providing a sequential structure to parallel brain processes. ToM is the ability to attribute mental states (i.e., beliefs, intents, desires, pretending, knowledge, etc.) to oneself and others and to understand that others have beliefs, desires, and intentions that are different from one's own [39]. Some features of ToM involve eye gaze and emotion interpretation: they are viewed to be language independent [40]. In contrast, it has been claimed that ToM reasoning, such as reasoning on a 'changed content task', depends upon language, specifically upon the possession of syntactic structures such as those that allow embedding false proposition within true statements. In a typical changed content task the experimenter shows to Anne a chocolate box with an unusual content (e.g., a set of colour pencils). Then the box is closed and Anne is requested to say what a person who has not seen the contents would say is inside the box. Varley and Siegal [41] have reported the case of a patient with agrammatic aphasia of such severity that language proposition were not apparently available at an explicit processing level in any modality of language use. Despite the severe grammatical impairment, he displayed ToM understanding and simple causal reasoning. This observation, along with a few similar case studies [42], demonstrates that reasoning about causes and beliefs involve processes that are independent of propositional language.

ERROR MONITORING AND ANOSOGNOSIA IN APHASIC PATIENTS

There are few opportunities to know the subjective experience of being affected by aphasia associated with severe comprehension deficit. Among the few available anecdotal reports, I found particularly interesting the interview with neuroanatomist Dr Jill Bolte Taylor (http://soundmedicine.iu.edu/podcast/012807_7.mp3) who in 1996 suffered a brain haemorrhage from a left hemisphere arteriovenous malformation. From her report it is clear that, from the beginning, she was perfectly aware of what was going on: that she was having a stroke, that she was unable to speak, and that she was producing meaningless utterances. At the same time she clearly noted a disturbance in her 'inner speech' (it was like someone was pushing the pause button to the dialogue that goes inside the brain).

Lazar *et al.* [43] provided a more systematic and controlled account of the experience from the viewpoint of the patient. During angiography, they induced a transient Wernicke's aphasia in a patient with left frontal arteriovenous malformation by super selective injection of anaesthetics (amobarbital sodium and lidocaine) exclusively into the lower division of the left middle cerebral artery. During the procedure the patient underwent examination of fluency, comprehension, naming, repetition, and oral reading. At baseline and 15 minutes after anaesthetic injection all aspects of language function were entirely normal. After the procedure, the patient had no recollection of some of the tasks that had been administered to him. By his account, however, there was a more systematic attempt to respond appropriately than could be inferred from his overt behaviour. His description indicated not only that he could think, but also that he could recall afterwards what it was he was trying to do.

Yet, not all aphasic patients seem aware of their deficits while they are aphasics. The phenomenon of anosognosia for aphasia presents a particularly striking failure of the normal monitoring functions for speech and, in some cases, seems to require the postulation of a more fundamental alteration of consciousness of the language processing systems [44].

Several sorts of language monitoring processes have been suggested, including those internal to the production system itself and those that depend on comprehension system [45–47]. Note that normal speakers (and listeners), not only aphasic patients, are often 'unaware' of their language errors, so that extremely focused attention may be necessary to pick up certain phonological and syntactic deviations [48]. Indeed, insensitivity to language errors in normal subjects depends on the circumstances and priorities. Perceptual correction mechanisms are often necessary to automatically penetrate the haze of false starts, repetitions, and occasional ungrammaticalities that are on the surface of most well formed intended messages [49].

Schlenck, Huber, and Willmes [50] looked for two types of speech behaviour in aphasic patients: repairs and anticipatory adjustments (prepairs). They found that repairs occurred far less frequently than 'prepairs', which indicates impaired postarticulatory as opposed to intact prearticulatory monitoring. 'Prepairs' were found to be most frequent in patients with relatively good comprehension, in patients with poor production, and in those who had both good comprehension and poor production. This finding indicates that good comprehension may be related to successful anticipation of production difficulties. Also, the relatively low frequency of repairs in all aphasics' groups may also point out to poor functioning of monitoring relying on comprehension abilities. Oomen, Postma, and Kohl [51] found that, contrary to normal controls, Broca's aphasic patients were not impaired in a noise-masked condition, such as confirming the greater reliance of Broca's aphasics on prearticulatory rather than on postarticulatory monitoring.

Anosognosia of linguistic deficit is present whenever an aphasic patient does not attempt to correct an error and, confronted with that error, denies its occurrence. Such unawareness of language disturbance is most often associated to specific forms of abnormal speech such as jargon, stereotypy, or echolalia. Typically, patients with anosognosia for aphasia produce a great amount of meaningless utterance, phonemic and semantic paraphasias, and neologisms. They show few of the hesitations, pauses, and self-correction found in most of the aphasic patients. However, there are also several patients with severe auditory comprehension deficit and blatant jargon aphasia who seem perfectly aware that they are aphasics [44, 52]. On the opposite side there has been also reports of lack of error awareness in a patient with relatively preserved auditory comprehension [53].

There are several possible theories to account for anosognosia for aphasia. Some authors argued for a psychodynamic explanation [54]. However, the observation that lack of awareness often does not extend to the accompanying motor disorders strongly argues against this hypothesis. Furthermore, double disso-ciation between jargon aphasia and awareness of the deficit indicates that simple monitoring failure cannot provide a general account of this kind of anosognosia.

Shuren *et al.* [55] have also reported an anosognosic aphasic patient that, although apparently unaware of his production errors, could detect his own speech errors when played back. The authors explained this dissociation as caused by the patient's inability to per-form speaking and listening at the same time, due to a reduced attentional capacity. However, the patient described by Maher *et al.* [53] not only recognized more of his errors in a recording of his voice than he did while speaking, but he also recognized more errors in a recording of the examiner making errors than he did when listening to the recordings of his own speech, a dissociation that cannot be accounted by reduced attentional capacity. With a series of exper-iments on four patients with jargon aphasia Marshall *et al.* [56] ruled out explanation of monitoring fail-ure in jargon aphasia based on deficit of auditory feedback or to resource limitation which prevents concurrent speaking and monitoring. The authors demonstrated that, at least for one of the four patients, monitoring difficulties arose when he was accessing phonology from semantics. They concluded that mon-itoring failure could arise from deficits within the pro-duction process, which preclude comparison of actual with intended output. However, while this theory might explain monitoring failure in jargon aphasic, it cannot account for double dissociation between jargon aphasia and anosognosia for aphasia.

In conclusion, there is clearly the need of a more systematic study of error monitoring in aphasia. However, while most aphasic patients have diffi-culty speaking and monitoring their own speech, lack of awareness of speech deficit (i.e., anosognosia) seems to go beyond speech monitoring. As suggested by Rubens and Garret [44] this points to the need to develop an account of monitoring processes that treat different classes of language structure as having dis-tinct access to conscious report. The possibility that the ability for flexible attentional focus can decline during the act of speaking as well as the effect of familiarity of one's own voice should also be taken into account.

CONCLUSION

Language is not only instrumental to inter-indi-vidual communication but it is likely to be a powerful tool to structure and to constraint the content of our consciousness. Yet, most of the neuropsychological literature on aphasia has been focused more on dem-onstrating the independence of thinking from language rather than on studying the effects of different language impairments on the functioning of working memory. A reason for this omission might have been the lack of theoretical models incorporating language components in the functional architecture of the working memory.

Baddeley's model of working memory appears to be a framework for a new research programme that can treat consciousness as an empirical, biological, and psychological phenomenon. However, we need a more detailed specification of the model, especially for what concerns the integration of information within the episodic buffer where the relatively auto-matic binding of properties that occur in the processes of normal perception should be considered separately from the more active and attentionally demanding integrative processes typical of the executive proc-esses of chunking [5].

Any possible role of the lexical, semantic, and gram-matical impairment of the content of consciousness should be also better investigated. On the other side, a better insight on the relationship between language and consciousness might be obtained by studying the nature of brain activation associated with growing awareness of conversation and communicative intention.

References

1. Bisiach, E. (1988) The (haunted) brain and consciousness. In Marcel, A.J. and Bisiach, E. (eds.) *Consciousness in Contemporary Science*, pp. 101–120. Oxford, UK: Clarendon Press.
2. Block, N. (1995) On a confusion about a function of conscious-ness. *Behav Brain Sci* 18:227–287.
3. Repovs, G. and Baddeley, A. (2006) The multi-component model of working memory: Explorations in experimental cognitive psychology. *Neuroscience* 139:5–21.
4. Baddeley, A.D. and Hitch, G. (1974) Working memory. In Bower, G.A. (ed.) *Recent Advances in Learning and Motivation*, pp. 47–90. New York, USA: Academic Press.
5. Baddeley, A. (2000) The episodic buffer: A new component of working memory? *Trends Cogn Sci* 4:417–423.
6. Baddeley, A. (2003) Working memory and language: An over-view. *J Comm Disord* 36:189–208.
7. Vallar, G. and Papagno, C. (2002) Neuropsychological impair-ment of verbal short-term memory. In Baddeley, A. *et al.*, (eds.) *Handbook of Memory Disorders*, 2nd Edition. pp. 249–270. Hoboken, New Jersey: Wiley.
8. Singer, W. (1999) Binding by neural synchrony. In Wilson, R.A. and Keil, F.C. (eds.) *The MIT Encyclopedia of the Cognitive Sciences*, pp. 81–84. Cambridge, MA, USA: MIT Press.
9. Baddeley, A.D. (1986) *Working Memory*, Oxford, UK: Oxford University Press.
10. Salamè, P. and Baddeley, A.D. (1982) Disruption of short-term memory by unattended speech: Implication for the structure of working memory. *J Verb Learn Verb Behav* 21:150–164.
11. Vallar, G. and Baddeley, A.D. (1984) Fractionation of work-ing memory: Neuropsychological evidence for a phonological short-term store. *J Verb Learn Verb Behav* 23:151–161.

12. Conrad, R. (1964) Acoustic confusion in immediate memory. *Br J Psychol* 55:75–84.

13. Baddeley, A.D., *et al.* (1975) Word length and the structure of working memory. *J Verb Learn Verb Behav* 14:575–589.

14. Alan Baddeley, Vivien Lewis and Giuseppe Vallar (1984) Exploring the articulatory loop. *Quart J Exp Psychol* 36A:233–252. New York, USA

15. Levine, D.N., *et al.* (1982) Language in the absence of inner speech. *Neuropsychologia* 20:391–409.

16. Baddeley, A.D. and Wilson, B. (1985) Phonological coding and short-term memory in patients without speech. *J Mem Lang* 24:490–502.

17. Bishops, D. and Robson, J. (1989) Unimpaired short-term memory and rhyme judgement in congenitally speechless individuals: Implication for the notion of 'articulatory coding'. *Quart J Exp Psychol* 41A:123–140.

18. Vallar, G. and Baddeley, A.D. (1987) Phonological short term memory and sentence processing. *Cogn Neuropsychol* 4:417–438.

19. Cubelli, R. and Nichelli, P. (1992) Inner speech in anarthria: Neuropsychological evidence of differential effects of cerebral lesions on subvocal articulation. *J Clin Exp Neuropsychol* 14:499 517.

20. Cubelli, R., *et al.* (1993) Anarthria impairs subvocal counting. *Percept Mot Skills* 77:971–978. New York, USA

21. Goldstein, K. (1948) *Language and Language Disorders*, New York: Grune & Stratton.

22. Feinberg, T.E., *et al.* (1986) 'Inner speech' in conduction aphasia. *Arch Neurol* 43:591–593. New York, USA.

23. Bartha, L. and Benke, T. (2003) Acute conduction aphasia: An analysis of 20 cases. *Brain Lang* 85:93–108.

24. Basso, A., *et al.* (1982) Left hemisphere damage and selective impairment of auditory verbal short-term memory. A case study. *Neuropsychologia* 20:263–274.

25 Baddeley, A.D., *et al.* (1988) When long-term learning depends on short-term storage. *J Mem Lang* 27:627–635.

26. Lichtheim, L., (1885) On aphasia. *Brain* 7:433–484.

27. Luria, A.R. (1970) *Traumatic Aphasia*, Mouton de Gruyter, Berlin, Germany

28. Luria, A.R. and Tsvetkova, L.S. (1967) The mechanism of 'dynamic aphasia'. *Found Lang* 4:296–307.

29. Costello, A.D. and Warrington, E.K. (1987) The dissociation of visuospatial neglect and neglect dyslexia. *J Neurol Neurosurg Psychiatr* 50:1110–1116.

30. Robinson, G., *et al.* (2006) Dynamic aphasia in progressive supranuclear palsy: A deficit in generating a fluent sequence of novel thought. *Neuropsychologia* 44:1344–1360.

31. Robinson, G., Blair, J. and Cipolotti, L. (1998) Dynamic aphasia: An inability to select between competing verbal responses? *Brain* 121 (Pt 1):77–89.

32. Levelt, W.J.M. (1989) *Speaking: From Intention to Articulation*, New York, USA: MIT Press.

33. Willem, J.M. Levelt, (1999) Producing spoken language: A blueprint of the speaker. In Brown, C.M. and Hagoort, P. (eds.) *The Neurocognition of Language*, pp. 83–122. Oxford: Oxford University Press.

34. Grosz, B.J. and Sidner, C.L. (1986) Attention, intentions, and the structure of discourse. *Comput Ling* 12:175–204.

35. McKeown, K.R. (1992) *Text Generation*, Cambridge, UK: Cambridge University Press.

36. Carruthers, P. (1996) *Language Thought and Consciousness: An Essay in Philosophical Psychology*, Cambridge, UK: Cambridge University Press.

37. Segal, G. (1996) Representing representations. In Carruthers, P. and Boucher, J. (eds.) *Language and Thought: Interdisciplinary Themes*, pp. 146–161. Cambridge, UK: Cambridge University Press.

38. Clark, A. (1996) *Being There: Putting Brain, Body and World Together Again*, New York, USA: MIT Press.

39. Premack, D.G. and Woodruff, G. (1978) Does the chimpanzee have a theory of mind? *Behav Brain Sci* 1:515–526.

40. Tiger-Flusberg, H. and Sullivan, K. (2000) A componential theory of mind: Evidence from Williams syndrome. *Cognition* 76:59–89.

41. Varley, R. and Siegal, M. (2000) Evidence for cognition without grammar from causal reasoning and 'theory of mind' in an agrammatic aphasic patient. *Curr Biol* 10:723–726.

42. Varley, R., *et al.* (2001) Severe impairment in grammar does not preclude theory of mind. *Neurocase* 7:489–493.

43. Lazar, R.M., *et al.* (2000) The experience of Wernicke's aphasia. *Neurology* 55:1222–1224.

44. Rubens, A.B. and Garret, M.F. (1991) Anosognosia of linguistic deficits in patients with neurological deficits. In Prigatano, G.P. and Schacter, D.L. (eds.) *Awareness of Deficit After Brain Injury: Clinical and Theoretical Issues*, pp. 40–52. Oxford, UK: Oxford University Press.

45. Levelt, W.J.M. (1989) *Speaking*, MIT Press. New York, USA

46. Postma, A. (2000) Detection of errors during speech production: A review of speech monitoring models. *Cognition* 77:97–131.

47. Hartsuiker, R.J., *et al.* (2005) Phonological encoding and monitoring in normal and pathological speech. In Hartsuiker, R.J., *et al.*, (eds.) *Phonological Encoding and Monitoring in Normal Speech and Pathological Speech*, pp. 1–14. . New York, USA: Psychology Press.

48. Cutler, A. (1981) The reliability of speech error data. *Linguistics* 19. 7(8): p. 561–582. Berlin, Germany: Mouton de Gruyter.

49. Foster, K.I. (1979) Levels of processing and the structure of the language processors. In Cooper, W.E. and Walker, E.C.T. (eds.) *Sentence Processing: Psycholinguistics Studies Presented to Merrill Garrett*, pp. 27–85. New York, USA: Erlbaum.

50. Schlenck, K.J., *et al.* (1987) 'Prepairs' and repairs: Different monitoring functions in aphasic language production. *Brain Lang* 30:226–244.

51. Oomen, C.C., *et al.* (2001) Prearticulatory and postarticulatory self-monitoring in Broca's aphasia. *Cortex* 37:627–641.

52. Lecours, A.R. and Joanette, Y. (1980) Linguistic and other psychological aspects of paroxysmal aphasia. *Brain Lang* 10:1–23.

53. Maher, L.M., *et al.* (1994) Lack of error awareness in an aphasic patient with relatively preserved auditory comprehension. *Brain Lang* 46:402–418.

54. Weinstein, E.A. and Lyerly, O.G. (1976) Personality factors in jargon aphasia. *Cortex* 12:122–133.

55. Shuren, J.E., *et al.* (1995) Attention and anosognosia: The case of a jargonaphasic patient with unawareness of language deficit. *Neurology* 45:376–378.

56. Marshall, J., *et al.* (1998) Why does monitoring fail in jargon aphasia? Comprehension, judgment, and therapy evidence. *Brain Lang* 63:79–107.

CHAPTER

27

Blindness and Consciousness: New Light from the Dark

Pietro Pietrini, Maurice Ptito and Ron Kupers

If we could splice the nerves so that the excitation of the ear fed the brain centre concerned with seeing, and vice versa, we would 'hear the lightning and see the thunder'

William James (1890)

ABSTRACT

How what we perceive is transformed into a coherent and integrated representation of the world around us is a question that has fascinated humans since the early days. What happens in our brain that enables us to make sense of what we see, hear, touch, smell or taste? How does the brain of someone who has never had any visual perception form an image of the external world? Do brains from sighted and blind individuals differ and how? In this chapter we discuss recent findings from research in animals as well from functional brain imaging studies in sighted and blind individuals that are shedding new light on how the brain works.

WHAT CAN WE LEARN ABOUT CONSCIOUSNESS FROM THE BLIND BRAIN?

The study of brain function in individuals with congenital blindness provides a powerful approach to understand how consciousness develops in the absence of sight. Classically, sight has always been regarded as the most important sense for humans to interact with the environment. Let us not forget that in the ancient Greek language the verb 'to know' (oi\da) was the past tense of the verb 'to see' (oJravw), that is, *'I saw and thus I know'*. The relevance of sight is also clearly reflected in the mental attitude senses of the lexicon of vision. Consider everyday linguistic uses such as *'can you see my point?'*, *'I see what you mean'*, etc. At the same time, the brain surface devoted to visual function in primates is quite remarkable, accounting for almost one-third of the whole cortex.

These few considerations are sufficient to raise some critical questions. How do individuals with congenital blindness form a conscious representation of a world that they have never seen? How do their brains behave? What happens to visual-devoted brain structures in individuals who are born deprived of sight or who lose vision at different ages? What does the study of blind individuals teach us about the functional organization of the brain in physiological conditions?

In this chapter we review evidence from studies conducted in animals and in humans in an attempt to shed new light on these questions.

STUDIES IN ANIMALS

The cerebral cortex has a remarkable capacity for plasticity and reorganization, both in animals and humans [1, 2]. Following loss of a particular sense, input from other modalities invades the cortical area that is deprived of its normal inputs. These intermodal connections result from a phenomenon called cross-modal plasticity. As early as 1977, Rebillard and colleagues [3] reported that the primary auditory cortex can be driven by visual stimuli in congenitally deaf cats. Conversely, studies on the microphthalmic mole rat (*Spalax ehrenbergi*) have shown that auditory stimulations can drive cells in the primary visual cortex [4]. Cells in the primary visual cortex of visually deprived cats, rats or mice can be driven by somatosensory or auditory inputs, suggesting cross-modal reorganization [5]. Peripheral inputs play a pivotal role in the organization of the neocortex, as cortical territories usually involved in visual processing are invaded by the auditory and somatosensory system. It seems therefore that the visual cortex is capable of rewiring in order to accommodate these non-visual inputs. However in case of early brain damage, abnormal neuronal connectivity patterns can be produced and an alternative approach to study cross-modal plasticity resides in the tampering with 'blue prints' during prenatal development. Relevant to this approach are the numerous studies on 'rewiring' in hamsters [6] and in ferrets (reviewed in [7]).

When the Brain of Hamsters Is 'Rewired'

If brain damage occurs during development, abnormal neuronal connectivity patterns can be produced. It is thus possible to induce, by lesioning central retinal targets, the formation of new and permanent retinofugal projections into non-visual thalamic sites such as the auditory nucleus [8, 9] (Figure 27.A1). These surgically induced retinal projections are retinotopically organized and make functional synapses [10]. Neurons in the somatosensory cortex (SI) of animals with ectopic retinal projections have visual response properties similar to those of neurons in the primary visual cortex of normal animals [10]. Ferrets with retinofugal projections to the auditory thalamus but no visual cortex appear to perceive light stimuli as visual [11]. The question concerning the parallelism between a different brain organization (produced by lesions) and a behavioural recovery is still debated although recent experiments both in rewired ferrets and hamsters seem to indicate a large degree of recovery in visual functions (reviewed in [9]). For example, responses to visual stimuli have been observed in the auditory cortex of hamsters with robust and permanent projections to the auditory thalamic nucleus (medial geniculate nucleus, MGB) lacking a visual cortex. Single neurons in the auditory cortex of these animals respond to visual stimuli and some of them respond equally well to visual as to auditory stimuli (Figure 27.B1). Moreover, cells responding to visual stimuli show orientation selectivity (Figure 27.C1), and motion and direction sensitivity (Figure 27.D1). These receptive field properties compare favourably well with those obtained from cells in the visual cortex of normal hamsters.

At the behavioural level, rewired hamsters can learn visual discrimination tasks as well as normal animals and a lesion of the auditory cortex abolishes this function (Figure 27.2) [12]. In fact, rewired hamsters with auditory cortex lesions exhibit cortical blindness similar to non-rewired hamsters with visual cortex lesions.

These results provide strong evidence for sensory substitution where a given sensory modality acquires

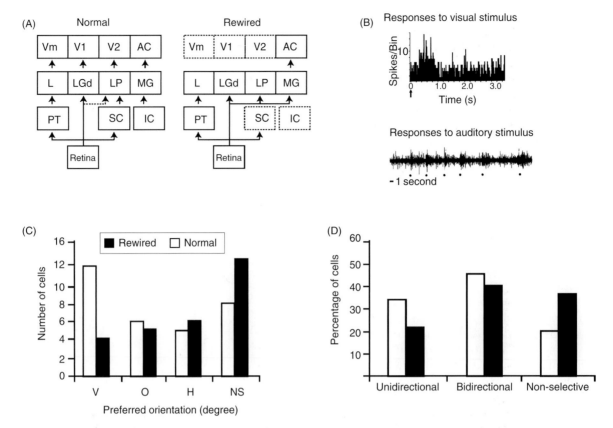

FIGURE 27.1 Visual properties of cells in the auditory cortex of rewired hamsters. (A) The visual system of normal and rewired hamsters. Examples of receptive field properties: (B) a bimodal neuron (audio-visual), (C) orientation and (D) direction selectivity.

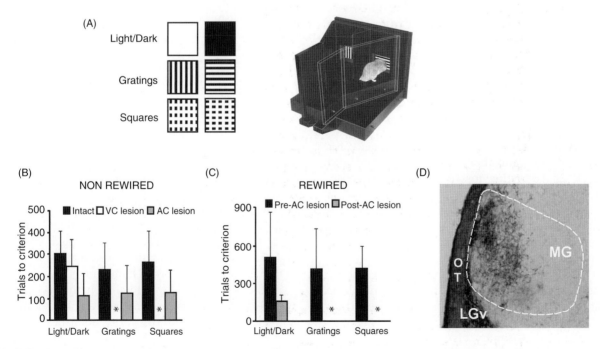

FIGURE 27.2 Visually guided behaviour of rewired hamsters. (A) Stimuli and apparatus. (B) Histograms showing trials to criterion on the visual discrimination tasks in non-rewired hamsters before and after ablation of visual (VC) and auditory (AC) cortices.*: Means and standard deviations cannot be calculated because only one animal learned the grating discrimination and none learned the squares discrimination. (C) Behaviour of rewired hamsters before and after AC lesions.* indicates that no animals with complete VC lesions learned the grating or squares discriminations when the AC was also ablated. (D) Video micrograph showing retino-MG projections in rewired hamsters. Lgv: ventral lateral geniculate nucleus.

the functional properties of a missing one. Most brain imaging studies in humans have addressed the question of cross-modal plasticity by studying Braille reading or sound perception in the blind. These studies have shown in a convincing manner that early blind subjects show augmented activity in the visual cortex evoked by tactile or auditory tasks compared to late blind or normal seeing subjects. Brain imaging studies in Braille readers have concluded that the brain of the blind is not only functionally reorganized (see reviews by [6, 13–15]) but also anatomically [16–19]. This raises questions about plastic mechanisms that take place in both the visually deprived and the normal brain as well as about the subjective character associated with activity in these 'rewired' areas.

STUDIES IN SIGHTED AND BLIND HUMAN SUBJECTS

How Do We Make Sense of the External World?

If we look around us, no matter how many different things unfold in front of our eyes, we are able to recognize all of them, to perceive their moving up and down or side by side, to distinguish even the more subtle shadows of colour and so on. That is, we seem to have the ability to recognize an infinite number of distinct objects. How this may happen has been a matter of fascinating debates for philosophers and scientists since the early days. Even if the 'visual brain' is widely distributed, the cortical surface responsible for integrating all the pieces of information and for recognizing all these object categories is rather limited. Single-cell recording in non-human primates and functional brain imaging studies in humans have suggested the existence of a 'fusiform face area' and of a 'parahippocampal place area' [20, 21]. While for these categories, and perhaps a few more, one could even speculate that evolution might have led to the selection of specialized subgroups of neurons given the biological relevance that both face and place recognition have for survival, this certainly cannot be true for the vast majority of object categories. According to an alternative model, different areas in the extrastriate ventro-temporal cortex are specialized for different types of perceptual processes. For instance, the fusiform face area would be responsible for expert recognition of items from any category, not merely faces [22, 23]. Thus, the peak response to faces shown by this region would be due to the fact that all of us are 'face-experts' as we begin to look at faces since

the very first days after birth. A few years ago, Haxby and colleagues [24] proposed a third model, called *Object Form Topology*, that may explain how a limited portion of the brain, such as the extrastriate visual cortex in the inferior surface of the temporal lobe, is capable of distinguishing an infinite number of object categories. The authors examined brain responses by using functional magnetic resonance imaging (fMRI) in a group of healthy young subjects while they viewed items from different object categories, including human faces, cats, houses and man-made objects such as bottles and shoes. The authors found that neural responses to the different object categories were not restricted to specific subregions within the extrastriate ventro-temporal cortex but were rather widely distributed and overlapping. That is, there was not such a thing as a specific response to a given category, say human faces or chairs, limited to a specific neuronal group. Rather, it looked as if most of this cortical area contributed to the elaboration of any of the object categories taken into exam. The authors reasoned that the specificity of the response was not due to the all-or-none activation of a given group of cells, but rather to the specificity of the whole pattern of neural activity elicited by that given category. In other words, this area of the cortex would be able to produce an infinite number of neural response patterns specific for each category of objects being viewed. Indeed, response patterns were so specific that they made it possible to predict what the subject was actually looking at. Moreover, the specificity of the patterns changed only minimally even when the voxels with the maximal response to a given category had been removed from the analysis. On the other hand, all the voxels with maximal response to a given category also responded to the presentation of the other categories. That is, the specificity of the response was not driven by smaller subgroups with the strongest activation within a wider cortical region, but was rather linked to the whole distributed pattern of neural activity [24]. Object form topology provides an explicit account for how the ventral temporal cortex can generate unique patterns of neural responses for a virtually unlimited number of categories.

Is Visual Cortex Just for Vision?

The demonstration that the representation of a face or object occurs through the concerted neural activity in a widely distributed cortical area within the ventral temporal cortex raises further questions. Is object form topology in these cortical areas strictly visual or does it represent a more abstract, supramodal functional organization? Furthermore, is visual experience a necessary prerequisite for this functional organization to develop?

Tactile Recognition Studies

We addressed this question in a new series of fMRI studies in sighted and congenitally blind individuals, using finger tactile recognition of the same object categories [24] or tactile recognition of geometric shapes through electrotactile stimulation of the tongue [25]. In the first series of studies, we tested whether the response patterns elicited by tactile recognition of face-masks and man-made objects of daily use (plastic bottles and shoes) in blindfolded sighted young subjects are distinct and to what extent response patterns during tactile recognition are similar to those elicited by visual recognition of the same object categories [26]. In the second series of experiments, we evaluated the ability of sighted and blind individuals to recognize shapes designed on their

tongue in the form of electrotactile pulses delivered by a tongue display unit (TDU) [25, 27].

Tactile recognition activated a large distributed cerebral network that included visual extrastriate regions in the inferior temporal and the ventral temporal cortices. In sighted subjects, the temporal areas activated by tactile recognition were also activated by visual recognition of the same object categories and the neural response patterns in these extrastriate cortical regions were category specific (Figure. 27.3A). Furthermore, the neural response patterns elicited by tactile perception of bottles or shoes were significantly correlated with the response patterns evoked by visual perception of the same object category, indicating that neural responses for these objects categories in those cortical regions are supramodal in nature; that is, that they are not merely restricted to visual perception [26]. Interestingly, the response pattern during tactile recognition of face-masks was not related to the response pattern evoked by visual recognition of faces. This is likely due to the fact that during tactile recognition subjects were not able to form an image of the whole face

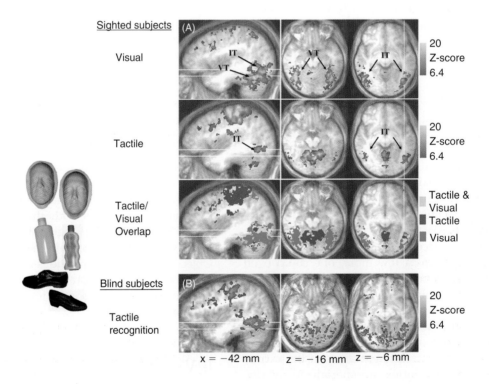

FIGURE 27.3 Supramodal neural response in extrastriate ventral temporal cortex in the human brain. On the left, examples of stimuli (life masks of faces, plastic bottles and shoes) used during tactile and visual recognition of different object categories in sighted and congenitally blind subjects. On the right side, brain areas that responded during tactile and/or visual object perception in sighted subjects and during tactile perception in blind individuals. The inferior temporal (IT) and ventral temporal (VT) regions activated by tactile and visual object perception are indicated. The tactile/visual overlap map shows the areas activated by both tactile and visual perception (shown in yellow), as well as the areas activated only by tactile (red) and visual (green) perception. The white lines correspond to the locations of the sagittal and axial slices. *Source*: Modified from [26].

but rather focused on single features, such as the chin or nose. This suggests that during tactile recognition of face-masks, subjects processed the faces more like other objects than like holistic face configurations [28]. Even within the visual modality, face inversion compromises configural face processing [29] and is associated with neural activation in extrastriate cortical regions that respond more to non-face objects than to faces [30].

Our results in sighted subjects confirm and extend the finding from other laboratories that visual and tactile object perception activate the dorsal part of the lateral occipital cortex (LO proper) [31–33] by showing a cross-modal correlation of response patterns between the two sensory modalities. Although findings in normal subjects cannot rule out the possibility that activation in the ventral temporal extrastriate cortex in blindfolded sighted individuals is due to visual imagery during tactile object recognition, this possibility is certainly less likely in congenitally blind individuals who never experienced sight. In this respect, the results of our fMRI study with a sensory substitution device deserve attention [34]. This study showed that congenitally blind subjects trained in tactile shape recognition with a tactile-to-vision sensory substitution device activate the inferotemporal cortex during a tactile object recognition task.

Is Vision Necessary to See What We Perceive?

Independent studies have shown that seeing an object or recalling the image of that object through visual imagery leads to similar responses in the brain [35, 36]. To determine the potential role of visual imagery in the activation of area LO during haptic object exploration, we examined brain responses to tactile recognition of the same object categories in congenitally blind or early blind subjects with no recollection of visual experience who, by definition, do not have any visually based imagery (though they do have imagery!).

Congenital/early blind subjects showed similar category-specific neural response patterns in the temporal extrastriate cortex as our sighted controls (Figure 27.3B). These findings are crucial in demonstrating that activation evoked by tactile recognition of distinct object categories in ventral temporal extrastriate cortex cannot be explained by visual imagery [25, 33, 35, 37]. These results also suggest that the development of topographically-organized, category-related representations in the extrastriate visual cortex does not require visual experience. Experience with objects acquired through other sensory modalities appears to be sufficient to support the development of these patterns.

Supramodal Cortical Organization Extends Beyond the Ventral Stream

Visual functions in the brain of human and non-human primates are primarily subdivided into a ventral 'what' pathway devoted to recognition of different object categories and a dorsal 'where' pathway that is responsible for spatial processing [38, 39]. The converging evidence discussed above favouring a supramodal functional organization in the ventral temporal cortex of the 'what' pathway in the brain has prompted us to ask whether a similar supramodal organization also exists in the 'where' pathway of the dorsal stream.

To answer this question, we have studied brain responses to tasks known to activate areas within the dorsal visual pathway, including spatial working memory, mental rotation and perception of translational motion and optic flow. *Optic flow* results from the perception of coherent changes in visual images caused by object or viewer movement [40]. *Tactile flow* involves analogous changes in tactile stimuli caused by object or subject movement. Both optic and tactile motion provide information about object form, position, orientation, consistency and movement, as well as information about the position and movement of the self in the environment [41]. Perception of visual motion activates the human extrastriate cortical region, hMT+ [9, 42]. Perception of tactile motion also results in the activation of hMT+ [43, 44], suggesting that this area is not merely visual but plays a more general role in the supramodal representation of sensory flow. Since mental imagery of visual movement also activates the hMT+ complex [45], the question arises again whether activation during tactile motion perception is mediated by visual mental imagery.

We therefore compared brain responses in sighted subjects and in individuals with congenital or early blindness during passive perception of visual and/or tactile motion. Optic motion stimuli consisted of grey dots on a black background whereas tactile motion stimuli were made of raised dots on a plastic surface moving horizontally or rotationally [46]. In sighted subjects, optic flow perception induced activation in the hMT+ complex in the posterior inferior temporal cortex bilaterally. Tactile flow perception activated the anterior part but deactivated a more posterior part of the hMT+ complex. In blind subjects, tactile flow perception activated a much more extensive region in the inferior temporal cortex that also included the more posterior part of the hMT+ complex, which was activated by visual motion and deactivated by tactile motion in sighted subjects (Figure 27.4). Similarly, using motion detection and motion discrimination tasks in positron emission tomography (PET) and fMRI studies, we were able to demonstrate that motion stimuli applied to the tongue resulted in a significant activation of the dorsal visual pathway, specifically area middle temporal (MT) [Cortex][34, 47] (Figure 27.5).

The observation that the hMT+ complex can be activated by perception of tactile motion even in subjects with congenital blindness demonstrates that recruitment of the hMT+ cortex is not mediated by

visual-based mental imagery and that visual experience is not necessary for the development of this cortical system. Visual experience, however, seems to play a crucial role in determining the functional segregation of hMT+ into a more anterior part that is involved in the representation of both optic and tactile motion and a more posterior part that is uniquely involved in the representation of optic flow. If the case that hMT+ develops in the absence of visual

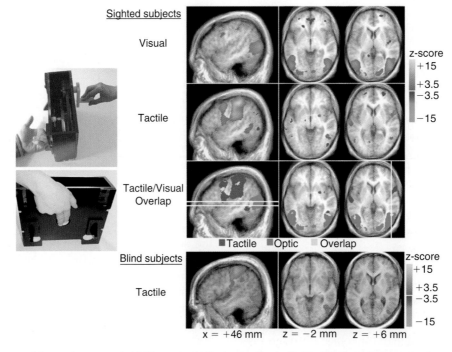

FIGURE 27.4   Supramodal neural response in hMT+ cortex in the human brain. Braille-like dot patterns moved on a plastic surface to provide translational (A) and rotational (B) tactile flow stimulation. Subjects' hands lay on the table with the index and middle fingers touching the plastic surface with dot patterns, as shown in the pictures on the left side. Brain areas are shown that responded during tactile or optic flow perception in sighted subjects and during tactile flow perception in blind subjects. The tactile/visual overlap map shows the areas activated by both tactile and optic flow perception (shown in yellow), as well as the areas activated only by tactile (red) and optic (green) perception. *Source*: Modified from [46].

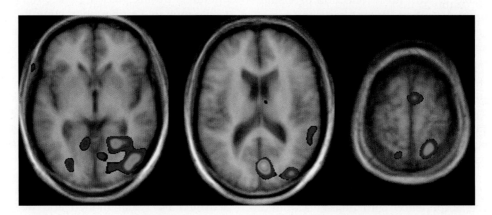

FIGURE 27.5   PET images showing activation of the dorsal visual pathway in congenital blind subjects during a motion direction discrimination task.

experience, the entire structure is involved in the representation of tactile motion. These results suggest that competitive interactions between visual and tactile inputs in normal development lead to functional specialization in hMT+ that does not develop without visual input.

Recently, hMT+ activation was shown in both sighted and congenitally blind individuals also while they listened to auditory stimuli that elicited the apparent perception of sounds moving right-to-left, front-to-back and self-rotating [48, 49].

This supramodal organization extends beyond area MT in the dorsal pathway. Indeed, spatial working memory and mental rotation tasks with visually or tactilely prompted stimuli evoked neural activity in the posterior parietal cortex in sighted subjects [50–53] as well as in individuals with congenital or early blindness [54]. In the latter study, we measured brain activity while sighted and congenital/early blind subjects performed a one-back spatial discrimination task of visually and/or tactilely presented matrices. Tactile matrices were wooden squares and cubes with three or five Velcro-covered target squares/cubes. White squares and rotating cubes with three or five black target squares/cubes represented the two- and three-dimensional visual stimuli. During both the visual and tactile spatial detection tasks, sighted subjects recruited a common fronto-parietal network that extended bilaterally from dorsolateral prefrontal and anterior cingulate cortex towards fronto-parietal sensorimotor and posterior parietal cortices, including precuneus and intraparietal sulci. During the tactile spatial discrimination task, the blind individuals showed a similar cortical activation pattern extending from the fronto-parietal network towards the sensorimotor cortex, the lateral occipito-temporal cortex and the cerebellum.

Given that spatial visual perception and visual imagery activate common cortical areas in the parietal lobes, we addressed the question whether spatial imagery might also rely on supramodal neural mechanisms. We studied brain activity in a group of sighted and congenital/early blind subjects while they performed a modified version of the mental clock task in three distinct conditions: auditory imagery, tactile discrimination and, for the sighted subjects, visual discrimination [55]. During the auditory imagery condition, subjects were asked to imagine two analogue clock faces showing the times that were indicated verbally by the examiner, and to judge in which case the clock hands formed the wider angle. During the visual and tactile angle discrimination conditions, participants compared pairs of clock faces visually or tactilely to decide which hand set formed the wider

angle. During the auditory imagery condition, both sighted and congenitally blind individuals activated posterior parietal areas, including the intraparietal sulcus and the inferior parietal lobule. The same areas were activated during the tactile and visual angle discrimination conditions. These findings therefore demonstrate that spatial imagery representation occurs in the posterior parietal extrastriate cortex also when spatial stimuli are not visual in nature.

Altogether, the results of these studies strongly indicate that 'visual' association cortical regions are capable of processing and interpreting information carried by non-visual sensory modalities. This is not merely the consequence of a phenomenon of plastic functional reorganization in the brain of subjects deprived of sight since birth or soon afterwards, as this ability also exists in sighted subjects. Not surprisingly, however, sighted and congenitally blind individuals do show differences in the extension and magnitude of the activation of the recruited areas that are likely due to the effects of rearrangements that follow the lack of sight, as discussed in details below. The supramodal nature of this functional cortical organization may explain how individuals who never had any visual experience are able to acquire normal knowledge about objects and their position in space, form mental representations of and interact effectively with the external world [26].

UNDERSTANDING WITHOUT SEEING

Understanding actions carried out by other individuals is crucial for survival and for social organization in human and non-human primates. A particular class of visuomotor neurons, originally discovered in area F5 of the monkey premotor cortex and called *mirror neurons*, discharge both when an animal performs a goal-directed action and observes another individual performing the same or a similar action [56]. The fact that this mirror neuron system is able to transform visual information into motor knowledge raises the hypothesis that this system may also have a significant role in action understanding. This has been confirmed by several animal studies showing that the mirror neuron system is recruited when monkeys receive a sufficient amount of non-visual clues which allows them to understand the meaning, and create a mental representation of the occurring actions, such as when listening to sounds of actions [57]. In fact, a subclass of auditory–visual mirror neurons responds both while monkeys perform hand or mouth actions and while they listen to sounds of similar actions.

Neurophysiological, behavioural and brain functional studies strongly support the existence of an observation–execution matching system in humans similar to the monkey mirror neuron system, that may enable humans not only to understand the actions of others but also to learn by imitation [58]. The human mirror neuron system is activated during the observation of actions done by others and recruits a complex network formed by occipital, temporal and parietal areas, and the inferior frontal gyrus. Auditory–visual mirror neurons that allow to understand the actions of others by hearing their sound have been described also in humans [59].

We recently asked whether an efficient mirror neuron system exists in individuals who have never had any visual experience, and whether this action recognition-oriented network shares common neural patterns in sighted and blind individuals. We measured neural response patterns in congenitally or early blind and sighted volunteers during the auditory presentation of hand-executed action or environmental sounds. Preliminary fMRI findings show that a left premotor–temporo-parietal network subserves action recognition through hearing in blind individuals, and that this network clearly overlaps with the left-lateralized network of the auditory mirror neuron system in sighted subjects [60]. These findings indicate that visual experience is not a necessary precondition for the functional development of the mirror neuron system and that a more abstract representation of actions done by others may take place also through non-visual sensory modalities. This may help to explain the ability of congenitally blind individuals to learn by imitation of others.

SUBJECTIVE EXPERIENCE ASSOCIATED WITH ACTIVATION OF THE VISUAL CORTEX

We next addressed the question of the subjective character of this visual cortex activation in the blind, by studying the subjective responses induced by transcranial magnetic stimulation (TMS) of the visually deprived and cross-modally responsive occipital cortex. In a first study, we exploited a tactile-to-vision sensory substitution model to examine the subjective character of experience associated with the activation of occipital cortex before and after the establishment of cross-modal plasticity [47]. More specifically, we wanted to test the possibility whether stimulation of the occipital cortex can induce subjective sensations or qualia associated with the new (tactile) input. We

stimulated the occipital cortex with TMS in a systematic manner before and after training with the TDU in a group of blind and blindfolded seeing control subjects. The TDU is a device that captures a visual image, taken by a camera, and translates it into electrotactile stimulation which is applied to the tongue [61]. With sufficient training, subjects learn to use the TDU to discriminate orientation, detect motion and form. As expected, TMS of the occipital cortex in control subjects only elicited phosphenes. Only two late blind subjects but none of the early blind subjects reported some fugitive central sparks following occipital TMS [62]. In sharp contrast, following a 1-week training period with the TDU, some blind subjects reported 'tactile sensations' on the tongue following occipital TMS. These tactile sensations were described as short-lasting experiences of distinct tingling, varying in intensity, extent and topography depending on the locus of the occipital cortex which was stimulated (Figure 27.6).

None of the trained blindfolded subjects reported TMS-induced tactile sensations on the tongue. TMS over the primary SI did not induce any subjective sensations, neither in blind nor in control subjects. Only few reports have described TMS-induced tactile sensations when stimulating SI [63–64]. This may be explained by the fact that excitation of the postcentral gyrus requires prolonged repetitive stimulation for accessing the perceptual system [65]. Not all blind subjects reported TMS-induced tactile sensations following training with the TDU. Although we have no definitive explanation for this intersubject variability, we found a positive correlation between the amount of occipital cortex activated in the PET study during a sensory substitution task and the number of occipital sites from which TMS-induced tactile sensations could be induced.

If tactile sensations referred to the tongue can be induced by stimulating the occipital cortex already following a 1-week training period with the TDU, what about TMS-induced tactile sensations in blind subjects who read Braille since childhood? Should not a daily experience with Braille reading also induce tactile sensations referred to the fingertips in proficient Braille readers? An anecdotal observation by Cohen and co-workers [66] already mentioned that TMS over the occipital cortex in blind Braille readers was able to induce occasional distorted somatosensory perceptions (missing dots, extra dots…) during Braille reading. We therefore addressed the question of remapping of the fingers onto the visual cortex in a subsequent study [67]. Participants were blind subjects who all read Braille on a daily basis and Braille-naive normal sighted controls. Like in the previous study, TMS of the

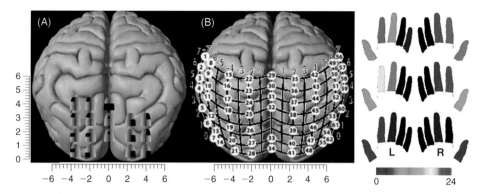

FIGURE 27.6 TMS of the visual cortex in congenitally blind subjects induces tactile sensations. (A) TMS-induced tactile sensations referred to the tongue in a congenitally blind subject following a 1-week training with the TDU. (B) TMS-induced tactile sensations referred to the fingertips in a congenitally blind proficient Braille reader. The colour map to the right indicates the fingers in which the subject experienced TMS-induced tactile sensations. The number of visual cortex sites from which paresthesiae could be induced in a particular finger is colour coded. On the colour scale, red indicates the highest number of cortical sites that induced paresthesiae in a particular finger and purple the lowest number.

occipital cortex in control subjects evoked only phosphenes. As predicted, blind subjects reported tactile sensations in the fingers that were described as short-lasting tingling sensations, varying in intensity, extent and topography depending on the stimulated locus of the occipital cortex (Figure 27.6). We found again important interindividual differences with respect to the number of sites from which tactile sensations could be induced and in the topography of the referred sensations. The blind subjects with paresthesiae in the fingers following occipital TMS where the ones with the highest amount of Braille reading hours/day and with the highest word reading speed. Like in the previous study, no subjective sensations were produced by TMS over SI in any of the subjects.

Cortical Reorganization or Unmasking?

The results of the experiments described above constitute the first direct demonstration that the subjective experience of activity in the visual cortex after sensory remapping is tactile, not visual. These results provide new insights into the long-established scientific debate on cortical dominance or deference [68, 69]. What is the experience of a subject in whom areas of cortex receive input from sensory sources not normally project to those areas? Our studies suggest that the qualitative character of the subject's experience is not determined by the area of cortex that is active (cortical dominance), but by the source of input to it (cortical deference). Our results are also in line with recent evidence that sensory cortical areas receive input from multiple sensory modalities early in development [70–72]. What is the neural mechanism driving this type of cross-modal plasticity? Two competing hypotheses have been put

forward. According to the *cortical reorganization* hypothesis, cross-modal brain responses are mediated by the formation of new pathways in the sensory-deprived brain. When the brain is deprived of visual input at an early age, tactile (and other non-visual) information is rerouted to visual cortex. For instance, electrophysiological recording studies in behaving monkeys following early visual deprivation showed that neurons in visual cortical area 19 respond to somatic inputs such as manipulating the experimenter's hand to search for food [73]. This is in sharp contrast with the findings obtained in normal seeing animals, in which area 19 neurons respond exclusively to visual inputs. This implies that following early visual deprivation tactile information reaches the visual cortex. This claim is largely supported by results of functional brain imaging studies showing activation of visual cortex in early blind subjects during Braille reading [15, 74–76] and other forms of tactile stimulation [27, 77]. The importance of visual deprivation early in early life is further underscored by the observation that brain activity patterns in occipital cortex evoked by tactile stimulation are significantly stronger in early blind compared to late blind subjects [75, 78]. According to the *unmasking* hypothesis, loss of a sensory input induces unmasking and strengthening of existing neuronal connections. Although the results of the second experiment are compatible with both hypotheses, the rapid onset of cross-modal responses in the TDU experiments (within 1 week) excludes the possibility of mediation by the establishment of new anatomical connections and therefore favours the unmasking hypothesis. One possibility is that training unmasks and strengthens pre-existing connections between the parietal and the occipital cortices. There is indeed electrophysiological [79] and anatomical [71, 72] evidence that primary visual cortex in normal mammals receives input not only from the visual thalamus, but also from somatosensory and auditory modalities. Single unit recordings in the visual cortex in unanaesthetized cats have shown that neurons in areas 17 and 18 receive both visual and auditory input [79]. Anatomical tracing studies have further shown that there are direct projections from the auditory cortex to area 17 of the macaque monkey [71]. Direct projections from parietal association areas to areas V1 and V2 in the calcarine fissure have also been described [72]. These non-visual inputs conveying tactile and auditory inputs to occipital cortex may modulate the processing of visual information [80], while not giving rise to subjective non-visual sensations under normal circumstances due to masking by the dominant visual input. In this respect it is interesting to mention the results of a TMS study which showed that disrupting the function of the visual cortex by TMS impairs tactile discrimination of grating orientation in normal seeing subjects [81]. This confirms that although the visual cortex receives tactile input, this normally does not lead to subjective tactile sensations. Thus, in our trained control subjects, TMS over occipital cortex produced only phosphenes, without tactile sensations. However, under certain circumstances, non-visual processing in the occipital cortex can be strengthened or unmasked. In line with the dynamic sensorimotor hypothesis, training with the TDU device results in new highly specific learned dynamic interaction patterns between sensory stimulation and active movement [82], thereby further strengthening and unmasking existing connections between the parietal and occipital cortices.

HOW BLINDNESS SHAPES THE BRAIN

What is the effect of visual deprivation on the gross anatomical organization of the brain and by which pathways does non-visual information reach the occipital cortex in the visually deprived brain? In recent years, modern brain imaging tools such as voxel-based morphometry (VBM) and diffusion tensor imaging (DTI) and diffusion tensor tractography (DTT) have been used to investigate alterations in grey and white matter of the brain of the blind *in vivo* [16, 18, 19, 83, 84]. The results of these studies seem to concur that there is a significant atrophy of all structures belonging to the visual pathways, including the lateral geniculate and the posterior pulvinar nuclei [19], the striate and extrastriate visual areas [18, 19, 83] and the inferior temporal gyrus and lateral orbital cortex, areas that are part of the ventral stream which is involved in object recognition [19]. Reductions also occur in non-visual structures such as the posterior hippocampus [19, 84]. Changes in white matter include atrophy of the optic tracts and optic chiasm, the optic radiations, the splenium of the corpus callosum [16, 18, 19, 82] and the inferior longitudinal fasciculus, a fibre bundle that connects the occipital cortex with the temporal lobe [19]. The latter pathway is involved in several visual functions and lesions of it may induce visual agnosia, prosopagnosia and disturbances in visual recent memory [85, 86]. In general, no studies reported direct evidence for the establishment of new pathways but only volume increases in existing cortico-cortical pathways. We reported a significant enlargement of the occipito-frontal fasciculus, the superior longitudinal fasciculus and the anterior portion (genu) of the corpus callosum (Figure 27.7). However, there seems to be indirect evidence for increased functional connectivity between parietal and visual areas in the blind.

For instance, a combined TMS–PET study reported that TMS of SI induces a significant blood flow increase in the occipital cortex in early blind but not in blindfolded control subjects [87]. In addition, we showed that functional connectivity between the

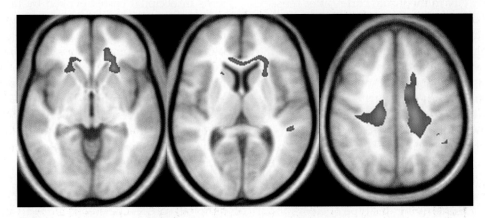

FIGURE 27.7   Increases in the white matter in the brain of congenitally blind subjects as revealed by VBM.

dorsal intraparietal sulcal area and the cuneus is increased in blind (but not in control) subjects trained with the TDU [27]. Moreover, somatosensory evoked potentials induced by electrical stimulation of the tongue after training with the TDU revealed in addition to the short latency (13–18 ms) N1–P1 complex over the parietal cortex, a second peak over the occipital cortex after 48–60 ms, suggesting a mediation by a cortico-cortical pathway [47]. Taken together, since no additional tracts have been demonstrated so far in early blind subjects, the data suggest that cross-modal functionality of the visual cortex in early blindness is primarily mediated by preserved or strengthened cortico-cortical connections. These cortico-cortical connections involve a pathway from SI to either VIP (ventral intraparietal area) or area 7 (or both), then to areas MT and V3 to finally reach the visual cortex.

A DARWINIAN STRUGGLE FOR SURVIVAL?

Although the majority of the studies have focused on the rerouting of tactile input to the visual cortex, the occipital cortex in the blind is involved in many more functions than just tactile processing. There is now a wealth of data showing that this cortex is activated in tasks involving lexical and phonological processing [88, 89], verbal memory [90, 91], repetition priming [92], auditory discrimination [93, 94] and selective attention [95]. This seems to suggest that the visually deprived occipital cortex is involved in a bewildering diverse compensatory plasticity. How to understand this multiplicity of cognitive functions of the occipital cortex in the blind? Does it reflect some kind of Darwinian principle of struggle for survival? As humans, we are living in a very visual world. This is already reflected by the fact that the visual cortex in primates covers about 30% of the total cortical surface. Therefore, the loss of vision is one of the most incapacitating events that can overcome to a person. In order to survive in our very visual world, blind subjects have to rely on other senses and develop these in a supranormal manner. As a result, they develop superior tactile and auditory discriminatory capacities as well as superior verbal memory functions to compensate for their loss of vision. Many functional brain imaging studies have shown that enhanced practice leads to an enlargement of cortical representations [96, 97]. In the normal brain, this is always reflected by an enlargement of the cortex that is normally involved in the execution of the task (e.g., an expansion of the motor cortex in musicians [97, 98]) and not by the recruitment of novel cortex. In case of loss of a sensory input, the opposite occurs. Rather than getting an expansion of the cortex proper for the execution of the task, the brain recruits de novo cortex which is normally not involved in execution of this particular task. This may represent a Darwinian reflex for survival. Recruitment of the visually deprived occipital cortex is a much more cost-effective computational solution since it does not put extra demands on the cortex which is normally used for executing this task, thereby leaving sufficient resources available for situations of increased demand. The pathways through which this occurs are available since birth but in the normal brain, activity is masked by the dominant specific afferent input to a particular cortical region.

How does the rewired cortex cope with this multitude of new inputs? Is there some kind of segregation of functions or does the visually deprived cortex become genuinely multimodal? It is difficult to answer this question since most studies only investigated one or at best a few cognitive functions in the same subjects. One of the few studies that investigated the cortical representation of multiple cognitive functions in the occipital cortex of the blind suggest that different functions may indeed be segregated anatomically [99]. However, more studies are needed to confirm these preliminary findings. The idea that different functions are anatomically segregated in the cortex of the blind may also provide an answer to a prominent question raised by our TMS studies. How is it possible that TMS of the occipital cortex induces tactile sensations referred to the tongue after a 1-week training period and in the fingertips in Braille readers but that it never evoked any auditory sensations or lexical or semantic thoughts? A possible explanation is that these rewired functions are located more anteriorly and hence further away from the TMS coil which makes them more difficult to evoke by stimulating at submaximal intensities.

FINAL CONSIDERATIONS

The study, in animals and in humans, of the dark-reared brain has shed a bright light on many questions regarding not only the plastic rearrangements that take place when vision is absent but also on the functional organization of the sighted brain itself. In this respect, the availability of novel non-invasive methodologies for the functional exploration of the brain in the past 25 years has made it possible to begin to understand the neural mechanisms that enable awareness of the surrounding world and make sense of it [100]. In this chapter, we reviewed and discussed some new findings from studies from our own labs as well as from others. We are well aware that the issues that we have considered are only a few among the many more that an ambitious topic such as the relation between blindness and consciousness may raise. For instance, we have completely omitted to discuss cortical blindness, as well as the effects of congenital blindness vs. blindness acquired at different ages, or the effects of monocular vision. Moreover, we have only briefly touched upon the 'blind social brain', a topic that merits a whole book by itself, not to mention emotional life and its disturbances. As was shown in this chapter, we have already learned a lot and we can still learn much more about the sighted brain by observing the blind brain.

A final important thought prompted by the many different findings from studies in animal and humans is that the blind brain should not be considered as a 'disabled' brain but rather as a truly 'differentially able' brain.

ACKNOWLEDGEMENTS

Research work reported in this article has been supported by the European Union (Grant IST-2001-38040} and IST-2006-027141 to Pietro Pietrini), by the Italian Ministry of Education, University and Research (PRIN RBNE018ET9-003, 200411841 and 2006117208 to Pietro Pietrini), by Fondazione IRIS, Castagneto Carducci (Livorno, Italy to Pietro Pietrini), by the Harland Sanders Foundation (to Maurice Ptito) and by the Lundbeck Foundation (to Ron Kupers). Pietro Pietrini wishes to thank the Unione Italiana Ciechi for its support to the blindness research programme, and the MRI Laboratory at the CNR Research Area 'San Cataldo' (Pisa, Italy). We thank Emiliano Ricciardi for comments on an earlier version of this chapter.

References

1. Kaas, J.H. (2002) Sensory loss and cortical reorganization in mature primates. *Prog Brain Res* 138:167–176.
2. Pascual-Leone, A., *et al.* (2005) The plastic human brain cortex. *Annu Rev Neurosci* 28:377–401.
3. Rebillard, G., *et al.* (1977) Enhancement of visual responses on the primary auditory cortex of the cat after an early destruction of cochlear receptors. *Brain Res* 129:162–164.
4. Bronchti, G., *et al.* (2002) Auditory activation of 'visual' cortical areas in the blind mole rat (Spalax ehrenbergi). *Eur J Neurosci* 16:311–329.
5. Toldi, J., *et al.* (1994) Neonatal monocular enucleation-induced cross-modal effects observed in the cortex of adult rat. *Neuroscience* 62:105–114.
6. Ptito, M. and Desgent, S. (2006) Sensory input-based adaptation and brain architecture. In Baltes, P., Reuter-Lorenz, P. and Rösler, F. (eds.) *Lifespan Development and the Brain*, pp. 111–113. New York, NY: Cambridge University Press.
7. Lyckman, A.W. and Sur, M. (2002) Role of afferent activity in the development of cortical specification. *Results Probl Cell Differ* 39:139–156.
8. Frost, D.O. and Metin, C. (1985) Induction of functional retinal projections to the somatosensory system. *Nature* 317:162–164.
9. Ptito, M., *et al.* (2001) When the auditory cortex turns visual. *Prog Brain Res* 134:447–458.
10. Metin, C. and Frost, D.O. (1989) Visual responses of neurons in somatosensory cortex of hamsters with experimentally induced retinal projections to somatosensory thalamus. *Proc Natl Acad Sci (USA)* 86:357–361.
11. Von Melchner, L., *et al.* (2000) Visual behaviour mediated by retinal projections directed to the auditory pathway. *Nature* 404:871–876.
12. Frost, D.O., *et al.* (2000) Surgically created neural pathways mediate visual pattern discrimination. *Proc Natl Acad Sci USA* 97:11068–11073.
13. Sathian, K. (2005) Visual cortical activity during tactile perception in the sighted and the visually deprived. *Dev Psychobiol* 46:279–286.
14. Merabet, L.B., *et al.* (2005) What blindness can tell us about seeing again: Merging neuroplasticity and neuroprostheses. *Nat Rev Neurosci* 6:71–77.
15. Sadato, N., *et al.* (1996) Activation of the primary visual cortex by Braille reading in blind subjects. *Nature* 380:526–528.
16. Shimony, J.S., *et al.* (2006) Diffusion tensor imaging reveals white matter reorganization in early blind humans. *Cereb Cortex* 16:1653–1661.
17. Liu, Y., *et al.* (2007) Whole brain functional connectivity in the early blind. *Brain* 130 (Pt 8):2085–2096.
18. Noppeney, U., *et al.* (2005) Early visual deprivation induces structural plasticity in gray and white matter. *Curr Biol* 15:488–490.
19. Ptito, M., *et al.* (2008b) Alterations of the visual pathways in congenital blindness. *Exp Brain Res* 187(1):41–9.
20. Kanwisher, N., *et al.* (1997) The fusiform face area: A module in human extrastriate cortex specialized for face perception. *J Neurosci* 17:4302–4311.
21. McCarthy, G., *et al.* (1997) Face-specific processing in the human fusiform gyrus. *J Cogn Neurosci* 9:605–610.
22. Gauthier, I., *et al.* (1999) Activation of the middle fusiform 'face area' increases with expertise in recognizing novel objects. *Nat Neurosci* 2:568–573.
23. Gauthier, I., *et al.* (2000) Expertise for cars and birds recruits brain areas involved in face recognition. *Nat Neurosci* 3:191–197.
24. Haxby, J.V., *et al.* (2001) Distributed and overlapping representations of faces and objects in ventral temporal cortex. *Science* 293:2425–2430.
25. Matteau, I., *et al.* (2008) Activation of the ventral visual pathway in congenital blindness. Vision. *Vis Impair Res* (Suppl) (in press).
26. Pietrini, P., *et al.* (2004) Beyond sensory images: Object-based representation in the human ventral pathway. *Proc Natl Acad Sci (USA)* 101:5658–5663.
27. Ptito, M., *et al.* (2005) Cross-modal plasticity revealed by electro-tactile stimulation of the tongue in the congenitally blind. *Brain* 128:606–614.
28. Kilgour, A.R. and Lederman, S.J. (2002) Face recognition by hand. *Percept Psychophys* 64:339–352.
29. Yin, R.K. (1969) Looking at upside-down faces. *J Exp Psychol* 81:141–145.

30. Haxby, J.V., *et al.* (1999) The effect of face inversion on activity in human neural systems for face and object perception. *Neuron* 22:189–199.

31. Amedi, A., *et al.* (2001) Visuo-haptic object-related activation in the ventral visual pathway. *Nat Neurosci* 4:324–330.

32. Amedi, A., *et al.* (2002) Convergence of visual and tactile shape processing in the human lateral occipital complex. *Cereb Cortex* 12:1202–1212.

33. James, T.W., *et al.* (2002) Differential effects of viewpoint on object-driven activation in dorsal and ventral streams. *Neuron* 35:793–801.

34. Matteau, I., *et al.* (2006) Tactile motion discrimination through the tongue in blindness. *Neuroimage* 31 (Suppl 1):132.

35. Ishai, A., *et al.* (2000) Distributed neural systems for the generation of visual images. *Neuron* 28:979–990.

36. O'Craven, K.M. and Kanwisher, N. (2000) Mental imagery of faces and places activates corresponding stimulus-specific brain regions. *J Cogn Neurosci* 2:1013–1023.

37. Sathian, K. and Zangaladze, A. (2002) Feeling with the mind's eye: Contribution of visual cortex to tactile perception. *Behav Brain Res* 135:127–132.

38. Ungerleider, L.G. and Mishkin, M. (1982) Two cortical visual systems. In Ingle, D.J., Goodale, M.A. and Mansfield, R.J.W. (eds.) *Analysis of Visual Behavior,* pp. 549–586. Cambridge, MA: MIT Press.

39. Haxby, J.V., *et al.* (1994) The functional organization of human extrastriate cortex: A PET-rCBF study of selective attention to faces and locations. *J Neurosci* 14:6336–6353.

40. Gibson, J.J. (1950) *The perception of the visual world,* Boston: Houghton Mifflin.

41. Bicchi, A., *et al.* (2008) Tactile flow explains haptic counterparts of common visual illusions. *Brain Res Bull* 75:737–741.

42. Watson, J.D., *et al.* (1993) Area V5 of the human brain: Evidence from a combined study using positron emission tomography and magnetic resonance imaging. *Cereb Cortex* 3:79–94.

43. Hagen, M.C., *et al.* (2002) Tactile motion activates the human middle temporal/V5 (MT/V5) complex. *Eur J Neurosci* 16:957–964.

44. Blake, R., *et al.* (2004) Neural synergy between kinetic vision and touch. *Psychol Sci,* 15:397–402.

45. Goebel, R., *et al.* (1998) The constructive nature of vision: Direct evidence from functional magnetic resonance imaging studies of apparent motion and motion imagery. *Eur J Neurosci* 10:1563–1573.

46. Ricciardi, E., *et al.* (2007) The effect of visual experience on the development of functional architecture in hMT+. *Cereb Cortex* 17:2933–2939.

47. Kupers, R., *et al.* (2006) Transcranial magnetic stimulation of the visual cortex induces somatotopically organized qualia in blind subjects. *Proc Natl Acad Sci (USA)* 103:13256–13260.

48. Poirier, C., *et al.* (2006) Auditory motion perception activates visual motion areas in early blind subjects. *Neuroimage* 31:279–285.

49. Ricciardi, E., *et al.* (2006b) Brain response to visual, tactile and auditory flow in sighted and blind individuals supports a supramodal functional organization in hMT+ complex. *NeuroImage* 31 (Suppl 1):512 TH-PM.

50. Prather, S.C., *et al.* (2004) Task-specific recruitment of dorsal and ventral visual areas during tactile perception. *Neuropsychologia* 42:1079–1087.

51. Reed, C.L., *et al.* (2005) What vs. where in touch: An fMRI study. *Neuroimage* 25:718–726.

52. Ricciardi, E., *et al.* (2006a) Neural correlates of spatial working memory in humans: A functional magnetic resonance imaging study comparing visual and tactile processes. *Neuroscience* 139:339–349.

53. Zhang, M., *et al.* (2005) Tactile discrimination of grating orientation: fMRI activation patterns. *Hum Brain Mapp* 25:370–377.

54. Bonino, D., *et al.* (2005) Supramodal cortical organization of the dorsal stream during visual and tactile spatial discrimination in sighted and congenitally-blind subjects. *NeuroImage* 26 (Suppl 1):1406, .

55. Bonino, D., *et al.* (2007) Neural correlates of mental representation of space in sighted and congenitally blind individuals as measured by fMRI. *NeuroImage* 36 (Suppl 1):208 TH-PM, .

56. Gallese, V., *et al.* (1996) Action recognition in the premotor cortex. *Brain* 119:593–609.

57. Kohler, E., *et al.* (2002) Hearing sounds, understanding actions: Action representation in mirror neurons. *Science* 297:846–848.

58. Rizzolatti, G. and Craighero, L. (2004) The mirror neuron system. *Annu Rev Neurosci* 27:169–192.

59. Gazzola, V., *et al.* (2006) Empathy and the somatotopic auditory mirror system in humans. *Curr Biol* 16:1824–1829.

60. Emiliano Ricciardi, Daniela Bonino, Lorenzo Sani, Tomaso. E.Vecchi, Mario Guazzelli, James V. Haxby, Luciano Fadiga, Pietro Pietrini. (2008) *Fuctional development of the mirror neuron system does not require visual experience: an fMRI study in sighted and congenitally blind individuals.* 14th Annual Meeting of the Human Brain Mapping Organization, June 15–19, Melbourne, Australia. Available on CD-Rom in NeuroImage, Vol. 41 Suppl. 1:696T-PM.

61. Bach-y-Rita, P. and Kercel, S. (2003) Sensory substitution and the human-machine interface. *Trends Cogn Sci* 7:541–546.

62. Cowey, A. and Walsh, V. (2000) Magnetically induced phosphenes in sighted, blind and blindsighted observers. *Neuroreport* 11:3269–3273.

63. Sugishita, M. and Takayama, Y. (1993) Paraesthesia elicited by repetitive magnetic stimulation of postcentral gyrus. *Neuroreport* 4:569–570.

64. Tegenthoff, M., *et al.* (2005) Improvement of tactile discrimination performance and enlargement of cortical somatosensory maps after 5 Hz rTMS. *PLoS Biol* 3:e362.

65. Libet, B., *et al.* (1964) Production of threshold levels of conscious sensation by electrical stimulation of human somatosensory cortex. *J Neurophysiol* 27:546–578.

66. Cohen, L.G., *et al.* (1997) Functional relevance of cross-modal plasticity in the blind. *Nature* 389:180–183.

67. Ptito, M., *et al.* (2008a) TMS of the occipital cortex induces tactile sensations in the fingers of blind Braille readers. *Exp Brain Res* 184:193–200.

68. James, W. (1890) *Principles of psychology,* New York: Dover.

69. Hurley, S.L. and Noë, A. (2003) Neural plasticity and consciousness. *Biol Philos* 18:131–168.

70. Wallace, M.T., *et al.* (2004) A revised view of sensory cortical parcellation. *Proc Natl Acad Sci (USA)* 101:2167–2172.

71. Falchier, A., *et al.* (2002) Anatomical evidence of multimodal integration in primate striate cortex. *J Neurosci* 22:5749–5759.

72. Rockland, K.S. and Ojima, H. (2003) Multisensory convergence in calcarine visual areas in macaque monkey. *Int J Psychophysiol* 50:19–26.

73. Hyvarinen, J., *et al.* (1991) Modification of parietal association cortex and functional blindness after binocular deprivation in young monkeys. *Exp Brain Res* 42:1–8.

74. Buchel, C., *et al.* (1998) Different activation patterns in the visual cortex of late and congenitally blind subjects. *Brain* 121:409–419.

75. Burton, H., *et al.* (2002) Adaptive changes in early and late blind: A fMRI study of Braille reading. *J Neurophysiol* 87:589–607.

76. Gizewski, E.R., *et al.* (2003) Cross-modal plasticity for sensory and motor activation patterns in blind subjects. *Neuroimage* 19:968–975.

77. Burton, H., *et al.* (2004) Cortical activity to vibrotactile stimulation: An fMRI study in blind and sighted individuals. *Hum Brain Mapp* 23:210–228.

78. Cohen, L.G., *et al.* (1999) Period of susceptibility for cross-modal plasticity in the blind. *Ann Neurol* 45:451–460.

79. Fishman, M.C. and Michael, P. (1973) Integration of auditory information in the cat's visual cortex. *Vision Res* 13:1415–1419.

80. Macaluso, E., *et al.* (2000) Modulation of human visual cortex by crossmodal spatial attention. *Science* 289:1206–1208.

81. Zangaladze, A., *et al.* (1999) Involvement of visual cortex in tactile discrimination of orientation. *Nature* 401:587–590.

82. O'Regan, J.K. and Noe, A. (2001) A sensorimotor account of vision and visual consciousness. *Behav Brain Sci* 24:939–973.

83. Pan, W.J., *et al.* (2007) Progressive atrophy in the optic pathway and visual cortex of early blind Chinese adults: A voxel-based morphometry magnetic resonance imaging study. *Neuroimage* 37:212–220.

84. Chebat, D.R., *et al.* (2007) Alterations in right posterior hippocampus in early blind individuals. *Neuroreport* 18:329–333.

85. Tusa, R.J. and Ungerleider, L.G. (1985) The inferior longitudinal fasciculus: A reexamination in humans and monkeys. *Ann Neurol* 18:583–591.

86. Catani, M., *et al.* (2003) Occipito-temporal connections in the human brain. *Brain* 126:2093–2107.

87. Wittenberg, G.F., *et al.* (2004) Functional connectivity between somatosensory and visual cortex in early blind humans. *Eur J Neurosci* 20:1923–1927.

88. Röder, B., *et al.* (2002) Speech processing activates visual cortex in congenitally blind humans. *Eur J Neurosci* 16:930–936.

89. Burton, H., *et al.* (2003) Dissociating cortical regions activated by semantic and phonological tasks: A FMRI study in blind and sighted people. *J Neurophysiol* 90:1965–1982.

90. Amedi, A., *et al.* (2004) Transcranial magnetic stimulation of the occipital pole interferes with verbal processing in blind subjects. *Nat Neurosci* 7:1266–1270.

91. Raz, N., *et al.* (2005) V1 activation in congenitally blind humans is associated with episodic retrieval. *Cereb Cortex* 15:1459–1468.

92. Kupers, R., *et al.* (2007) rTMS of the occipital cortex abolishes Braille reading and repetition priming in blind subjects. *Neurology* 68:691–693.

93. Weeks, R., *et al.* (2000) A positron emission tomographic study of auditory localization in the congenitally blind. *J Neurosci* 20:2664–2672.

94. Gougoux, F., *et al.* (2005) A functional neuroimaging study of sound localization: Visual cortex activity predicts performance in early-blind individuals. *PLoS Biol* 3 (2):e27.

95. Stevens, A.A., *et al.* (2007) Preparatory activity in occipital cortex in early blind humans predicts auditory perceptual performance. *J Neurosci* 27:10734–10741.

96. Draganski, B., *et al.* (2004) Neuroplasticity: Changes in grey matter induced by training. *Nature* 427:311–312.

97. Bengtsson, S.L. (2005) Extensive piano practicing has regionally specific effects on white matter development. *Nat Neurosci* 8:1148–1150.

98. Lotze, M., *et al.* (2003) The musician's brain: Functional imaging of amateurs and professionals during performance and imagery. *Neuroimage* 20:1817–1829.

99. Amedi, A., *et al.* (2003) Early 'visual' cortex activation correlates with superior verbal memory performance in the blind. *Nat Neurosci* 6:758–766.

100. Pietrini, P. (2003) Toward a biochemistry of the mind? *Am J Psychiatr* 160:1907–1908.

The Neurology of Consciousness: An Overview

Giulio Tononi and Steven Laureys

OUTLINE

ABSTRACT

This final chapter provides the reader with an overview of the neurological and neurobiological literature on the neural substrate of consciousness. First, the chapter reviews the evidence suggesting that consciousness can be dissociated from other brain functions, such as responsiveness to sensory inputs, motor control, attention, language, memory, reflection, spatial frames of reference, the body and perhaps even the self. The chapter then summarizes what has been learned by studying global changes in the level of consciousness, such as sleep, anesthesia, seizures, and vegetative states. Next, it asks what can be said at this point about the role of different brain structures in generating experience. Then dynamic aspects of neural activity are discussed, such as sustained vs. phasic activity, feedforward vs. reentrant activity, and the role of neural synchronization. The chapter ends by briefly considering how a theoretical analysis of the fundamental properties of consciousness can complement neurobiological studies.

Many chapters of this book present a composite picture of the relationship between consciousness and the brain, as seen from several different angles by many different authors. Can one discern, from such a fragmented perspective, the contours of the neural process underlying consciousness, the ghost in the machine? Not yet, a sceptical reader casting a cold eye on this book might conclude; or perhaps something is beginning to emerge, though dimly. But at least, this volume should have made clear that neurological investigations, often forgotten by philosophers and neuroscientists alike because what they offer is often rough, dirty, and idiosyncratic, still provide the fundamental empirical evidence concerning the physical substrate of consciousness: it is by examining how human consciousness is drastically changed by anatomical or functional changes in the brain, and conversely by considering which changes in brain structure and dynamics do not seem to affect consciousness much, that over the past 100 years or so we have been learning the lay of the land.

This final chapter attempts to provide the reader with an overview of the neurological and neurobiological literature, stating what seems to be reasonably established and what is instead still open or unknown. First, the chapter reviews the evidence suggesting that consciousness can be dissociated from other brain functions, such as responsiveness to sensory inputs, motor control, attention, language, memory, reflection, spatial frames of reference, the body and perhaps even the self. The chapter then summarizes what has been learned by studying global changes in the level of consciousness, such as sleep, anesthesia, seizures, and vegetative states. Next, it asks what can be said at this point about the role of different brain structures in generating experience. Then dynamic aspects of neural activity are discussed, such as sustained vs. phasic activity, feed-forward vs. reentrant activity, and the role of neural synchronization. The chapter ends by briefly considering how a theoretical analysis of the fundamental properties of consciousness can complement neurobiological studies.

CONSCIOUSNESS AND OTHER BRAIN FUNCTIONS

Many suggestions have been ventured in the hope to alleviate the puzzle of subjective experience. Perhaps consciousness emerges somehow when an organism is immersed in some complex sensorimotor loop that includes the environment. Another common idea is that consciousness may arise when one part of the brain, acting as the 'subject' (typically the front), looks upon another part as its object (typically the back), and evaluates or reflects upon its activity. It is often thought that in the end consciousness may reduce to attention and its brain mechanisms, since we are usually conscious of what we attend. Much could be said about each of these suggestions. Here, we briefly consider some recent results (and some very old evidence) indicating that consciousness – in the sense of having an experience – does not require sensorimotor loops involving the body and the world, does not require language, introspection or reflection, can do without spatial frames of reference and perhaps even without a sense of the body and the self, and does not reduce to attention or memory. Due to space limitations, we will not discuss the relationship between consciousness and time, between consciousness and emotion, or the notion of conscious access.

Consciousness and Sensory Input/Motor Output

We are usually conscious of what goes on around us, and occasionally of what goes on within our body. So it is only natural to think that consciousness may be tightly linked to the ongoing interaction we maintain with the world and the body. However, there are many examples to the contrary. We are conscious of our thoughts, which do not seem to correspond to anything out there; we can also imagine things that are not out there. When we do so, sensory areas can be activated from the inside [1], though there are some differences [2]. Also, stimulus-independent conscious-ness is associated with its own patterns of activation within cortex and thalamus [3]. During dreams, we are virtually disconnected from the environment [4] – hardly anything of what happens around us enters consciousness, and our muscles are paralyzed (except for eye muscles and diaphragm). Nevertheless, we are vividly conscious: all that seems to matter is that the corticothalamic system continues to function more or less like in wakefulness, as shown by unit record-ing, electroencephalography (EEG) and neuroimag-ing studies performed during rapid eye movement (REM) sleep, when dreams are most intense [5]; [6]. Interestingly, certain regions of the corticothalamic sys-tems, such as dorsolateral prefrontal cortex, are deac-tivated in REM sleep, which likely accounts for some peculiarities of dreaming experiences, such as the reduction of voluntary control.

Neurological evidence also indicates that neither sensory inputs nor motor outputs are needed to gener-ate consciousness. For instance, retinally blind people can both imagine and dream visually if they become blind after 6–7 years of age or so [7, 8]), (see also Chapter 27). Patients with the locked-in syndrome can be almost completely paralyzed, and yet they are just as conscious as healthy subjects [9] (Chapter 15), and can compose eloquent accounts of their condition [10]. A transient form of paralysis is one of the characteris-tic features of narcolepsy. Severe cataplectic attacks can last for minutes and leave the patient collapsed on the floor, utterly unable to move or to signal, but fully aware of her surroundings [11, 12]. Drug addicts known as *frozen addicts* who show symptoms of severe Parkinson's disease due to MPTP-induced damage to the dopaminergic system are also fully conscious, yet unable to move or speak [13]. Thus, consciousness here and now seems to depend on what certain parts of the brain are doing, without requiring any obligatory inter-action with the environment or the body.

Consciousness and Language

There have been claims that consciousness only emerges with language [14], though it seems prepos-terous to suggest that infants and animals are uncon-scious automata. Neurological evidence from adult humans can help settle the issue by asking whether consciousness is preserved in patients with aphasia. Nichelli (Chapter 26) reviews the evidence indicat-ing that even deep aphasia does not seem to interrupt the flow of experience, though it may alter or abolish certain aspects of it, such as inner speech. He points to the remarkable interview with Dr. Jill Bolte-Taylor, a

neuroanatomist who was struck with a left hemisphere haemorrhage. Over the course of 3–4 hours, she lost her inner speech, became hemiparetic, and soon real-ized that her utterances did not make sense, nor did those of others. In her retrospective recall of that time, she experienced the loss of function of a good part of the left hemisphere, language included, and remained fully conscious, though things felt differently from a 'right hemisphere perspective.' Her account not only confirms that consciousness continues in the absence of language – or at least left hemisphere specializa-tions having to do with comprehension and produc-tion, but that thought and self-reflection continue too. Another extraordinary report is from a patient who underwent an anesthetic injection into the lower divi-sion of the left middle anterior artery. The anesthetic presumably led to the inactivation of posterior tem-poral, inferior parietal, and lateral temporo-occipital region of the left hemisphere, and caused as expected a deep Wernicke aphasia indistinguishable from that due to strokes, except that is was temporary (a few minutes) and fully reversible [15]. From the patient's recollections of the experience, it is clear not only that he was conscious and thinking, but that he also had a much better understanding of the situation than appeared from the language tests being administered. Moreover, he could usually recall what happened and what he was trying to do, especially when presented with pictures rather than with spoken or written material. For instance, he recalled that he was desper-ately trying to identify the picture of a tennis racket, of which he was fully aware, but all that came out was 'perkbull.' He wanted to add that he owned one, but thought to have said instead that he had just bought one – in reality, he had said nothing. These examples leave little doubt that experience continues after the loss of the left hemisphere's language functions.

Consciousness and Introspection/Reflection

Consciousness is usually evaluated by verbal reports, and questions about consciousness ('Did you see anything on the screen?') are answered by 'looking inside' retrospectively and reporting what one has just experienced. So it is perhaps natural to suggest that consciousness may arise through the ability to reflect on our own perceptions: our brain would form a scene of what it sees, but we would become conscious of it – experience it subjectively – only when we, as a subject of experience, watch that scene from the inside. This suggestion is often framed in a neurobiological context by assuming that patterns of activity corresponding to 'unconscious' or 'subconscious' percepts form in posterior regions of the cerebral cortex involved in the categorization/association of sensory stimuli. These percepts then become conscious when mainly anterior prefrontal and cingulate regions involved in self-representations interact with posterior cortex, perhaps by reading in signals through forward connections and selectively amplifying them through back-connections (more on this later).

There is of course no doubt that the brain categorizes its own patterns of activity, in the sense that neurons respond mainly to the activity of other neurons, so the brain is constantly 'looking at itself.' However, this is not necessarily in terms of a 'subject' (the front) looking at an 'object' represented in sensory cortices (the back). Leaving aside the mystery of why reflecting on something should make it conscious, this scenario is made less plausible by a common observation: when we become absorbed in some intense perceptual task, for example watching an engrossing movie, playing a fast-paced video game, or rushing through the woods at high speed, we are vividly conscious – we are immersed in the rapid flow of experience – without any need for reflection or introspection. Often, we become so immersed in such flow that we may lose the sense of self, the inner voice. Perhaps the habit of thinking about consciousness makes the experts forget that much of experience is unreflective.

A recent neuroimaging study by Malach *et al.* [16] throws some interesting light on these old observations. Subjects were scanned with functional magnetic resonance imaging (fMRI) in three conditions. In the slow categorization task, subjects were asked to categorize pictures into animal/no-animal categories. During the introspective task, subjects viewed the images and then self-introspected about their emotional response (strong/neutral). Finally, the fast categorization task was identical to the 'slow' condition but at triple the stimulation rate. Thus, 'slow' and 'introspection' conditions were identical in terms of sensory stimuli and motor output but differed in the cognitive task. On the other hand, 'slow' and 'rapid' conditions were similar in the cognitive task but differed in the sensorimotor processing and attentional loads. Behavioural measurements confirmed that self-awareness was high during the introspection task, and virtually abolished during rapid categorization. The neuroimaging results were clear: during rapid categorization there was an activation of prefrontal regions, whereas sensory cortex was strongly activated during rapid categorization. Crucially, during introspection self-related cortex was deactivated below the rest condition. This deactivation of prefrontal regions was thus the neural correlate of 'losing oneself' in the task. To the extent that these prefrontal regions were indeed involved in self-representation,

these findings suggest that their activation is not necessary for the emergence of perceptual consciousness, but only to reflect upon it and report it to others. Indeed, it appears that self-related activity is actually shut off during highly demanding sensory tasks.

Consciousness and Attention

Attention and consciousness often go hand-in-hand: when we pay attention to an object, our experience of it becomes more vivid, and when we shift our attention, it fades from consciousness. Attention can be bottom-up, as when a salient stimulus – say a flash or a sound turn our gaze or a colored letter in the middle of a black text pops out at us, capturing attention. Top-down attention instead is willingly deployed towards a particular position in space, a particular feature, or a particular object. It is often assumed that attention is a necessary prerequisite for consciousness [17–19]. For example, if we do not attend to it, we may fail to see a large, stable stimulus at the very centre of the visual display – the phenomenon appropriately known as inattentional blindness [20]. However, already Wundt and James argued that attention was a mechanism for selecting within consciousness, and several recent papers have reinforced this view (see [21–23]). Tsuchiya and Koch (Chapter 6) make an especially strong case for a double dissociation between visual attention and visual consciousness. After briefly considering examples where attention and consciousness coincide (we attend to something and we see it, or we do not attend to it and do not see it), they examine the two critical dissociations: situations in which events or objects are attended to without being consciously perceived; and situations in which events or objects can be consciously perceived in the near absence of top-down attention. For example, invisible words (through masking) can produce priming only if the subject was attending to the invisible prime-target pair; without attention, the same word failed to elicit priming [24]. There are by now several reports, both in blindsight patients and healthy subjects, indicating that attention can facilitate responses to unseen stimuli [25, 26]. More generally, when we are looking for something laying just in front of us (the purloined letter), we are paying attention to something we do not see. Indeed, the very act of paying attention may inhibit access to consciousness. The tip-of-the-tongue phenomenon may be another familiar demonstration that attention may actually interfere with consciousness. Thus, selective attention does not necessarily result in conscious experience, and may even be counterproductive. Some neurophysiological evidence also seems consistent with this view. For instance, an event-related potential component (N2pc) that appears to be a correlate of top-down attention can be elicited by stimuli that remain invisible [27]; also, attention to an invisible stimulus can increase the activation of primary visual cortex [28]. Finally, a recent magnetoencephalography (MEG) study showed that consciously seen stimuli induced increased mid-frequency gamma-band activity over contralateral visual cortex whether attended or not, whereas spatial attention modulated high-frequency gamma-band activity in response to both consciously seen and unseen stimuli [29].

On the other hand, we can be conscious of something without deploying attention to it. When we contemplate an empty blue sky, there is no need for selective attention, and yet the experience is vivid. Conversely, when we attend intensely onto something, the world outside the focus of attention does not disappear from consciousness: we still experience the gist or context of the overall visual scene that faces us. Indeed, as observed by Tsuchiya and Koch, gist is immune from inattentional blindness [20] – when a photograph covering the entire background is briefly and unexpectedly flashed onto the screen, subjects can accurately report a summary of its content. In the 30 ms necessary to apprehend the gist of a scene, top-down attention cannot play much of a role. Similarly, a subject engaged in a task that requires focusing attention on the centre of the visual field can still perceive the difference between a background scene containing an animal from one that does not [30]. Or think of when driving home on a familiar segment of the highway: top-down, one may be attending the radio, or to the plans for the evening. Despite claims to the contrary, it is not that we do not experience at all the monotonous road that does not claim our attention: we simply do not have to think about how to navigate it as long as things are predictable, and presumably do not form explicit memories. Finally, as indicated by neuroimaging studies mentioned above, consciousness without attention and consciousness with attention may have different neural correlates: Victor Lamme has suggested that consciousness without attention could be generated by interactions among posterior regions of the cortex, whereas when top-down attention boosts conscious experience prefrontal cortex enters the game through reentrant interactions with posterior cortex [31]. We will return to this distinction when considering the role of the front vs. the back of the brain in generating consciousness.

Consciousness and Memory

Considerations similar to those just reviewed for attention are likely to apply to working memory – the ability to keep things in mind for a few seconds. Indeed, attention and working memory are closely related and may be conceptualized as two different aspects of the same process [32]: attention selects some aspects of an existing scene, whereas working memory selects the same aspects in the absence of the stimulus. Indeed, the ability to imagine things is itself closely related to working memory. Moreover, the neural structures subserving working memory and top-down attention overlap to a large degree both anatomically and functionally [33]. Should one then expect a double dissociation also between working memory and consciousness? To this date, this question has not received much attention. Moreover, the question is complicated by the need to distinguish between the targets of attention, working memory, and imagery, typically located in posterior cortex, where activity is either enhanced in response to a stimulus, or else maintained or even generated in its absence, and control mechanisms, typically located in anterior cortex, which are responsible for directing attention, manipulating contents of working memory, and generate images [34]. Given the close relationship between working memory and attention, it is perhaps conceivable that working memory may be maintained for items of which the subject is not currently conscious, just like attention can be. But it is undisputable that one can be conscious of something without exercising any working memory, as when we follow the rapid flow of images in a movie. Indeed, there are disorders, typically associated with prefrontal lesions, in which working memory is severely compromised but consciousness is clearly preserved.

The relationship between consciousness and episodic memory (also known as autonoetic memory) is complex, but there is little doubt that consciousness can be present even when episodic memory is impaired (the converse would seem to be out of the question). In syndromes of transient amnesia (Chapter 25), patients are obviously conscious – they engage in conversations, carry out complex tasks, but later show no memory of what they did (anterograde amnesia). Butler and Zeman discuss a case described by Hughlings-Jackson in which a doctor suffering from epileptic transient amnesia visited a patient, correctly diagnosed pneumonia, and wrote down prescriptions and notes without remembering anything about the episode. Perhaps the amnesia for a stretch of familiar highway is a normal example of the same dissociation: under normal circumstances, if our attention is engaged elsewhere, and if there is no particular reason to engage it on the scene we face when driving, we may simply not burden hippocampal circuits to lay down useless memories. In transient amnesia, the hippocampus may not be capable of laying down memories, either due to some kind of trauma (transient global amnesia) or because it is preempted by seizure activity (transient epileptic amnesia). When damage to the hippocampal formation is permanent, as with the bitemporal resection suffered by H.M. and similar patients, anterograde amnesia is permanent, and the patient is limited to the immediate present and to the content of his working memory. Yet as described by Postle (Chapter 24), when interacting with H.M. there was little doubt that he was conscious.

On the other hand, when amnesia is deep, consciousness is altered in peculiar ways. Usually, patients with transient amnesia appear to be confused and uncertain about the past (retrograde amnesia). H.M. and other patients recounted by Postle (Chapter 24) describe an unsettling feeling of entering the world as from deep sleep, when we may be briefly unsure about who we are and where we are, except that feeling in their case is permanent. Possibly, this deficit may also reduce the window of time over which the conscious present flows. Also, recent studies have shown that patients with damage to the hippocampal formation also show a deficit in imagination, not just in memory, and their account of the world, both remembered, experienced in the present, and imagined, appears to be less rich, lacking in color, detail, and spatial coherence [35–37]. This view fits nicely with evidence for a role of the hippocampal formation in responding to as well as storing relations among objects in a context-dependent (episodic) manner [38]. Over time and over multiple episodes of retrieval the memory is transformed to one that is more schematic (semantic) and independent of the hippocampus [39, 40]. Thus, while consciousness remains in the absence of episodic memory and of the hippocampal formation, it does seem to lose not just an external sketchpad for writing down memories, but actually a part of itself.

Consciousness and Space: Balint's Syndrome

We all have the strong impression that much of experience is situated in an outside, external space. In turn, this external space is centred on an internal space, that of the body. And, whenever we think about our own experience, nothing is stronger than the feeling that it is centred somewhere within the head, roughly between the eyes. Can consciousness even exist without any representation of space, or of our own body, or without our 'first-person' perspective, centred somewhere behind the eyes? These questions are hard to answer on the basis of neurological evidence because representations of space and of the body are widespread, and lesions that eliminate all such representations would have to be so wide as to

make any firm conclusion unwarranted. Nevertheless, a few lessons can still be learned.

Neurophysiological studies have demonstrated that the brain employs multiple maps of external space, some unimodal, some multimodal, many in the cerebral cortex, especially but not exclusively in parietal lobes, but some also in thalamus and colliculi. Parietal areas receive converging visual, auditory, and touch inputs, as well as proprioceptive and vestibular signals about the position of the eyes, head, and limbs. These maps implement different frames of reference, so there are eye-centred, head-centred, and body-centred maps, maps for distant space and maps for peri-personal space [41]. Attention can rapidly shift between one frame of reference and the other, and there are indications that more global frames of reference may be a speciality of right hemisphere maps, whereas more local maps are a speciality of the left. It is also clear that, under normal conditions, many different maps are kept in register for smooth functioning, and that posterior parietal cortex, especially on the right side, is important in coordinating these various maps, perhaps through what has been called a master map. Indeed, studies in monkeys have identified neurons that respond only to the stimulus that is being selected as the current target for attention – a kind of a winner-takes-all principle over space, and do so in a stable manner, in line with the need of a stable perceptual representation of a target for action. This fits with the finding that parietal neurons are involved not only in multimodal spatial integration of sensory input, but also in the early stages of planning spatial movements. Multimodal neurons in different parietal areas are also well-suited to mediate smooth transformations between different frames of reference, showing responses to one stimulus modality (e.g., visual) that are influenced in a multiplicative manner by stimuli in other modalities (e.g., proprioceptive or vestibular) – an effect called gain modulation [42].

How much of the information about external space that is constantly being updated within and across these many maps leads to experience, and how much instead remains unconscious? Conscious experience of space is so pervasive that it seems to provide a general framework for much of what we experience, at least in the visual and auditory domain. In fact, Kant thought that space was an essential substrate for all experience. And yet, there is neurological evidence that the capacity to experience external space may be lost, while at the same time most other aspects of experience are preserved, and unconscious aspects of space representation continue to function [41]. The evidence comes primarily from a rare syndrome, Balint's syndrome, characterized by the triad of (i) simultagnosia (the inability to see more than one object at a time, also known as tunnel vision); (ii) optic apraxia (inability to reach for objects in space; and (iii) paralysis of gaze (the eyes usually stare straight ahead, though they are not paralyzed, as shown for instance by reflex movements). Simultagnosia is the most relevant component: it means that all experience of external space is lost, so that objects cannot be located at different places, and therefore at any given time only one object is experienced, outside any spatial framework. By contrast, experience of the body is intact. Balint patients behave as if they were blind, but in reality their visual experience is preserved – they can see and report objects, shapes, faces, colors, and all kinds of visual features. However, at any given time they will only experience one particular object, the one that happens to grab their fixation point, at the exclusion of everything else. Most notably, while they can easily recognize and describe the object they are experiencing, they have no idea of where it might be in space: left, right, up and down are impossible for them to say, and of course spatial relationships among objects are out of the question. So, just as one can lose the experience of color, one can lose the experience of external space. (Balint patients have problems also with auditory space, though less marked, at least in the single case that was studied [43].) They also have a problem binding colors with shapes, as indicated by frequent illusory conjunctions, in which the color of another object is mistakenly attributed to the one they are experiencing. In the few cases studied in detail, the site of the lesion was bilateral inferior parietal cortex, centred around the angular gyrus (area 39). Balint patients seem to indicate, then, that we can lose selectively the experience of external space without losing consciousness – specifically visual consciousness of objects – thus proving that an external spatial framework is not a prerequisite for experience. However, they still seem to know that space exists (see [41, p. 162]), (perhaps because they still experience it in reference to their own body – in other words, they do not seem to have anosoagnosia (see below)).

Consciousness and Space: Neglect

While Balint's syndrome is exceedingly rare, presumably because it involves bilateral, symmetric parietal lesions, neglect is a common occurrence, especially early on after acute brain lesions on the right side (Chapter 21). A patient with neglect acts as if he is inattentive to one half of the world – most often the left half. He may not notice people and objects on the left side, may read only the right side of a map, may eat only the right

side of the food on his plate, or shave only one side of his face. In the clinic, neglect can be revealed by simple paper-and-pencil tests. For example, asked to mark all lines on a page, the patient marks only those on the right side. Asked to mark the middle of a line, he errs towards the right side. Asked to draw a figure, he leaves out the left side of it. Nevertheless, a typical neglect patient is definitely not blind: if an isolated object is shown on the left, the patient can see it and pick it up. Indeed, neglect is most apparent in competitive situations, a phenomenon called 'extinction.' The same stimulus on the left side that is reported if presented alone, is ignored if presented simultaneously with a stimulus on the right side. Importantly, patients may also show neglect for imagined or remembered left space: asked to imagine the buildings lining the main piazza in Milan, a patient would only recall those on the right side of where he imagined himself standing [43]. In short, a patient with neglect behaves as if his attention were pathologically locked onto events and things on the right side and pathologically inattentive to events and things on the left side. It is attention, rather than perception, that appears to be hampered in neglect. This attentional problem may explain why, as a rule, a patient with neglect remains unaware of his problem, especially early on. Later on, he may admit that he tends to ignore things on the left side, but continues to do so.

Neglect can occur in sensory modalities besides vision, including audition, touch, proprioception, and smell, and it can affect various aspects of space, from one's own body (personal space) to nearby objects (peri-personal space) to distant objects. For example, one patient may neglect objects on the left side that are out of reach but not objects nearby, another one may neglect only objects that are within reach, and yet another may neglect his own left face. Or a patient may ignore his left arm and leg, trying to climb out of bed without them even though he is not at all paralyzed. Finally, some patients may show predominantly motor neglect, in that their eye or hand movements are biased towards the right. Presumably, the specific form of neglect suffered by every individual patient depends on the precise localization of the underlying brain lesion.

Many brain lesions can produce some kind of neglect in humans, but the most typical and long-lasting syndromes are produced by lesions involving the right inferior parietal lobe. These lesions produce the common neglect syndrome, which is for the left side of space. Neglect for the right side, which is very rare and usually much milder, can occasionally be produced by lesions of the left parietal lobe. Lesions that produce neglect are often widespread, but by examining the anatomical overlap in many different patients, the critical cortical areas appear to be the right angular gyrus at the temporo-parietal junction, corresponding to Brodmann areas 39, although another important region seems to be the right parahippocampal cortex [45, 46]). As will be discussed later, the right temporo-parietal junction, together with right ventral frontal areas, constitutes the ventral attention network, which is necessary for target detection and reorienting towards salient, unexpected events either right or left of the midline [47]. The ventral attention network is strongly connected, by way of the right middle frontal gyrus, to the dorsal attention network of the same side, which controls the allocation of spatial attention to extrapersonal space and the selection of stimuli and responses primarily to contralateral space. In this way, right temporo-parietal lesions would lead to a functional imbalance in posterior parietal cortex that secondarily causes a rightward bias with detection deficits to the left of the midline [48].

An intriguing finding in neglect is that, though patients fail to report stimuli on the left side (e.g., visual stimuli in the left visual field), signals related to those stimuli can still be detected using fMRI not only within early visual areas of the occipital lobe, but also along the right ventral visual pathway into the temporal lobe, which is often intact [49, 50]. On the other hand, the degree of activation for undetected stimuli in the neglected field is weaker than for those that can be detected, and it fails to engage a larger fronto-parietal network, a difference that is also reflected in EEG evoked responses. These findings suggest that the activation of the ventral visual system in isolation, even up to the level of semantics of words and pictures, is not sufficient for conscious detection [51], as is also suggested by studies of inattentional and change blindness (see below, and Chapters 5 and 21).

Consciousness, Body, and Self

Balint's syndrome suggests that consciousness can exist even in the absence of awareness of external space – after all, many modalities of consciousness are not spatial at all. But what about awareness of the self, or even of our own body? Can consciousness exist in the complete absence of a sense of self or of a body? The self is a multilayered concept, and different people or disciplines tend to conceptualize it in very different ways.

In a neurological context, it is useful to keep a few distinctions in mind. First and foremost is the *narrative, autobiographical self* – the one that characterizes in a fundamental sense who we are. As important as this self may be for each of us, it seems clear that an autobiographical self is not a prerequisite for

experience – just think of how it may take some time to reconnect with it when awakening in the morning, though experience is already present.

Then there is the *feeling of agency*: experiencing that one is the source of one's action. There is a growing neurological literature about the neural substrate of agency, and about how agency may be altered in pathological conditions [52–55]. Again, however, experience of agency is not necessary for consciousness – one can be completely passive and still experience the flow of images.

At a more basic level then there is the *feeling of ownership* – the knowledge that your body and its parts are indeed yours. The body is heavily represented in the brain, and not only in the cerebral cortex. There are maps of the body already in the brainstem, in the thalamus, and in multiple cortical areas, especially primary and secondary somatosensory cortex, right posterior insular cortex, and portions of the parieto-temporal junction (Chapter 1). The representations deal with touch, proprioception, and vestibular signals, which very soon become integrated into multi-modal maps. The hypothalamus and brainstem have access to many other inputs from the body and the viscera, although much of what is recorded there does not seem to make it to consciousness.

Like the experience of external space, the experience of our own body might appear as an integral, obligatory aspect of all experience. Usually, awareness of the body is discrete and stays in the background, perhaps because it is always there and is relatively stable compared to the awareness of external circumstances. But is a complete loss of body awareness impossible, perhaps even unconceivable? A few intriguing phenomena may speak to the issue.

Recent experiments, exploiting for instance the so-called rubber hand illusion, have shown that our sense of ownership can be altered, and we may feel like we own a hand that is not ours [56]. The sense that our body is ours appears to depend on neural circuits centred in right posterior insula. Then there is asomatognosia, a condition in which patients may claim that the left arm and leg may be missing, or that it may disappear. In such cases the site of lesions is usually in right posterior parietal areas, though premotor cortex may also play a role [57]. Asomatognosia suggests that certain brain lesions may selectively eliminate awareness of the body without compromising consciousness. However, asomatognosia is usually for just a part of the body, so firm conclusions are not possible.

A more global phenomenon is the out-of-body experience [58] (Chapter 23). In its full manifestation, a subject may feel that he is disembodied, that is, he does not feel located within his own body. Instead, the subject feels that he – his experiencing self – is located or centred somewhere else with respect to his body, typically hovering over it at some distance. Moreover, he may be able to contemplate his own body from this new perspective (autoscopy). Out-of-body experiences, which can be triggered by brain lesions, seizures, anesthesia and some drugs, and sometimes occur when falling asleep, are associated with an altered functioning of the temporo-parietal junction, including the insula, especially on the right side. This brain region combines tactile, proprioceptive, and visual signals in a coordinated reference frame, and receives abundant vestibular projections. It is activated when subjects imagine to change perspective and see the world from somewhere else [59]. Compellingly, focal electrical stimulation in the same area can produce full-fledged out-of-body experiences [60]. Clinical data and a further electrical stimulation study in humans suggest that disembodiment and autoscopy (and change in perspective) can be dissociated: disembodiment would be due to perturbations of the junction between right supramarginal and angular gyri, leading to somatosensory–vestibular disintegration, whereas autoscopy/change in perspective would be obtained by perturbing a slightly more posterior region of the right angular gyrus involving visual pathways [61]. An extrastriate body areas is also thought to be involved in perception of the body [62, 63]. It remains to be clarified whether disembodiment can indeed be construed as a true lack of experience of the body, or rather as a dislocation of such experience. But altogether, asomatognosia and out-of-body experiences suggest that it may be possible to lose one's bodily self without losing consciousness.

What seems to be left if we take away the bodily self is the centredness of any experience: even in the out-of body experience, experience seems to be localized somewhere behind the eyes, even if such disembodied self is not associated with any physical simulacrum. But it is centred somewhere. One could argue that what is centred in this case is just the visual experience of space – since subjects report seeing their own body from such altered first-person perspective. Conceivably, however, one could have an out-of-body experience induced in a patient with Balint's syndrome, in which case there would be simultagnosia – the loss of a spatial reference frame for experience, together with a loss of a reference to the body. What kind of experience would this be, or would experience vanish? Though such thought experiments are always dangerous, a reasonable guess would be that experience would still persists: like a Balint patient, one would experience a single object, or say an intense smell, not located in space, and not associated to a body. Perhaps states achieved thorough transcendental meditation techniques can approximate a loss of awareness of space, body, and self: experts reports a feeling of silence, no bodily feelings, unboundedness (no space, and possibly no self), and no time. Even in such cases, though, the experience would still be happening to one particular entity – it would be 'centred,' if you wish, but not in the conventional spatial sense. This last sense of 'self', which we may call the 'intrinsic' or 'subjective' self – would be one and the same as the experience, not further dissociable.

Consciousness, Perception, Imagination, and Absolute Agnosia

Neuropsychology provides perhaps the most compelling evidence concerning which brain areas are *necessary* for experiencing particular conscious modalities. In principle, compiling a list of the areas whose lesion eliminates the experience of colors, shapes, visual motion, faces, places, and so on, should yield the anatomical substrate of conscious vision. Completing the list for other modalities and submodalities would yield the anatomical substrate of consciousness in its entirety. However, such a list is hard to come by, and not just because brain lesions are rarely selective and symptoms change with time: a more fundamental reason is that, to ascertain that the neural substrate of a conscious modality, say a sensory modality, has truly been eliminated, one must be able to demonstrate a complete loss of: (i) the corresponding sensory experiences; (ii) the ability to imagine, remember, or dream any such experience; (iii) the first-hand understanding of what is missing.

To see why, consider first a simple thought experiment concerning a hypothetical sixth sense – let's say echolocation. Obviously, we are not endowed with neural hardware appropriate for generating echolocation qualia. Not surprisingly, when we move around our house, we do not experience any echolocation-like quale. But it is not just a matter of not having the appropriate sensors or sensory pathways: we cannot even imagine what such a quale would feel like, or dream that we are echolocating. Finally, we do not really understand first-hand what we are missing, even though we may know a lot about how bats, for example, make use of echolocation, and some of us can talk about echolocation in great detail. Equipping us with a bat-like sonar (say with a visual or auditory output) might help us to navigate in the dark, but it would not generate echolocation qualia.

To make things a bit more concrete, consider a conscious submodality we are familiar with, namely color. Assume that a cortical area C is the one actually responsible for providing us with color qualia (in association with other areas that ensure a proper level of consciousness); another cortical area A provides 'processed' sensory input to area C – say by computing color constancy – so that the appropriate activity patterns are triggered in C when a surface of a certain reflectance is viewed; finally, a cortical area B can generate similar patterns (maybe less effectively) in C in a top-down manner, implementing the ability to imagine colors.

Given such a scenario, a lesion of area A would lead to what might be called pure achromatopsia: a patient would not be able to discriminate among colors and would not experience colors when presented with colored stimuli. However, the patient would still be able to imagine, remember, or dream of colors. Moreover, he would be perfectly aware that he is missing color, that is, things would look strangely black and white. Such patients have indeed been described [64, 65]. For example, patient E.H. [64] was impaired at color perception: he could not recognize colored characters in the Ishihara pseudoisochromatic plates, could not arrange patches in terms of their hue, and could not match objects with the proper colored swatch. On the other hand, he could imagine colored objects and say the appropriate color, and respond correctly if asked, for example, which of a plum and an eggplant had more red in it.

By contrast, a lesion of area B would lead to the isolated loss of the ability to imagine colors, with no deficit in color perception, and a preserved understanding of what color means. Again, such patients have been described [66], case II [67], case KQu [68], see also [69]. An especially selective example is that of patient QP [70], who had an isolated deficit in color imagery and color memory secondary to a concussive episode. QP had normal color perception, would properly name colors, could even dream in color, but since the time of the injury she had trouble imagining colors or remembering most colors, both short and long term (intriguingly, she had little problem with shades of blue).

Continuing along these lines, a combined lesion of both areas A and B (or of their connections) would produce a patient who not only does not experience the color of objects but, in addition, cannot imagine or remember color. However, he would be fully aware that his world has turned black and white, and would complain about missing color. Such achromatopsic patients with no color imagery have also been described. For example, the painter I, recounted by Oliver Sacks [71], described his symptoms after a car accident thus: 'My vision was such that everything appeared to me as a black and white television screen ... I can see a worm wiggling a block away ... But-I AM TOTALLY COLOUR-BLIND.' To him it made no difference if he was looking with his eyes open, or attempting to imagine colors, or remembering scenes that he knew had color, or whether he was dreaming – he only saw 'awful and disgusting' shades of grey. Being a painter, he could discuss the 256 colors of the Pantone chart and the finer aspects of hues without being able to see them. Obviously, patient I understood perfectly what colors meant, and was overwhelmed by its loss. In such cases, one could speculate that area C, being deafferented from areas A and B, would have no opportunity to become activated, but it would still be functional (for example, direct stimulation with transcranial magnetic stimulation (TMS) might produce colored phosphenes). The inactivity of area C would then constantly signal to upstream areas that the current visual input is achromatic, just as when watching black and white movies.

However, feeling of an absence is not the same as an absence of feeling – having a functional but inactive area C is very different from not having it at all. Indeed, with damage to area C, there should be a complete loss of color consciousness, whether seen, imagined, remembered or dreamt and, crucially, the patient would not understand first-hand what color really means (just as we do not understand echolocation first-hand) and what he is missing. Nevertheless, he could certainly talk about color second-hand, just as we can talk about echolocation. A patient possibly similar to this ideal case has also been described [72]. Patient MAH seems to have a pure form of color agnosia: he cannot name the color of colored pencils (though he has no problem with color naming *per se*), and he cannot tell whether an object is shown with its proper color (as opposed to, say, a purple banana). Moreover, he fails to group colored tokens according to their color, and is clearly not sure about what he is trying to do. When asked to color line drawings of common objects, he produced an orange cherry with a purple stick, or a blue meadow with pink daffodils. On the other hand, MAH can respond to color unconsciously, as demonstrated by priming tasks and a Stroop task, and he performed flawlessly and rapidly on the Ishihara test (he could easily see the characters as being different from the background). He could also discriminate between different hues, although slowly and with little confidence about what he was doing. But when asked about the color of a bright green bag, he hesitated, and then said it was a bright color, perhaps yellow or orange. His condition was apparently congenital (and possibly hereditary, as his mother and one of his daughters showed similar deficits), and he had no relevant neurological problem. MAH is highly educated and knows about the physics of color, but it would seem that he knows about color second-hand, as a biologist may know about echo-location. Uneasily, he admits that he may be color blind 'or something like that,' though occasionally he claims to like colors (especially Fauve paintings). It may be that, though he does see differences between differently colored objects, these may be in terms of brightness or other achromatic attributes, and that he may lack color qualia. In that case, he may not really understand color first-hand the way normal subjects do, or the way pure achromatopsic patients do: we might call his condition one of *absolute agnosia* for color. Absolute agnosia would automatically imply loss of conscious perception for that modality, as well as loss of imagery, memory, and dreaming. What MAH is missing, then, would truly be the neural substrate for the qualia pertaining to the color submodality, due to the absence of the relevant circuits. Thus, at least in principle, identifying patients with absolute agnosia for different modalities and submodalities of consciousness, as well as the underlying dysfunction (the equivalent of 'area C') would reveal the true neural substrate of the corresponding qualia.

Consciousness and Anosognosia

Given the above definition of absolute agnosia (lack of first-hand understanding) as essential to the lack of consciousness in a given modality, it is natural to ask whether examples of anosognosia (unawareness of deficit) in the neuropsychological literature may represent a similar lack of first-hand understanding, and thus of consciousness for that modality. Patients with anosognosia often seem to deny their loss without understanding what they are talking about. For instance, patients with Anton's syndrome can be completely blind due to cortical lesions (to the point that they may not be able to tell whether the light is on or off), yet they insist that they do see, and make up excuses as to why they fail in the simplest visual tasks. It could be that such patients, besides being blind, have indeed absolute agnosia for vision, having lost all sense of what seeing (and not seeing) means: they may merely resort to vision-related words and memories without actually being able to experience anything visual, not even in their imagination or their dreams. However, there are cases of Anton's syndrome that suggest a different interpretation. Careful testing of patient H.S., a cortically blind lady with bilateral damage to primary visual cortex who denied her blindness, suggests that she may actually have had visual experiences, only these were imagined ones – given the lack of competition from retinal input, these images may have convinced her that

she could see [73]. After all, during dreams we are all anosognosic: we generate visual images which we think veridical and falsely attribute to the environment, without realizing that our eyes are closed and we are blind. Thus, anosognosia may not necessarily imply absolute agnosia, as long as a patient with anosognosia can generate images in the affected modality, and gives the impression of understanding first-hand what he is talking about when he describes his experiences.

Examples of selective anosognosia for color blindness are hard to come by, but there are examples of selective unawareness of deficits in other visual submodalities, such as anosognosia for face perception [74], and in other modalities, such as anosognosia for hemi-anaesthesia, for unilateral neglect, for language comprehension and production, and so on. A dramatic example of anosognosia is unawareness of motor deficit, whereby patients deny that their left arm or leg is paralyzed, and usually ignore requests to move it (often in the absence of sensory loss and intellectual impairment). Recent studies have indicated that unawareness of (left) paralysis may result from lesions of (right) premotor cortex, especially areas 6 and 44, sensorimotor cortex, and right insula [75]. These lesions would compromise the comparison between signals representing the intended actions and those monitoring the actual action [76]. In this way, the area responsible for motor awareness ('area C') would receive the motor intention signals (presumably from supplementary motor area) but no mismatch signal, and would thus not be able to tell that the movement was not executed. Alternatively, the input layer to 'area C' from the sensory stream may be dysfunctional, so the patient cannot tell anymore whether activity patterns in 'area C' are triggered by extrinsic or intrinsic sources.

These examples not only highlight the importance of neuropsychological investigations – above and beyond what can be established with neuroimaging alone – but they also indicate how difficult it is to determine, in each patient, what exactly is amiss within a given modality of consciousness: does he lack the relevant aspects of conscious perception as well as imagination, memory, dreaming and, crucially, first-hand understanding of what he is missing? Does he have a selective anosognosia because of an absolute agnosia, or conversely because he can still concoct conscious images in the absence of sensory input? And can he still make covert (unconscious) use of relevant information? All of these questions must be addressed before cortical 'nodes' for individual modalities and submodalities of consciousness can be identified with some confidence.

GLOBAL ALTERATIONS OF CONSCIOUSNESS

In neurology, a distinction is traditionally drawn between the level of consciousness and the content of consciousness. When you fall asleep, for example, the level of consciousness decreases to the point that you become virtually unconscious – the degree to which you are conscious (of anything) becomes progressively less and less. The content of consciousness, instead, refers to the particular experience you are having at any given time, for a similar level of consciousness. This distinction is useful when considering alterations of consciousness. On one side there are localized brain lesions that lead to the loss of specific dimensions of consciousness – defined above as absolute agnosia – without any major change in the level of consciousness. On the other side there are global alterations in the level of consciousness, such as occur, besides certain stages of sleep, in anesthesia, coma, vegetative states, and generalized seizures. It is to these that we now turn.

Sleep

The most commonplace, daily demonstration that the level of consciousness can change dramatically is provided by sleep (see Chapter 8). In the laboratory, a subject is awakened during different stages of sleep and asked to report 'anything that was going through your mind just before waking up.' What is most noteworthy for the present purposes is that a number of awakenings from non-rapid eye movement (NREM) sleep, especially early in the night when EEG slow waves are prevalent, can yield no report whatsoever. Thus, early slow wave sleep is the only phase of adult life during which healthy human subjects may deny that they were experiencing anything at all. When present, reports from NREM sleep early in the night are often short and thought-like. However, especially later in the night, reports from NREM sleep can be longer, more hallucinatory and, generally speaking, more dream-like. On the other hand, awakenings during REM sleep almost always yield dreams–vivid conscious experiences, sometimes organized within a complex narrative structure [4, 77].

What are the processes underlying the fading of the level of consciousness during early slow wave sleep? Metabolic rates do decrease in many cortical areas, especially frontal and parietal areas, and related thalamic nuclei, as is seen in other conditions characterized by reduced consciousness, such as coma, vegetative states, and anesthesia. By contrast, primary sensory cortices are not deactivated compared to resting wakefulness [6, 78]. However, neural activity in the corticothalamic system is far from shutting down. Instead, triggered by a decrease in acetylcholine and other modulators, cortical and thalamic neurons undergo slow oscillations (1 Hz or less) between up- and down-state [79]. During the up-state cortical cells remain depolarized at waking levels for around a second and fire at waking rates, often in the gamma range [80]. However, the up-state of NREM sleep is not stable as in wakefulness and REM sleep, but it is inherently bistable. The longer neurons remain depolarized, the more likely they become to precipitate into a hyperpolarized down-state – a complete cessation of synaptic activity that can last for a tenth of a second or more – after which they revert to another up-state. The transition from up- to down-state appears to be due to depolarization-dependent potassium currents and to short-term synaptic depression, both of which increase with the amount of prior activation [81]. The slow oscillation is found in virtually every cortical neuron, and is synchronized across the cortical mantle by cortico-cortical connections, which is why the EEG records high-voltage, low-frequency waves.

An intriguing possibility is that changes in the level of consciousness during sleep may be related to the degree of bistability of corticothalamic networks, leading to a breakdown of cortical integration – loosely defined as the ability of different cortical regions to talk to each other [82] (Chapter 8). Alternatively, deep sleep may impair consciousness by leading to bistable, stereotypic cortical responses associated with a loss of information [82, 83].

Consider first the loss of integration. In a recent study, TMS was used in conjunction with high-density EEG to record cortical evoked responses to direct stimulation in waking and sleep [83, 84]. During wakefulness, TMS induced a sustained response made of rapidly changing patterns of activity that persisted until 300 ms and involved the sequential activation of specific brain areas, depending on the precise site of stimulation. During early NREM sleep, however, the brain response to TMS changed markedly. When applied to lateral cortical regions, the activity evoked by TMS remained localized to the site of stimulation, without activating connected brain regions, and lasted for less than 150 ms [84]. This finding indicates that during early NREM sleep, when the level of consciousness is reduced, effective connectivity among cortical regions breaks down, implying a corresponding breakdown of cortical integration. Computer simulations suggest that this breakdown of effective connectivity may be due to the induction of a local down-state (S. Esser and G. Tononi, in preparation).

Further experiments with TMS/EEG suggest that deep sleep may be associated with a loss of information even when the brain can produce global responses. When applied over centromedian parietal regions, each TMS pulse triggered a stereotypical response implying the induction of a global down-state: a full-fledged, high-amplitude slow wave [83] that closely resembled spontaneous ones and that travelled through much of the cortex [85]. Such stereotypical responses could be induced even when, for the preceding seconds, there were no slow waves in the spontaneous EEG, indicating that perturbations can reveal the potential bistability of a system irrespective of its observed state. Altogether, these TMS-EEG measurements suggest that the sleeping brain, despite being active and reactive, becomes inherently bistable: it either breaks down in causally independent modules or bursts into a global, stereotypical response. By contrast, during REM sleep late in the night, when dreams become long and vivid and the level of consciousness returns to levels close to those of wakefulness, the responses to TMS also recover and come to resemble more closely those observed during wakefulness: evoked patterns of activity become more complex and spatially differentiated, although some late components are still missing (Tononi and Massimini, unpublished results).

Anesthesia

The most common among exogenous manipulations of the level of consciousness is general anesthesia. Anesthetics come in two main classes: intravenous agents used for induction, such as propofol and ketamine, generally administered together with sedatives such as midazolam and dexmedetomidine; and inhaled agents such as isoflurane, sevoflurane and desflurane, or the gases xenon and nitrous oxide. The doses of inhaled anesthetics are usually referred to their minimum alveolar concentration (MAC): a MAC value of 1 is the dose that prevents movement in 50% of subjects in response to a painful surgical stimulation. At low MAC values (0.1–0.2) anesthetics produce amnesia, first explicit and then implicit. Frequently there are distortions of time perception, such as slowing down and fragmentation, and a feeling of disconnection from the environment. Also, at low MAC values anesthetics produce increasing sleepiness and make arousal progressively more difficult, suggesting that to some extent they can mimic neurophysiological events underlying sleep. At around 0.3 MAC people experience a decrease in the level of consciousness, also described as a 'shrinking' in the field of consciousness, as if they were kept on the verge of falling asleep. MAC-awake, usually around

0.3–0.4 MAC, is the point at which response to verbal command is lost in 50% of patients, and is considered the point at which consciousness is lost (LOC). The transition to unconsciousness (LOC) appears to be rather brusque, not unlike the collapse of muscle tone that usually accompanies it, suggesting that neural processes underlying consciousness change in a non-linear manner. At concentrations above LOC, movements are still possible, especially partially coordinated responses to painful stimuli, suggesting that some degree of 'unconscious' processing is still possible. Complete unresponsiveness is usually obtained just above MAC 1.0.

At the cellular level, many anesthetics have mixed effects, but the overall result is a decrease in neuronal excitability by either increasing inhibition or decreasing excitation. Most anesthetics act by enhancing gamma-amino-butyric-acid (GABA) inhibition or by hyperpolarizing cells through an increase of potassium leak currents. They can also interfere with glutamatergic transmission and antagonize acetylcholine at nicotinic receptors [86, 87]. But what are critical circuits mediating the LOC induced by anesthetics?

A considerable number of neuroimaging studies in humans have recently shed some light on this issue [88]. A common site of action of several anesthetics is posterior cingulate cortex and medial parietal cortical areas, as well as lateral parietal areas [88] (Chapter 10), but so far it is not possible to conclude whether anesthetics produce unconsciousness when they affect a particular set of areas, as opposed to by producing a widespread deactivation of corticothalamic circuits. The most consistent effects produced by most anesthetics at LOC is a reduction of thalamic metabolism and blood flow, suggesting the possibility that the thalamus may serve as a consciousness switch [89]. However, both positron emission tomography (PET) and fMRI signals mostly reflect synaptic activity rather than cellular firing, and the thalamus receives a massive innervation from cortex. Moreover, the relative reduction in thalamic activity occurs on a background of a marked decrease in global metabolism (30–60%) that involves many cortical regions. Thus, thalamic activity as recorded by neuroimaging may represent an especially sensitive, localized readout of the extent of widespread cortical deactivation, rather than the final common pathway of unconsciousness [90]. In fact, spontaneous thalamic firing in animal models of anesthesia is mostly driven by corticothalamic feedback [91], and the metabolic effects of enflurane on the thalamus can be abolished by an ipsilateral cortical ablation [92], suggesting that the switch in thalamic unit activity is driven primarily through a reduction in afferent corticothalamic feedback more than by a direct effect of anesthesia on thalamic neurons. Recently, thalamic activity was recorded using depth electrodes in a patient undergoing anesthesia for the implant of a deep brain stimulator [93]. With either propofol or sevoflurane, when the patient lost consciousness, the cortical EEG changed dramatically. However, there was little change in the thalamic EEG until almost 10 minutes later. This result implies that the deactivation of cortex alone is sufficient for loss of consciousness, and conversely that thalamic activity alone is insufficient to maintain it (see below).

Whatever the ultimate target of anesthetics, loss of consciousness may not necessarily require that neurons in these structures be inactivated. In fact, it may be sufficient that subtler, dynamic aspects of neural activity be affected. As with sleep, some evidence indicates that anesthetic agents may impair consciousness by disrupting cortical integration. Alternatively, anesthetics may impair consciousness by leading to bistable, stereotypic cortical responses associated with a loss of information.

Consider first large-scale integration. Anesthetics are known to slow down neural responses [94–96]. As this effect may not occur uniformly across the cortex, it is likely to disrupt synchronization among distant areas. Indeed, when consciousness fades there is a drop in coherence in the gamma range (usually 20 to 80 Hz) between right and left frontal cortices as well as between frontal and occipital regions [97]. Animal experiments also show that anesthetics suppress fronto-occipital gamma coherence, both under visual stimulation and at rest. The effect is gradual and much stronger for long-range than local coherence [98]. The loss of front-to-back interactions between anterior and posterior regions of the cortex may be especially critical: at anesthetic concentrations leading to unresponsiveness in rats, transfer entropy, which provides a directional measure of information flow, decreases in the front-to-back direction – from frontal to parietal and from frontal or parietal to occipital cortex – when feed-forward transfer entropy is still high [99]. In line with these observations, at hypnotic concentrations the anesthetic desflurane suppresses selectively the late component of neuronal firing (>100 ms), presumably due to reentrant connections, but not the early (~40 ms), feed-forward component, in rat visual cortex (Hudetz, in preparation). Unit recording studies in animals also show that feed-forward responses persist during anesthesia (in fact, that is how they were traditionally investigated), but contextual modulation of firing, associated for instance with attention and presumably mediated by back-connections, are abolished [100–102]. Anesthetic agents may be especially effective at disrupting integration because the corticothalamic system

seems to be organized like a small-world network – mostly local connectivity augmented by comparatively few long-range connections [103]. Thus, anesthetics need only disrupt a few long-range connections to produce a set of disconnected components [104]. Indeed, computer simulations demonstrate a rapid state transition at a critical anesthetic dose [105, 106].

Consider now the information aspect. When the number of differentiated activity patterns that can be produced by the corticothalamic system shrinks, neural activity becomes less informative, even though it may be globally integrated [82]. Several general anesthetics produce a characteristic burst-suppression pattern in which a near-flat EEG is interrupted every few seconds by brief, quasi-periodic bursts of global activation that are remarkably stereotypic. It has now been shown that such stereotypic bursts can also be elicited by visual, auditory, and even micromechanical stimuli [107–110]. Whether evoked or spontaneous, this stereotypic burst-suppression pattern indicates that during deep anesthetic unconsciousness the corticothalamic system can still be active – in fact hyperexcitable – and can produce global, integrated responses. However, the repertoire of responses has shrunk to a stereotypic burst-suppression pattern, with a corresponding loss of information.

Coma and Vegetative States

While consciousness may nearly fade during certain phases of sleep, and be kept at very low levels for a prescribed period during general anesthesia, coma and vegetative states are characterized by a loss of consciousness that is hard or impossible to reverse [111]. Coma – an enduring sleep-like state of immobility with eyes closed from which the patient cannot be aroused – represents the paradigmatic form of pathological loss of consciousness (Chapter 11). Typically, coma is caused by a suppression of corticothalamic function by drugs, toxins, or internal metabolic derangements. Other causes of coma are head trauma, strokes, or hypoxia due to heart failure, which again cause a widespread destruction of corticothalamic circuits. Smaller lesions of the reticular activating system can also cause unconsciousness, presumably by deactivating the corticothalamic system indirectly.

Patients who survive a coma may recover while others enter the so-called vegetative state, in which eyes reopen, giving the appearance of wakefulness, but unresponsiveness persists (Chapter 13). Soon, regular sleep/waking cycles follow. Respiration, other autonomic functions, and brainstem functions are relatively preserved, and stereotypic, reflex-like responses can occur, including yawning and grunting, but no purposeful behaviour. Patients may remain vegetative for a long time, or may emerge to a 'minimally conscious state'. This is distinguished from the vegetative state because of the occasional occurrence of some behaviours that do not appear to be purely reflexive, suggesting that some degree of consciousness may be present.

Postmortem analysis in vegetative patients reveals that the brainstem and hypothalamus, and specifically the reticular activating system, are largely spared, which explains why patients look awake. Usually the vegetative state is due to widespread lesions of grey matter in neocortex and thalamus, to widespread white matter damage and diffuse axonal injury, or to bilateral thalamic lesions, especially of the paramedian thalamic nuclei [111]. Thalamic damage can be secondary to diffuse cortical damage due to retrograde degeneration (just like in metabolic studies of anesthesia, changes in the thalamus are much more concentrated and therefore easier to document that in cortex). However, isolated paramedian thalamic damage can cause persistent unconsciousness. Indeed, recovery from a vegetative state was associated with the restoration of functional connectivity between intralaminar thalamic nuclei and prefrontal and anterior cingulate cortices [112]. A recent study by Niko Schiff *et al.* shows the role of the thalamus even more dramatically: bilateral deep brain electrical stimulation of the central thalamus restored a degree of behavioural responsiveness in a patient who had remained in a minimally conscious state for 6 year following brain trauma [113]. In an older study, a state of akinetic mutism was associated with hypersynchronous spike-and-wave activity in paramedian thalamus. After an induced Phenobarbital coma, seizures activity resolved and the patients began to speak [114].

In vegetative states, brain metabolism is globally reduced by 50% to 60%, most notably in regions such as the posterior cingulate cortex and the precuneus [115, 116]. These are also the areas that reactivate most reliably if a patient regains consciousness. A recent case study reported an extraordinary recovery of verbal communication and motor function in a patient who had remained in a minimally conscious state for 19 years [117]. Diffusion tensor MRI showed increased fractional anisotropy (assumed to reflect myelinated fiber density) in posteromedial cortices, encompassing cuneus, and precuneus. These same areas showed increased glucose metabolism as studied by PET scanning, likely reflecting the neuronal regrowth paralleling the patient's clinical recovery.

This and other neuroimaging studies of vegetative or minimally conscious patients are demonstrating ever more clearly that a purely clinical diagnosis of persistent loss of consciousness may at times be dramatically inaccurate. Several imaging studies have now shown that, even in completely unresponsive patients, as long as significant portions of the corticothalamic system are preserved, cognitive stimuli can induce patterns of activation similar to those seen in healthy subjects [115, 118]. Since stimuli that are not perceived consciously can still activate appropriate brain areas (see below and Chapters 5 and 21), inferring the presence of consciousness may be unwarranted. However, in a recent, thought-provoking study, a clinically vegetative, seemingly unresponsive patient was put in the scanner and asked to imagine playing tennis or navigating through her room. Remarkably, the patient showed fMRI activation patterns of the appropriate cortical regions, exactly like healthy subjects. Obviously, these activations could not be due to unconscious processing of stimuli [119]. Of note, this patient had widespread frontal lesions, while posterior cortex was largely preserved.

Seizures

The abnormal, hypersynchronous discharge of neurons is a frequent cause of short-lasting impairments of consciousness. Consciousness is lost or severely affected in so-called generalized seizures, such as absence and tonic-clonic seizures, and to a lesser extent in complex partial seizures (Chapters 2 and 19). Absence seizures, which are more frequent in children, are momentary lapses of consciousness during which a child stops what she was doing and stares straight ahead blankly. Absence seizures are accompanied by spike-and-wave complexes at around 3 Hz in the EEG, reflecting cycles of synchronous firing and silence of large number of neurons. There is great variability in the degree of unresponsiveness both across subjects and, within the same subject, between seizures. Sometimes, simple behaviours such as repetitive tapping or counting, can proceed unimpaired during the seizures, but more complex tasks come to a halt.

Generalized convulsive seizures usually comprise a tonic phase of muscle stiffening, followed by a clonic phase with jerking of the arms and legs. After the convulsion the person may be lethargic or in a state of confusion for minutes up to hours. During the tonic phase of a convulsive seizure neural activity is greatly increased, as indicated by high-frequency activity in the EEG. The clonic phase is accompanied by synchronous spikes and waves in the EEG, corresponding to millions of neurons alternately firing in strong bursts and turning silent. Loss of consciousness during the tonic phase of generalized seizures is noteworthy because it occurs at times when neuronal activity is extremely high and synchronous.

Partial complex seizures often begin with strange abdominal sensations, fears, premonitions, or automatic gestures. The person progressively loses contact with the environment, exhibits a fixed stare and is unable to respond adequately to questions or commands. Stereotyped, automatic movements are common. Complex partial seizures usually last from 15 seconds to 3 minutes. Seizure activity is usually localized to the medial temporal lobe.

The diagnosis of seizures is made through clinical observation and EEG recordings. In absence and tonic–clonic seizures the scalp EEG shows diffuse abnormalities, suggesting a generalized involvement of brain networks, whereas in partial complex seizures the abnormalities are confined to a medial temporal focus on one side. However, neuroimaging studies using single photon emission computed tomography (SPECT), PET, and fMRI, and depth EEG recordings in humans and animals have revealed that generalized seizures do not affect all brain areas indiscriminately, whereas complex partial seizures alter brain activity less focally than initially thought [120–123]. In fact, it now appears that all seizures causing an impairment of consciousness are associated with changes in activity in three sets of brain areas (Chapters 2 and 19), namely: (i) increased activity in the upper brainstem and medial thalamus; (ii) decreased activity in the anterior and posterior cingulate, medial frontal cortex, and precuneus; (iii) altered activity in the lateral and orbital frontal cortex and in the lateral parietal cortex. In tonic–clonic seizures, fronto-parietal association areas show increased activity, while the pattern is more complex and variable in absence seizures, though parietal areas are usually deactivated. Complex partial seizures show decreased activity in frontal and parietal association cortex, which is associated with the onset of slow waves similar to those of sleep or anesthesia (rather than to epileptiform discharges).

At this stage, it is not clear which of these three sets of areas, alone or in combination, are crucial for the loss of consciousness. However, two things are clear: first, the areas involved in the loss of consciousness associated with seizures correspond to those affected in sleep, anesthesia, and the vegetative state, pointing to a common substrate for the most common forms of loss of consciousness; second, especially during the tonic phase of convulsive seizures, it would seem that consciousness is lost when neurons are excessively and synchronously active, rather than inactive. Perhaps, as with the bistable, hypersynchronous transitions between down- and up-states during sleep, and with the hypersynchronous burst-suppression patterns during deep anesthesia, consciousness fades when the repertoire of available neural states shrinks, and with it the information capacity of the system (see below, and [82]).

THE NEUROANATOMY OF CONSCIOUSNESS

Despite the wealth of evidence reviewed in this book, it is still difficult to converge on a circumscribed set of brain structures that are 'minimally sufficient and jointly necessary' for consciousness [124] (Chapter 1). It is also important to keep in mind that, at this stage, we have no idea whether the elementary neural units that contribute to consciousness are local groups of neurons, such as cortical minicolumns, or individual neurons, and perhaps only neurons located in certain layers or belonging to a particular class. What is undisputed, and certainly not new, is that broad lesions or inactivations of the corticothalamic system abolish consciousness, whereas lesions of other parts of the brain do not. Beyond this, it is still difficult to be more precise with a sufficient degree of confidence. Recent developments, however, make it at least possible to ask some pertinent questions and suggest comparisons that may help to sharpen scientific inquiry.

Below, we briefly review, without any pretence at completeness: (i) the evidence that establishes the central role of the corticothalamic system and rules out other areas of the brain; (ii) the role of the thalamus vs. that of the cortex; (iii) that of primary areas vs. higher order visual areas; (iv) the ventral vs. the dorsal stream; (v) fronto-parietal networks vs. the default system; and finally (vi) posterior vs. anterior (prefrontal) cortices.

The Corticothalamic System vs. the Rest of the Brain

As we just mentioned, the only conclusion that can be drawn for sure about the neural substrate of consciousness is that it includes parts of the corticothalamic system. The evidence comes from many different sources, and it constitutes the true bedrock of the neurology of consciousness. Unambiguous examples of persistent vegetative state demonstrate that the loss of consciousness is usually associated with widespread lesions of the grey or white matter of the cortex, and most of the time with a significant thalamic involvement [111].

The evidence is just as persuasive that patients remain conscious after lesions of brain structures outside the corticothalamic system, first among them the spinal cord, which can be severed without affecting consciousness in any direct manner. Brainstem structures (and their hypothalamic extensions) offer a more instructive example: every neurologist knows that if the brainstem is damaged or compressed, coma is likely to ensue – even minor lesions affecting the reticular activating system can produce unconsciousness. However, as demonstrated by patients who awaken from coma and enter the vegetative state, a functioning brainstem is insufficient for consciousness in the absence of a functioning corticothalamic system – there is wakefulness (eyes open), but no experience. Whether the corticothalamic system can resume its function and sustain consciousness if the brainstem reticular activating system is permanently damaged is unclear but, as suggested by the dramatic effects on consciousness of deep cortical stimulation in the median thalamus, the reticular activating system appears to have the role of an on-off switch, rather than of a generator of consciousness. Animal experiments indicate that as long as some activating systems remain, for example both cholinergic and non-cholinergic cells in the basal forebrain [125, 126], consciousness may be possible. Hypothalamic lesions in isolation seem to produce somnolence rather than unconsciousness.

The cerebellum offers another interesting case study. Even widespread cerebellar lesions or ablations hardly affect consciousness, yet the cerebellum has even more neurons that the cerebral cortex, is richly endowed with connections, neurotransmitters and neuromodulators, receives inputs from the sensory periphery, controls motor outputs, contains maps of the body and the outside space, is strongly connected in both directions with thalamus and cortex, and often shows selective activation during cognitive tasks and in relation to emotion [127, 128]. As we shall briefly discuss in a later section, the cerebellum can be usefully contrasted to the corticothalamic complex to evince which aspects of neural organization are important for generating consciousness.

Concerning other brain structures the evidence is more complex. A case has been made for the claustrum as a key structure for consciousness [129]. To this day selective lesions have not been reported, but claustral lesions associated with widespread striatal lesions do not necessarily cause unconsciousness [130]. Selective, bilateral lesions of the basal ganglia are rare, although there are cases of selective bilateral necrosis of the striatum and related structures, including the claustrum [130, 131–134], as well as several instances of bilateral pallidotomy for the control of movement disorders [135–137]. Also, a case can be made for a virtual blockade of basal ganglia function in extreme Parkinson's disease and perhaps in catatonic states [138, 142]. Such cases show some

degree of cognitive impairment, but most problems have to do with movement initiation and control, dysphonia progressing to aphonia, dysarthria and finally mutism, and or with the execution of abnormal (athetoid) or automatic movements. Consciousness, however, appears to be preserved – children affected before 3 years of age may not speak but respond to sensory stimuli and communicate with their parents [130]; adults may develop cognitive problems, including a frontal syndrome, but are clearly conscious [134]. However, lesions involving portions of the basal ganglia as well as the anterior cingulate can result in akinetic mutism (see below) or in the 'slow syndrome' [111]. In the latter case, patients are slow and somnolent, but communications is possible. Circuits involving the basal ganglia originate mostly from anterior cortex, the portion of the corticothalamic complex whose necessity for consciousness is more questionable, as discussed below. Thus, despite being an integral component of at least five parallel cortico–subcortico–cortical circuits, the basal ganglia may not contribute directly to consciousness. Rather, basal ganglia (and cerebellar circuits) are thought to play an important role in transforming hard, slow, error-prone sequences of movements that are performed under conscious control, into smooth, fast, and error-free routines that are executed automatically [140–141].

Finally, we have seen above, on the section on memory, that bilateral hippocampal lesions that abolish episodic, autobiographical memory do not abolish consciousness. However, what consciousness remains is less rich – there is a deficit in imagination- and it may be especially constricted in its temporal dimension – the duration of the conscious present (see Chapter 24).

Cortex vs. Thalamus

The thalamus is sometimes considered as a seventh layer of cortex, so contrasting its role with that of the cortex proper may be a useless enterprise. Nevertheless, it has been suggested that the thalamus, and especially the intralaminar nuclei, may constitute a 'centrencephalic system' where consciousness resides [142]. Very few patients in a persistent vegetative state or minimally conscious state have circumscribed brain lesions. As we have seen however, those who do often have bilateral damage in a region including paramedian thalamic nuclei [111], though such lesions usually include neighbouring fiber tracts. Moreover, the restoration of functional connectivity between paramedian thalamus and cingulate cortices is an early sign of recovery from the vegetative state [112], and bilateral deep brain electrical stimulation of the central thalamus restored behavioural responsiveness in a patient who had remained in a minimally conscious state for 6 years [113]. In animals, acute thalamic manipulations can have major effects. For example, an infusion of GABA agonists (mimicking anesthetic action) into central medial intralaminar nuclei causes animals to fall 'asleep' and the EEG to slow down [143, 147]. Conversely, rats kept under an anesthetic concentration of sevoflurane can be awakened by a minute injection of nicotine in the same area [145]. Perhaps, then, the thalamus plays a special role in generating consciousness.

Alternatively, the role of the thalamus may be indirect, by facilitating cortico–cortical interactions. For instance, consistent with the role of the thalamus as a seventh layer of cortex, efficient communication between cortical areas might requires a thalamic relay [146–148] (but see [149, 150]): in that case thalamic lesions would lead to a functional disconnection despite an activated cortex. The anatomy is consistent with such a role: -positive matrix cells, which are especially concentrated within some of the intralaminar thalamic nuclei [150, 151], project diffusely to many areas of the cortex, where they provide a more superficial innervations (layers I, II, and upper III). Also, matrix cells receive collaterals mostly from cortical cells in layer V, which in turn have much wider intracortical collaterals than layer VI cells, (and are especially sensitive to anesthetics). Cells within intralaminar thalamic nuclei are capable of firing in the gamma range and can provide NDMA receptor activation, subthreshold depolarization and coherent oscillatory bias to distant cortical areas [152], thereby potentially facilitating long range interactions. Also, intralaminar nuclei are ideally poised to work as an anatomical hub connecting many cortical regions [153], and are a prominent target of inputs from the reticular activating system of the brainstem. For these reasons, matrix cells can be conceptualized as a veritable thalamic activating system capable of facilitating effective interactions among many cortical areas and thereby of sustaining consciousness.

On the other hand, other evidence suggests a closer link between cortex and consciousness, whether or not the thalamus is involved. As we have seen above, when a patient with depth electrodes in the thalamus was anesthetized, the cortical EEG changed dramatically the instant the patient lost consciousness, but the thalamic EEG remained unchanged until almost 10 minutes later [93]. A complementary result is provided by another study in epileptic patient: during REM sleep – a state usually associated with dreaming – the cortical EEG was duly activated, but the thalamic EEG in the medial pulvinar nucleus showed slow wave activity [154]. Though only a small portion of

the thalamus was recorded in these studies, it would seem that deactivating cortex is sufficient for losing consciousness, whereas thalamic activation may not be necessary for maintaining it. Indeed, it was reported long ago that, following a complete ablation of the thalamus, the cortex can still produce an activated EEG [155, 156]. A more effective consciousness switch may be located in the basal forebrain, as long as both cholinergic and noncholinergic cells are targeted [125]. For example, brainstem stimulation that produces an arousal reaction and the activation of the EEG [157] becomes ineffective when the local anesthetic lidocaine is injected into the basal forebrain, but not so much when it is injected into the thalamus.

Primary Areas vs. Higher Order Areas

Since the suggestion by Crick and Koch that primary visual cortex may not be part of the 'neural correlate of consciousness ' [158], a remarkable amount of refined neuroscience has attempted to settle the question whether this brain area is 'in' or 'out.' That is, does primary visual cortex contribute directly to visual consciousness, or only indirectly – a sort of larger, higher-up retina? Consider retinal neurons. Though they certainly rely information to all parts of the visual system, and their activity usually determines what we see when we open our eyes, they do not seem to contribute directly to conscious experience. For example, their rapidly shifting firing patterns do not correspond well with what we perceive, which is much more stable. Moreover, during blinks and eye movements retinal activity changes dramatically, but visual perception does not. Also, the retina has a blind spot at the exit of the optic nerve where there are no photoreceptors, and it has low spatial resolution and no color sensitivity at the periphery of the visual field, but we are not aware of any of this. More importantly, lesioning the retina does not prevent conscious visual experiences. As we have seen, a person who becomes retinally blind as an adult continues to have vivid visual images and dreams. Conversely, stimulating the retina during sleep by keeping the eyes open and presenting various visual inputs does not yield any visual experience and does not affect visual dreams.

What is the situation with primary visual cortex? Psychophysical experiments indicate that several stimuli known to affect the activity of V1 neurons have no perceptual counterpart [95, 159, 160]. Also, single neuron recordings from the monkey, using paradigms such as binocular rivalry, find that activity in V1 tends to follow the physical stimulus, rather than the percept, unlike neurons higher up in the visual hierarchy [161–163]. On the other hand, a number of fMRI BOLD studies have found that activity in human V1, and even in the lateral geniculate nucleus (LGN), was correlated with perception (Chapter 5) [164–166]. Perhaps the reason for the discrepancy has to do with how well one controls for attention, which is often tightly bound with perception and is known to activate V1 [23] (Chapter 6). Indeed, a recent study employing a dual-task paradigm has shown that, once attention is accounted for, there is no residual correlation of V1 hemodynamic activity with perception [167]. Similarly, V1 fMRI signals associated with unperceived line drawings were modulated by visual attention [28]. Finally, it is possible to decode from V1 BOLD activity the orientation of a masked stimulus, even though subjects could not guess its orientation [168].

Additional evidence against a direct contribution of not only V1 but other primary sensory cortices comes from studies of sensory stimulation during slow wave sleep (Chapter 8) and in vegetative patients (Chapter 3). Using evoked responses or neuroimaging, these studies show the localized activation of primary areas in the absence of any indication of consciousness. However, it should be remembered that areas higher up in the cortical hierarchy, often considered to be contributing to experience, can also be activated, at least at the fMRI level, in the absence of conscious perception, as shown by studies of backward masking [169], inattention [170, 171], and neglect [172]. Perhaps in some of these instances the activation that reaches higher areas is merely insufficient, for instance in masking. Alternatively, the fMRI signal may be strong, as in inattention and neglect, but it may lack some other features that would only be evident with units recordings, such as fast oscillations or synchronization with other areas, or it may be that higher areas must respond to inputs from lower areas for their activation to contribute to consciousness. Finally, less is known about the possible contribution to consciousness of other primary cortices such as motor cortex. However, some evidence exists to show, for example, that masked visual stimuli can elicit motor cortex activation and increase its excitability as probed with TMS, and yet remain unperceived. Of course, demonstrating that activation or changes in excitability in primary cortices do not translate in reportable changes in experience does not prove that no activation pattern would be able to elicit experience – just think of the fact that even high intensity TMS or direct electrical stimulation usually fail to affect consciousness, no matter what brain area is the target, with only a few exceptions [173].

Current evidence thus seems to support the hypothesis that V1 does not contribute directly to visual experience. However, it is hard to say whether this applies to all visual attributes, such as precise topography, detailed contours, or luminosity, as has been argued by some [174, 175]. Also, lesions of primary visual cortex lead to the striking phenomenon of 'blindsight,' in which patients claim to have no conscious perception of stimuli, though they perform better than chance on forced-choice tasks where they are asked to detect stimuli, locate them, decide on their orientation and direction of motion [176] (see also Chapter 21). Compelling evidence supports the idea that blindsight is subserved by subcortical visual pathways that originate from the superior colliculus and bypass primary visual cortex. The subjective blindness of blindsight patients may perhaps be explained purely in terms of insufficient feedforward activation of higher visual areas, denying any direct role to V1 *per se* in generating experience. But it is hard to be sure: would the activation of extrastriate cortex, in the absence of a functional V1, be sufficient for visual experience, and of what kind? Some experiments using TMS in both blindsight patients and healthy subjects [177–179] leave at least the door open for a more direct contribution by V1.

Ventral vs. Dorsal Stream

Based on previous work indicating a subdivision between a ventral and a dorsal visual stream diverging from primary visual cortex, a case has been made for distinguishing between a ventral stream for perception and a dorsal stream for action [180, 181]. The ventral stream includes a number of areas in ventral temporal and lateral occipital cortex (the lateral occipital complex); the dorsal stream includes areas V3A, V5, V7 and intraparietal areas in the posterior parietal cortex. According to the initial account [180], which was subsequently refined [181], activity in the ventral stream gives rise to conscious experience, extracting invariant features that subserve object identification, as well as the relationships among objects within the context of a visual scene. This system would allow us to construct a lasting representation of the word, categorize objects and events, talk about them, form explicit memories, and plan long-term actions. By contrast, the dorsal stream deals with the moment-to-moment information about the precise size, shape, location, and disposition of objects for the rapid visual control of skilled actions, such as tracking, reaching, and grasping the object. It has little memory and its activity remains unconscious. There is in fact neurological evidence for a double dissociation between the two systems: some patients with ventral stream lesions have a 'visual object agnosia' in which they lack the conscious experience of the shape of objects, but can unconsciously adapt the reaching and grasping to the unperceived object just as well as healthy controls. Other patients with dorsal stream lesions have an 'optic ataxia' in which they perceive the objects but cannot execute the appropriate skilled movements (see also Chapter 21). Some visual illusions can also be used to show a dissociation between the two systems. One sees here the another aspect of the dichotomy between the slow, consciously controlled actions when first learning a new skill, and the rapid, effortless executed skill after it has been learned: in the first case, the brain calls on a large and diverse amount of information, specifying a wide context, whereas in the latter case it employs only the minimum amount of information that is required to execute the movement at hand.

Recently, however, it was shown that areas in the dorsal stream respond not only to the location of objects but also to their identity, and that hierarchically higher intraparietal areas in the dorsal stream do so in a viewpoint- and size-invariant manner, just as ventral areas do [182], and as required by perceptual constancies that are characteristic of conscious experience. These selective, invariant responses to objects could be elicited irrespective of any requirement for action, and were not due to attentional confounds. As we have seen, areas in posterior parietal cortex implement a detailed map of space, so both spatial and object information are available in close proximity. Indeed, given that visual objects can activate ventral areas in neglect syndromes and inattentional blindness without giving rise to conscious experience, one wonders which set of object-selective areas is more important for experience.

Posterior vs. Anterior (Prefrontal) Cortex

Lesion studies support the notion that consciousness does not require prefrontal cortex and, by inference, the functions it performs. Early studies showed that large, bilateral prefrontal resections did not abolish consciousness. For instance, Hebb reported that removal of large portions of the frontal cortex had little effect on intelligence: Penfield had resected one-third or more of each frontal lobe of patient K.P. to eliminate epileptic foci, yet K.P. showed 'a striking postoperative improvement in personality and intellectual capacity' [183]. Psychosurgery led to the widespread adoption of prefrontal lobotomy and leucotomy, in which prefrontal cortex was deafferented from its thalamic inputs, again with no major

impairment of consciousness [184, 185] (with the exception of anterior cingulotomy, which could result in akinetic mutism, see below). A number of psychiatric patients also underwent the bilateral resection of prefrontal cortical areas, either in isolation or in combination, according to Brodmann's atlas ('topectomy') [186]. Yet even patients receiving a bilateral resection of, say, areas 10, 11, 45–47, or 8–10, or 44–46,10, or area 24 (ventral anterior cingulate), showed no gross behavioural change and certainly maintained consciousness. Some received both topectomy and lobotomy, again with no gross effects on consciousness.

Patients with widespread, bilateral damage to prefrontal cortex remain rare, but two recent clinical studies provide additional, intriguing evidence. A young man who had fallen on an iron spike that completely penetrated through both of his frontal lobes, nevertheless went on to live a stable family life – marrying and raising two children – in an appropriate professional and social setting. Although displaying many of the typical frontal lobe behavioural disturbances, he never complained of loss of sensory perception nor did he show visual or other deficits [187]. Another case is that of a young woman with massive bilateral prefrontal damage of unclear aetiology [188]. While manifesting grossly deficient scores in frontal lobe tests, she showed no abnormal perceptual abilities, and there was no issue whether she was conscious (that is not to say that such patients do not suffer from subtle visual deficits [189]).

The evidence is more ambiguous with medial prefrontal lesions, especially those involving anterior cingulate cortex and supplementary motor areas, often due to ruptured aneurysms of the anterior communicating artery. The presentation of such patients has been described as *akinetic mutism* [190], which is usually categorized as a variant of minimally conscious states (Chapter 14, [191]). Although the term akinetic mutism has been sometimes used to denote different clinical conditions having different pathology (e.g., the so-called slow syndrome), the classic presentation is that of a patient who lies indeed immobile and mute, but gives the impression of hypervigilance, following actions and objects with conjugated eye movements. However, it is generally impossible to elicit any responses, establish contact (though in some patients, occasionally, monosyllabic answers are reported), and there is no spontaneous purposive activity. In a few cases, clinicians have the impression that such patients may understand what is going on (which is why they are considered to be mute rather than vegetative), implying that consciousness is present (though possibly impaired), but not evidenced in behaviour due to a complete lack of motivation or block of executive function (as opposed to paralysis, as in the locked-in syndrome, Chapter 15). Others instead consider such patients as essentially unconscious. The interpretation is complicated by the fact that, in the rare instance in which such patients recover, there is usually amnesia for the akinetic episode, as in the original case of Cairns, though one patient who eventually recovered reported that she remembered the questions posed by the doctor but did not see a reason to respond (Laureys, personal communication). Cases in which the syndrome resolves through dopaminergic therapy, as well as acute akinesia in Parkinsonism, are also difficult to interpret, and may or may not resemble classic akinetic mutism from a functional point of view. Perhaps the most intriguing results have been obtained in such patients by using event-related potentials. Such studies have shown that, while several aspects of the EEG responses may be altered, there can be a differential response to semantically meaningful stimuli, for example in oddball paradigms [192–194]. Similar findings have been obtained in a number of vegetative patients, usually when the background EEG contained frequencies above 4 Hz. Though these preserved responses are hard to interpret, they support the possibility that at least some degree of consciousness may be preserved after medial anterior lesions and possibly also in other instances of clinical unresponsiveness.

Contrast these examples of widespread anterior damage with patients with bilateral posterior damage resulting in a syndrome of *hyperkinetic mutism* [191, 195–197]: such patients are engaged in a whirlwind of motor activity, coordinated but without purpose. There is no indication that they have any awareness of self or environment (and of course they do not speak). An extreme case was described by Niko Schiff *et al.* ([198], Patient 1). The patient exhibited continuous, spontaneous, non-directed choreiform movements of head, body, and extremities when awake. He was mute and his movements had no relationship to visual, auditory, or tactile stimuli. A PET study showed a profound hypometabolism of posterior forebrain regions, whereas anterior, cortico-striato-pallido–thalamo–cortical circuits showed comparatively high metabolism. Is there any experience left in such patients? Is a self-despairing in complete nothingness, experiencing thoughts of action with no object? Or is this condition associated with a complete disappearance of the world and the self, and thus of consciousness? Intriguingly, a late posterior positivity having a parietal peak is the event-related potential component that is most reliably impaired in states of seeming unconsciousness, and which distinguishes best between consciously detected vs. undetected stimuli [193].

Altogether, at present it would seem that consciousness abides mostly in the back of the corticothalamic complex (though maybe not in the very back), rather than in the front, and that the front may not be strictly required for experience to be present. Also, there is no doubt that the bulk of experience is sensory, and as such resides in posterior cortex. As we have seen, neuroimaging experiments do some justice to this view, showing that prefrontal cortex is deactivated when self-reflection is abolished by task demand, but experience is vividly present [16]. However, that anterior cortex may not be necessary for consciousness does not entail that it does not contribute directly to it in any aspect [199]. After all, being self-conscious (reflecting upon what one perceives) is different from being conscious (perceiving it), yet both are experiences. Perhaps feelings of thought, reflection, effort, will, emotion and so on are generated by anterior cortex, though no firm evidence exists. Also, premotor cortex may contribute to specific aspects of consciousness, such as the awareness of movement [200] and the feeling of agency [201]. Alternatively, prefrontal cortex may provide unconscious plans, strategies, skills and memories, as well as attention. If this were the case, we would need to know what is wrong with this large portion of the cortex. Is it wired in radically different way from posterior cortex? Is it broken up into segregated loops encompassing the basal ganglia? At the very least, the study of the contribution of anterior cortical areas to consciousness is one of the ripest areas for future investigations.

Lateral Fronto-Parietal Network vs. (Medial) Default System

An orthogonal way of slicing the cortical cake is to distinguish between the relative contribution to consciousness of lateral vs. mesial regions. In fact, there is increasing evidence for the existence of two corticothalamic networks usually characterized by antagonistic activation patterns in fMRI studies [202–204] (Chapter 7). One is a lateral 'attention' network, the other a predominantly mesial 'default' system. The lateral attention network is further subdivided into a dorsal and a ventral attentional system [205]. The dorsal system is bilateral and composed of the intraparietal sulcus and frontal eye field at the junction of the precentral and superior frontal sulcus. It is involved in voluntary (top-down) orienting and shows activity increases after presentation of cues indicating where, when, or to what subjects should direct their attention. The ventral system is right-lateralized and composed of the right temporal-parietal junction and the right ventral frontal cortex. This system shows activity increases upon detection of salient targets and after abrupt changes in sensory stimuli. The dorsal and ventral lateral attentional systems also appear in functional connectivity maps during spontaneous activity, and their function can be coordinated by other prefrontal regions [206]. Not surprisingly, since attention and consciousness often go together, many neuroimaging studies show an activation of this lateral network, usually with the addition of anterior cingulate areas, in paradigms contrasting perceived vs. unperceived stimuli [19, 207] (Chapter 5). For instance, these regions are more active for unmasked vs. masked words and images; detected vs. undetected changes during change blindness; reported vs. missed stimuli during the attentional blink, seen vs. extinguished stimuli in neglect patients.

The 'default' network [202, 203] includes primarily medial cortical areas such as the medial prefrontal cortex, the posterior cingulate cortex, and the precuneus. However, it also includes a lateral parietal component posterior to the intraparietal sulcus. The default network was identified because it typically shows decreased activity when subjects perform cognitive tasks. In resting functional connectivity studies, regions of the default network show strong positive correlations among themselves, presumably due to the high density of anatomical connections [203]. Posteromedial cortex appears to be a particularly important area of the brain, since it happens to have higher levels of baseline energy consumption (the precuneus) than the rest of the cortex (see Chapter 1). Nevertheless, the functional role of posteromedial cortex is only partially understood, as selective, bilateral lesions of these areas are hardly ever reported. Therefore, evidence comes mostly from neuroimaging studies and transient, incomplete disruption through TMS. Regions within posteromedial cortex, especially the precuneus, are activated during visuo-spatial imagery, retrieval of episodic memories, spontaneous thought, and during tasks that refer to the self and require a first-person perspective [208]. While these studies suggest a role in conscious processes focusing on internal signals rather than on external ones, other studies point to a more direct relevance to consciousness *per se*. Activity in posteromedial areas is altered during generalized seizures, and a strong deactivation is observed in hypnosis, sleep, general anesthesia with both propofol and inhalation agents, and in the vegetative state. As we have seen, recovery of function in posteromedial cortex and reestablishment of functional connectivity with thalamus and frontal cortex are among the early signs of recovery of consciousness. However, it should be noted that posteromedial cortex appear to be deactivated to a similar extent in both NREM and REM sleep [5, 6, 78]. Given that REM sleep

is usually associated with vivid dreams, it is questionable whether the activation of posteromedial cortex is necessary for consciousness *per se* or rather for certain aspects of self-consciousness and related cognitive activities. For instance, at intermediate doses certain anesthetics such as xenon produces a selective deactivation of posterior mesial cortex, yet subjects report depersonalization and out-of-body experiences, rather than unconsciousness. Moreover, a patient with bilateral hypometabolism in the precuneus and superior temporal lobe, as well as in right posterior cingulate gyrus, was demented and psychotic, with delusions and hallucinations, but evidently conscious [209] (but see [210] and Chapter 1, for the view that posteromedial lesions may compromise consciousness).

Despite the temptation to assign consciousness to either the lateral or medial component given their task-on vs. task off activation pattern, and their anticorrelated functional connectivity, there are reasons to wonder whether these two subdivisions may actually be jointly involved in generating experience. For example, the anticorrelated functional connectivity emerges only after regressing out a large, correlated component [211]. Moreover, there is evidence that both medial and lateral areas may be part of a larger, anatomically defined 'structural core'. Recently, the application of graph-theoretical methods to diffusion spectrum imaging of fiber tracts in humans has revealed the existence of a structural core of heavily interconnected cortical regions [212]. This core is centred on a prominent medial 'backbone' that includes the posterior cingulate cortex, the precuneus, the cuneus, as well as the paracentral lobule, and the isthmus of the cingulate (retrosplenial) cortex. The structural core thus overlaps in part with the 'default network,' although the medial prefrontal cortex is conspicuously absent. There is, however, an important lateral component of this structural core, which includes the bank of the superior temporal sulcus, the temporo–parieto–occipital junction, and the inferior and superior parietal cortex. Thus, the structural core also includes the posterior portion of the lateral attentional system. The structural core extends symmetrically to both hemispheres, and all its constituent areas have strong bilateral connections to associative (non-primary) nuclei of the thalamus, as well as to diffusely projecting thalamic cells.

Neuroimaging studies also point to a joint involvement of both lateral and medial regions: in vegetative patients, minimally conscious patients, seizures associated with alterations of consciousness, general anesthesia, and sleeping subjects, there is a remarkably similar set of regions that are deactivated compared to control conditions: these include both the lateral fronto-parietal network and medial regions such as medial prefrontal cortex and precuneus. Another interesting case is that of a man emerging from a minimally conscious state (due to diffuse axonal injury) after the administration of the GABA agonist zolpidem [213, 214]. In this case, blood flow as measured by SPECT increased by almost 40% bilaterally in medial frontal cortex as well as in lateral areas such as middle frontal and supramarginal gyri. So perhaps both the medial and lateral contingents are important. Given the evidence just reviewed that posterior cortex is more important than anterior cortex reviewed in the previous section, it may be that a *posterior complex of associative areas* comprising the lateral temporo–parieto–occipital junction and perhaps a posteromesial backbone currently represents the safest bet as to the brain regions that are most likely to be necessary for the bulk of conscious experience. Alternatively, consciousness may depend on a more circumscribed set of associative cortical areas, such as those lesioned in hyperkinetic mutism, but when consciousness is gone, naturally attention, self-monitoring and similar function also collapse, as reflected in a more generalized pattern of deactivation.

Left vs. Right Hemisphere

Finally, one should consider the most traditional of dichotomies: the one between the left and the right brain. As discussed by Gazzaniga and Miller (Chapter 20), the evidence from split-brain patients, and even more so the results of right hemispherectomy operations, show beyond any doubt that the isolated left hemisphere, whether alone or disconnected from the right hemisphere, can support a conscious self that is similar to that supported by of an intact, fully equipped brain. Importantly, after a hemispherectomy or split-brain operation, the patient (speaking through the left hemisphere) is anosognosic and feels in no way changed, although for example the left half of the visual field is no longer available.

People familiar with split-brain patients have little doubt that the isolated right hemisphere can support a second consciousness (Chapter 20). Long-term observations make it clear that the disconnected right hemisphere not only has its own private sensory and motor channels with which it can communicate with the environment, but it has its specific perceptual skills, can have a word lexicon, has its own memories and may even have its own characteristic preferences and dislikes. After spending some time testing split-brain patients, examiners spontaneously refer to the two hemispheres as if they were distinct people.

Naturally enough, being limited in language and reasoning skills, under usual circumstances the right hemisphere is literally dominated by the left hemisphere – it is usually passive, and does not complain or cause trouble, just as in some highly asymmetric marriages. Also, its cognitive style seems to be very different. As we have seen, it is much more literal in its recognition of images and events, and thereby often more accurate, in contrast with a left hemisphere that is constantly formulating hypotheses and trying to make sense of what happens. Also, in some tests the right hemisphere's cognitive style is strangely 'un-human'. For example, in a guessing game in which a stimulus is red say 75% of the time, and green 25% of the time, and the occurrence of stimuli is entirely at random, humans respond by trying to match the probability of red and green, thereby making many mistakes. By contrast, animals such as rats and goldfish respond red all the time, and in this way maximize their success rate. In such a game, the left hemisphere behaves just like a human, probably because it is a characteristic human feature to try and find a pattern even in random events. The right hemisphere, by contrast, behaves just like a rat or a goldfish would. Michael Gazzaniga has also shown that the right hemisphere fails in certain simple reasoning and classification tasks that are solved both by 12-month-old children as well as by monkeys.

On the other hand, the extraordinary patient P.S., studied by Joseph Ledoux and Michael Gazzaniga, who had a remarkable ability to comprehend words with the right hemisphere, and went on to develop a limited ability to speak through it, leaves little doubt that the right hemisphere can at times even have an individual sense of self. The rare cases of left hemispherectomy in right-handed adolescents also indicate that the right hemisphere can sustain a consciousness and a self, although when the right hemisphere is left alone after the operation it is certain to undergo a variety of plastic changes that may partly modify its original functioning. It seems inconceivable, however, that consciousness would return in a left hemispherectomized patient only when and to the extent that language is recovering – it is much more plausible that consciousness and self are already there, and it is just language skills that are being added, just as in a recovering aphasic patient (see above).

Despite the remarkable evidence that the disconnected right hemisphere has its own conscious experience and perhaps at times even its own self, it is worth considering the alternative possibility that the isolated right hemisphere may actually be just an unconscious 'zombie'. Could it be that its responses are not dissimilar from those provided by a patient with blindsight? Or by the 'unconscious action system' of Miller and Goodale? Several considerations cast doubt on this possibility. Unlike blindsight patients, the isolated right hemisphere does not respond just in forced-choice tests, but can exhibit spontaneous choices. It is capable not just of adjusting behaviour for action, but can master perceptual tasks that are impossible for patients with temporal lesions that lack explicit object recognition. It can do much more than just 'automatic routines', and can initiate purposeful behaviours if properly asked. It is far more lucid that a sleepwalker or a patient with a partial complex seizure. Finally, the isolated right hemisphere can even express individual preference and goals, and recognize a picture of itself (although less easily than the left hemisphere). Thus, the kind of consciousness associated with the isolated right hemisphere could be comparable, and in some cases more sophisticated, with that of other primates lacking language.

THE NEUROPHYSIOLOGY OF CONSCIOUSNESS

The studies discussed above indicate that, even within the cerebral cortex, changes in neural activity do not necessarily correlate with changes in conscious experience. Also, we saw earlier that most of the cortex is active during early NREM sleep and anesthesia, not to mention during generalized seizures, but subjects have little conscious content to report. Thus, it is natural to suggest that some additional dynamic feature of neural activity must be present to generate conscious content. Here we consider the role of: (i) sustained vs. phasic activity; (ii) reentrant vs. feed-forward activity; and (iii) synchronous or oscillatory activity.

Sustained vs. Phasic Activity

A plausible idea is that neural activity may contribute to consciousness only if it is sustained for a minimum period of time, perhaps around a few hundred milliseconds. At the phenomenological level, there is no doubt that the 'now' of experience unfolds at a time scale comprised between tens and several hundred milliseconds [215], and in some aspects may even stretch to 1 or 2 seconds [216]. Other experiments have made use of the attentional blink phenomenon: when an observer detects a target in a rapid stream of visual stimuli, there is a brief period of time during which the detection of subsequent targets is impaired. Remarkably, targets that directly follow the first target are less impaired than those that follow after 200–400 ms [217]. By manipulating attention, identical visual stimuli can be made conscious

or unconscious. In such studies, event-related potentials reflecting early sensory processing (the P1 and N1 components) were identical for seen and unseen stimuli, but quickly diverged around 270 ms, suggesting that stimuli only become visible when a sustained wave of activation spreads through a distributed network of cortical association areas [171, 218].

More generally, the requirement for sustained discharge might account for why fast, reflex responses of the kind mediated by, say, the spinal cord, do not seem to contribute to consciousness. Fast, reflex-like responses also take place in the cerebral cortex. For example, the action-oriented dorsal visual stream rapidly adjusts movements that remain outside of consciousness [181]. Perhaps these reflex-like adjustments to fast-changing aspects of the environment that must be tracked on-line are incompatible with the development of sustained discharge patterns. By contrast, such sustained patterns may be necessary for the ventral stream to build a stable representation of a visual scene. By the same token, if the ventral stream could be forced to behave in a reflex-like manner, it should cease to be part of the neural substrate of consciousness. Indeed, this can be achieved by pushing the ventral system to perform ultra-rapid categorizations such as deciding whether a natural image contains an animal or not [219–221]. In such cases, a sweep of activity travels from the retina through several stages of feed-forward connections along the hierarchy of ventral visual areas, until it elicits an appropriate categorization response. This process takes as little as 150 ms, which leaves only about 10 ms of processing per stage. Thus, only a few spikes can be fired before the next stage produces its output, yet they are sufficient to specify selective responses for orientation, motion, depth, color, shape, and even animals, faces, or places, conveying most of the relevant information about the stimulus [222]. While this fast feed-forward sweep within the ventral system is sufficient for the near-automatic categorization of stimuli and a behavioural response, it seems insufficient to generate a conscious percept [223]. For example, if another image (the mask) is flashed soon after the target image, subjects are still able to categorize the target, though they may deny having seen it consciously. Thus, consciousness would seem to require that neural activity in appropriate brain structures lasts for a minimum amount of time, perhaps as much as is needed to guarantee interactions among multiple areas.

On the other hand, other data would seem to suggest that it may actually be the phasic, onset- or offset discharge of neurons that correlates with experience. The most stringent data come again from studies of visual masking (for a review see [224]). To be effective, masking stimuli must either precede (forward masking) or follow (backward masking) target stimuli at appropriate time intervals, and usually need to be spatially contiguous. Macknik, Martinez-Conde and collaborators showed, using a combination of psychophysics, unit recordings in animals, and neuroimaging in humans, that for simple, unattended target stimuli, masking stimuli suppress visibility if their 'spatiotemporal edges' overlap with the spatiotemporal edges of the targets, that is, if they begin or end when target stimuli begin or end, in space and time. They confirmed that such spatiotemporal edges correspond to transient bursts of spikes in primary visual cortex. If these bursts are inhibited, for example if the offset discharge elicited by the target stimulus is obliterated by the onset of the mask, the target becomes invisible. Most likely, these spatiotemporal edges of increased firing are both generated (target stimuli) and suppressed (masking stimuli) by mechanisms of lateral inhibition, which are ubiquitous in sensory systems [224].

Additional evidence for the importance of phasic, transient activation of neurons in determining the visibility of stimuli comes from studies of microsaccades – the small, involuntary movements that our eyes make continually [225]. If microsaccades are counteracted by image stabilization on the retina, stationary objects fade and become completely invisible. In a recent study [226], subjects were asked to fixate a central dot (which tends to reduce microsaccades) while attending to a surrounding circle. Soon, the circle fades and merges into the background (the Troxler illusion). It was found that before a fading period, the probability, rate, and magnitude of microsaccades decreased. Before transitions toward visibility, the probability, rate, and magnitude of microsaccades increased, compatible with the hypothesis that microsaccades are indeed necessary for visibility. Importantly, in macaque monkeys, when an optimally oriented line was centred over the receptive field of cells in V1, the cell's activity increased after microsaccades, and tended to emit bursts [227], suggesting again that phasic activity may be crucial for visibility.

One should remember, however, that the importance of phasic discharges for stimulus awareness has only been demonstrated for early visual cortex but, as we saw above, the neural substrate of consciousness is more likely to lie elsewhere. Psychophysically, masking is similarly effective when masking stimuli are presented monoptically (through the same eye as the target) and dichoptically (through the other eye). The analysis of fMRI data in humans show that a correlate of monoptic visual masking can be found in all retinotopic visual areas, whereas dichoptic masking is only seen in retinotopic areas downstream of V2 within the occipital lobe [228], suggesting an anatomical lower bound for the neural substrate of consciousness. Thus, it could be that phasic onset- and offset discharges are important not in and of themselves, but because they are particularly effective in activating downstream areas that directly support consciousness. In these downstream areas, perhaps, consciousness may actually require sustained firing. Indeed, the duration of the activation of face-selective neurons in IT is strongly correlated with the visibility of masked faces [229].

Reentrant vs. Feed-forward Activity

Another possibility is that it is not so much sustained firing that triggers the awareness of a stimulus, but rather the occurrence of a 'reentrant' wave of activity (also described as recurrent, recursive, or reverberant) from higher to lower cortical areas. In this view, when a stimulus evokes a feed-forward sweep of activity, it is not seen consciously, but it becomes so when the feed-forward sweep is joined by a reentrant sweep [102]. This logic could apply both to early sensory areas such as V1 as well as to higher areas such as IT. For example, when face neurons in the fusiform face area are first activated, we would not see a face consciously, although we could turn our eyes towards it or press a button to indicate our unconscious categorization as a face. However, when face-selective neurons receive a backward volley from some higher area, for example frontal cortex, the face would become visible.

This view is based on several considerations. An important one, though rarely confessed, is that a mere sequence of feed-forward processing steps seems far too 'straightforward' and mechanical to offer a substrate for subjective experience. Reentrant processes, by 'closing the loop' between past- and present activity, or between predicted and actual versions of the input, would seem to provide a more fertile substrate for giving rise to reverberations [230], generating emergent properties through cell assemblies [231], implementing hypothesis testing through resonances [232], linking present with past [233, 234], and subject with object [210].

A more concrete reason why reentrant activity is an attractive candidate for the neural substrate of consciousness is that it travels through back-connections, of which the cerebral cortex is extraordinarily rich [235]. In primates, feed-forward connections originate mainly in supragranular layers and terminate in layer 4. Feedback connections instead originate in both superficial and deep layers, and usually terminate outside of layer 4. The sheer abundance of back-connections in sensory regions suggests that they ought to serve some important purpose, and giving rise to a conscious percept might just fit the bill. However, back-connections, and associated reentrant volleys, are just as numerous between V1 and visual thalamus, which is usually denied any direct contribution to awareness. Also, there does not seem to be any lack of back-connections within the dorsal stream. It should be emphasized that the strength and termination pattern of back-connections seem more suited to a modulatory/synchronizing role than to driving their target neurons. For example, the focal inactivation of area 18 can slightly increase or decrease discharge rates of units in area 17, but does not change their feature selectivity for location and orientation [236]. Also, the numerosity of backward connections is a natural consequence of the hierarchical organization of feed-forward ones. For instance, cells in the LGN are not oriented, while cells in area 17 are. To be unbiased, feedback to any one LGN cell should come from area 17 cells of all orientations, which requires many connections; on the other hand, since at any given time only area 17 cells corresponding to a given orientation would be active, feedback effects would not be strong. If they were, properties of area 17 cells, such as orientation selectivity, would be transferred upon LGN cells, which they are not (to a first approximation). Backward signals certainly play a role in sensory function: for instance, they can mediate some extra-classical receptive field effects, provide a natural substrate for both attentional modulation and imagery, and can perhaps dynamically route feed-forward processing according to prior expectations. But are backward signals really critical for consciousness?

The most intriguing data in support of a role for reentrant activity in conscious perception have come from neurophysiological experiments. In awake, monkeys trained to signal whether or not they saw a salient figure on a background, the early, feed-forward response of V1 neurons was the same, no matter whether or not the monkey saw the figure [237]. However, a later response component was suppressed when the monkey did not see the figure. Light anesthesia also eliminated this later component without affecting the initial response. Late components are thought to reflect reentrant volleys from higher areas, although other studies have disputed this claim [238]. The late response component crucial for the visibility of stimuli under backward masking might also be due to a reentrant volley [102]. In this case the timing of maximal backward masking should be independent of target duration, since it would be determined exclusively by the time needed for the early component to travel to higher areas and return to primary visual cortex. Instead, the timing of maximal masking

depends on the timing of target offset, suggesting that the component that is obliterated is a feedforward offset discharge, not a reentrant one [224]. Moreover, the late component can be dissociated from a behavioural response simply by raising the decision criterion [237], and it can occur in the absence of report during change- and inattentional blindness [239]. Perhaps in such cases subjective experience is present but, due to an insufficient involvement of frontal areas, it cannot be reported [30, 240, 241]? But then, by the same token, why should we rule out subjective experience during the feedforward sweep?

Another main source of evidence for a role of reentrant volleys in consciousness comes from experiments using TMS. In an early experiment, Pascual-Leone and Walsh applied TMS to V5 to elicit large, moving phosphenes [170]. They then applied another, subthreshold TMS pulse to a corresponding location in V1. When TMS to V1 was delivered after TMS to V5 (+5 to +45 ms), subjects often did not see the V5 phosphene, and when they saw one, it was not moving. Their interpretation was that disruption of activity in V1 at the time of arrival of a reentrant volley from V5 interferes with the experience of attributes encoded by V5. In a subsequent study [242], it was shown that, when a subthreshold pulse was applied over V5, followed 10–40 ms later by a suprathreshold pulse over V1, subjects reported a V5-like phosphene (large and moving), rather than a V1 phosphene (small and stationary). Their interpretation was that activity in V5 that, on its own, is insufficient to induce a moving percept, can produce such a percept if the level of induced activity in V1 is high enough.

In another study [243], subjects were shown either an oriented bar or a colored patch – stimuli that are processed in visual cortex. If, around 100 ms later, a TMS pulse was applied to V1, the stimulus became perceptually invisible, although on forced-choice subjects could still discriminate orientation or color. This result indicates that, without any overt participation of V1, stimuli can reach extrastriate areas without eliciting a conscious percept, just as in blindsight patients. It also suggests that, since the forward sweep reaches V1 after just 30 or 40 ms, the TMS pulse may abolish the awareness of the stimulus not so much by blocking feedforward transmission, but by interfering with the backward volley (see also [244]). On the other hand, it cannot be ruled out that the TMS pulse may act instead by triggering a cortical–thalamo–cortical volley that interferes with the offset discharge triggered by the stimulus, as may indeed be the case in backward masking.

Yet another study, this time using fMRI, examined the neural correlates of brightness (perceptual lightness) using backward masking. The psychometric visibility function was not correlated with the stimulated portion of V1, but with downstream visual regions, including fusiform cortex, parietal–frontal areas, and with the sectors of V1 responding to the unstimulated surround [168]. Remarkably, visibility was also correlated with the amount of coupling (effective connectivity) between fusiform cortex and the portion of V1 that responded to the surround. Once again, this result could be explained by the activation of reentrant connections, though fMRI cannot distinguish between forward and backward influences.

Synchronization and Oscillations

Another influential idea is that consciousness may require the synchronization, at a fine temporal scale, of large populations of neurons distributed over many cortical areas, in particular via rhythmic discharges in the gamma range (30–70 Hz and beyond) [245] (Chapter 4). The emphasis on synchrony ties well with the common assumption that consciousness requires the 'binding' together of a multitude of attributes within a single experience, as when we see a rich visual scene containing multiple objects and attributes that is nevertheless perceived as a unified whole [246]. According to this view, the neural substrate of such an experience would include two aspects: first, the underlying activation pattern (groups of neurons that have increased their firing rates) would be widely distributed across different areas of the cerebral cortex, each specialized in signalling a different object or attribute within the scene; second, the firing of these activated neurons would be synchronized on a fast time scale to signal their binding into a single percept. In this respect, synchrony seems ideally suited to signal relatedness: for example, in the presence of a red square, some neurons would respond to the presence of a square, while other would respond to the presence of the color red. If they synchronize at a fast time scale, they would indicate to other groups of neurons that there is a red square, 'binding' the two features together [247]. By contrast, signalling relatedness by increased firing rates alone would be more cumbersome and probably slower [246]. Also, fine temporal scale synchrony has the welcome property of disambiguating among multiple objects – if a green cross was present simultaneously with the red square, cross and green neurons would also be active, but false conjunctions would be avoided by precise phase locking [247]. Moreover, computational models predict that, for the same level of firing, synchronous input is more effective on target neurons than asynchronous input [247, 248], and indeed synchrony makes a difference to the outputs to the rest of the brain [249, 250].

Finally, large-scale models predict that synchrony in the gamma range occurs due to the reciprocal connectivity and loops within the corticothalamic system [251, 252], and indeed phase alignment between distant groups of neurons in the gamma range anticipates by a few millisecond increase in gamma-band power [253]. In this respect, oscillatory activity, even when subthreshold, could further facilitate synchronous interactions by biasing neurons to discharge within the same time frame [254].

Experimental evidence concerning the role of synchrony/synchronous oscillations in perceptual operations was initially obtained in primary visual areas of anesthetized animals (for a review see ([255], Chapter 4). For example, in primary visual cortex, neurons have been found that respond to a coherent object by synchronizing their firing in the gamma range. Stimulus-specific, gamma range synchronization is greatly facilitated when the EEG is activated by stimulating the mesencephalic reticular formation [256, 257], by attention [258], and increases for a dominant stimulus under binocular rivalry even though firing rates may not change [259, 260].

Other evidence has come from EEG studies of phase-locking in humans. A recent study compared the neural correlates of words that were consciously perceived with that of masked words that had been processed and semantically decoded but had remained unconscious [261]. The results show that consciously perceived words induced theta oscillations in multiple cortical regions until the test stimulus was presented and a decision reached, while a burst of gamma activity occurred over central and frontal leads just prior and during the presentation of the test stimulus. Importantly, the earliest event distinguishing conscious and unconscious processing was not visible in the power changes of oscillations but in their phase locking. About 180 ms after presentation of stimuli that were consciously perceived, induced gamma oscillations recorded from a large number of regions exhibited precise phase locking both within and across hemispheres for around 100 ms. These results have been interpreted to indicate that a transient event of gamma synchrony resets multiple parallel processes to a common time frame. The global theta rhythm that follows after this trigger event could provide the time frame for allowing a global integration of information provided by sensory inputs and internal sources. Or perhaps beta–gamma synchrony could enable the integration of activity patterns within local cortical areas, while theta synchrony would permit the integration of more globally distributed patterns: the more global the representation, the longer the time scale for the integration of distributed information.

It would be premature to conclude, however, that synchrony in one or another frequency band is necessarily a marker of consciousness. As revealed by an increasing number of EEG, MEG, electrocorticography, and multiunit recordings, cognitive tasks are associated with complex modes of synchronous coupling among populations of neurons that shift rapidly both within and across different frequency bands, within and between areas, and in relation to the timing of the task [253]. It would rather seem that, given the brain's remarkable connectivity, synchrony is an inevitable accompaniment of neural activity, and that it is bound to change just as activity patterns change, depending on the precise experimental conditions. Whether a particular kind of synchrony, for example in the gamma range, is uniquely associated with consciousness, is still unclear. For example, high-beta and gamma synchrony can be found in virtually every brain region investigated, including some that are unlikely to contribute directly to consciousness. Also, it is not yet clear whether synchrony in the gamma range vanishes during early NREM sleep, during anesthesia, or even during seizures. Human studies are still inconsistent on this point, whereas animal studies show a paradoxical increase in gamma synchrony when rats loose the righting reflex (thought to correspond more or less to the loss of consciousness in humans, see [99, 262]). It would seem that there can be synchrony without consciousness, though perhaps not consciousness without synchrony, at least in mammalian brains.

Finally, there are some difficult conceptual problems in characterizing synchrony as an essential ingredient that unifies perceptual states and thereby makes them conscious. While many experiences do indeed involve several different elements and attributes that are 'bound' together into a unified percept, there are many other experiences, equally conscious, that do not seem to require much binding at all: for instance, an experience of pure darkness or of pure blue, or a loud sound that briefly occupies consciousness and has no obvious internal structure – would merely seem to require the strong activation of the relevant neurons, with no need for signalling relatedness to other elements, and thus no need for synchrony. Also, the idea that the neural correlate of a given conscious experience are given by active neurons bound by synchrony discounts the importance of inactive ones: information specifying that particular unified experience must be conveyed both by which neurons are active and which are not, yet for inactive neurons there does not seem to be anything to bind. On the other hand, if most neurons in the cortex were to become active hypersynchronously, as is the case in generalized seizures, they should result in maximal 'binding,' but consciousness vanishes rather than become more vivid.

A THEORETICAL PERSPECTIVE

Progress in neuroscience will hopefully lead to a better understanding of what distinguishes neural structures or processes that are associated with consciousness from those that are not. But even if we come closer to this goal, we still need to understand *why* certain structures and processes have a privileged relationship with subjective experience. For example, why is it that neurons in corticothalamic circuits are essential for conscious experience, whereas cerebellar neurons, despite their huge numbers, are not? And what is wrong with many cortical circuits, including some in V1, that makes them unsuitable to yield subjective experience? Or why is it that consciousness wanes during slow wave sleep early in the night, despite levels of neural firing in the corticothalamic system that are comparable to those in quiet wakefulness? Other questions are even more difficult to address in the absence of a theory. For example, is consciousness present in animals that have a nervous system considerably different from ours? And what about computerized robots or other artefacts that behave intelligently but are organized in a radically different way from human brains?

Consciousness as Integrated Information

It would seem that, to address these questions, we need a theoretical approach that tries to establish, at the fundamental level, what consciousness is, how it can be measured, and what requisites a physical system must satisfy in order to generate it. The *integrated information theory* of consciousness represents such an approach [82].

According to the theory, the most important property of consciousness is that it is extraordinarily *informative*. This is because, whenever you experience a particular conscious scene, it rules out a huge number of alternative experiences. Classically, the reduction of uncertainty among a number of alternatives constitutes information [263, 264]. For example, you lie in bed with eyes open and experience pure darkness and silence. This is one of the simplest experiences you might have, one that may not be thought as conveying much information. One should realize, however, that the informativeness of what you just experienced lies not in how complicated it is to describe, but in how many alternatives were ruled out when you experienced it: you could have experienced any one frame from any of innumerable movies, or the smoke and flames of your room burning, or any other possible scene, but you did not – instead, you experienced darkness and silence. This means that when you experienced darkness and silence, whether you think or not of what was ruled out (and you typically don't), you actually gained access to a large amount of information. This point is so simple that its importance has been overlooked.

It is just as essential to realize that the information associated with the occurrence of a conscious state is *integrated* information. When you experience a particular conscious state, that conscious state is an integrated whole – it cannot be subdivided into components that are experienced independently. For example, the conscious experience of the particular phrase you are reading now cannot be experienced as subdivided into, say, the conscious experience of how the words look independently of the conscious experience of how they sound in your mind. Similarly, you cannot experience visual shapes independently of their color, or perceive the left half of the visual field of view independently of the right half.

Based on these and other considerations, the theory claims that the level of consciousness of a physical system is related to the repertoire of causal states (information) available to the system as a whole (integration). That is, whenever a system enters a particular state through causal interactions among its elements, it is conscious in proportion to how many system states it has thereby ruled out, provided these are states of the system as a whole, not decomposable into states of causally independent parts [82] (Balduzzi and Tononi, submitted). More precisely, the theory introduces a measure of integrated information called Φ, quantifying the reduction of uncertainty (i.e., the information) that is generated when a system enters a particular state through causal interactions among its parts, above and beyond the information that is generated independently within the parts themselves (hence integrated information). The parts should be chosen in such a way that they can account for as much non-integrated (independent) information as possible.

According to the theory, if a system has a positive value of Φ (and it is not included within a larger subset having higher Φ) it is called a *complex*. For a complex, and only for a complex, it is appropriate to say that when it enters a particular state, it generates an amount of integrated information corresponding to Φ. Since integrated information can only be generated *within* a complex and not outside its boundaries,

consciousness is necessarily subjective, private, and related to a single point of view or perspective [82, 265]. Some properties of complexes are worth pointing out. A given physical system, such as a brain, is likely to contain more than one complex, many small ones with low Φ values, and perhaps a few large ones. We suspect that in the brain there is at any given time a complex of comparatively much higher Φ, which we call the *main complex*. Also, a complex can be causally connected to elements that are not part of it through *ports-in* and *ports-out*. In that case, elements that are part of the complex contribute to its conscious experience, while elements that are not part of it do not, even though they may be connected to it and exchange information with it through *ports-in* and *ports-out*. One should also note that the Φ value of a complex is dependent on both spatial and temporal scales that determine what counts as a state of the underlying system. In general, the relevant spatial and temporal scales are those that jointly maximize Φ[82]. In the case of the brain, the spatial elements and time scales that maximize Φ may be local collections of neurons such as minicolumns and periods of time comprised between tens and hundreds of ms, respectively, though at this stage it is difficult to adjudicate between minicolumns and individual neurons.

Accounting for Neurobiological Observations

Measuring Φ and finding complexes is not easy for realistic systems, but it can be done for simple networks that bear some structural resemblance to different parts of the brain [81, 257]. For example, by using computer simulations, it is possible to show that high Φ requires networks that conjoin functional specialization (due to its specialized connectivity, each element has a unique functional role within the network) with functional integration (there are many pathways for interactions among the elements.). In very rough terms, this kind of architecture is characteristic of the mammalian corticothalamic system: different parts of the cerebral cortex are specialized for different functions, yet a vast network of connections allows these parts to interact profusely. And indeed, as we have seen, the corticothalamic system is precisely the part of the brain which cannot be severely impaired without loss of consciousness.

Conversely, Φ is low for systems that are made up of small, quasi-independent modules. This may be why the cerebellum, despite its large number of neurons, does not contribute much to consciousness: its synaptic organization is such that individual patches of cerebellar cortex tend to be activated independently of one another, with little interaction between distant patches [258, 259].

Computer simulations also show that units along multiple, segregated incoming or outgoing pathways are not incorporated within the repertoire of the main complex. This may be why neural activity in afferent pathways (perhaps as far as V1), though crucial for triggering this or that conscious experience, does not contribute directly to conscious experience; nor does activity in efferent pathways (perhaps starting with primary motor cortex), though it is crucial for reporting each different experience.

The addition of many parallel cycles also generally does not change the composition of the main complex, although Φ values can be altered. Instead, cortical and subcortical cycles or loops implement specialized subroutines that are capable of influencing the states of the main corticothalamic complex without joining it. Such informationally insulated cortico–subcortical loops could constitute the neural substrates for many unconscious processes that can affect and be affected by conscious experience [82, 269, 270], such as those that enable object recognition, language parsing, or translating our vague intentions into the right words. At this stage, however, it is hard to say precisely which cortical circuits may be informationally insulated. Are primary sensory cortices organized like massive afferent pathways to a main complex 'higher up' in the cortical hierarchy? Is much of prefrontal cortex, and the parallel loops originating there and going through basal ganglia and thalamic nuclei, organized like a massive efferent pathway? Do certain cortical areas, such as those belonging to the dorsal visual stream, remain partly segregated from the main complex? Do interactions *within* a cortico-thalamic minicolumn qualify as intrinsic mini-loops that support the main complex without being part of it? Unfortunately, answering these questions and properly testing the predictions of the theory requires a much better understanding of cortical neuroanatomy than is presently available [271].

Other simulations show that the effects of cortical disconnections are readily captured in terms of integrated information [82]: a 'callosal' cut produces, out of large complex corresponding to the connected cortico-thalamic system, two separate complexes, in line with many studies of split-brain patients [272]. However, because there is great redundancy between the two hemispheres, their Φ value is not greatly reduced compared to when they formed a single complex. Functional disconnections may also lead to a restriction of the neural substrate of consciousness, as is seen in neurological neglect phenomena, in psychiatric conversion and dissociative disorders, and possibly during

dreaming and hypnosis. It is also likely that certain attentional phenomena may correspond to changes in the composition of the main complex underlying consciousness. Phenomena such as the attentional blink, where a fixed sensory input may at times make it to consciousness and at times not, may also be due to changes in functional connectivity: access to the main corticothalamic complex may be enabled or not based on dynamics intrinsic to the complex [273]. Phenomena such as binocular rivalry may also be related, at least in part, to dynamic changes in the composition of the main corticothalamic complex caused by transient changes in functional connectivity [274]. Computer simulations confirm that functional disconnection can reduce the size of a complex and reduce its capacity to integrate information [82]. While it is not easy to determine, at present, whether a particular group of neurons is excluded from the main complex because of hard-wired anatomical constraints, or is transiently disconnected due to functional changes, the set of elements underlying consciousness is not static, but form a *'dynamic complex'* or *'dynamic core'* [265].

From the perspective of integrated information, a reduction of consciousness during early sleep would be consistent with the ensuing bistability of cortical circuits. As we have seen, studies using TMS in conjunction with high-density EEG show that early NREM sleep is associated either with a breakdown of the effective connectivity among cortical areas, and thereby with a loss of integration [83, 84], or with a stereotypical global response suggestive of a loss of repertoire and thus of information [83]. As we have also seen, similar changes are seen in animal studies of anesthesia [99, 109, 110]. Computer simulations also indicate that the capacity to integrate information is also reduced if neural activity is extremely high and near-synchronous, due to a dramatic decrease in the available degrees of freedom [265]. This reduction in degrees of freedom could be the reason why consciousness is reduced or eliminated in absence seizure and other conditions characterized by hypersynchronous neural activity.

Finally, we have seen that consciousness not only requires a neural substrate with appropriate anatomical structure and appropriate physiological parameters: it also needs time [215]. The theory predicts that the time requirement for the generation of conscious experience in the brain emerge directly from the time requirements for the build-up of an integrated repertoire among the elements of the corticothalamic main complex [82] (Balduzzi and Tononi, in preparation). To give an obvious example, if one has to perturb half of the elements of the main complex for less than a millisecond, no perturbations would produce any effect on the other half within this time window, and the repertoire measured by Φ would be equal to zero. After say 100 ms, however, there is enough time for differential effects to be manifested, and Φ should grow.

Some Implications

Naturally, the integrated information theory converges with other neurobiological frameworks [19, 124, 264] and cognitive theories [269] on certain key facts: that our own consciousness is generated by distributed corticothalamic networks, that reentrant interactions among multiple cortical regions are important, that the mechanisms of consciousness and attention overlap but are not the same, and that there are many 'unconscious' neural systems. Importantly, however, the examples discussed above show that the integrated information theory can begin to account, in a coherent manner, for several puzzling facts about consciousness and the brain. This goes beyond proposing a provisional list of candidate brain areas for the neural substrate of consciousness, and of seemingly important neural ingredients, such as synchronization, sustained or phasic firing, reentrant activity, or widespread 'broadcasting', without a principled explanation of why they would be important or whether they would be always necessary.

The integrated information theory also avoids the pitfalls associated with assigning conscious qualities to individual brain elements. For example, it is sometimes assumed loosely that the firing of specific corticothalamic elements (e.g., those for red) conveys some specific information (e.g., that there is something red), and that such information becomes conscious either as such, or perhaps if it is disseminated widely. However, a given corticothalamic element has no information about whether what made it fire was a particular color rather than a shape, a visual stimulus rather than a sound, a sensory stimulus rather than a thought. All it knows is whether it fired or not, just as each receiving element only knows whether it received an input or not. Thus, the information specifying 'red' cannot possibly be in the message conveyed by the firing of any neural element, whether it is located in a high-order cortical area, or whether it is broadcasting widely. According to the theory, that information resides instead in the reduction of uncertainty occurring when a whole complex enters one out of a large number of available states – the complex, and not its elements, are the locus of consciousness. Indeed, within a complex, both active and inactive neurons count, just as the sound of an orchestra is specified both by the instruments that are playing and by those

that are silent. Though it would be too long to address the issue here, the theory proposes that, just like the quantity of consciousness is given by the amount of integrated information generated within a complex, the particular quality of consciousness – including the redness of red – is given by the specific informational relationships among the elements of the complex [82].

The integrated information theory also predicts that consciousness depends exclusively on the ability of a system to integrate information, whether or not it has a strong sense of self, language, emotion, or is immersed in an environment, contrary to some common intuitions, but consistent, as reviewed in this overview, with the overall neurological evidence. Of course, the theory recognizes that these same factors are important historically because they favour the development of neural circuits forming a main complex of high Φ. For example, integrated information grows as that system incorporates statistical regularities from its environment and learns [276]. In this sense, the emergence of consciousness in biological systems is predicated on a long evolutionary history, on individual development, and on experience-dependent change in neural connectivity.

Finally, the integrated information theory says that the presence and extent of consciousness can be determined, in principle, also in cases in which we have no verbal report, such as infants or animals, or in neurological conditions such as minimally conscious states, akinetic mutism, psychomotor seizures, and sleepwalking. In practice, of course, measuring Φ accurately in such systems will not be easy, but approximations and informed guesses are certainly conceivable. The theory also implies that consciousness is not an all-or-none property, but is graded: specifically, it increases in proportion to a system's repertoire of available states. In fact, any physical system with some capacity for integrated information would have some degree of experience, irrespective of the constituents of which it is made, and independent of its ability to report.

Whether these and other predictions turn out to be compatible with future clinical and experimental evidence, a coherent theoretical framework should at least help to systematize a number of neuropsychological and neurobiological results that might otherwise seem disparate.

References

1. Kosslyn, S.M., Ganis, G. and Thompson, W.L. (2001) Neural foundations of imagery. *Nat Rev Neurosci* 2:635–642.
2. Amedi, A., Malach, R. and Pascual-Leone, A. (2005) Negative BOLD differentiates visual imagery and perception. *Neuron* 48:859–872.

3. Mason, M.F., Norton, M.I., Van Horn, J.D., Wegner, D.M., Grafton, S.T. and Macrae, C.N. (2007) Wandering minds: The default network and stimulus-independent thought. Science 315:393–395.

4. Hobson, J.A., Pace-Schott, E.F. and Stickgold, R. (2000) Dreaming and the brain: Toward a cognitive neuroscience of conscious states. Behav Brain Sci 23:793–842. discussion 904–1121.

5. Maquet, P., Péters, J., Aerts, J., Delfiore, G., Degueldre, C., Luxen, A. and Franck, G. (1996) Functional neuroanatomy of human rapid-eye-movement sleep and dreaming. Nature 383:163–166.

6. Braun, A.R., Balkin, T.J., Wesenten, N.J., Carson, R.E., Varga, M., Baldwin, P., Selbie, S., Belenky, G. and Herscovitch, P. (1997) Regional cerebral blood flow throughout the sleep-wake cycle. An H2(15)O PET study. Brain 120:1173–1197.

7. Hollins, M. (1985) Styles of mental imagery in blind adults. Neuropsychologia 23:561–566.

8. Buchel, C., Price, C., Frackowiak, R.S. and Friston, K. (1998) Different activation patterns in the visual cortex of late and congenitally blind subjects. Brain 121 (Pt 3):409–419.

9. Laureys, S., Pellas, F., Van Eeckhout, P., Ghorbel, S., Schnakers, C., Perrin, F., Berre, J., Faymonville, M.E., Pantke, K.H., Damas, F., Lamy, M., Moonen, G. and Goldman, S. (2005) The locked-in syndrome: What is it like to be conscious but paralyzed and voiceless? Prog Brain Res 150:495–511.

10. Bauby, J.-D. (1997) The Diving-Bell and the Butterfly: A Memoir of Life in Death. New York: Alfred A. Knopf.

11. Guilleminault, C. (1976) Cataplexy. In Guilleminault, C., Dennet, W. and Passouant, P. (eds.) Narcolepsy, pp. 125–143. New York: Spectrum.

12. Siegel, J. (2000) Narcolepsy. Sci Am 282:76–81.

13. Langston, J. and Palfreman, J. (1995) The Case of the Frozen Addicts., New York: Vintage Books.

14. Macphail, E.M. (1998) The Evolution of Consciousness. Oxford; New York: Oxford University Press.

15. Lazar, R.M., Marshall, R.S., Prell, G.D. and Pile-Spellman, J. (2000) The experience of Wernicke's aphasia. Neurology 55:1222–1224.

16. Hasson, U., Nir, Y., Levy, I., Fuhrmann, G. and Malach, R. (2004) Intersubject synchronization of cortical activity during natural vision. Science 303:1634–1640.

17. Posner, M.I. (1994) Attention: The mechanisms of consciousness. Proc Natl Acad Sci USA 91:7398–7403.

18. O'Regan, J.K. and Noe, A. (2001) A sensorimotor account of vision and visual consciousness. Behav Brain Sci 24:939–973. discussion 973–1031.

19. Dehaene, S., Changeux, J.P., Naccache, L., Sackur, J. and Sergent, C. (2006) Conscious, preconscious, and subliminal processing: A testable taxonomy. Trends Cogn Sci 10:204–211.

20. Mack, A. and Rock, I. (1998) Inattentional Blindness, Cambridge. MA: MIT Press.

21. Baars, B.J. (1997) Some essential differences between consciousness and attention, perception, and working memory. Conscious Cogn 6:363–371.

22. Lamme, V.A. (2003) Why visual attention and awareness are different. Trends Cogn Sci 7:12–18.

23. Koch, C. and Tsuchiya, N. (2007) Attention and consciousness: Two distinct brain processes. Trends Cogn Sci 11:16–22.

24. Naccache, L., Blandin, E. and Dehaene, S. (2002) Unconscious masked priming depends on temporal attention. Psychol Sci 13:416–424.

25. Kentridge, R.W., Heywood, C.A. and Weiskrantz, L. (1999) Attention without awareness in blindsight. Proc Biol Sci 266:1805–1811.

26. Kentridge, R.W., Nijboer, T.C. and Heywood, C.A. (2008) Attended but unseen: Visual attention is not sufficient for visual awareness. Neuropsychologia 46:864–869.

27. Woodman, G.F. and Luck, S.J. (2003) Dissociations among attention, perception, and awareness during object-substitution masking. Psychol Sci 14:605–611.

28. Bahrami, B., Lavie, N. and Rees, G. (2007) Attentional load modulates responses of human primary visual cortex to invisible stimuli. Curr Biol 17:509–513.

29 Wyart, V. and Tallon-Baudry, C. (2008) Neural Dissociation between Visual Awareness and Spatial Attention. J Neurosci 28:2667–2679.

30. Li, F.F., VanRullen, R., Koch, C. and Perona, P. (2002) Rapid natural scene categorization in the near absence of attention. Proc Natl Acad Sci USA 99:9596–9601.

31. Lamme, V.A. (2006) Towards a true neural stance on consciousness. Trends Cogn Sci 10:494–501.

32. Olivers, C.N. (2008) Interactions between visual working memory and visual attention. Front Biosci 13:1182–1191.

33. Mayer, J.S., Bittner, R.A., Nikolic, D., Bledowski, C., Goebel, R. and Linden, D.E. (2007) Common neural substrates for visual working memory and attention. Neuroimage 36:441–453.

34. Postle, B.R. (2006) Working memory as an emergent property of the mind and brain. Neuroscience 139:23–38.

35. Lee, A.C., Bussey, T.J., Murray, E.A., Saksida, L.M., Epstein, R.A., Kapur, N., Hodges, J.R. and Graham, K.S. (2005) Perceptual deficits in amnesia: Challenging the medial temporal lobe 'mnemonic' view. Neuropsychologia 43:1–11.

36. Barense, M.D., Gaffan, D. and Graham, K.S. (2007) The human medial temporal lobe processes online representations of complex objects. Neuropsychologia 45:2963–2974.

37. Hassabis, D., Kumaran, D., Vann, S.D. and Maguire, E.A. (2007) Patients with hippocampal amnesia cannot imagine new experiences. Proc Natl Acad Sci USA 104:1726–1731.

38. Hannula, D.E., Tranel, D. and Cohen, N.J. (2006) The long and the short of it: relational memory impairments in amnesia, even at short lags. J Neurosci 26:8352–8359.

39. Nadel, L. and Moscovitch, M. (1997) Memory consolidation, retrograde amnesia and the hippocampal complex. Curr Opin Neurobiol 7:217–227.

40. Winocur, G., Moscovitch, M. and Sekeres, M. (2007) Memory consolidation or transformation: Context manipulation and hippocampal representations of memory. Nat Neurosci 10:555–557.

41. Robertson, L.C. (2004) Space, Objects, Minds, and Brains. New York: Psychology Press.

42. Cohen, Y.E. and Andersen, R.A. (2002) A common reference frame for movement plans in the posterior parietal cortex. Nat Rev Neurosci 3:553–562.

43. Phan, M.L., Schendel, K.L., Recanzone, G.H. and Robertson, L.C. (2000) Auditory and visual spatial localization deficits following bilateral parietal lobe lesions in a patient with Balint's syndrome. J Cogn Neurosci 12:583–600.

44. Bisiach, E. and Luzzatti, C. (1978) Unilateral neglect of representational space. Cortex 14:129–133.

45. Mort, D.J., Malhotra, P., Mannan, S.K., Rorden, C., Pambakian, A., Kennard, C. and Husain, M. (2003) The anatomy of visual neglect. Brain 126:1986–1997.

46. Committeri, G., Pitzalis, S., Galati, G., Patria, F., Pelle, G., Sabatini, U., Castriota-Scanderbeg, A., Piccardi, L., Guariglia, C. and Pizzamiglio, L. (2007) Neural bases of personal and extrapersonal neglect in humans. Brain 130:431–441.

47. Corbetta, M. and Shulman, G.L. (2002) Control of goal-directed and stimulus-driven attention in the brain. Nat Rev Neurosci 3:201–215.

48. He, B.J., Snyder, A.Z., Vincent, J.L., Epstein, A., Shulman, G.L. and Corbetta, M. (2007) Breakdown of functional connectivity in frontoparietal networks underlies behavioral deficits in spatial neglect. *Neuron* 53:905–918.

49. Rees, G., Wojciulik, E., Clarke, K., Husain, M., Frith, C. and Driver, J. (2000) Unconscious activation of visual cortex in the damaged right hemisphere of a parietal patient with extinction. *Brain* 123 (Pt 8):1624–1633.

50. Rees, G., Wojciulik, E., Clarke, K., Husain, M., Frith, C. and Driver, J. (2002b) Neural correlates of conscious and unconscious vision in parietal extinction. *Neurocase* 8:387–393.

51. Driver, J. and Vuilleumier, P. (2001) Perceptual awareness and its loss in unilateral neglect and extinction. *Cognition* 79:39–88.

52. Ruby, P. and Decety, J. (2001) Effect of subjective perspective taking during simulation of action: A PET investigation of agency. *Nat Neurosci* 4:546–550.

53. Frith, C. (2002) Attention to action and awareness of other minds. *Conscious Cogn* 11:481–487.

54. Farrer, C., Franck, N., Georgieff, N., Frith, C.D., Decety, J. and Jeannerod, M. (2003) Modulating the experience of agency: A positron emission tomography study. *Neuroimage* 18:324–333.

55. David, N., Bewernick, B.H., Cohen, M.X., Newen, A., Lux, S., Fink, G.R., Shah, N.J. and Vogeley, K. (2006) Neural representations of self versus other: Visual-spatial perspective taking and agency in a virtual ball-tossing game. *J Cogn Neurosci* 18:898–910.

56. Tsakiris, M., Hesse, M.D., Boy, C., Haggard, P. and Fink, G.R. (2007) Neural signatures of body ownership: A sensory network for bodily self-consciousness. *Cereb Cortex* 17:2235–2244.

57. Arzy, S., Overney, L.S., Landis, T. and Blanke, O. (2006a) Neural mechanisms of embodiment: Asomatognosia due to premotor cortex damage. *Arch Neurol* 63:1022–1025.

58. Lenggenhager, B., Smith, S.T. and Blanke, O. (2006) Functional and neural mechanisms of embodiment: Importance of the vestibular system and the temporal parietal junction. *Rev Neurosci* 17:643–657.

59. Vogeley, K., May, M., Ritzl, A., Falkai, P., Zilles, K. and Fink, G.R. (2004) Neural correlates of first-person perspective as one constituent of human self-consciousness. *J Cogn Neurosci* 16:817–827.

60. Blanke, O., Mohr, C., Michel, C.M., Pascual-Leone, A., Brugger, P., Seeck, M., Landis, T. and Thut, G. (2005) Linking out-of-body experience and self processing to mental own-body imagery at the temporoparietal junction. *J Neurosci* 25:550–557.

61. De Ridder, D., Van Laere, K., Dupont, P., Menovsky, T. and Van de Heyning, P. (2007) Visualizing out-of-body experience in the brain. *N Engl J Med* 357:1829–1833.

62. Downing, P.E., Jiang, Y., Shuman, M. and Kanwisher, N. (2001) A cortical area selective for visual processing of the human body. *Science* 293:2470–2473.

63. Arzy, S., Thut, G., Mohr, C., Michel, C.M. and Blanke, O. (2006b) Neural basis of embodiment: distinct contributions of temporoparietal junction and extrastriate body area. *J Neurosci* 26:8074–8081.

64. Shuren, J.E., Brott, T.G., Schefft, B.K. and Houston, W. (1996) Preserved color imagery in an achromatopsic. *Neuropsychologia* 34:485–489.

65. Bartolomeo, P., Bachoud-Levi, A.C. and Denes, G. (1997) Preserved imagery for colours in a patient with cerebral achromatopsia. *Cortex* 33:369–378.

66. De Vreese, L.P. (1991) Two systems for colour-naming defects: verbal disconnection vs colour imagery disorder. *Neuropsychologia* 29:1–18.

67. Goldenberg, G. (1992) Loss of visual imagery and loss of visual knowledge – a case study. *Neuropsychologia* 30:1081–1099.

68. Luzzatti, C. and Davidoff, J. (1994) Impaired retrieval of object-colour knowledge with preserved colour naming. *Neuropsychologia* 32:933–950.

69. Bartolomeo, P. (2002) The relationship between visual perception and visual mental imagery: A reappraisal of the neuropsychological evidence. *Cortex* 38:357–378.

70. Jakobson, L.S., Pearson, P.M. and Robertson, B. (2008) Hue-specific colour memory impairment in an individual with intact colour perception and colour naming. *Neuropsychologia* 46:22–36.

71. Sacks, O.W. (1995) *An Anthropologist on Mars: Seven Paradoxical Tales*, 1st Edition. New York: Knopf.

72. van Zandvoort, M.J., Nijboer, T.C. and de Haan, E. (2007) Developmental colour agnosia. *Cortex* 43:750–757.

73. Goldenberg, G., Mullbacher, W. and Nowak, A. (1995) Imagery without perception – a case study of anosognosia for cortical blindness. *Neuropsychologia* 33:1373–1382.

74. Young, A.W., de Haan, E.H. and Newcombe, F. (1990) Unawareness of impaired face recognition. *Brain Cogn* 14:1–18.

75. Berti, A., Bottini, G., Gandola, M., Pia, L., Smania, N., Stracciari, A., Castiglioni, I., Vallar, G. and Paulesu, E. (2005) Shared cortical anatomy for motor awareness and motor control. *Science* 309:488–491.

76. Spinazzola, L., Pia, L., Folegatti, A., Marchetti, C. and Berti, A. (2008) Modular structure of awareness for sensorimotor disorders: Evidence from anosognosia for hemiplegia and anosognosia for hemianaesthesia. *Neuropsychologia* 46:915–926.

77. Hobson, J.A. and Pace-Schott, E.F. (2002) The cognitive neuroscience of sleep: Neuronal systems, consciousness and learning. *Nat Rev Neurosci* 3:679–693.

78. Maquet, P., Degueldre, C., Delfiore, G., Aerts, J., Péters, J.M., Luxen, A. and Franck, G. (1997) Functional neuroanatomy of human slow wave sleep. *J Neurosci* 17:2807–2812.

79. Steriade, M., Timofeev, I. and Grenier, F. (2001) Natural waking and sleep states: A view from inside neocortical neurons. *J Neurophysiol* 85:1969–1985.

80. Destexhe, A., Hughes, S.W., Rudolph, M. and Crunelli, V. (2007) Are corticothalamic 'up' states fragments of wakefulness? *Trends Neurosci* 30:334–342.

81. Steriade, M. (2003) The corticothalamic system in sleep. *Front Biosci* 8:D878–D899.

82. Tononi, G. (2004a) An information integration theory of consciousness. *BMC Neurosci* 5:42.

83. Massimini, M., Ferrarelli, F., Esser, S.K., Riedner, B.A., Huber, R., Murphy, M., Peterson, M.J. and Tononi, G. (2007) Triggering sleep slow waves by transcranial magnetic stimulation. *Proc Natl Acad Sci USA* 104:8496–8501.

84. Massimini, M., Ferrarelli, F., Huber, R., Esser, S.K., Singh, H. and Tononi, G. (2005) Breakdown of cortical effective connectivity during sleep. *Science* 309:2228–2232.

85. Massimini, M., Huber, R., Ferrarelli, F., Hill, S. and Tononi, G. (2004) The sleep slow oscillation as a traveling wave. *J Neurosci* 24:6862–6870.

86. Campagna, J.A., Miller, K.W. and Forman, S.A. (2003) Mechanisms of actions of inhaled anesthetics. *N Engl J Med* 348:2110–2124.

87. Franks, N.P. (2006) Molecular targets underlying general anaesthesia. *Br J Pharmacol* 147 (Suppl 1):S72–81.

88. Alkire, M.T. and Miller, J. (2005) General anesthesia and the neural correlates of consciousness. *Prog Brain Res* 150:229–244.

89. Alkire, M.T., Haier, R.J. and Fallon, J.H. (2000) Toward a unified theory of narcosis: Brain imaging evidence for a thalamocortical switch as the neurophysiologic basis of anesthetic-induced unconsciousness. *Conscious Cogn* 9:370–386.

90. Ori, C., Dam, M., Pizzolato, G., Battistin, L. and Giron, G. (1986) Effects of isoflurane anesthesia on local cerebral glucose utilization in the rat. Anesthesiology 65:152–156.

91. Vahle-Hinz, C., Detsch, O., Siemers, M. and Kochs, E. (2007) Contributions of GABAergic and glutamatergic mechanisms to isoflurane-induced suppression of thalamic somatosensory information transfer. Exp Brain Res 176:159–172.

92. Nakakimura, K., Sakabe, T., Funatsu, N., Maekawa, T. and Takeshita, H. (1988) Metabolic activation of intercortical and corticothalamic pathways during enflurane anesthesia in rats. Anesthesiology 68:777–782.

93. Velly, L.J., Rey, M.F., Bruder, N.J., Gouvitsos, F.A., Witjas, T., Regis, J.M., Peragut, J.C. and Gouin, F.M. (2007) Differential dynamic of action on cortical and subcortical structures of anesthetic agents during induction of anesthesia. Anesthesiology 107:202–212.

94. Munglani, R., Andrade, J., Sapsford, D.J., Baddeley, A. and Jones, J.G. (1993) A measure of consciousness and memory during isoflurane administration: the coherent frequency. Br J Anaesth 71:633–641.

95. Andrade, J., Sapsford, D.J., Jeevaratnum, D., Pickworth, A.J. and Jones, J.G. (1996) The coherent frequency in the electro-encephalogram as an objective measure of cognitive function during propofol sedation. Anesth Analg 83:1279–1284.

96. Plourde, G., Villemure, C., Fiset, P., Bonhomme, V. and Backman, S.B. (1998) Effect of isoflurane on the auditory steady-state response and on consciousness in human volunteers. Anesthesiology 89:844–851.

97. John, E.R., Prichep, L.S., Kox, W., Valdes-Sosa, P., Bosch-Bayard, J., Aubert, E., Tom, M., di Michele, F. and Gugino, L.D. (2001) Invariant reversible QEEG effects of anesthetics. Conscious Cogn 10:165–183.

98. Imas, O.A., Ropella, K.M., Wood, J.D. and Hudetz, A.G. (2006) Isoflurane disrupts anterio-posterior phase synchronization of flash-induced field potentials in the rat. Neurosci Lett 402:216–221.

99. Imas, O.A., Ropella, K.M., Ward, B.D., Wood, J.D. and Hudetz, A.G. (2005a) Volatile anesthetics disrupt frontal-posterior recurrent information transfer at gamma frequencies in rat. Neurosci Lett 387:145–150.

100. Lamme, V.A., Super, H. and Spekreijse, H. (1998b) Feedforward, horizontal, and feedback processing in the visual cortex. Curr Opin Neurobiol 8:529–535.

101. Lamme, V.A., Zipser, K. and Spekreijse, H. (1998a) Figure-ground activity in primary visual cortex is suppressed by anesthesia. Proc Natl Acad Sci USA 95:3263–3268.

102. Lamme, V.A. and Roelfsema, P.R. (2000) The distinct modes of vision offered by feedforward and recurrent processing. Trends Neurosci 23:571–579.

103. Buzsaki, G., Geisler, C., Henze, D.A. and Wang, X.J. (2004) Interneuron Diversity series: Circuit complexity and axon wiring economy of cortical interneurons. Trends Neurosci 27:186–193.

104. Rozenfeld, H.D. and Ben-Avraham, D. (2007) Percolation in hierarchical scale-free nets. Phys Rev E Stat Nonlin Soft Matter Phys 75:061102.

105. Steyn-Ross, D.A., Steyn-Ross, M.L., Wilcocks, L.C. and Sleigh, J.W. (2001) Toward a theory of the general-anesthetic-induced phase transition of the cerebral cortex. II. Numerical simulations, spectral entropy, and correlation times. Phys Rev E Stat Nonlin Soft Matter Phys 64:011918.

106. Steyn-Ross, M.L., Steyn-Ross, D.A., Sleigh, J.W. and Wilcocks, L.C. (2001) Toward a theory of the general-anesthetic-induced phase transition of the cerebral cortex. I. A thermodynamics analogy. Phys Rev E Stat Nonlin Soft Matter Phys 64:011917.

107. Hartikainen, K., Rorarius, M., Makela, K., Perakyla, J., Varila, E. and Jantti, V. (1995) Visually evoked bursts during isoflurane anaesthesia. Br J Anaesth 74:681–685.

108. Makela, K., Hartikainen, K., Rorarius, M. and Jantti, V. (1996) Suppression of F-VEP during isoflurane-induced EEG suppression. Electroencephalogr Clin Neurophysiol 100:269–272.

109. Hudetz, A.G. and Imas, O.A. (2007) Burst activation of the cerebral cortex by flash stimuli during isoflurane anesthesia in rats. Anesthesiology 107:983–991.

110. Kroeger, D. and Amzica, F. (2007) Hypersensitivity of the anesthesia-induced comatose brain. J Neurosci 27:10597–10607.

111. Posner, J.B. and Plum, F. (2007) Plum and Posner's Diagnosis of Stupor and Coma, 4th Edition. Oxford; New York: Oxford University Press.

112. Laureys, S., Faymonville, M.E., Luxen, A., Lamy, M., Franck, G. and Maquet, P. (2000) Restoration of thalamocrotical connectivity after recovery from persistent vegetative state. Lancet 355:1790–1791.

113. Schiff, N.D., Giacino, J.T., Kalmar, K., Victor, J.D., Baker, K., Gerber, M., Fritz, B., Eisenberg, B., O'Connor, J., Kobylarz, E.J., Farris, S., Machado, A., McCagg, C., Plum, F., Fins, J.J. and Rezai, A.R. (2007) Behavioural improvements with thalamic stimulation after severe traumatic brain injury. Nature 448:600–603.

114. Williams, D. and Parsons-Smith, G. (1951) Thalamic activity in stupor. Brain 74:377–398.

115. Laureys, S., Owen, A.M. and Schiff, N.D. (2004) Brain function in coma, vegetative state, and related disorders. Lancet Neurol 3:537–546.

116. Schiff, N.D. (2006b) Multimodal neuroimaging approaches to disorders of consciousness. J Head Trauma Rehabil 21:388–397.

117. Voss, H.U., Uluc, A.M., Dyke, J.P., Watts, R., Kobylarz, E.J., McCandliss, B.D., Heier, L.A., Beattie, B.J., Hamacher, K.A., Vallabhajosula, S., Goldsmith, S.J., Ballon, D., Giacino, J.T. and Schiff, N.D. (2006) Possible axonal regrowth in late recovery from the minimally conscious state. J Clin Invest 116:2005–2011.

118. Schiff, N.D. (2006) Measurements and models of cerebral function in the severely injured brain. J Neurotrauma 23:1436–1449.

119. Owen, A.M., Coleman, M.R., Boly, M., Davis, M.H., Laureys, S. and Pickard, J.D. (2006) Detecting awareness in the vegetative state. Science 313:1402.

120. Blumenfeld, H. and Taylor, J. (2003) Why do seizures cause loss of consciousness? Neuroscientist 9:301–310.

121. Blumenfeld, H., Westerveld, M., Ostroff, R.B., Vanderhill, S.D., Freeman, J., Necochea, A., Uranga, P., Tanhehco, T., Smith, A., Seibyl, J.P., Stokking, R., Studholme, C., Spencer, S.S. and Zubal, I.G. (2003) Selective frontal, parietal, and temporal networks in generalized seizures. Neuroimage 19:1556–1566.

122. Blumenfeld, H., McNally, K.A., Vanderhill, S.D., Paige, A.L., Chung, R., Davis, K., Norden, A.D., Stokking, R., Studholme, C., Novotny, E.J.Jr., Zubal, I.G. and Spencer, S.S. (2004) Positive and negative network correlations in temporal lobe epilepsy. Cereb Cortex 14:892–902.

123. Blumenfeld, H. (2005) Consciousness and epilepsy: Why are patients with absence seizures absent? Prog Brain Res 150:271–286.

124. Crick, F. and Koch, C. (2003) A framework for consciousness. Nat Neurosci 6:119–126.

125. Buzsaki, G., Bickford, R.G., Ponomareff, G., Thal, L.J., Mandel, R. and FH Gage, F.H. (1988) Nucleus basalis and thalamic control of neocortical activity in the freely moving rat. J Neurosci 8:4007–4026.

126. Dringenberg, H.C. and Olmstead, M.C. (2003) Integrated contributions of basal forebrain and thalamus to neocortical

activation elicited by pedunculopontine tegmental stimulation in urethane-anesthetized rats. *Neuroscience* 119:839–853.

127. Glickstein, M. (2007) What does the cerebellum really do? *Curr Biol* 17:R824–827.

128. Schmahmann, J.D., Weilburg, J.B. and Sherman, J.C. (2007) The neuropsychiatry of the cerebellum – insights from the clinic. *Cerebellum* 6:254–267.

129. Crick, F.C. and Koch, C. (2005) What is the function of the claustrum? *Philos Trans R Soc Lond B Biol Sci* 360:1271–1279.

130. Straussberg, R., Shorer, Z., Weitz, R., Basel, L., Kornreich, L., Corie, C.I., Harel, L., Djaldetti, R. and Amir, J. (2002) Familial infantile bilateral striatal necrosis: Clinical features and response to biotin treatment. *Neurology* 59:983–989.

131. Leuzzi, V., Favata, I. and Seri, S. (1988) Bilateral striatal lesions. *Dev Med Child Neurol* 30:252–257.

132. Leuzzi, V., Bertini, E., De Negri, A.M., Gallucci, M. and Garavaglia, B. (1992) Bilateral striatal necrosis, dystonia and optic atrophy in two siblings. *J Neurol Neurosurg Psychiatr* 55:16–19.

133. Craver, R.D., Duncan, M.C. and Nelson, J.S. (1996) Familial dystonia and choreoathetosis in three generations associated with bilateral striatal necrosis. *J Child Neurol* 11:185–188.

134. Caparros-Lefebvre, D., Destee, A. and Petit, H. (1997) Late onset familial dystonia: could mitochondrial deficits induce a diffuse lesioning process of the whole basal ganglia system? *J Neurol Neurosurg Psychiatr* 63:196–203.

135. Scott, R., Gregory, R., Hines, N., Carroll, C., Hyman, N., Papanasstasiou, V., Leather, C., Rowe, J., Silburn, P. and Aziz, T. (1998) Neuropsychological, neurological and functional outcome following pallidotomy for Parkinson's disease. A consecutive series of eight simultaneous bilateral and twelve unilateral procedures. *Brain* 121 (Pt 4):659–675.

136. Ghika, J., Ghika-Schmid, F., Fankhauser, H., Assal, G., Vingerhoets, F., Albanese, A., Bogousslavsky, J. and Favre, J. (1999) Bilateral contemporaneous posteroventral pallidotomy for the treatment of Parkinson's disease: neuropsychological and neurological side effects. Report of four cases and review of the literature. *J Neurosurg* 91:313–321.

137. York, M.K., Lai, E.C., Jankovic, J., Macias, A., Atassi, F., Levin, H.S. and Grossman, R.G. (2007) Short and long-term motor and cognitive outcome of staged bilateral pallidotomy: A retrospective analysis. *Acta Neurochir (Wien)* 149:857–866. discussion 866.

138. Northoff, G. (2002) What catatonia can tell us about 'top-down modulation': A neuropsychiatric hypothesis. *Behav Brain Sci* 25:555–577. discussion 578–604.

139. Northoff, G., Kotter, R., Baumgart, F., Danos, P., Boeker, H., Kaulisch, T., Schlagenhauf, F., Walter, H., Heinzel, A., Witzel, T. and Bogerts, B. (2004) Orbitofrontal cortical dysfunction in akinetic catatonia: A functional magnetic resonance imaging study during negative emotional stimulation. *Schizophr Bull* 30:405–427.

140. Debaere, F., Wenderoth, N., Sunaert, S., Van Hecke, P. and Swinnen, S.P. (2004) Changes in brain activation during the acquisition of a new bimanual coodination task. *Neuropsychologia* 42:855–867.

141. Floyer-Lea, A. and Matthews, P.M. (2004) Changing brain networks for visuomotor control with increased movement automaticity. *J Neurophysiol* 92:2405–2412.

142. Bogen, J.E. (1997) Some neurophysiologic aspects of consciousness. *Semin Neurol* 17:95–103.

143. Miller, J.W. and Ferrendelli, J.A. (1990) Characterization of GABAergic seizure regulation in the midline thalamus. *Neuropharmacology* 29:649–655.

144. Miller, J.W., Gray, B.C., Turner, G.M. and Bardgett, M.E. (1993) An ascending seizure-controlling pathway in the medial brainstem and thalamus. *Exp Neurol* 121:106–112.

145. Alkire, M.T., McReynolds, J.R., Hahn, E.L. and Trivedi, A.N. (2007) Thalamic microinjection of nicotine reverses sevoflurane-induced loss of righting reflex in the rat. *Anesthesiology* 107:264–272.

146. Guillery, R.W., Feig, S.L. and Van Lieshout, D.P. (2001) Connections of higher order visual relays in the thalamus: A study of corticothalamic pathways in cats. *J Comp Neurol* 438:66–85.

147. Guillery, R.W. and Sherman, S.M. (2002) Thalamic relay functions and their role in corticocortical communication: Generalizations from the visual system. *Neuron* 33:163–175.

148. Sherman, S.M. and Guillery, R.W. (2002) The role of the thalamus in the flow of information to the cortex. *Philos Trans R Soc Lond B Biol Sci* 357:1695–1708.

149. Shipp, S. (2003) The functional logic of cortico-pulvinar connections. *Philos Trans R Soc Lond B Biol Sci* 358:1605–1624.

150. Jones, E.G. (2007) *The Thalamus*, 2nd Edition. Cambridge, UK; New York: Cambridge University Press.

151. Jones, E.G. (1998) A new view of specific and nonspecific thalamocortical connections. *Adv Neurol* 77:49–71. discussion 72–43.

152. Llinas, R.R., Leznik, E. and Urbano, F.J. (2002) Temporal binding via cortical coincidence detection of specific and nonspecific thalamocortical inputs: A voltage-dependent dye-imaging study in mouse brain slices. *Proc Natl Acad Sci USA* 99:449–454.

153. Scannell, J.W., Burns, G.A., Hilgetag, C.C., O'Neil, M.A. and Young, M.P. (1999) The connectional organization of the cortico-thalamic system of the cat. *Cereb Cortex* 9:277–299.

154. Magnin, M., Bastuji, H., Garcia-Larrea, L. and Mauguière, F. (2004) Human thalamic medial pulvinar nucleus is not activated during paradoxical sleep. *Cereb Cortex* 14:858–862.

155. Villablanca, J. and Salinas-Zeballos, M. E. Sleep-wakefulness, EEG and behavioural studies of chronic cats without the thalamus: the 'athalamic' cat. *Arch Ital Biol* 110, 383–411.

156. Vanderwolf, C.H. and Stewart, D.J. (1988) Thalamic control of neocortical activation: a critical re-evaluation. *Brian Res Bull* 20:529–538.

157. Moruzzi, G. and Magoun, H.W. (1949) Brain stem reticular formation and activation of the EEG. *Electroencephalogr Clin Neuro* 1:455–473.

158. Crick, F. and Koch, C. (1995) Are we aware of neural activity in primary visual cortex? *Nature* 375:121–123.

159. He, S. and MacLeod, D.I. (2001) Orientation-selective adaptation and tilt after-effect from invisible patterns. *Nature* 411:473–476.

160. Jiang, Y., Zhou, K. and He, S. (2007) Human visual cortex responds to invisible chromatic flicker. *Nat Neurosci* 10:657–662.

161. Logothetis, N.K. (1998) Single units and conscious vision. *Philos Trans R Soc Lond B Biol Sci* 353:1801–1818.

162. Leopold, D.A. and Logothetis, N.K. (1999) Multistable phenomena: Changing views in perception. *Trends Cogn Sci* 3:254–264.

163. Blake, R. and Logothetis, N.K. (2002) Visual competition. *Nat Rev Neurosci* 3:13–21.

164. Tong, F., Nakayama, K., Vaughan, J.T. and Kanwisher, N. (1998) Binocular rivalry and visual awareness in human extrastriate cortex. *Neuron* 21:753–759.

165. Lee, S.H., Blake, R. and Heeger, D.J. (2005) Traveling waves of activity in primary visual cortex during binocular rivalry. *Nat Neurosci* 8:22–23.

166. Rees, G. (2007) Neural correlates of the contents of visual awareness in humans. *Philos Trans R Soc Lond B Biol Sci* 362:877–886.

167. Lee, S.H., Blake, R. and Heeger, D.J. (2007) Hierarchy of cortical responses underlying binocular rivalry. *Nat Neurosci* 10:1048–1054.

168. Haynes, J.D., Driver, J. and Rees, G. (2005) Visibility reflects dynamic changes of effective connectivity between V1 and fusiform cortex. *Neuron* 46:811–821.

169. Dehaene, S., Naccache, L., Cohen, L., Bihan, D.L., Mangin, J.F., Poline, J.B. and Riviere, D. (2001) Cerebral mechanisms of word masking and unconscious repetition priming. *Nat Neurosci* 4:752–758.

170. Marois, R., Yi, D.J. and Chun, M.M. (2004) The neural fate of consciously perceived and missed events in the attentional blink. *Neuron* 41:465–472.

171. Sergent, C., Baillet, S. and Dehaene, S. (2005) Timing of the brain events underlying access to consciousness during the attentional blink. *Nat Neurosci* 8:1391–1400.

172. Vuilleumier, P., Sagiv, N., Hazeltine, E., Poldrack, R.A., Swick, D., Rafal, R.D. and Gabrieli, J.D. (2001) Neural fate of seen and unseen faces in visuospatial neglect: A combined event-related functional MRI and event-related potential study. *Proc Natl Acad Sci USA* 98:3495–3500.

173. Penfield, W. (1975) *The Mystery of the Mind: A Critical Study of Consciousness and the Human Brain*. Princeton, NJ: Princeton University Press.

174. Zeki, S. (1993) *A Vision of the Brain*. Oxford; Boston: Blackwell Scientific Publications.

175. Pollen, D.A. (1999) On the neural correlates of visual perception. *Cereb Cortex* 9:4–19.

176. Weiskrantz, L. (1996) Blindsight revisited. *Curr Opin Neurobiol* 6:215–220.

177. Cowey, A. and Walsh, V. (2000) Magnetically induced phosphenes in sighted, blind and blindsighted observers. *Neuroreport* 11:3269–3273.

178. Pascual-Leone, A. and Walsh, V. (2001) Fast backprojections from the motion to the primary visual area necessary for visual awareness. *Science* 292:510–512.

179. Silvanto, J., Cowey, A., Lavie, N. and Walsh, V. (2007) Making the blindsighted see. *Neuropsychologia* 45:3346–3350.

180. Milner, A.D. and Goodale, M.A. (1995) *The Visual Brain in Action*. Oxford; New York: Oxford University Press.

181. Goodale, M. and Milner, A. (2005) *Sight Unseen: An Exploration of Conscious and Unconscious Vision*. Oxford, UK: Oxford University Press.

182. Konen, C.S. and Kastner, S. (2008) Two hierarchically organized neural systems for object information in human visual cortex. *Nat Neurosci*.

183. Hebb, D.O. and Penfield, W. (1940) Human behavior after extensive bilateral removal from the frontal lobes. *Arch Neurol Psychiatr* 42:421–438.

184. Fulton, J.F. (1949) *Functional Localization in Relation to Frontal Lobotomy*. New York: Oxford University Press.

185. Mashour, G.A., Walker, E.E. and Martuza, R.L. (2005) Psychosurgery: past, present, and future. *Brain Res Brain Res Rev* 48:409–419.

186. Mettler F.A. (1949). Columbia University. Dept. of Neurology., Greystone Park Psychiatric Hospital. Selective partial ablation of the frontal cortex, a correlative study of its effects on human psychotic subjects. [New York]: Hoebar.

187. Mataro, M., Jurado, M.A., Garcia-Sanchez, C., Barraquer, L., Costa-Jussa, F.R. and Junque, C. (2001) Long-term effects of bilateral frontal brain lesion: 60 years after injury with an iron bar. *Arch Neurol* 58:1139–1142.

188. Markowitsch, H.J. and Kessler, J. (2000) Massive impairment in executive functions with partial preservation of other cognitive functions: The case of a young patient with severe degeneration of the prefrontal cortex. *Exp Brain Res* 133:94–102.

189. Barcelo, F., Suwazono, S. and Knight, R.T. (2000) Prefrontal modulation of visual processing in humans. *Nat Neurosci* 3:399–403.

190. Cairns, H., Oldfield, R.C., Pennybacker, J.B. and Whitteridge, D. (1941) Akinetic mutism with an epidermoid cyst of the 3rd ventricle. *Brain* 64:273–290.

191. Schiff, N.D. and Plum, F. (2000) The role of arousal and 'gating' systems in the neurology of impaired consciousness. *J Clin Neurophysiol* 17:438–452.

192. Kotchoubey, B., Schneck, M., Lang, S. and Birbaumer, N. (2003) Event-related brain potentials in a patient with akinetic mutism. *Neurophysiol Clin* 33:23–30.

193. Kotchoubey, B. (2005) Event-related potential measures of consciousness: Two equations with three unknowns. *Prog Brain Res* 150:427–444.

194. Kotchoubey, B., Lang, S., Mezger, G., Schmalohr, D., Schneck, M., Semmler, A., Bostanov, V. and Birbaumer, N. (2005) Information processing in severe disorders of consciousness: Vegetative state and minimally conscious state. *Clin Neurophysiol* 116:2441–2453.

195. Fisher, C.M. (1983) Honored guest presentation: Abulia minor vs. agitated behavior. *Clin Neurosurg* 31:9–31.

196. Inbody, S. and Jankovic, J. (1986) Hyperkinetic mutism: Bilateral ballism and basal ganglia calcification. *Neurology* 36:825–827.

197. Mori, E. and Yamadori, A. (1989) Rejection behaviour: A human homologue of the abnormal behaviour of Denny-Brown and Chambers' monkey with bilateral parietal ablation. *J Neurol Neurosurg Psychiatr* 52:1260–1266.

198. Schiff, N.D., Ribary, U., Moreno, D.R., Beattie, B., Kronberg, E., Blasberg, R., Giacino, J., McCagg, C., Fins, J.J., Llinas, R. and Plum, F. (2002) Residual cerebral activity and behavioural fragments can remain in the persistently vegetative brain. *Brain* 125:1210–1234.

199. Stuss, D.P.T. and Alexander, M. (2001) Consciousness, self-awareness and the frontal lobes. In Salloway S.M.P. and Duffy, J. (eds.), *The Frontal Lobes and Neuropsychiatric Illness*, pp 101–112. Washington: American Psychiatric Press.

200. Sarrazin, J.C., Cleeremans, A. and Haggard, P. (2007) How do we know what we are doing? Time, intention and awareness of action. *Conscious Cogn*.

201. Slachevsky, A., Pillon, B., Fourneret, P., Renie, L., Levy, R., Jeannerod, M. and Dubois, B. (2003) The prefrontal cortex and conscious monitoring of action: An experimental study. *Neuropsychologia* 41:655–665.

202. Raichle, M.E., MacLeod, A.M., Snyder, A.Z., Powers, W.J., Gusnard, D.A. and Shulman, G.L. (2001) A default mode of brain function. *Proc Natl Acad Sci USA* 98:676–682.

203. Fox, M.D. and Raichle, M.E. (2007) Spontaneous fluctuations in brain activity observed with functional magnetic resonance imaging. *Nat Rev Neurosci* 8:700–711.

204. Raichle, M.E. and Snyder, A.Z. (2007) A default mode of brain function: A brief history of an evolving idea. *Neuroimage* 37:1083–1090. discussion 1097–1089.

205. Corbetta, M., Kincade, J.M., Ollinger, J.M., McAvoy, M.P. and Shulman, G.L. (2000) Voluntary orienting is dissociated from target detection in human posterior parietal cortex. *Nat Neurosci* 3:292–297.

206. Fox, M.D., Corbetta, M., Snyder, A.Z., Vincent, J.L. and Raichle, M.E. (2006) Spontaneous neuronal activity distinguishes human dorsal and ventral attention systems. *Proc Natl Acad Sci USA* 103:10046–10051.

207. Rees, G., Kreiman, G. and Koch, C. (2002a) Neural correlates of consciousness in humans. *Nat Rev Neurosci* 3:261–270.

208. Cavanna, A.E. and Trimble, M.R. (2006) The precuneus: A review of its functional anatomy and behavioural correlates. *Brain* 129:564–583.

209. Le Ber, I., Marie, R.M., Chabot, B., Lalevee, C. and Defer, G.L. (2007) Neuropsychological and 18FDG-PET studies in a family with idiopathic basal ganglia calcifications. *J Neurol Sci* 258:15–122.

210. Damasio, A.R. (1999) *The Feeling of What Happens: Body and Emotion in the Making of Consciousness*, 1st Edition. New York: Harcourt Brace.

211. Fox, M.D., Snyder, A.Z., Vincent, J.L., Corbetta, M., Van Essen, D.C. and Raichle, M.E. (2005) The human brain is intrinsically organized into dynamic, anticorrelated functional networks. *Proc Natl Acad Sci USA* 102:9673–9678.

212. Hagmann, P., Cammoun, L., Gigandet, X., Meuli, R., Honey, C.J. et al. Mapping the structural core of human cerebral cortex. *PLoS Biol* 6: e159.

213. Clauss, R.P., van der Merwe, C.E. and Nel, H.W. (2001) Arousal from a semi-comatose state on zolpidem. *S Afr Med J* 91:788–789.

214. Clauss, R. and Nel, W. (2006) Drug induced arousal from the permanent vegetative state. *NeuroRehabilitation* 21:23–28.

215. Bachmann, T. (2000) *Microgenetic Approach to the Conscious Mind*. Amsterdam; Philadelphia: John Benjamins Pub. Co.

216. Poppel, E. and Artin, T. (1988) *Mindworks: Time and Conscious Experience*. Boston, MA, USA: Harcourt Brace Jovanovich, Inc.

217. Raymond, J.E., Shapiro, K.L. and Arnell, K.M. (1992) Temporary suppression of visual processing in an RSVP task: An attentional blink? *J Exp Psychol Hum Percept Perform* 18:849–860.

218. Vogel, E.K., Luck, S.J. and Shapiro, K.L. (1998) Electro-physiological evidence for a postperceptual locus of suppression during the attentional blink. *J Exp Psychol Hum Percept Perform* 24:1656–1674.

219. Thorpe, S., Fize, D. and Marlot, C. (1996) Speed of processing in the human visual system. *Nature* 381:520–522.

220. Bacon-Mace, N., Mace, M.J., Fabre-Thorpe, M. and Thorpe, S.J. (2005) The time course of visual processing: Backward masking and natural scene categorisation. *Vision Res* 45:1459–1469.

221. Kirchner, H. and Thorpe, S.J. (2006) Ultra-rapid object detection with saccadic eye movements: Visual processing speed revisited. *Vision Res* 46:1762–1776.

222. Hung, C.P., Kreiman, G., Poggio, T. and DiCarlo, J.J. (2005) Fast readout of object identity from macaque inferior temporal cortex. *Science* 310:863–866.

223. VanRullen, R. and Koch, C. (2003) Visual selective behavior can be triggered by a feed-forward process. *J Cogn Neurosci* 15:209–217.

224. Macknik, S.L. (2006) Visual masking approaches to visual awareness. *Prog Brain Res* 155:177–215.

225. Martinez-Conde, S., Macknik, S.L. and Hubel, D.H. (2004) The role of fixational eye movements in visual perception. *Nat Rev Neurosci* 5:229–240.

226. Martinez-Conde, S., Macknik, S.L., Troncoso, X.G. and Dyar, T.A. (2006) Microsaccades counteract visual fading during fixation. *Neuron* 49:297–305.

227. Martinez-Conde, S., Macknik, S.L. and Hubel, D.H. (2002) The function of bursts of spikes during visual fixation in the awake primate lateral geniculate nucleus and primary visual cortex. *Proc Natl Acad Sci USA* 99:13920–13925.

228. Tse, P.U., Martinez-Conde, S., Schlegel, A.A. and Macknik, S.L. (2005) Visibility, visual awareness, and visual masking of simple unattended targets are confined to areas in the occipital cortex beyond human V1/V2. *Proc Natl Acad Sci USA* 102:17178–17183.

229. Rolls, E.T., Tovee, M.J. and Panzeri, S. (1999) The neurophysiology of backward visual masking: Information analysis. *J Cogn Neurosci* 11:300–311.

230. Lorente de Nó, R. (1938) The cerebral cortex: Architecture, intracortical connections and motor projections. In Fulton, J. (ed.) *Physiology of the Nervous System*, London: Oxford University Press.

231. Hebb, D.O. (1949) *The Organization of Behavior: A Neuropsychological Theory*. New York: Wiley.

232. Grossberg, S. (1999) The link between brain learning, attention, and consciousness. *Conscious Cogn* 8:1–44.

233. Edelman, G.M. and Mountcastle, V.B. (1978) *The Mindful Brain: Cortical Organization and the Group-Selective Theory of Higher Brain Function*. Cambridge: MIT Press.

234. Edelman, G.M. (1989) *The Remembered Present: A Biological Theory of Consciousness*. New York, USA: Basic Books, Inc.

235. Felleman, D.J. and Van Essen, D.C. (1991) Distributed hierarchical processing in the primate cerebral cortex. *Cereb Cortex* 1:1–47.

236. Martinez-Conde, S., Cudeiro, J., Grieve, K.L., Rodriguez, R., Rivadulla, C. and Acuna, C. (1999) Effects of feedback projections from area 18 layers 2/3 to area 17 layers 2/3 in the cat visual cortex. *J Neurophysiol* 82:2667–2675.

237. Super, H., Spekreijse, H. and Lamme, V.A. (2001) Two distinct modes of sensory processing observed in monkey primary visual cortex (V1). *Nat Neurosci* 4:304–310.

238. Rossi, A.F., Desimone, R. and Ungerleider, L.G. (2001) Contextual modulation in primary visual cortex of macaques. *J Neurosci* 21:1698–1709.

239. Scholte, H.S., Witteveen, S.C., Spekreijse, H. and Lamme, V.A. (2006) The influence of inattention on the neural correlates of scene segmentation. *Brain Res* 1076:106–115.

240. Block, N. (2005) Two neural correlates of consciousness. *Trends Cogn Sci* 9:46–52.

241. Tsuchiya, N. and Koch, C. (2005) Continuous flash suppression reduces negative afterimages. *Nat Neurosci* 8:1096–1101.

242. Silvanto, J., Cowey, A., Lavie, N. and Walsh, V. (2005) Striate cortex (V1) activity gates awareness of motion. *Nat Neurosci* 8:143–144.

243. Boyer, J.L., Harrison, S. and Ro, T. (2005) Unconscious processing of orientation and color without primary visual cortex. *Proc Natl Acad Sci USA* 102:16875–16879.

244. Ro, T., Breitmeyer, B., Burton, P., Singhal, N.S. and Lane, D. (2003) Feedback contributions to visual awareness in human occipital cortex. *Curr Biol* 13:1038–1041.

245. Crick, F. and Koch, C. (1990) Some reflections on visual awareness. *Cold Spring Harbor Symposia on Quantitative Biology* 55:953–962.

246. Singer, W. (1999) Neuronal synchrony: A versatile code for the definition of relations? *Neuron* 24:49–65. 111–125.

247. Tononi, G., Sporns, O. and Edelman, G.M. (1992) Reentry and the problem of integrating multiple cortical areas: Simulation of dynamic integration in the visual system. *Cereb Cortex* 2:310–335.

248. Abeles, M. (1991) *Corticonics: Neural Circuits of the Cerebral Cortex*. Cambridge; New York: Cambridge University Press.

249. Brecht, M., Singer, W. and Engel, A.K. (1999) Patterns of synchronization in the superior colliculus of anesthetized cats. *J Neurosci* 19:3567–3579.

250. Schoffelen, J.M., Oostenveld, R. and Fries, P. (2005) Neuronal coherence as a mechanism of effective corticospinal interaction. *Science* 308:111–113.

251. Lumer, E.D., Edelman, G.M. and Tononi, G. (1997a) Neural dynamics in a model of the thalamocortical system 2. The role of neural synchrony tested through perturbations of spike timing. *Cereb Cortex* 7:228–236.

252. Lumer, E.D., Edelman, G.M. and Tononi, G. (1997b) Neural dynamics in a model of the thalamocortical system 1. Layers, loops and the emergence of fast synchronous rhythms. *Cereb Cortex* 7:207–227.

253. Womelsdorf, T., Schoffelen, J.M., Oostenveld, R., Singer, W., Desimone, R., Engel, A.K. and Fries, P. (2007) Modulation of neuronal interactions through neuronal synchronization. *Science* 316:1609–1612.

254. Engel, A.K., Fries, P. and Singer, W. (2001) Dynamic predictions: Oscillations and synchrony in top-down processing. *Nat Rev Neurosci* 2:704–716.

255. Singer, W. and Gray, C.M. (1995) Visual feature integration and the temporal correlation hypothesis. *Ann Rev Neurosci* 18:555–586.

256. Munk, M.H., Roelfsema, P.R., Konig, P., Engel, A.K. and Singer, W. (1996) Role of reticular activation in the modulation of intracortical synchronization. *Science* 272:271–274.

257. Herculano-Houzel, S., Munk, M.H., Neuenschwander, S. and Singer, W. (1999) Precisely synchronized oscillatory firing patterns require electroencephalographic activation. *J Neurosci* 19:3992–4010.

258. Roelfsema, P.R., Engel, A.K., Konig, P. and Singer, W. (1997) Visuomotor integration is associated with zero time-lag synchronization among cortical areas. *Nature* 385:157–161.

259. Fries, P., Roelfsema, P.R., Engel, A.K., Konig, P. and Singer, W. (1997) Synchronization of oscillatory responses in visual cortex correlates with perception in interocular rivalry. *Proc Natl Acad Sci USA* 94:12699–12704.

260. Fries, P., Neuenschwander, S., Engel, A.K., Goebel, R. and Singer, W. (2001) Rapid feature selective neuronal synchronization through correlated latency shifting. *Nat Neurosci* 4:194–200.

261. Melloni, L., Molina, C., Pena, M., Torres, D., Singer, W. and Rodriguez, E. (2007) Synchronization of neural activity across cortical areas correlates with conscious perception. *J Neurosci* 27:2858–2865.

262. Imas, O.A., Ropella, K.M., Ward, B.D., Wood, J.D. and Hudetz, A.G. (2005b) Volatile anesthetics enhance flash-induced gamma oscillations in rat visual cortex. *Anesthesiology* 102:937–947.

263. Jones, D.S. (1979) *Elementary Information Theory*. New York: Oxford University Press.

264. Cover, T.M. and Thomas, J.A. (2006) *Elements of Information Theory*, 2nd Edition. Hoboken, NJ: Wiley-Interscience.

265. Tononi, G. and Edelman, G.M. (1998) Consciousness and complexity. *Science* 282:1846–1851.

266. Tononi, G. (2005) Consciousness, information integration, and the brain. *Prog Brain Res* 150:109–126.

267. Cohen, D. and Yarom, Y. (1998) Patches of synchronized activity in the cerebellar cortex evoked by mossy-fiber stimulation: questioning the role of parallel fibers. *Proc Natl Acad Sci USA* 95:15032–15036.

268. Bower, J.M. (2002) The organization of cerebellar cortical circuitry revisited: Implications for function. *Ann NY Acad Sci* 978:135–155.

269. Baars, B.J. (1988) *A Cognitive Theory of Consciousness*. New York, USA: Cambridge University Press.

270. Tononi, G. (2004b) Consciousness and the brain: Theoretical aspects. In Adelman, G. and Smith, B. (eds.) *Encyclopedia of Neuroscience*, 3rd Edition. Elsevier.

271. Ascoli, G.A. (1999) Progress and perspectives in computational neuroanatomy. *Anat Rec* 257:195–207.

272. Gazzaniga, M.S. (1995) Principles of human brain organization derived from split-brain studies. *Neuron* 14:217–228.

273. Dehaene, S., Sergent, C. and Changeux, J.P. (2003) A neuronal network model linking subjective reports and objective physiological data during conscious perception. *Proc Natl Acad Sci USA* 100:8520–8525.

274. Lumer, E.D. (1998) A neural model of binocular integration and rivalry based on the coordination of action-potential timing in primary visual cortex. *Cereb Cortex* 8:553–561.

275. Balduzzi, D. and Tononi, G. (2008) Integrated information in discrete dynamical systems: motivation and theoretical framework. *PLoS Comput Biol* 13:e1000091.

276. Tononi, G., Sporns, O. and Edelman, G.M. (1996) A complexity measure for selective matching of signals by the brain. *Proc Natl Acad Sci USA* 93:3422–3427.

Index

CNS. *See* Central nervous system.
Cognitive consciousness. *See* Internal consciousness.
Cognitive impairment and disruption of brain functional integrity, in Alzheimer's disease, 205–207
Cognitive neuroscience, of NDEs, 320–321
Cognitive processing, in non-responsive patients, 228–230
Cognitive science, xi
Coma, 137–150
  comatose patient, 145–149
  definition of, 138
  differential diagnosis and, 145
  disorders as cause of, 138–145
    hyperthermia and hypothermia, 142–143
    metabolic, nutritional and toxic encephalopathies, 139–141, 140t, 141t
    structural brain lesions, 139, 139f
    systemic and CNS infections, 141–142
    trauma, 143–145
  neurological examination and consciousness relating to, 18f, 19t, 20–21t, 22–23
  pathophysiology of, 138, 138f
  vegetative state and, 388–389
  VS, MCS and, behavioural features comparison of, 175t
Comatose patient
  management of, 145–147
    care in, 147–148
    diagnostic steps in, 146–147
    future directions in, 149
    prognosis and ethical management of
      for anoxic-ischaemic encephalopathy, after cardiac arrest, 148
      for brain death, 148
      for traumatic brain injury, 148–149
Communication
  LIS relating to, 195, 196b, 196f
  in paralyzed patients. *See* Brain-computer interfaces, for communication, in paralysed patients.
Complete locked-in state (CLIS), 219, 221, 222, 224, 225b, 226, 228
Complex partial seizures, 253–255
Concussion, 143
Conduction aphasia, inner speech in, 355
Conscious awareness, in VS, assessment of, 163–172
Conscious but unremembered behaviour, automatism and, 348–349

Conscious perception, synchronized gamma oscillations and, 45–46, 49–50
Conscious processing, 44
Conscious reportability, 272–273
Consciousness, x. *See also* DOC, NCC, Visual consciousness.
  in absence
    of attention, 68–69
    of sensory inputs and self-reflection, 98–101
  anosognosia and, 262–264, 385
  without attention, 68
    neuronal substrate to, 73
  attention and, 378–379
    dissociations between, 69–72
  attention and, relationship between
    functional considerations relating to, 64–66
    introduction to, 63–64
    other conceptual distinctions, relationship to, 72–73
    visual events and behaviours, four-fold processing way of, 66–67
  attention in opposition of, 69, 69n1, 70–71b
  behavioural. *See* External consciousness
  blindness and, 360–374
    animal studies relating to, 361, 362f
    brain shaped by, 370–371, 370f
    human studies relating to, 363–367, 366f
    understanding of, 367–368
  body, self, and, 382–383
  brain and, xi-xii, 44
  brain functions and, 376
  content of, 18, 43–44
  correlates of, 329–331
  definition of, 44
  dementia and: how the brain loses its self, 204–216
    brain loosening relating to, 212–214
    cognitive impairment and disruption of brain functional integrity in Alzheimer's disease, 205–207
    degenerative dementia, 207
    delusional misidentification syndromes, 212
    hallucinations, 210–212
    loss of insight, loss of sight v., 207–210
  disorders of. *See* Brain-computer interfaces, for communication, in paralysed patients.

epilepsy and
  absence seizures, 250–251
  complex partial seizures, 253–255
  consciousness system, 249–250, 249f
  generalized tonic-clonic seizures, 251–253
  impaired, 248t
  introduction to, 247–249
external (behavioural), 6
global alterations of, 386–390
hippocampus, memory, and, 326–338
human, understanding biological basis of, ix
impaired states of. *See* Consciousness, neurological examination of.
as integrated information, 402–403
internal (cognitive, mental), 6
intrinsic brain activity and
  activity, decrease of, 82–85, 84f
  background of, 81–82
  brain imaging, 82
  conceptual framework for, 86
  future questions relating to, 86–87
  "noise" in the fMRI BOLD signal, 85–86
introspection/reflection and, 377–378
language and, 377
level of, 18, 50
memory and, 379–380
MTL amnesia relating to, 331–335
network for, 249–250, 249f, 253–254, 253f
neuroanatomy of, 390–398
neurology of, 375–412
  implications of, 405
  theoretical perspective, 402–405
neurophysiology of, 398–402
overview of phenomenon and possible neural basis, 3–14
  definition of, 4–6
  deriving neuroanatomy from clinical neurological evidence, 9–11
  evolutionary perspective relating to, 12
  neuroanatomical and neurophysiological considerations relating to, 7–9
perceptions relating to, 43–44, 48
  imagination, absolute agnosia, and, 383–385
processing, without top-down attention and, 69
of self, 348
sensory input/motor output and, 376–377
in sleep, 95–102, 97f
space and